UTERINE PATHOLOGY

CAMBRIDGE ILLUSTRATED SURGICAL PATHOLOGY

Series Editor: Lawrence Weiss, MD
City of Hope National Medical Center, Duarte, California

Other Books in the Series

Intraoperative Consultation in Surgical Pathology, Mahendra Ranchod, MD

Modern Immunohistochemistry, Peiguo Chu, MD, and Lawrence Weiss, MD

Nervous System, Hannes Vogel, MD

Lymph Nodes, Lawrence Weiss, MD

Head and Neck, Margaret Brandwein-Gensler, MD

UTERINE PATHOLOGY

CAMBRIDGE ILLUSTRATED SURGICAL PATHOLOGY

Robert A. Soslow and Teri A. Longacre

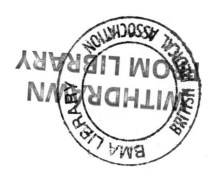

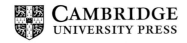
CAMBRIDGE
UNIVERSITY PRESS

CAMBRIDGE UNIVERSITY PRESS
Cambridge, New York, Melbourne, Madrid, Cape Town,
Singapore, São Paulo, Delhi, Mexico City

Cambridge University Press
The Edinburgh Building, Cambridge CB2 8RU, UK

Published in the United States of America by Cambridge University Press, New York

www.cambridge.org
Information on this title: www.cambridge.org/9780521509800

First published 2012

Printed in the United Kingdom at the University Press, Cambridge

A catalog record for this publication is available from the British Library

Library of Congress Cataloguing-in-Publication data

Soslow, Robert A.
  Uterine pathology : Cambridge illustrated surgical pathology / Robert A. Soslow, Teri Longacre.
    p.   cm. – (Cambridge illustrated surgical pathology)
  Includes bibliographical references and index.
  ISBN 978-0-521-50980-0 (Hardback)
  1. Uterus–Cancer–Diagnosis.   2. Cervix uteri–Cancer–Diagnosis.   3. Pathology, Surgical.
I. Longacre, Teri.   II. Title.
  RC280.U8S665 2012
  616.99′466–dc23

2011039826

ISBN 978-0-521-50980-0 Hardback

CONTENTS

CONTRIBUTORS

Mika Fujiwara, MD
Fellow, Department of Pathology
Stanford University School of Medicine
Stanford, CA, USA

Claudia Haynes, MD
Staff Pathologist, Department of Pathology
Kaiser Permanente Santa Clara Medical Center
Santa Clara, CA, USA

Christina S. Kong, MD
Associate Professor, Department of Pathology
Stanford University School of Medicine
Stanford, CA, USA

PREFACE

Uterine pathology represents one of the most important parts of any anatomic pathology practice, both in quantitative terms and in complexity. Discussion in this book is built around major pathologic entities in the uterus and cervix while highlighting the diverse and complex spectrum of alterations encountered in daily practice. The book's primary goal is to lay the foundation for diagnostic accuracy, relevance and reproducibility by emphasizing clear description and problem solving throughout. We have also sought to dispel common misconceptions and encourage an intelligent and thoughtful approach to diagnostic problems using all the tools available to the modern pathologist. Through this, we hope the book stimulates curiosity and excitement about the field of gynecologic pathology.

The first four chapters cover cytology and surgical pathology of the uterine cervix. Highlights here are the in-depth coverage of the diagnostic use of biomarkers in cervical pathology and practical guidelines that can be used for staging and reporting cervical neoplasia. The non-neoplastic endometrium and chapters devoted to tumors of the uterine corpus follow. Examples of problematic differential diagnoses that are discussed include: complex atypical hyperplasia versus endometrioid adenocarcinoma; FIGO grade 3 endometrioid adenocarcinoma versus clear cell, serous and undifferentiated carcinomas; carcinosarcoma (MMMT) versus endometrioid adenocarcinoma with spindle cell features; adenofibroma versus adenosarcoma; atypical smooth muscle tumor versus leiomyosarcoma; and primary versus metastatic carcinomas involving the uterus. New developments in gestational trophoblastic disease and Lynch syndrome are also presented. It is our sincere hope that this book will serve as a comprehensive and practical resource in uterine pathology for the general and gynecologic subspecialist pathologist.

ACKNOWLEDGMENTS

This work would not have been possible without the help and inspiration of a number of individuals, especially our mentors and our spouses. We acknowledge the visionary leadership of Richard Kempson and Michael Hendrickson that helped shape our philosophies about morphological interpretation, classification, terminology and clinico-pathological correlation and research. We hope to convey that spirit of thoughtful inquiry to the next generation of pathologists. A large debt of gratitude is owed to Richard Hildebrandt (Teri Longacre's spouse), and Michael Ogborn (Rob Soslow's spouse), for their patient and loving support as we worked on this project.

Our colleagues and trainees deserve particular acknow-ledgment: we continue to learn from them every day. Finally, we sincerely thank Norm Cyr at Stanford and Kin Kong and Allyne Manzo at Memorial for their assistance in preparation of the figures and diagrams in the book – Norm did a magnificent job with the endometrial cancer diagram in Chapter 7 – and Daniel Chiappetta for his help proofreading the galleys.

1 CYTOLOGY OF THE UTERINE CERVIX AND CORPUS

M. Fujiwara and C. S. Kong

INTRODUCTION

Cervical cytology is a screening tool that helps to categorize patients for their risk of cervical neoplasm depending on the degree of shift from normal cervical cytology and the amount of the abnormal change seen. Since the cervix is subject to hormonal effects, the clinical context (exogenous estrogens, pregnancy, etc.) should be considered when evaluating cervical cytology specimens.

The first cervical cytology screen is recommended for women starting at age 21, or 3 years after the onset of sexual intercourse, whichever comes first[1,2]. Women under the age of 30 should be screened annually with conventional cytology, or biennially using liquid-based methods. For women over the age of 30, human papillomavirus (HPV) testing can be used in conjunction with cytology, and if both tests are negative, screening can be reduced to every 3 years[3]. After the age of 70, women may choose to stop screening if no abnormal results were found in three or more consecutive cervical cytology specimens over the prior 10 years. Cervical cytology results are reported according to the 2001 Bethesda System (Table 1.1)[4].

Cervical cytology screening allows for evaluation of exfoliated cells from the transformation zone, where most cervical cancers arise. Traditionally, cervical cytology samples have been smeared directly onto a slide, fixed with ethanol, and Papanicolaou stained. These conventional smears are rapidly being replaced by liquid-based methods such as ThinPrep and SurePath. For liquid-based preparations, the cervical sample is rinsed directly into a vial of proprietary fixative solution – methanol-based CytoLyt® for ThinPrep (Hologic, Bedford, MA) and ethanol-based CytoRich® for SurePath (BD Diagnostics, Burlington, NC). Both ThinPrep and SurePath utilize proprietary methods for minimizing obscuring material such as blood, mucus, and debris to produce a thin layer of evenly distributed cells on a slide. Although some studies have shown fewer unsatisfactory specimens with the liquid-based method,

Table 1.1 2001 Bethesda System

Specimen type	Conventional Liquid-based (specify type, e.g., ThinPrep, SurePath) Other
Specimen adequacy	Satisfactory for evaluation Unsatisfactory for evaluation
General categorization (optional)	Negative for intraepithelial lesion or malignancy Epithelial cell abnormality Other: endometrial cells in a woman over 40 years of age
Interpretation/result	Negative for intraepithelial lesion or malignancy (specify organisms, other non-neoplastic findings)
Squamous	Atypical squamous cells – of undetermined significance (ASC-US) – cannot exclude HSIL (ASC-H) Low-grade squamous intraepithelial lesion High-grade squamous intraepithelial lesion Squamous cell carcinoma
Glandular	Atypical endocervical, endometrial *or* glandular cells (NOS or favor neoplastic) Endocervical adenocarcinoma in situ Adenocarcinoma
Other	Endometrial cells in a woman over 40 years of age Other malignant neoplasms
Ancillary testing	Human papillomavirus (HPV), gonorrhea (GC), chlamydia: include description of test method(s) and results
Automated review	Specify device and result, if slide is examined by an imaging system
Educational notes and suggestions (optional)	Based on ASCCP Management Guidelines

the performance of conventional and liquid-based methods in detecting high-grade lesions is similar[5,6]. Lower cost is an advantage for the conventional method, whereas the ability to use the same specimen for HPV and gonorrhea (GC)/chlamydia testing is an advantage for the liquid-based method. In addition, automated imaging systems such as the ThinPrep Imager or BD FocalPoint are optimized for liquid-based preparations. The American College of Obstetricians and Gynecologists (ACOG) accepts both conventional and liquid-based methods[7].

Despite the effectiveness of cervical cytology as a screening tool for cervical dysplasia, the reported false-negative rate of cervical cytology varies greatly, ranging from 0 to 94% (average of 51.9%)[8]. Human papillomavirus testing is a more sensitive method compared to cytology, although it is less specific[9].

PROGNOSIS

Cervical squamous intraepithelial lesion

The risk of harboring at least cervical intraepithelial neoplasia (CIN) 2 based on an abnormal cervical cytology result is as follows: 27% for HPV-positive atypical squamous cells of undetermined significance (ASC-US) or low-grade squamous intraepithelial lesion (LSIL); 50% for atypical squamous cells – cannot exclude high-grade squamous intraepithelial lesion (ASC-H); and over 70% for high-grade squamous intraepithelial lesion (HSIL)[10].

Atypical glandular cells

Atypical glandular cells (AGC) are diagnosed in about 0.2–0.9% of cervical cytology specimens, with significant disease present in 12–36% of the cases. The risk of finding a significant lesion on follow-up is 9–41% for atypical glandular cells NOS (not otherwise specified) and 27–96% for atypical glandular cells, favor neoplastic[13,14]. High-grade squamous intraepithelial lesion is the most common abnormality found on follow-up[15,16]. Other abnormalities detected on biopsy include endocervical adenocarcinoma in situ (AIS), invasive carcinomas (cervical, endometrial, and extrauterine), and other benign endometrial pathology. In patients whose cervical cytology test also detected a squamous abnormality, such as high-grade squamous intraepithelial lesion, ASC-H, or ASC-US, in addition to the atypical glandular cells, it is significantly more likely

that the glandular abnormality originated from the cervix and not from a non-cervical site (e.g., endometrium)[17].

Postmenopausal women have a higher rate of significant abnormality, with up to 50% of the cases showing cervical or endometrial lesions, including 15–20% endometrial carcinoma and 5% invasive cervical carcinoma. In women under 40, the most common precancerous or malignant lesions detected are high-grade squamous intraepithelial lesion and adenocarcinoma in situ[17].

MANAGEMENT AND TREATMENT

The American Society for Colposcopy and Cervical Pathology (ASCCP) first published consensus guidelines for the management of women with abnormal cervical cancer screening tests in 2001, and revised the guidelines in 2006[3]. There are also similar consensus guidelines for the management of intraepithelial neoplasia and adenocarcinoma in situ diagnosed histologically[3]. The guidelines specify different management algorithms for the general population vs. special populations, as the risk of high-grade squamous intraepithelial lesion or cancer differs in these various groups. A significant change with the 2006 guidelines is the identification of adolescents (defined as women 20 years and younger) as a special population that should be treated less aggressively than the general population. Human papillomavirus testing as specified in the guidelines refers to testing for high-risk types only. Currently, there are two high-risk HPV assays approved by the US Food and Drug Administration (FDA) – Digene Hybrid Capture 2 (used in the ASCUS-LSIL Triage Study) and Cervista HPV HR. (See the *Ancillary diagnostic tests* section.)

Negative cervical cytology

For women aged 30 years and older, HPV testing can be used in conjunction with cervical cytology for screening. If the cervical cytology and HPV tests are both negative, routine screening can be decreased to every three years. If the HPV test is positive, the patient can be followed with repeat cervical cytology and HPV testing at 12 months or, if HPV genotyping is available, the sample can be further evaluated to determine if HPV types 16/18 are present[3,18]. If the cervical cytology sample is positive for HPV16/18, immediate colposcopy is indicated. If the HPV16/18 test is negative, then the patient can be followed with repeat cytology and HPV testing in 12 months. Genotyping can be performed with Cervista HPV 16/18 (Hologic, Bedford, MA) or with HPV polymerase chain reaction (PCR). There are currently no FDA-approved HPV PCR systems available in the United States, but PCR can be internally validated by individual pathology laboratories.

For women under the age of 30, HPV testing is contra-indicated given the high prevalence of HPV infections and spontaneous clearance rates of up to 90%[19]. These patients should be followed with cytology only.

Atypical squamous cells of undetermined significance

Based on data from the ASCUS-LSIL Triage Study, there are three acceptable methods for managing ASC-US in the general population: (1) reflex testing for high-risk HPV; (2) immediate colposcopy; or (3) repeat cervical cytology at 6 and 12 months[3,20]. It should be noted that performing reflex HPV testing together with repeat cervical cytology at 6 months is not recommended; when the two tests are combined for follow-up, sensitivity remains the same while specificity drops. If the HPV test or colposcopy is negative, the patient can be followed with a repeat cervical cytology test at 12 months. However, if the HPV test is positive, the patient should be referred for immediate colposcopy with biopsy of visible lesions. If no visible lesions are identified or colposcopy is unsatisfactory, endocervical curettage is recommended. If cervical dysplasia is not identified, rec-ommended follow-up is HPV testing at 12 months or cervical cytology at 6 and 12 months. Colposcopy is rec-ommended if the subsequent HPV test is positive or at least ASC-US is identified on the cervical cytology. Human papillomavirus testing should not be performed more fre-quently than once every 12 months.

In adolescent women, HPV infection and minor cytologic abnormalities are common, but the risk of invasive cervical cancer is very low, and most HPV infections clear within two years without treatment. Consequently, it is recommended that adolescent women with ASC-US be managed less aggres-sively, with repeat cervical cytology at 12 and 24 months. Immediate colposcopy and reflex HPV testing are considered unacceptable. Only patients with high-grade squamous intraepithelial lesion at the 12-month cervical cytology test or at least ASC-US at the 24-month cervical cytology test should be referred for colposcopy.

Immunosuppressed (including HIV-positive), postmeno-pausal, and pregnant women should be managed the same as patients in the general population, except endocervical curettage is contraindicated in pregnant patients. In addition, for pregnant women, colposcopy can be deferred until at least six weeks postpartum.

Atypical squamous cells, cannot exclude high-grade squamous intraepithelial lesion (ASC-H)

Colposcopic examination with biopsy is recommended for ASC-H. If high-grade squamous intraepithelial lesion is not identified on biopsy, there are two options for follow-up: HPV testing at 12 months or repeat cervical cytology at 6 and 12 months. If the HPV test is positive or if cervical cytology shows ASC-US or above, colposcopy is recommended. If the HPV test is negative or both the follow-up cervical cytology tests are negative, the patient can resume routine yearly screening.

Low-grade squamous intraepithelial lesion

Women with a cytologic diagnosis of low-grade squamous intraepithelial lesion have the same risk of harboring high-grade squamous intraepithelial lesion as high-risk HPV-positive ASC-US, and should be managed similarly, i.e., with immediate colposcopy and biopsy of visible lesions. If no visible lesions are identified or colposcopy is unsatisfactory, endocervical curet-tage is recommended. If squamous intraepithelial lesion (SIL) is not identified, recommended follow-up is HPV testing at 12 months or cervical cytology at 6 and 12 months. Human papillomavirus triage of low-grade squamous intraepithelial lesion is not indicated, except in postmenopausal women.

For adolescents, the recommended management is follow-up with annual cytology testing and referral to colposcopy only if at least high-grade squamous intra-epithelial lesion is found at the 12-month cervical cytology or at least ASC-US at the 24-month cervical cytology.

Preferred management for pregnant women is immediate colposcopy, but it is also acceptable to defer colposcopy until at least six weeks postpartum. If the initial colposcopy does not show any colposcopic, histologic, or cytologic features to suggest high-grade squamous intraepithelial lesion or cancer, the patient can be further evaluated postpartum; additional exams are considered unacceptable. Endocervical curettage is also contraindicated in pregnant women.

High-grade squamous intraepithelial lesion

In the general population, high-grade squamous intra-epithelial lesion can be managed by colposcopy with endocervical sampling or immediate loop electrosurgical excision procedure (LEEP) of visible lesions. If colposcopy is satisfactory and high-grade squamous intraepithelial lesion is not identified histologically, the options for further evaluation are (1) diagnostic excision or (2) follow-up with colposcopy and cervical cytology at 6 and 12 months. Review of the cytology, histology, and colposcopy results should always be done in cases where there is a major discrepancy between the cytologic and histologic diagnosis, and management revised if any diagnoses are changed. If colposcopy is not satisfactory and high-grade squamous intraepithelial lesion is not identified on biopsy, diagnostic excision is recommended. Human papillomavirus triage or follow-up by repeat cervical cytology is unacceptable for the management of high-grade squamous intraepithelial lesion cytology.

Adolescent women with a cytologic diagnosis of high-grade squamous intraepithelial lesion should be evaluated with colposcopy and endocervical sampling. Immediate loop electrosurgical excision procedure is not acceptable. If colposcopy is satisfactory and high-grade squamous intraepithelial lesion is not identified histologically, preferred management is to follow the patient with colposcopy and cervical cytology at 6 month intervals for up to 24 months. Biopsy is recommended if a high-grade lesion is identified on colposcopy or if there is persistent high-grade squamous intraepithelial lesion by cytology for a year; diagnostic excision is recommended if high-grade squamous intraepithelial lesion persists by cytology for 24 months without identification of high-grade squamous intraepithelial lesion on biopsy. Patients can return to routine screening after two consecutive negative cervical cytology results, if no high-grade lesions are identified by colposcopy.

In pregnant women, endocervical sampling and loop electrosurgical excision procedure are unacceptable unless invasive cancer is suspected. They should be evaluated with colposcopy and biopsy of lesions suspicious for high-grade squamous intraepithelial lesion or cancer. If high-grade squamous intraepithelial lesion is not identified, repeat colposcopy and cervical cytology should be deferred until at least six weeks postpartum.

Endometrial cells in a woman over 40

Endometrial cells are found in 0.5–1.8% of cervical cytology specimens in women over 40 years. Endometrial sampling is recommended in all postmenopausal women with endometrial cells in their cervical cytology sample. However, if they are premenopausal, asymptomatic, and

without risk factors, no further evaluation is needed; if they are symptomatic or have risk factors for endometrial neoplasms, such as unexplained vaginal bleeding or chronic anovulation, endometrial sampling is recommended.

Atypical glandular cells

The diagnosis of "atypical glandular cells (AGC)" is often associated with benign, reactive conditions, but there is also a significant risk of underlying high-grade squamous intraepithelial lesion, endocervical adenocarcinoma in situ and invasive adenocarcinoma. Consequently, colposcopy with endocervical curettage is recommended for all categories of atypical glandular cells (i.e., atypical glandular cells NOS; atypical endocervical cells NOS; atypical glandular cells, favor neoplasia; atypical endocervical cells, favor neoplasia), except for "atypical endometrial cells." Endometrial sampling is also indicated in women over the age of 35 years or in younger women with risk factors for endometrial pathology (e.g., vaginal bleeding or chronic anovulation).

For a diagnosis of "atypical endometrial cells," endocervical and endometrial sampling are recommended; colposcopy can be performed at the initial evaluation or deferred. If no endometrial pathology is identified then colposcopy is indicated. For all categories of atypical glandular cells, HPV testing should be performed at the time of colposcopy, if not previously obtained. However, it is unacceptable to triage atypical glandular cells with HPV testing or to follow with repeat cytology.

MORPHOLOGY

Low-grade squamous intraepithelial lesion

Low-grade squamous intraepithelial lesion (LSIL) is characterized by nuclear enlargement (three times the size of intermediate cell nuclei), hyperchromasia, and irregular nuclear membranes (Figure 1.1). Binucleation and multinucleation are common. Koilocytes, which have a sharply defined, irregularly shaped perinuclear halo with a peripheral rim of thickened cytoplasm, are characteristic of low-grade squamous intraepithelial lesion but are not required for the diagnosis. Of note, cells seen in low-grade squamous intraepithelial lesion have abundant cytoplasm with low nuclear-to-cytoplasmic (N:C) ratios.

Atypical squamous cells of undetermined significance (ASC-US) are defined as squamous cells with nuclei that are 2.5–3 times the size of an intermediate cell nucleus, minimal

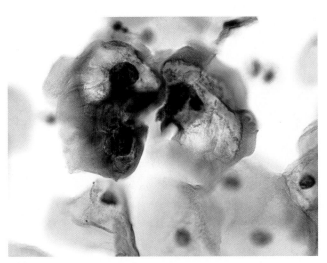

Figure 1.1 Low-grade squamous intraepithelial lesion (LSIL). Koilocytes with sharply punched-out, irregular halos surrounding enlarged, hyperchromatic, irregular nuclei.

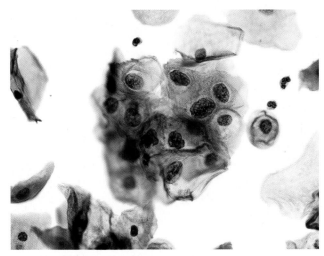

Figure 1.2 Atypical squamous cells, of undetermined significance (ASC-US). Atypical squamous cells with mild nuclear enlargement, minimal hyperchromasia, and slight nuclear membrane irregularities.

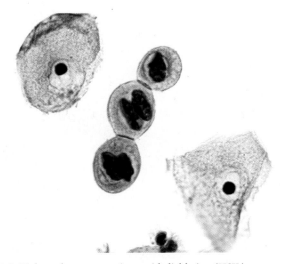

Figure 1.3 High-grade squamous intraepithelial lesion (HSIL). Cluster of cells with hyperchromatic, irregular nuclei, and high nuclear-to-cytoplasmic ratios.

nuclear hyperchromasia, and slightly irregular nuclear membranes (Figure 1.2). Halos, if present, lack the characteristic punched-out appearance of koilocytes or appear regular in shape without a thickened rim of cytoplasm. Cells with dark, pyknotic nuclei and dense orangeophilic cytoplasm (atypical parakeratosis) may also be seen. The diagnosis of ASC-US is best applied to cases where the atypical cells have some but not all the features of low-grade squamous intraepithelial lesion.

High-grade squamous intraepithelial lesion

High-grade squamous intraepithelial lesion is characterized by single cells, syncytial aggregates, and clusters of cells with irregular nuclear contours and high nuclear-to-cytoplasmic ratios of at least 1:1 (Figure 1.3). The nuclei are larger than an intermediate cell nucleus and, while they vary in size, they are not as large as those seen with low-grade squamous intraepithelial lesion. The cytoplasm varies from delicate to dense. The cells are typically hyperchromatic. However, with non-imaged ThinPrep slides, the cells may lack significant hyperchromasia. This is seen when the standard Richard-Allan hematoxylin or cyto-stain is used. However, it is not an issue with the proprietary ThinPrep Imager stain, which is a quantitative nuclear stain that allows computerized assessment of DNA content. With both Sure-Path and ThinPrep, dispersed abnormal single cells are more common and the cells may appear smaller and less abnormal. It is important to screen for single cells with high nuclear-to-cytoplasmic ratios and irregular nuclear membranes.

The diagnosis of "atypical squamous cells, cannot exclude HSIL" should be used for cases where the features raise concern for, but fall short of, a definitive diagnosis of high-grade squamous intraepithelial lesion (Figure 1.4). These are often cases where it is difficult to distinguish high-grade squamous intraepithelial lesion from one of its mimics, such as endometrial cells or squamous metaplastic cells.

Squamous cell carcinoma

Cervical squamous cell carcinoma (SCC) is commonly non-keratinizing, but keratinizing squamous cell carcinoma can also occur. Non-keratinizing squamous cell carcinoma can appear similar to high-grade squamous intraepithelial

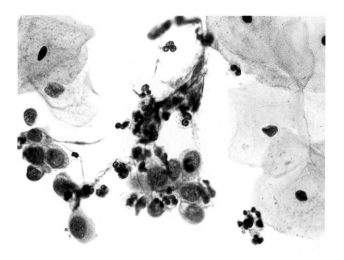

Figure 1.4 Atypical squamous cells, cannot exclude high-grade squamous intraepithelial lesion (ASC-H). High nuclear-to-cytoplasmic-ratio cells with slight nuclear membrane irregularities and minimal hyperchromasia.

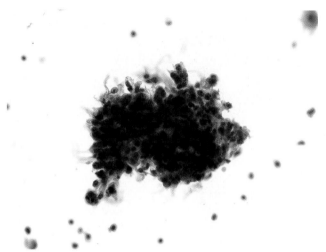

Figure 1.5 Squamous cell carcinoma (SCC). Syncytial aggregates of hyperchromatic cells with dense cytoplasm. Necrosis appears as granular debris along the edges of cell clusters on liquid-based preparations.

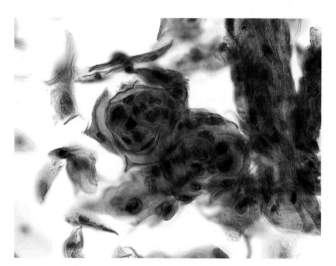

Figure 1.6 Keratinizing squamous cell carcinoma. Squamous pearls and dysplastic cells with high nuclear-to-cytoplasmic ratios help distinguish keratinizing squamous cell carcinoma from low-grade squamous intraepithelial lesion.

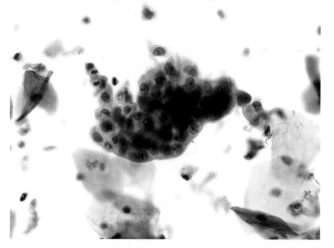

Figure 1.7 Atypical endocervical cells NOS. Crowded group of endocervical cells with enlarged nuclei and mitotic activity.

Atypical endocervical cells

lesion, with syncytial aggregates of hyperchromatic cells, but with squamous cell carcinoma the cells will also exhibit macronucleoli and occur in a background of necrotic debris and degenerating blood (Figure 1.5). On liquid-based preparations, tumor diathesis appears as granular debris clinging to the edges of cell clusters.

Keratinizing squamous cell carcinoma can appear similar to low-grade squamous intraepithelial lesion, with heavily keratinized low N:C ratio cells. The presence of keratin pearls, tadpole or spindled cells, and isolated single cells with scant cytoplasm and marked nuclear pleomorphism will support a diagnosis of squamous cell carcinoma (Figure 1.6).

The diagnosis of "atypical endocervical cells NOS" applies to endocervical cell atypia which exceeds that of reactive or reparative changes, but does not meet criteria for a definitive diagnosis of endocervical adenocarcinoma in situ (AIS) or invasive adenocarcinoma. In general, the atypical features are mild but reflect the types of changes that are seen with glandular neoplasia; for example, nuclear crowding, oval-to-cigar-shaped nuclei, nuclear membrane irregularities, nuclear enlargement (3–5 times normal), hyperchromasia, and nucleoli (Figure 1.7). Mitotic figures are typically rare, but if mitotic activity is identified within a group of glandular cells, it is best to issue a diagnosis of

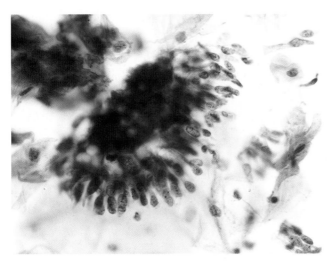

Figure 1.8 Atypical glandular cells, favor neoplastic. Atypical endocervical cells with feathering but only minimal nuclear membrane irregularities and minimal crowding.

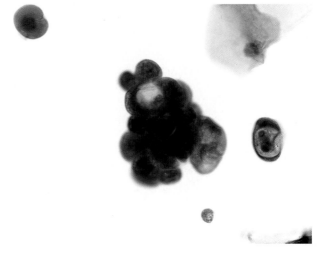

Figure 1.9 Atypical endometrial cells. Cluster of endometrial cells with nuclear enlargement and prominent nucleoli.

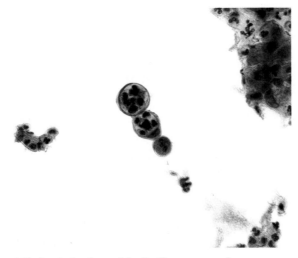

Figure 1.10 Atypical endometrial cells. The presence of cytoplasmic vacuoles filled with neutrophils is an abnormal finding in endometrial cells.

atypical endocervical cells. The distinction between benign endocervical glands and a minimal deviation or well-differentiated endocervical adenocarcinoma can be difficult even on histologic sections, and mitotic activity can be a helpful feature in detecting these well-differentiated carcinomas.

The diagnosis of "atypical endocervical cells, favor neoplastic" applies to cases where the degree of endocervical atypia is more pronounced but continues to fall qualitatively or quantitatively short of a definitive diagnosis of endocervical adenocarcinoma. In addition to the features described above, the cell groups may also show rosetting or feathering, with splaying of the cytoplasm at the edges of the cell clusters (Figure 1.8).

Atypical endometrial cells

Atypical endometrial cells will be recognizable as endometrial in origin but should exhibit atypia beyond what is expected for normal exfoliated endometrial cells. The cell clusters have slightly enlarged nuclei, mild hyperchromasia, and small nucleoli (Figure 1.9). The presence of numerous neutrophils within a cytoplasmic vacuole of an endometrial cell is an abnormal finding that should lead to a diagnosis of "atypical endometrial cells" (Figure 1.10).

Atypical glandular cells

If atypical glandular cells are present but it cannot be determined whether they are endocervical or endometrial in origin, a diagnosis of "atypical glandular cells NOS" or "atypical glandular cells, favor neoplastic" may be used.

Endocervical adenocarcinoma

The distinction between endocervical adenocarcinoma in situ and adenocarcinoma may not be clear cut on cervical cytology and, in many instances, clinical and radiographic correlation and a tissue specimen are required to differentiate the two. Adenocarcinoma in situ is characterized by strips of cells with crowded, palisading nuclei that are enlarged, elongate, and irregular (Figure 1.11). Nuclear-to-cytoplasmic ratios are increased and the chromatin is coarse and dark. On conventional smears, the apical cytoplasm frequently strips away, giving the impression of a row of feathers

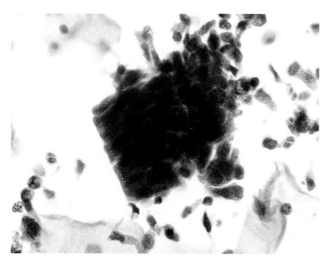

Figure 1.11 Endocervical adenocarcinoma in situ: Strips of abnormal endocervical cells with elongate, markedly irregular nuclei and nuclear crowding.

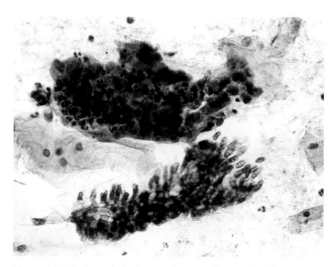

Figure 1.12 Endocervical adenocarcinoma. Cluster of malignant glandular cells (upper) would not be classifiable as endocervical in origin without the strip of adenocarcinoma in situ cells (lower).

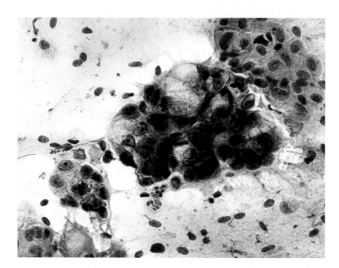

Figure 1.13 Endometrial adenocarcinoma. Three-dimensional clusters of malignant cells with pleomorphic nuclei, prominent nucleoli, and large cytoplasmic vacuoles are characteristic of serous carcinoma.

("feathering"). This is less commonly seen with liquid-based preparations. Apoptotic bodies and mitotic figures may also be identified but are not specific or required. Finding single atypical glandular cells is uncommon.

With invasive endocervical adenocarcinoma, the cells are clearly malignant with enlarged, pleomorphic nuclei and finely vacuolated cytoplasm; macronucleoli may also be seen. The tumor cells occur as syncytial aggregates and three-dimensional clusters (Figure 1.12). Tumor diathesis is a useful indicator of invasion but is less prominent on liquid-based preparations, where it will appear as granular debris along the edges of the tumor cell clusters.

While these features are diagnostic of adenocarcinoma, they are non-specific as to site of origin. The only way that a diagnosis of invasive endocervical adenocarcinoma can be made on a cervical cytology specimen is if these findings are present along with features of endocervical adenocarcinoma in situ.

Endometrial adenocarcinoma

Endometrial adenocarcinoma is frequently indistinguishable from endocervical adenocarcinoma based on cytology. However, there are certain features that are characteristic of endometrial origin, such as malignant cells with numerous intracytoplasmic neutrophils, or papillary clusters of cells with large cytoplasmic vacuoles and markedly pleomorphic nuclei (typically seen with serous carcinomas) (Figure 1.13). Cases that lack features characteristic of endometrial origin should be classified as adenocarcinoma NOS, with determination of primary site deferred to the resection specimen, as well as clinical and radiographic findings.

Metastatic carcinoma

Metastatic adenocarcinoma should be suspected when the morphology is unusual for a uterine primary or the background lacks a tumor diathesis. Common sites that metastasize to the cervix include the urinary bladder, breast, ovary and fallopian tube, kidney, and gastrointestinal tract (e.g., colon, stomach) (Figure 1.14).

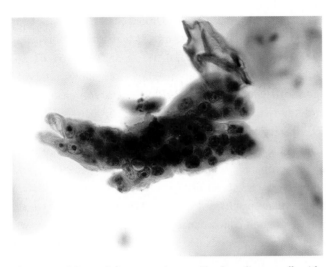

Figure 1.14 Metastatic breast carcinoma. Clearly malignant cells with enlarged nuclei and a cytoplasmic vacuole compressing the nucleus that do not resemble usual Mullerian tract primaries; the background also lacks tumor diathesis.

ANCILLARY DIAGNOSTIC TESTS

Digene Hybrid Capture 2

Digene Hybrid Capture 2 (HC2) (Qiagen, Valencia, CA) is FDA approved for triaging patients with a diagnosis of ASC-US and for co-testing in women aged 30 years and older. It is the assay that was used in the ASCUS-LSIL Triage Study that led to the current recommendation for HPV triage of ASC-US[20]. Two probes are available – low risk and high risk – but only the high-risk probe has clinical utility. It targets 13 high-risk HPV types (16, 18, 31, 33, 35, 39, 45, 51, 52, 56, 58, 59, 68).

Digene HC2 has a detection limit of 5000 copies of HPV DNA (1 pg/ml) and has good interlaboratory reproducibility. However, the HC2 is unable to specifically type HPV, and lacks an internal control to assure specimen adequacy. It also has poor reproducibility near the 1 pg/ml cutoff. Results near the cutoff are best reported as equivocal; a significant number of these borderline cases are negative by HPV polymerase chain reaction.

The overall false-positive rate of HC2 is 6.2%. This is due to both cross-hybridization and signal leak. Cross-hybridization with low-risk HPV types has been reported to occur at a rate of 1.9%. Although this can lead to false-positive results, it also increases the clinical sensitivity of the assay and allows detection of high-risk HPV types that are not directly targeted by the test probe (e.g., HPV66)[21]. Signal leak in contiguous samples has been observed in 4.3% of cases.

Cervista

Cervista HPV HR and Cervista HPV 16/18, formerly known as Invader, (Third Wave Technologies, Hologic, Bedford, MA) are two signal-amplification HPV assays that were FDA approved in 2009. Cervista requires a smaller sample volume (2 ml vs. 4 ml) than HC2 and has an internal control which detects human histone 2 gene (*H2be*) that allows for evaluation of specimen adequacy. Cervista HPV HR targets 14 high-risk HPV types (16, 18, 31, 33, 35, 39, 45, 51, 52, 56, 58, 59, 66, 68), which are the same as those targeted by Digene HC2 with the addition of HPV66. It is approved for ASC-US triage and for co-testing in women aged 30 years and older. Cervista HPV 16/18 targets HPV types 16 and 18, which are more oncogenic and responsible for the majority of cervical cancers. It is approved for use in conjunction with Cervista HPV HR, specifically for further evaluation of patients who are HPV positive.

The clinical validation study for Cervista HPV HR showed 93% clinical sensitivity for the detection of >CIN2 and 100% for >CIN3; negative predictive value was 99.1% for >CIN2 and 100% for >CIN3[22]. Analytic sensitivity ranges from 1250–7500 copies, and analytic specificity is high with no cross-reactivity reported when tested with seven non-oncogenic HPV types[23]. A separate population-based study in China showed similar sensitivity and specificity of Cervista HPV HR and HC2 for the detection of >CIN3: sensitivity 95.1% Cervista vs. 97.9% HC2; specificity 90.3% Cervista vs. 87.8% HC2[24]. However, in a study where Cervista HPV HR was used to evaluate 65 samples with borderline Digene HC2 results, there was a 6.1% false-positive rate[25] (line blot genotyping assay as gold standard).

The clinical validation study for Cervista HPV 16/18 showed a detection rate of 68.8% for >CIN2 and 77.3% for >CIN3, which correlates with the estimated prevalence of HPV16 and HPV18[22]. When stratified by age, Cervista HPV 16/18 showed similar sensitivity and negative predictive value (NPV) for women under 30 and over 30, but lower specificity (61.9 vs. 79.9%) and lower positive predictive value (15.2 vs. 21.9%) for women under 30[26]. Cervista HPV 16/18 has high analytic specificity with no reported cross-reactivity with low-risk types. Cross-reactivity with high-risk HPV type 31 has been reported when using high concentrations of HPV31 cloned DNA samples; however, when HPV31-positive clinical samples were tested, no cross-reactivity was observed[27].

Kinney *et al.* evaluated the test performance data in the package inserts for Cervista HPV HR and Cervista HPV

16/18, and raised concerns about the assays being overly sensitive, with 2–4 times more positive results than were reported in the premarketing approval trial[28]. Increased analytic sensitivity is not always desirable since the goal is detecting clinically relevant infections. Overly sensitive assays can lead to overtreatment of patients and increased cost of care. While Kinney *et al.* raised this concern, they also note that post-marketing studies evaluating Cervista will be important in determining the clinical sensitivity of these assays in actual practice.

Slide-based assays

Human papillomavirus in situ hybridization (ISH) and immunohistochemistry (IHC) stains for p16 and ProEx C, surrogate markers for high-risk HPV, can be performed on cervical cytology slides. However, these assays are limited by the need for manual screening of the stained slide and the difficulty in interpreting the stains. While specificity is usually better with these assays than with HC2, the limited amount of material evaluated negatively impacts sensitivity. Various studies comparing Ventana Inform in situ hybridization with HC2 have shown insufficient sensitivity for Ventana in situ hybridization to be used for ASC-US triage (43–61% in situ hybridization vs. 97–100% HC2)[29–31].

In addition to staining cells with integrated high-risk HPV, p16 and ProEx C can show focal staining of benign squamous metaplastic cells and endocervical cells[32]. This makes it difficult to interpret the stain, since only positive cells that are cytologically atypical cells should be scored as positive. Consequently, sensitivity and specificity will vary depending on the skill of the pathologist reading the slide.

Human papillomavirus polymerase chain reaction

Polymerase chain reaction (PCR) is the traditional gold standard for detecting HPV, and can identify the specific type of HPV. Human papillomavirus PCR for types 16 and 18 can be used for triaging women over 30 with negative cervical cytology but positive HPV test. Currently, there are no commercially available platforms in the United States, but individual clinical laboratories have internally validated "home-brewed" HPV PCR assays.

Roche has developed two HPV detection systems – Amplicor (consensus) and LinearArray (type specific) – that are available in Europe but have not yet received FDA approval for use in the United States. The Amplicor consensus assay detects the same 13 high-risk HPV types as Digene HC2 (i.e., types 16, 18, 31, 33, 35, 39, 45, 51, 52, 56, 58, 59, 68), while the LinearArray assay allows for type-specific detection of 37 high-risk (same as consensus assay) and low-risk (6, 11, 26, 40, 42, 53, 54, 55, 56, 61, 64, 66, 67, 69, 70, 71, 72, 73, 81, 82, 83, 84, CP6108, IS39) HPV types. Using LinearArray genotyping as the gold standard, Sandri *et al.* compared Roche Amplicor with Digene HC2 and showed increased sensitivity (100% vs. 85% for HC2) and similar specificity (95% vs. 93% for HC2)[33]. Overall, there was good concordance (83%) between the two assays, but Amplicor was positive in significantly more cases that were cytologically normal. This indicates that the increased sensitivity of Amplicor reflects a higher analytic sensitivity and corresponding lower clinical specificity. Improved sensitivity is not necessarily desirable since not all HPV infections lead to the development of a high-grade squamous intraepithelial lesion.

Imaging

Imaging systems can be used for primary screening or quality control (QC) review. The goals are to improve quality by decreasing screening and interpretative error and to increase productivity. These systems are most useful in labs with poor sensitivity and are less useful in labs with a high degree of accuracy. The US Clinical Laboratory Improvement Amendment (CLIA) limits the number of slides screened by a cytotechnologist to 100 per 8-hour minimum workday. With location-guided screening, the Centers for Medicare and Medicaid Services (CMS) allows up to 200 slides. Actual productivity is less than the allowable maximum. The actual time savings of the imaging system depends on the experience of the cytotechnologist and whether the laboratory requires rapid QC rescreening[5,34,35]. For experienced cytotechnologists, the imaging system may decrease productivity.

There are currently three FDA-approved imaging systems: ThinPrep Imaging System (Hologic), FocalPoint GS (BD), and FocalPoint Slide Profiler (BD). The ThinPrep and FocalPoint GS systems allow for location-guided screening of liquid-based preparations. In contrast, the FocalPoint Slide Profiler performs primary screening of SurePath or conventional cervical cytology specimens and allows for archiving of up to 25% of successfully processed slides from non-high-risk patients without manual review.

The ThinPrep® Imaging System was FDA approved in 2003 for dual review of ThinPrep. After the Imager screens the slide, a cytotechnologist reviews 22 fields of view using a review scope. If any abnormal cells are seen, a full slide screen must be performed. The sensitivity is equivalent or better for detection of low-grade and high-grade squamous intraepithelial lesion, and the specificity is higher for detection of high-grade squamous intraepithelial lesion when compared to manual screening alone. It has an improved false-negative rate of 0.012% versus 5.6% for conventional smears and 2.2% for non-imaged ThinPrep[36]. Although the Imager is limited in its ability to detect classic koilocytes, the miss rate is similar to manual screening[37]. In a study by Jayamohan et al., the Imager accurately selected fields of view with atypical glandular cells in 82% of cases; in all false-negative cases, reactive changes or endometrial cells were present which led to full manual review[38]. The unsatisfactory rate with the Imager is the same or decreased, but there is a reported 2–3% increase in the number of cases lacking a transformation zone component[39].

The BD FocalPoint™ Slide Profiler is FDA approved for primary screening of SurePath or conventional cervical cytology slides. Although this system lacks location guidance, it functions as a triage device and identifies cases that are more likely to contain significant abnormalities. Each slide is assigned a score based on a proprietary algorithm, and the slides are sorted into one of four categories: review (quintiles 1–5), no further review (NFR), process review, or QC review. The cases selected for manual review are further divided into one of five quintiles, with the highest suspicion for neoplasia placed in quintile 1 and the lowest suspicion in quintile 5. Unsatisfactory cases are automatically assigned to quintile 5 to ensure that a manual screen is performed. Up to 25% of successfully processed slides from non-high-risk patients categorized as NFR can be archived as negative without manual review. In the United States, the No Further Review function is disabled when the Slide Profiler is used in conjunction with the GS Imaging System. Process review applies to cases where there is a physical problem with the slide (e.g., coverslip and slide too thin; instrument unable to focus) or if there is an issue with the instrument (e.g., scanning interrupted). Quality control review uses the quintile ranking to select slides for directed QC review, thereby enriching the QC slides with cases more likely to be false negative. The Slide Profiler performs well, with 50% low-grade squamous intraepithelial lesion, 70% high-grade squamous intraepithelial lesion, and 69% squamous cell carcinoma placed in quintile 1; only rare high-grade squamous intraepithelial lesion and 4.5% low-grade squamous intraepithelial lesion were ranked as NFR[40]. No atypical glandular cells cases with abnormal histologic follow-up were categorized as NFR, but malignant cases did not preferentially rank into the higher quintiles[41].

The BD FocalPoint™ GS Imaging System was FDA approved in 2008 for SurePath slides only. Internationally, it can be used with both SurePath and conventional cervical cytology slides. This system works in conjunction with the automated screening function of the BD FocalPoint™ Slide Profiler and adds a location-guided screening system. The GS Review Station shows 11 fields of view: 10 selected for the greatest probability of showing an abnormality, with the most abnormal fields shown first, and 1 for location confirmation. In examining the fields of view, the cytotechnologists have to examine the entire field including the edges, since the abnormality could be anywhere in the field. This takes adjusting to, since screeners are accustomed to focusing on the center of the slide while moving the stage and examining overlapping fields. Compared to manual screening, this system had a 20% and 10% increase in detection of high-grade and low-grade squamous intraepithelial lesions, respectively, and a small but statistically significant decrease in specificity[42].

DIFFERENTIAL DIAGNOSIS

Low-grade squamous intraepithelial lesion

Glycogenation

Glycogenation of squamous cells can be confused with koilotypic change seen in low-grade squamous intraepithelial lesion. However, glycogen halos are not sharply demarcated and the nucleus is centrally located within the halo. The nuclei also lack atypia, with no enlargement or hyperchromasia. Glycogen can also give a yellow tinge to the cytoplasm within the area of perinuclear clearing (Figure 1.15).

Inflammatory/reactive changes

Inflammatory halos are less well demarcated than koilocytic halos. They are also uniform, with an equal distance between the edge of the halo and the edge of the nucleus. They are typically seen in association with an inflammatory background, and infectious organisms such as *Candida* or *Trichomonas* may also be present. These halos are also known as "trich halos" (Figure 1.16).

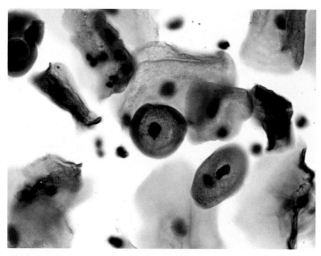

Figure 1.15 Glycogen halos. Cytoplasm within the halo often has a yellow tint and the nuclei lack atypia.

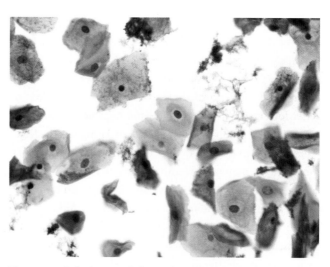

Figure 1.16 Inflammatory halos. Halos with indistinct borders and centrally placed nuclei that lack cytologic atypia.

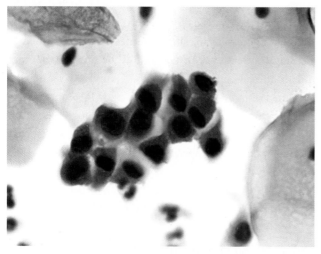

Figure 1.17 Squamous metaplasia. High nuclear-to-cytoplasmic-ratio cells with dense cytoplasm but nuclei that have even chromatin and smooth nuclear contours.

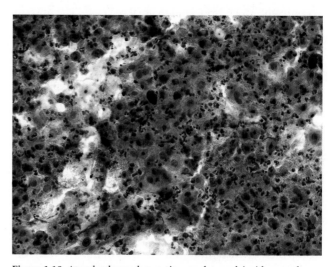

Figure 1.18 Atrophy: hyperchromatic, smudgy nuclei with smooth nuclear contours in a background of inflammation and granular debris.

High-grade squamous intraepithelial lesion and squamous cell carcinoma

Squamous metaplasia

Squamous metaplastic cells can have high nuclear-to-cytoplasmic ratios and are readily identified by their dense cytoplasm. However, some high-grade squamous intraepithelial lesion cells may have metaplastic cytoplasm. The distinction between reactive squamous metaplasia and high-grade squamous intraepithelial lesion depends on the appearance of the nucleus. Reactive metaplastic cells have nuclei with smooth nuclear membranes and even chromatin, while high-grade squamous intraepithelial lesion cells have marked nuclear membrane irregularities and are usually hyperchromatic (Figure 1.17). In cases where a definitive

distinction cannot be made, it is best to use the diagnosis of "atypical squamous cells, cannot exclude HSIL."

Atrophy

While hyperchromatic crowded groups of parabasal cells are characteristic of atrophy, it is important to evaluate these groups for nuclear pleomorphism, nuclear membrane irregularities, and mitotic activity. These features are clues to the presence of high-grade squamous intraepithelial lesion mimicking atrophy. Parabasal cells have generalized nuclear enlargement but should be relatively uniform in size and shape with smooth nuclear contours and even chromatin.

The background of granular debris and inflammation seen with severe atrophy can mimic the tumor diathesis of squamous cell carcinoma (Figure 1.18). However, karyorrhectic

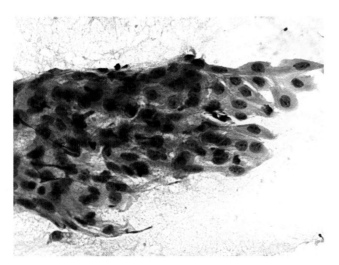

Figure 1.19 Repair: monolayer sheets of streaming cells with enlarged nuclei and prominent nucleoli but smooth nuclear contours.

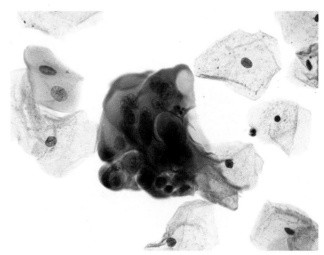

Figure 1.20 Radiation change: atypical nuclei but cells maintain normal nuclear-to-cytoplasmic ratios.

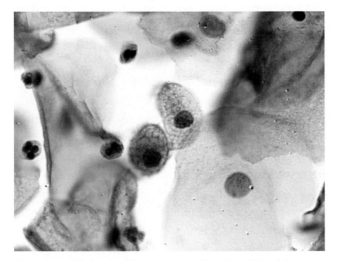

Figure 1.21 Histiocytes. Eccentric, bean-shaped nuclei and foamy cytoplasm.

nuclear debris should be seen with a true tumor diathesis. "Blue blobs" are collections of basophilic amorphous material that reflect degenerated parabasal cells or inspissated mucus. These collections should not be mistaken for tumor cells. In general, it is a good rule to never interpret cells that lack cytoplasm or exhibit degenerative changes as evidenced by the lack of chromatin detail.

Repair

Reparative changes can lead to marked cytologic atypia that raises concern for carcinoma in situ (high-grade squamous intraepithelial lesion) or squamous cell carcinoma. The cells can have enlarged nuclei with prominent nucleoli and increased nuclear-to-cytoplasm ratios. However, monolayer sheets of cells with distinct cell borders and streaming (cells

oriented in the same direction) are characteristic of repair (Figure 1.19). Although atypical, the cells will be relatively monomorphous, with smooth nuclear contours and prominent nucleoli in almost every cell. Neutrophils may also infiltrate the cell clusters. With liquid-based preparations, streaming of the cells may be less apparent.

Radiation-related change

With a history of prior radiation, caution should be exercised in making a definitive diagnosis of dysplasia or recurrent carcinoma. Radiation effect can produce cells with bizarre nuclear shapes and enlarged nuclei. However, the cells maintain normal nuclear-to-cytoplasmic ratios; as the nuclei enlarge, the cytoplasm correspondingly increases in amount (Figure 1.20). Cytoplasmic vacuoles are also commonly seen with radiation change. In cases where the atypia exceeds what is expected for radiation change but the cells are not overtly dysplastic or malignant, it is best to issue a diagnosis of atypical squamous cells. This will lead to further evaluation with colposcopy, biopsy, and HPV testing.

Histiocytes

Histiocytes may be seen in chronic inflammatory processes as well as in postmenopausal and postpartum women. Although histiocytes may be seen as single cells, they are typically present in a streaming pattern on conventional smears. They exhibit round-to-oval or bean-shaped nuclei that are eccentrically placed. In contrast to the smooth or dense cytoplasm of squamous cells, histiocytes have moderate amounts of foamy, often vacuolated cytoplasm (Figure 1.21). On liquid-based preparations, the nuclei tend to be rounder in shape

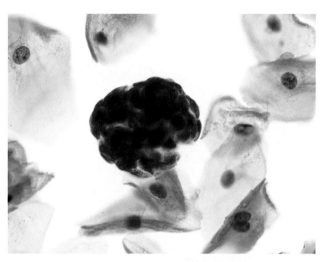

Figure 1.22 Endometrial cells. Tight, three-dimensional ball of cells with small nuclei, scant cytoplasm, and nuclear molding.

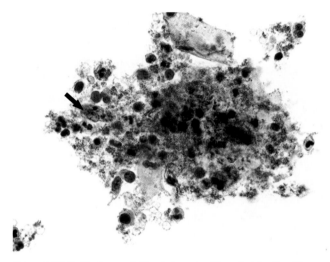

Figure 1.23 Follicular cervicitis. Aggregate of lymphoid cells with tingible-body macrophages (arrow).

and can be difficult to distinguish from hypochromic high-grade squamous intraepithelial lesion on thinprep slides.

Endometrial cells

Endometrial cells occur as tight, three-dimensional, ball-like clusters, and are rarely seen as single cells. The cells have scant cytoplasm and small nuclei that are round, but can also exhibit irregular nuclear contours and nuclear molding (Figure 1.22). On liquid-based preparations, endometrial cells can appear atypical, since nucleoli, cytoplasmic vacuoles, and apoptotic bodies are more readily seen. Single cells are also more common. However, endometrial cells can be distinguished from high-grade squamous intraepithelial lesion by the small size of the nuclei, which are the same size or smaller than intermediate cell nuclei. In contrast, high-grade squamous intraepithelial lesion nuclei are larger.

Follicular cervicitis

On liquid-based preparations, lymphoid cells from follicular cervicitis tend to aggregate, and the clumps can mimic high-grade squamous intraepithelial lesion (Figure 1.23). However, on closer examination, it will become apparent that the aggregates consist of a mixed population of lymphocytes, including plasma cells. Tingible-body macrophages may also be seen and are a useful feature for avoiding an overdiagnosis[43].

High-grade squamous intraepithelial lesion vs. squamous cell carcinoma

It can be difficult to distinguish high-grade squamous intra-epithelial lesion from invasive squamous cell carcinoma based on cytologic features alone. Prominent nucleoli are not a useful distinguishing feature since they can be seen with

both in situ and invasive carcinomas. Unless a clear tumor diathesis is present in the background, it is best to avoid a definitive diagnosis of squamous cell carcinoma.

Low-grade squamous intraepithelial lesion

Low-grade squamous intraepithelial lesion is characterized by dysplastic cells with low nuclear-to-cytoplasmic ratios, while high-grade squamous intraepithelial lesion has high nuclear-to-cytoplasmic ratios of greater than 1:1. In practice, this distinction is not always clear cut, especially when a handful of cells with increased nuclear-to-cytoplasmic ratios are seen in a background of numerous low-grade squamous intraepithelial lesion cells. In these cases, a diagnosis of "low-grade squamous intraepithelial lesion, cannot exclude high-grade squamous intraepithelial lesion" can be used to alert the treating physician that immediate colposcopy should be performed instead of following the patient with repeat cytology[44–47].

Keratinizing squamous cell carcinoma can be mistaken for low-grade squamous intraepithelial lesion. Malignant keratinizing cells have low nuclear-to-cytoplasmic ratios with abundant orangeophilic cytoplasm, which can be mistaken for koilocytes. However, noting the presence of keratin pearls, tadpole cells and malignant cells with high nuclear-to-cytoplasmic ratios should prevent an underdiagnosis of low-grade squamous intraepithelial lesion (Figure 1.6).

Endocervical adenocarcinoma in situ

Tubal metaplasia

Tubal metaplasia occurs as strips of glandular cells with round-to-oval nuclei, smooth nuclear membranes, and even chromatin. In contrast to adenocarcinoma in situ, they lack nuclear stratification and crowding, but the impression of palisading can lead to a diagnosis of atypical glandular cells. Although not always apparent, the presence of cilia is characteristic of tubal metaplasia (Figure 1.24)[48,49].

Endometriosis or direct endometrial sampling

If the possibility of endometriosis or direct endometrial sampling is not recognized, proliferative endometrial glands can be mistaken for endocervical adenocarcinoma in situ. Endometrial glands occur as sheets or strips of columnar cells with mild to severe nuclear pleomorphism and hyperchromasia (Figure 1.25). Feathering and rosette formation, as well as mitotic activity, can also be seen. However, the nuclei usually have smooth nuclear contours

and lack the crowding and stratification seen with adenocarcinoma in situ. Finding smaller clusters of endometrial stromal cells can also be helpful[50].

Direct sampling of the lower uterine segment or endometrial cavity can also occur, especially in women with a shortened cervix due to prior loop electrosurgical excision procedure or cone procedures. The findings are similar to what is seen with endometriosis. Identifying biphasic tissue fragments of endometrial glands embedded within stroma is a useful distinguishing feature (Figure 1.26)[51].

With an exodus pattern, a dark core of endometrial stromal cells surrounded by glandular cells may be seen. If the core of stromal cells is not recognized, the columnar endometrial glandular cells may be overdiagnosed as atypical glandular cells (Figure 1.27).

High-grade squamous intraepithelial lesion involving endocervical glands

High-grade squamous intraepithelial lesion involving endocervical glands can give the appearance of atypical glandular cells, and it is the most frequent abnormality found in follow-up for a cytologic diagnosis of atypical glandular cells. While high-grade squamous intraepithelial lesion and adenocarcinoma in situ can coexist, features that will help distinguish high-grade squamous intraepithelial lesion from a glandular abnormality include identifying areas of clear squamous differentiation, or finding single cells with high nuclear-to-cytoplasmic ratios and irregular nuclear membranes. Single cells are uncommonly seen with adenocarcinoma in situ. In addition, endocervical glands involved by high-grade squamous intraepithelial lesion tend to show

Figure 1.24 Tubal metaplasia. Strips of glandular cells with oval nuclei; cilia are characteristic but not always present.

(A)

(B)

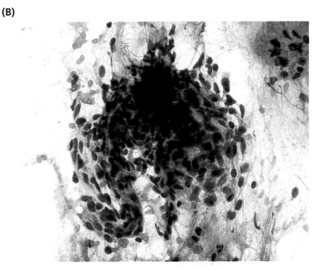

Figure 1.25 Endometriosis. Atypical glandular cells with coarse chromatin and feathering (A); noting the presence of endometrial stromal cells is helpful (B).

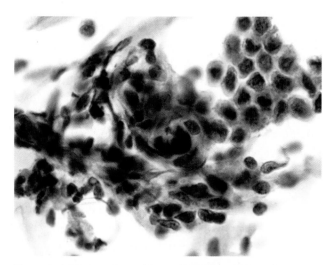

Figure 1.26 Direct endometrial sampling. Biphasic tissue fragments with endometrial glands embedded, associated with endometrial gland embedded in stroma.

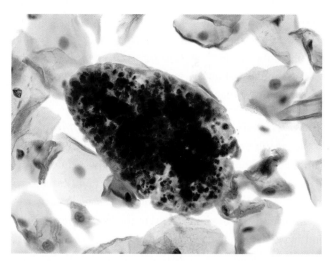

Figure 1.27 Endometrial stromal cells surrounded by glandular cells.

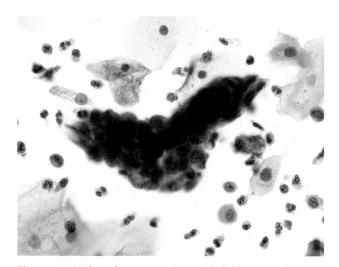

Figure 1.28 High-grade squamous intraepithelial lesion involving endocervical glands. Circumferential arrangement of nuclei along the periphery is characteristic of high-grade squamous intraepithelial lesion.

circumferentially arranged nuclei along the periphery, in contrast to the radial, stratified arrangement of nuclei with adenocarcinoma in situ (Figure 1.28). If both glandular and squamous abnormalities are indentified, this can be indicated in the cytology report by providing two separate diagnoses.

REFERENCES

1. Saslow D, Runowicz CD, Solomon D, *et al.* American Cancer Society guideline for the early detection of cervical neoplasia and cancer. *J Low Genit Tract Dis* 2003;**7**:67–86.

2. Smith RA, Cokkinides V, Brooks D, *et al.* Cancer screening in the United States, 2011: a review of current American Cancer Society guidelines and issues in cancer screening. *CA Cancer J Clin* 2011;**61**:8–30.

3. Wright TC, Jr., Massad LS, Dunton CJ, *et al.* 2006 Consensus guidelines for the management of women with abnormal cervical cancer screening tests. *Am J Obstet Gynecol* 2007;**197**:346–55.

4. Solomon D, Davey D, Kurman R, *et al.* The 2001 Bethesda System: terminology for reporting results of cervical cytology. *Jama* 2002;**287**:2114–19.

5. Davey E, d'Assuncao J, Irwig L, *et al.* Accuracy of reading liquid based cytology slides using the ThinPrep Imager compared with conventional cytology: prospective study. *BMJ* 2007;**335**:31.

6. Siebers AG, Klinkhamer PJ, Grefte JM, *et al.* Comparison of liquid-based cytology with conventional cytology for detection of cervical cancer precursors: a randomized controlled trial. *JAMA* 2009;**302**:1757–64.

7. ACOG Committee on Practice Bulletins—Gynecology. ACOG Practice Bulletin no. 109: Cervical cytology screening. *Obstet Gynecol* 2009;**114**:1409–20.

8. DeMay RM. Cytopathology of false negatives preceding cervical carcinoma. *Am J Obstet Gynecol* 1996;**175**:1110–13.

9. Cuzick J, Mayrand MH, Ronco G, Snijders P, Wardle J. Chapter 10: New dimensions in cervical cancer screening. *Vaccine* 2006; **24**(Suppl 3):S90–7.

10. Cox JT, Schiffman M, Solomon D. Prospective follow-up suggests similar risk of subsequent cervical intraepithelial neoplasia grade 2 or 3 among women with cervical intraepithelial neoplasia grade 1 or negative colposcopy and directed biopsy. *Am J Obstet Gynecol* 2003;**188**:1406–12.

11. Sherman ME, Castle PE, Solomon D. Cervical cytology of atypical squamous cells-cannot exclude high-grade squamous intraepithelial lesion (ASC-H): characteristics and histologic outcomes. *Cancer* 2006;**108**:298–305.

12. Evans MF, Adamson CS, Papillo JL, *et al.* Distribution of human papillomavirus types in ThinPrep Papanicolaou tests classified according to the Bethesda 2001 terminology and correlations with patient age and biopsy outcomes. *Cancer* 2006;**106**:1054–64.

13. Levine L, Lucci JA, 3rd, Dinh TV. Atypical glandular cells: new Bethesda Terminology and Management Guidelines. *Obstet Gynecol Surv* 2003;**58**:399–406.

14. Westin MC, Derchain SF, Rabelo-Santos SH, *et al.* Atypical glandular cells and adenocarcinoma in situ according to the Bethesda 2001 classification: cytohistological correlation and clinical implications. *Eur J Obstet Gynecol Reprod Biol* 2008; **139**:79–85.

15. Mathers ME, Johnson SJ, Wadehra V. How predictive is a cervical smear suggesting glandular neoplasia? *Cytopathology* 2002;**13**: 83–91.

16. Chhieng DC, Gallaspy S, Yang H, Roberson J, Eltoum I. Women with atypical glandular cells: a long-term follow-up study in a high-risk population. *Am J Clin Pathol* 2004;**122**:575–9.

17. Zhao C, Florea A, Onisko A, Austin RM. Histologic follow-up results in 662 patients with Pap test findings of atypical glandular cells: results from a large academic womens hospital laboratory employing sensitive screening methods. *Gynecol Oncol* 2009; **114**:383–9.

18. ASCCP. HPV Genotyping Clinical Update; 2011. (Accessed Oct 14 2011, at http://www.asccp.org/ConsensusGuidelines/HPVGenotyping ClinicalUpdate/tabid/5963/Default.aspx.)

19. Ho GY, Bierman R, Beardsley L, Chang CJ, Burk RD. Natural history of cervicovaginal papillomavirus infection in young women. *N Engl J Med* 1998;**338**:423–8.

20. Solomon D, Schiffman M, Tarone R. Comparison of three management strategies for patients with atypical squamous cells of undetermined significance: baseline results from a randomized trial. *J Natl Cancer Inst* 2001;**93**:293–9.

21. de Cremoux P, Coste J, Sastre-Garau X, et al. Efficiency of the hybrid capture 2 HPV DNA test in cervical cancer screening. A study by the French Society of Clinical Cytology. *Am J Clin Pathol* 2003;**120**:492–9.

22. Einstein MH, Martens MG, Garcia FA, et al. Clinical validation of the Cervista HPV HR and 16/18 genotyping tests for use in women with ASC-US cytology. *Gynecol Oncol* 2010;**118**:116–22.

23. Day SP, Hudson A, Mast A, et al. Analytical performance of the Investigational Use Only Cervista HPV HR test as determined by a multi-center study. *J Clin Virol* 2009;**45**(Suppl 1):S63–72.

24. Belinson JL, Wu R, Belinson SE, et al. A population-based clinical trial comparing endocervical high-risk HPV testing using hybrid capture 2 and Cervista from the SHENCCAST II study. *Am J Clin Pathol* 2011;**135**:790–5.

25. Galan-Sanchez F, Rodriguez-Iglesias MA. Use of Cervista HPV HR assay for detection of human papillomavirus in samples with hybrid capture borderline negative results. *Apmis* 2010; **118**:681–4.

26. Einstein MH, Garcia FA, Mitchell AL, Day SP. Age-stratified performance of the Cervista HPV 16/18 genotyping test in women with ASC-US cytology. *Cancer Epidemiol Biomarkers Prev* 2011; **20**:1185–9.

27. Bartholomew DA, Luff RD, Quigley NB, Curtis M, Olson MC. Analytical performance of Cervista HPV 16/18 genotyping test for cervical cytology samples. *J Clin Virol* 2011;**51**:38–43.

28. Kinney W, Stoler MH, Castle PE. Special commentary: patient safety and the next generation of HPV DNA tests. *Am J Clin Pathol* 2010;**134**:193–9.

29. Davis-Devine S, Day SJ, Freund GG. Test performance comparison of inform HPV and hybrid capture 2 high-risk HPV DNA tests using the SurePath liquid-based Pap test as the collection method. *Am J Clin Pathol* 2005;**124**:24–30.

30. Hesselink AT, van den Brule AJ, Brink AA, et al. Comparison of hybrid capture 2 with in situ hybridization for the detection of high-risk human papillomavirus in liquid-based cervical samples. *Cancer* 2004;**102**:11–18.

31. Kurtycz DF, Smith M, He R, Miyazaki K, Shalkham J. Comparison of methods trial for high-risk HPV. *Diagn Cytopathol* 2010; **38**:104–8.

32. Siddiqui MT, Hornaman K, Cohen C, Nassar A. ProEx C immunocytochemistry and high-risk human papillomavirus DNA testing in Papanicolaou tests with atypical squamous cell (ASC-US) cytology: correlation study with histologic biopsy. *Arch Pathol Lab Med* 2008;**132**:1648–52.

33. Sandri MT, Lentati P, Benini E, et al. Comparison of the Digene HC2 assay and the Roche AMPLICOR human papillomavirus (HPV) test for detection of high-risk HPV genotypes in cervical samples. *J Clin Microbiol* 2006;**44**:2141–6.

34. Bentz JS. Liquid-based cytology for cervical cancer screening. *Expert Rev Mol Diagn* 2005;**5**:857–71.

35. Passamonti B, Bulletti S, Camilli M, et al. Evaluation of the FocalPoint GS system performance in an Italian population-based screening of cervical abnormalities. *Acta Cytol* 2007;**51**: 865–71.

36. Chivukula M, Saad RS, Elishaev E, et al. Introduction of the Thin Prep Imaging System (TIS): experience in a high volume academic practice. *Cytojournal* 2007;**4**:6.

37. Zhang FF, Banks HW, Langford SM, Davey DD. Accuracy of ThinPrep Imaging System in detecting low-grade squamous intraepithelial lesions. *Arch Pathol Lab Med* 2007;**131**: 773–6.

38. Jayamohan Y, Karabakhtsian RG, Banks HW, Davey DD. Accuracy of Thinprep Imaging System in detecting atypical glandular cells. *Diagn Cytopathol* 2009;**37**:479–82.

39. Papillo JL, St John TL, Leiman G. Effectiveness of the ThinPrep Imaging System: clinical experience in a low risk screening population. *Diagn Cytopathol* 2008;**36**:155–60.

40. Kardos TF. The FocalPoint System: FocalPoint slide profiler and FocalPoint GS. *Cancer* 2004;**102**:334–9.

41. Chute DJ, Lim H, Kong CS. BD FocalPoint slide profiler performance with atypical glandular cells on SurePath Papanicolaou smears. *Cancer Cytopathol* 2010;**118**:68–74.

42. Wilbur DC, Black-Schaffer WS, Luff RD, et al. The Becton Dickinson FocalPoint GS Imaging System: clinical trials demonstrate significantly improved sensitivity for the detection of important cervical lesions. *Am J Clin Pathol* 2009;**132**:767–75.

43. Halford JA. Cytological features of chronic follicular cervicitis in liquid-based specimens: a potential diagnostic pitfall. *Cytopathology* 2002;**13**:364–70.

44. Al-Nourhji O, Beckmann MJ, Markwell SJ, Massad LS. Pathology correlates of a Papanicolaou diagnosis of low-grade squamous intraepithelial lesion, cannot exclude high-grade squamous intraepithelial lesion. *Cancer* 2008;**114**:469–73.

45. Difurio MJ, Mailhiot T, Sundborg MJ, Nauschuetz KK. Comparison of the clinical significance of the Papanicolaou test interpretations LSIL cannot rule out HSIL and ASC-H. *Diagn Cytopathol* 2010;**38**:313–17.

46. Owens CL, Moats DR, Burroughs FH, Gustafson KS. "Low-grade squamous intraepithelial lesion, cannot exclude high-grade squamous intraepithelial lesion" is a distinct cytologic category: histologic outcomes and HPV prevalence. *Am J Clin Pathol* 2007;**128**:398–403.

47. Elsheikh TM, Kirkpatrick JL, Wu HH. The significance of "low-grade squamous intraepithelial lesion, cannot exclude high-grade squamous intraepithelial lesion" as a distinct squamous abnormality category in Papanicolaou tests. *Cancer* 2006;**108**: 277–81.

48. Ducatman BS, Wang HH, Jonasson JG, Hogan CL, Antonioli DA. Tubal metaplasia: a cytologic study with comparison to other

neoplastic and non-neoplastic conditions of the endocervix. *Diagn Cytopathol* 1993;**9**:98–103; discussion –5.

49. Novotny DB, Maygarden SJ, Johnson DE, Frable WJ. Tubal metaplasia. A frequent potential pitfall in the cytologic diagnosis of endocervical glandular dysplasia on cervical smears. *Acta Cytol* 1992;**36**:1–10.

50. Szyfelbein WM, Baker PM, Bell DA. Superficial endometriosis of the cervix: a source of abnormal glandular cells on cervicovaginal smears. *Diagn Cytopathol* 2004;**30**:88–91.

51. Sauder K, Wilbur DC, Duska L, Tambouret RH. An approach to post-radical trachelectomy vaginal-isthmus cytology. *Diagn Cytopathol* 2009;**37**:437–42.

2 CERVIX: SQUAMOUS CELL CARCINOMA AND PRECURSORS

M. Fujiwara and C. S. Kong

INTRODUCTION

Cervical carcinoma is the second most common cancer in women worldwide and is the third leading cause of cancer-related deaths[1]. In the United States, although the incidence and mortality rates have significantly decreased since the introduction of the Papanicolaou smear (cervical cytology test) as a screening test in 1941, it is still sixth in cancer incidence and tenth in mortality rate for women of African-American and Hispanic descents[2]. The discrepancy in rates worldwide and within the United States is largely due to differences in availability of cervical cancer screening programs.

Squamous cell carcinomas comprise the majority of the cancers of the cervix (~80%) and are the type that has benefitted most from cervical cytology screening. Infection with high-risk types of HPV has been shown to be a necessary but not sufficient cause of cervical cancer[5]. There are 15 high-risk types (16, 18, 31, 33, 35, 39, 45, 51, 52, 56, 58, 59, 68, 73, and 82), with HPV16 as the most common type in squamous cell carcinomas[6]. Carcinogenesis involves progression from intraepithelial and in situ lesions to invasive carcinoma.

Two vaccines against HPV have been approved by the FDA. Gardasil (Merck, Whitehouse Station, NJ) is a quadrivalent vaccine against HPV types 6, 11, 16, and 18, and is approved for females aged 9–26 for prevention of cervical, vaginal and vulvar cancer caused by HPV types 16 and 18, and for females and males aged 9–26 for the prevention of anal cancer and genital warts caused by HPV types 6 and 11. Cervarix (GlaxoSmith Kline, London, England) is a bivalent vaccine against HPV types 6, 11, 16 and 18 for use in females aged 9–25 for the prevention of cervical cancer. Both Gardasil and Cervarix are administered in three doses over a six-month period and are most effective in preventing high-grade dysplasia when given before an infection[9]. They have been shown to provide at least 5–6 years of immunity and protection, and studies are underway to determine the role

of booster vaccines[10]. Although HPV types 16 and 18 account for the majority of cervical cancers, the vaccines do not target the other high-risk HPV types, and it is unknown if there will be cross-protection. Women who have been vaccinated will continue to require cervical cytology screening.

CLINICAL CHARACTERISTICS

The median age for the diagnosis of cervical cancer is 48 years, with no appreciable difference for squamous cell carcinoma and adenocarcinoma[11]. The risk factors for the development of squamous cell carcinoma and adenocarcinomas are similar, and the risk increases with increased number of sexual partners, earlier age of first intercourse, earlier age at first birth, and increase in duration of oral contraceptive use. Immunocompromised patients, such as those with human immunodeficiency virus (HIV) and transplant recipients, are also at increased risk for HPV-related dysplasia[12]. Smoking appears to increase risk for squamous cell carcinoma only, and not for adenocarcinoma[11]. Most of the risk factors are related to a woman's chance of exposure to high-risk HPV types. Although cervical cancer is frequently asymptomatic, the most common symptoms include abnormal vaginal bleeding, postcoital bleeding, and vaginal discharge.

Preoperative assessment

Cervical cytology and human papillomavirus testing

Cervical cytology is an effective screening tool that allows for the evaluation of exfoliated cells from the transformation zone where most cervical dysplasias and cancers arise. Since high-risk HPV is necessary for the development of cervical cancer, HPV testing plays an important role in the management of cervical cytology abnormalities. (See Chapter 1.)

Colposcopy with biopsy

Colposcopy with biopsy and endocervical curettage is an additional tool used preoperatively after an abnormal cervical cytology screen or HPV test result. The false-negative rate of colposcopy ranges from 2.7 to 23%[15].

Prognosis

Cervical squamous intraepithelial lesion

Low-grade squamous intraepithelial lesion (LSIL) represents a heterogeneous group of lesions with a high rate of regression and uncommon progression to high-grade squamous intraepithelial lesion within the first 24 months. Only 2.1% of women with low-grade squamous intraepithelial lesion progress to high-grade squamous intraepithelial lesion or invasive carcinoma; the risk for progression is higher if a woman tests positive for high-risk HPV or is older than 30 years of age[19,20]. In contrast, the incidence of invasive cervical cancer in patients with untreated high-grade squamous intraepithelial lesion is 31% over the course of 30 years vs. 0.7% for those with adequate treatment[21].

Squamous cell carcinoma

The overall five-year survival rate for patients with squamous cell carcinoma is 70.5%[22]. Although prognosis is excellent when detected early (International Federation of Gynecology and Obstetrics [FIGO] stage IA1, IA2) with a five-year survival rate of 97.5%, patients presenting with distant metastasis (FIGO stage IVB) have an abysmal five-year survival rate of 9.3%. Tumor size and depth of tumor invasion are independent prognostic factors[23]. Narrowly defined microinvasive squamous cell carcinoma is associated with a negligible risk for lymph node metastasis (1–2%), risk of recurrence (0.9%), and risk of death (0.5%)[24,25]. Although vascular invasion was initially thought to be associated with a worse prognosis, more recent studies have not found it to be an independent prognostic indicator[26,27]. In immunocompromised patients, cervical carcinoma is associated with a very aggressive course and poor outcome[28,29].

Management and treatment

The ASCCP 2006 Consensus Guidelines for the Management of Intraepithelial Neoplasia and Adenocarcinoma in Situ reflect different management algorithms for the general population vs. special populations, as the risk of high-grade squamous intraepithelial lesion or cancer differs in these various groups[30]. A significant change with the 2006 guidelines is the identification of adolescents (defined as women 20 of years and younger) as a special population that should be treated less aggressively than the general population.

Low-grade squamous intraepithelial lesion

The recommended management for patients with low-grade squamous intraepithelial lesion (CIN1) on biopsy depends on the prior cytologic diagnosis. With a prior diagnosis of ASC-US, ASC-H, or low-grade squamous intraepithelial lesion, the patient can be followed with HPV testing every 12 months or repeat cytology at 6 and 12 months. Colposcopy is indicated if HPV testing is positive or if repeat cytology shows ASC-US or worse. With a prior cytologic diagnosis of high-grade squamous intraepithelial lesion or atypical glandular cells NOS, acceptable options include observation with colposcopy and cytology at 6 and 12 months or immediate loop electrosurgical excision procedure (LEEP). Whenever there is a major discrepancy between the cytologic and histologic diagnoses, the prior cytology slide should be reviewed in conjunction with the biopsy, and level sections of the biopsy examined.

All adolescent women (≤ 20 years of age) with CIN1 on biopsy should be managed conservatively with follow-up cytology at 12 months. Colposcopy is recommended only if cytology at 12 months shows at least high-grade squamous intraepithelial lesion, or if cytology at 24 months shows at least ASC-US. Follow-up with HPV testing is not acceptable in the adolescent population. Pregnant women should also be managed conservatively with no treatment.

High-grade squamous intraepithelial lesion

Women with a histologic diagnosis of high-grade squamous intraepithelial lesion (CIN2–3) and satisfactory colposcopy can be treated with either excision or ablation. Ablation is not acceptable if the colposcopy is unsatisfactory or if the CIN2–3 is recurrent. Hysterectomy is also unacceptable as primary therapy. Given the significant risk for progression to invasive squamous cell carcinoma, observation with colposcopy and cytology is unacceptable.

If CIN2–3 is present at the resection margin, it is preferable to follow with cytology and endocervical sampling at 4–6 months, but it is also acceptable to re-excise. Acceptable post-treatment follow-up includes HPV testing at 6 and 12 months, cytology alone at 6 months, or cytology and colposcopy at 6 months. Colposcopy with endocervical sampling is recommended for women who are HPV positive or have cytology results of ASC-US or higher. Repeat treatment or hysterectomy based on a positive HPV result is unacceptable. However, repeat excision or hysterectomy is acceptable for recurrent or persistent CIN2–3.

In adolescent women diagnosed with CIN2–3, it is acceptable to either treat or follow with colposcopy and cytology for up to 24 months. However, if the lesion is specified as CIN2, observation is preferred, while treatment is recommended for CIN3 or if colposcopy is unsatisfactory.

Pregnant women should be followed with colposcopy and cytology at intervals of no more than every 12 weeks. Postponing further evaluation until 6 weeks postpartum is also acceptable. Unless invasive cancer is suspected, repeat biopsy and treatment are unacceptable.

Microinvasive squamous cell carcinoma

Narrowly defined microinvasive squamous cell carcinoma (i.e., ≤ 3 mm depth of invasion; ≤ 7 mm horizontal extent; no lymphatic-vascular invasion) can be treated conservatively with cold knife conization or large loop excision in women who wish to preserve fertility, or with simple hysterectomy. For low-stage lesions that do not meet these strict criteria, the standard treatment has been radical hysterectomy with lymph node dissection.

Invasive squamous cell carcinoma

The management of women with invasive squamous cell carcinoma depends on the FIGO stage at diagnosis[31]. In 2002, the American Congress of Obstetricians and Gynecologists developed clinical management guidelines for patients with cervical carcinoma[32]. Cervical cancer can largely be divided into two categories of early stage (IA1–IIA) and late-stage (IIB–IVB) disease (Table 2.1).

Modified radical hysterectomy with regional lymph node dissection is recommended for patients with FIGO stage IA2 tumors and above. However, a subset of patients with FIGO stage IA2 and IB1 tumors can undergo fertility-preserving treatment with radical trachelectomy[33]. Although this spares the uterus, the live birth rate for women after trachelectomy is low (17%), and the rate of second-trimester losses and preterm births is high[33].

Women with FIGO stage IB–IIA tumors may be treated non-surgically with external beam radiation therapy and brachytherapy. Although five-year survival rates are comparable between the surgical and non-surgical approaches,

Table 2.1 American Joint Committee on Cancer (AJCC)/International Federation of Gynecology and Obstetrics (FIGO) staging for cervical carcinomas

TNM[a]	FIGO	Description
TX	n/a	Primary tumor cannot be assessed
T0	n/a	No evidence of primary tumor
Tis	n/a	Carcinoma in situ
T1	I	Cervical carcinoma confined to uterus
T1a	IA	Invasive carcinoma diagnosed only by microscopy. Stromal invasion ≤ 5.0 mm depth of invasion and ≤ 7.0 mm horizontal spread. Vascular space involvement does not affect staging
T1a1	IA1	Stromal invasion ≤ 3.0 mm depth of invasion and ≤ 7.0 mm horizontal spread
T1a2	IA2	Stromal invasion > 3.0 mm but ≤ 5.0 mm, with ≤ 7.0 mm horizontal spread
T1b1	IB1	Clinically visible lesion ≤ 4.0 cm in greatest dimension
T1b2	IB2	Clinically visible lesion > 4.0 cm in greatest dimension
T2	II	Cervical carcinoma invades beyond uterus but does not extend to pelvic wall or lower third of vagina
T2a	IIA	Tumor without parametrial invasion
T2a1	IIA1	Clinically visible lesion ≤ 4.0 cm in greatest dimension
T2a2	IIA2	Clinically visible lesion > 4.0 cm in greatest dimension
T2b	IIB	Tumor with parametrial invasion
T3	III	Tumor extends to pelvic wall and/or involves lower third of vagina, and/or causes hydronephrosis or non-functioning kidney
T3a	IIIA	Tumor involves lower third of vagina without extension to pelvic wall
T3b	IIIB	Tumor extends to pelvic wall and/or causes hydronephrosis or non-functioning kidney
T4	IVA	Tumor invades mucosa of bladder or rectum, and/or extends beyond true pelvis
N0		No regional lymph node metastasis
N1	IIIB	Regional lymph node metastasis
M0		No distant metastasis
M1	IVB	Distant metastasis (includes peritoneal spread, involvement of supraclavicular or mediastinal lymph nodes, lung, liver, or bone)

n/a: not applicable.

[a] The tumor, node, metastasis (TNM) system of the AJCC and the Union for International Cancer Control (UICC).

there is a difference in the types of complications[34]. Surgery enables the preservation of sexual and ovarian function, while radiation therapy may be better suited for women unable to tolerate a surgical procedure.

Women with late-stage disease (FIGO IIB–IVB) are generally treated with external beam radiation therapy, brachytherapy, and concurrent cisplatin-based chemotherapy. There is no difference in treatment recommendations for squamous cell carcinoma based on the different histologic subtypes.

Follow-up for recurrences is performed every three months for one year, every four months for the second year, every six months for years three to five, and then annually with direct examinations and cervical cytology.

MORPHOLOGY

Gross pathology

Precursor lesions and early invasive carcinomas may only be visible by colposcopic examination after application of 3–5% acetic acid to the cervix. Low-grade squamous intraepithelial lesions often take on a whitish appearance, whereas high-grade squamous intraepithelial lesions tend to demonstrate changes such as punctation, mosaicism, and atypical vessels. More advanced invasive carcinomas can be either exophytic, endophytic, or ulcerative. Care should be taken with hysterectomy specimens to determine macroscopic tumor size, depth of invasion, and, if present, involvement of vaginal, endometrial, and parametrial tissue.

Microscopic pathology

Low-grade squamous intraepithelial lesion (CIN1)

Low-grade squamous intraepithelial lesion (LSIL) is characterized by thickened mucosa with hyperchromatic enlarged nuclei in the upper layers. Normal squamous cell nuclei typically become smaller as they mature and move towards the surface. In contrast, dysplastic nuclei are enlarged and are similar in size or larger than the basal cell nuclei. The nuclei of the dysplastic cells are darker than those of the uninvolved squamous mucosa. Binucleated cells are present in 90% of low-grade squamous intraepithelial lesion, and when surrounded by a cytoplasmic halo are termed koilocytes. Koilocytic halos should be sharply punched out and irregularly shaped with a variable distance from the edge of the halo to the edge of the nucleus (Figure 2.1). Parakeratosis may also be present.

Flat condylomas commonly occur in the transformation zone and are associated with high-risk HPV.

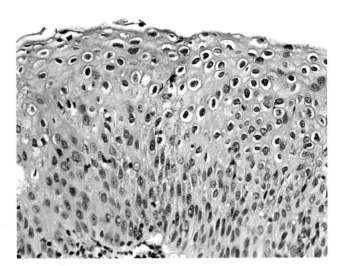

Figure 2.1 Low-grade squamous intraepithelial lesion (CIN1). Koilocytes are notable in the upper layers of the thickened squamous mucosa.

Immature condylomas (squamous papilloma) also occur in the transformation zone but are less common. They exhibit a filiform, papillary growth pattern and are associated with low-risk HPV types 6 and 11. Exophytic condylomas, or condyloma acuminatum, are also associated with low-risk HPV types but are typically found in the vulva and occur less frequently in the cervix.

The ASCUS-LSIL Triage Study (ALTS) on interobserver variability found poor reproducibility for the histologic diagnosis of low-grade squamous intraepithelial lesion, with kappa statistics of 0.46–0.49[35]. There was agreement on the diagnosis of low-grade squamous intraepithelial lesion in 43% of cases, but 41% of the cases diagnosed by the staff pathologists as low-grade squamous intraepithelial lesion were downgraded by the QC pathologists to negative. Most of the downgraded cases were positive for high-risk HPV; the significance of this finding was not addressed.

High-grade squamous intraepithelial lesion (CIN2–3)

High-grade squamous intraepithelial lesion (HSIL) is characterized by atypical cells with high nuclear-to-cytoplasmic ratios (at least 1 : 1), irregular nuclear contours, and coarse chromatin. These abnormalities involve one-third to two-thirds of the mucosal thickness in CIN2 (Figure 2.2) and more than two-thirds in CIN3 (Figure 2.3). Mitotic figures are commonly found in the upper half of the epithelium, and the cells are crowded with loss of polarity, making cells at the basal layer indistinguishable from the surface. In contrast to low-grade squamous intraepithelial lesion, high nuclear-to-cytoplasmic-ratio cells involve

Table 2.2 Histologic features of low-grade (LSIL) vs. high-grade (HSIL) squamous intraepithelial lesion

	Low-grade squamous intraepithelial lesion	High-grade squamous intraepithelial lesion
Nuclei	Large; with or without binucleation or multinucleation	Small, similar in size to basal cell nuclei
Nuclear-to-cytoplasmic ratio of dysplastic cells	Low	$\geq 1:1$
Location of dysplastic cells	Upper layers of mucosa	Lower two-thirds for CIN2; full thickness for CIN3
Distribution of mitoses	Lower half of mucosa	Upper half of mucosa
Basal layer	Minimal changes	Loss of polarity

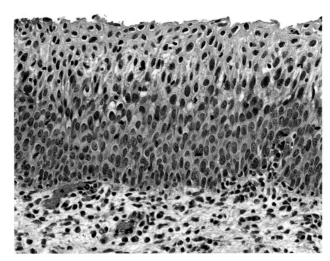

Figure 2.2 High-grade squamous intraepithelial lesion (CIN2). Atypical high nuclear-to-cytoplasmic-ratio cells involve more than one-third of the mucosal thickness; koilocytes are also present near the surface.

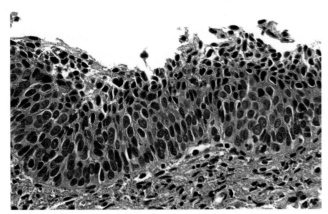

Figure 2.3 High-grade squamous intraepithelial lesion (CIN3). Full-thickness involvement of the mucosa by atypical high nuclear-to-cytoplasmic-ratio cells.

more than one-third of the mucosal thickness, and high mitotic figures can be seen (Table 2.2).

While a diagnosis of high-grade squamous intraepithelial lesion can be used to encompass CIN2 and CIN3, it is best to indicate in the diagnostic line whether the lesion represents CIN2 or CIN3. The ASCUS-LSIL Triage Study found poor interobserver agreement (43.4%) between clinical center pathologists and QC pathologists for the diagnosis of CIN2; a similar number of cases were downgraded or upgraded[36]. A large population-based study of patients from Guanacaste, Costa Rica also reported the diagnosis of CIN2 to be significantly less reproducible than CIN3[37]. Two review pathologists agreed with 13–31% of CIN2 diagnoses, and 81–84%, CIN3. CIN3 also showed a

higher correlation with high-risk HPV and with a diagnosis of high-grade squamous intraepithelial lesion on cytology. These studies support the concept of CIN2 as an equivocal diagnosis that encompasses a mixture of both CIN1 and CIN3. Recognizing the poor reproducibility of the diagnosis and the greater likelihood of regression, CIN2 can be treated less aggressively in the adolescent population (20 years of age or less)[30].

Microinvasive squamous cell carcinoma

Microinvasive squamous cell carcinomas arise in the background of high-grade squamous intraepithelial lesion and can be recognized from low power as a break in the usual smooth contours of the mucosal junction with the submucosa. Irregular tongues of epithelium with more abundant eosinophilic cytoplasm extend into the surrounding stroma, which is usually loose and may be associated with an inflammatory infiltrate. With invasion, the cells will typically appear more mature than dysplastic cells and will exhibit evidence of squamous differentiation such as keratinization or keratin pearl formation.

Microinvasive squamous cell carcinoma is also known as early invasive carcinoma or microcarcinoma, and is defined by the depth of stromal invasion and horizontal extent. Currently, the term is most commonly applied to completely excised squamous cell carcinomas with stromal invasion of 3 mm or less and horizontal spread of 7 mm or less, corresponding to FIGO stage IA1. (Figure 2.4) The applicability of the microinvasive term to completely excised squamous cell carcinomas with a depth of invasion >3 to ≤5 mm

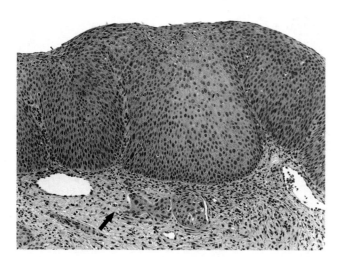

Figure 2.4 Microinvasive squamous cell carcinoma. Jagged fingers of tumor cells (arrow) invade to a depth of less than 3 mm and extend horizontally less than 7 mm.

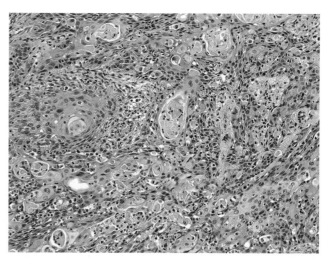

Figure 2.5 Keratinizing squamous cell carcinoma. Irregular nests of tumor cells with dense, eosinophilic cytoplasm and central collections of keratin debris invade into desmoplastic stroma.

(FIGO stage IA2) is more controversial. These carcinomas are associated with a higher risk of lymph node metastasis (7.8%) and death (2.4%)[24].

Measurement for depth of invasion should start at the basement membrane of the mucosa at the point of invasion. This can either be from the surface or from an endocervical gland. In cases where the origin is indeterminate, it is best to measure from the basement membrane of the surface mucosa. Measurement of horizontal extent is usually straightforward but can be problematic in the uncommon cases where discontinuous foci are present or where the invasive component extends over several blocks. There are no rules about how far apart each focus should be before it is considered distinct, and the literature does not address whether multiple foci of superficial invasion each measuring less than 7 mm in horizontal extent can still be defined as microinvasive. For clarity in reporting in these problematic cases, it is best to provide as much information as possible. Discontinuous foci should be measured and reported separately with a comment regarding the difficulty in classifying these lesions. In cases where the invasive focus extends over several blocks, the report should indicate the greatest horizontal extent in a single cross-section, the number of blocks involved, and the thickness of the specimen sections (usually 3 mm) which will allow for an estimate of extent of involvement. With this information, the gynecologist can then decide whether to treat the patient conservatively as a microinvasive carcinoma, or more aggressively.

Before defining a tumor as microinvasive, it is essential to evaluate the entire lesion. The term should not be applied to cases where the invasive component extends to a peripheral or deep margin, since in these cases the true extent of involvement cannot be determined. The presence or absence of lymphovascular invasion is not a criterion for the diagnosis of microinvasive carcinoma, but does play a role in management decisions.

Squamous cell carcinoma

Invasive squamous cell carcinoma can be subclassified into several different histologic types: keratinizing, non-keratinizing, basaloid, warty, papillary, lymphoepithelioma-like, squamo-transitional, and verrucous. Except for verrucous, all the types are associated with high-risk HPV.

Keratinizing squamous cell carcinomas are well-differentiated carcinomas characterized by keratin pearls (concentric whorls of squamous cells) and tumor cells with abundant, dense, eosinophilic cytoplasm surrounding central nests of keratin. Jagged nests of malignant cells and individual keratinizing cells invade into surrounding desmoplastic stroma (Figure 2.5).

In contrast, non-keratinizing carcinomas lack keratin pearls and appear less well differentiated, with higher nuclear-to-cytoplasmic ratios, increased nuclear pleomorphism, and more frequent mitotic figures (Figure 2.6). The cells will continue to exhibit evidence of squamous differentiation with dense eosinophilic cytoplasm and intercellular bridges. Non-keratinizing carcinomas are typically moderately differentiated.

Basaloid squamous cell carcinomas are poorly differentiated, with rounded nests of basal-type squamous cells with hyperchromatic nuclei, inconspicuous nucleoli, and

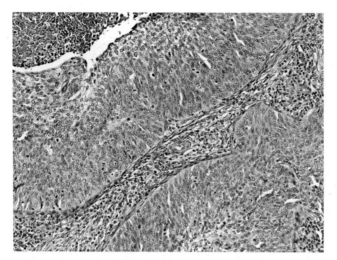

Figure 2.6 Non-keratinizing squamous cell carcinoma. Tumor cells are characterized by high nuclear-to-cytoplasmic ratios, increased nuclear pleomorphism and less evidence of squamous differentiation.

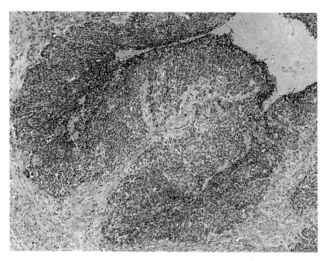

Figure 2.7 Basaloid squamous cell carcinoma. Rounded nests of tumor cells with hyperchromatic nuclei and scant cytoplasm.

scant cytoplasm (Figure 2.7). Comedo-type necrosis or keratinization can also occur within the nests.

The warty and papillary subtypes refer to the architectural pattern of the invasive squamous cell carcinoma. Warty carcinomas will superficially resemble a condyloma with koilocytes and hyperparakeratosis, while papillary carcinomas will exhibit fibrovascular cores lined by cells resembling high-grade squamous intraepithelial lesion. Superficial biopsies of either can lead to a mistaken impression of an in situ or dysplastic process. However, one should consider these special types if only condylomatous changes are seen in a biopsy of a large mass or if papillary architecture is noted (not typically seen with high-grade squamous intraepithelial lesion).

Lymphoepithelioma-like carcinoma resembles the undifferentiated type of nasopharyngeal carcinoma, consisting of syncytial nests of poorly differentiated epithelial cells with vesicular nuclei and prominent nucleoli in a background of an intense lymphocytic infiltrate. While some studies have shown an association with HPV and no association with the Epstein–Barr virus (EBV), others from Asia have detected EBV in a significant subset of cases[38]. A more recent study by Chao *et al.* found low copy numbers of EBV DNA in 9/9 cases of lymphoepithelioma-like carcinoma and 7/25 squamous cell carcinoma (no special type); high-risk HPV was detected in 8/9 cases of lymphoepithelioma-like carcinoma and all cases of squamous cell carcinoma[41]. Given the low copy numbers of EBV, it was postulated that EBV was present in tumor-infiltrating lymphocytes (TILs) and not in the tumor cells, arguing against an etiologic role for EBV.

Squamotransitional cell carcinoma is a rare variant that resembles transitional cell carcinomas of the urinary tract but is associated with high-risk HPV. Before diagnosing this variant, a bladder primary needs to be excluded.

Verrucous carcinoma is a special type of very well-differentiated squamous cell carcinoma that more commonly occurs in the vulva. The tumor is characterized by an exophytic warty growth that is mirrored by a bulbous endophytic component. The exophytic component projects above the mucosal surface as "church spires": pointy to slightly rounded fingers of cytologically bland mucosa with prominent hyperkeratosis. The endophytic squamous component invades as bulbous masses with chronic inflammation in the submucosa and a pushing border, rather than the irregular, ragged infiltration typically seen with invasive carcinomas. Although they do not metastasize, verrucous carcinomas have a tendency to recur locally.

Tumor grading

Squamous cell carcinomas of the cervix are graded as well differentiated (grade 1), moderately differentiated (grade 2), and poorly differentiated (grade 3). Well-differentiated tumors show cells with uniform nuclei, eosinophilic cytoplasm and easily identifiable squamous maturation such as keratin formation and intercellular bridges. Moderately differentiated tumors retain some of the features of squamous differentiation, but not to the degree of the well-differentiated carcinomas. Poorly differentiated tumors lack overt squamous differentiation and instead are composed of primitive-appearing cells with high nuclear to cytoplasmic ratios. Tumor grading is not thought to be predictive of prognosis.

Tumor staging

Cervical squamous cell carcinomas are staged according to the American Joint Committee on Cancer (AJCC) TNM classification system and the International Federation of Gynecology and Obstetrics (FIGO) system (Table 2.1)[42]. Since most patients are treated non-surgically, staging is frequently based on clinical evaluation, which can include physical examination (palpation, visual inspection, colposcopy), diagnostic procedures (endocervical curettage, hysteroscopy, cystoscopy, proctoscopy, intravenous urography), and radiologic studies (X-ray, computed tomography [CT], magnetic resonance imaging [MRI], and positron emission tomography [PET]).

Pathologic staging can be performed in cases where tissue is surgically removed. It is primarily pertinent in low-stage disease where depth of invasion and horizontal extent must be determined microscopically. Macroscopically visible disease is automatically at least T1b, and the determination of T2–4 is based upon extent of spread, which is typically by direct extension. Tumor also spreads through the lymphatic system, involving the peritoneum, lung, liver, bone, and distant lymph nodes (supraclavicular, mediastinal, and para-aortic).

Lymph nodes

The risk for lymph node involvement strongly correlates with stage. The obturator and iliac lymph nodes are most commonly involved by metastatic carcinoma[43]. The pattern of drainage leads to spread to the pelvic sidewall lymph nodes followed by common iliac then para-aortic.

ANCILLARY DIAGNOSTIC TESTS

p16 immunohistochemistry

p16 is a surrogate marker for detecting the presence of high-risk HPV that has integrated into the host genome. Immunohistochemical stain for p16 is useful for distinguishing high-grade squamous intraepithelial lesion from immature squamous metaplasia and atrophy, but the results should always be interpreted in the context of the morphologic findings.

Optimal specificity for the diagnosis of squamous dysplasia is obtained by requiring continuous ($\geq 80\%$), strong nuclear or nuclear and cytoplasmic staining of the basal layer for the stain to be interpreted as positive (Figure 2.8).

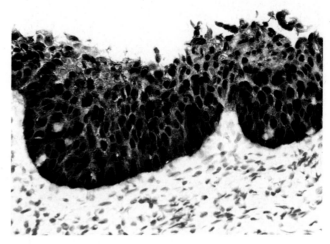

Figure 2.8 Diffuse, strong p16 reactivity correlates with integration of high-risk HPV into the host genome. (High-grade squamous intraepithelial lesion.)

Diffuse, strong staining has been shown by many studies to correlate with the presence of high-risk HPV[46]. Together with morphologic features that raise concern for dysplasia, it can be used to support a diagnosis of dysplasia. However, determination of grade should be based on morphologic features and not on the pattern of p16 reactivity. Although full-thickness p16 reactivity is more frequently seen with high-grade squamous intraepithelial lesion, and partial-thickness with low-grade squamous intraepithelial lesion, the thickness of mucosal p16 reactivity is not a reliable feature for grading dysplasia. Occasional cases of high-grade squamous intraepithelial lesion will exhibit staining that does not extend above half the mucosal thickness, and similarly low-grade squamous intraepithelial lesion can exhibit full-thickness reactivity[50]. p16 is most useful in evaluating problematic cases where the differential diagnosis is between high-grade squamous intraepithelial lesion and immature squamous metaplasia or atrophy. It is less useful where the differential diagnosis is between low-grade squamous intraepithelial lesion and a benign process, since not all low-grade squamous intraepithelial lesion cases are associated with high-risk HPV. Overexpression of p16 is only seen when HPV has integrated into the host genome, and this does not occur with low-risk HPV types. In cases of low-grade squamous intraepithelial lesion, a negative p16 stain does not exclude the possibility of dysplasia.

Focal (5–80%), strong p16 reactivity is less specific, and while it occurs in a subset of low-grade and high-grade squamous intraepithelial lesion, it can also be seen with benign squamous metaplasia and tubal metaplasia

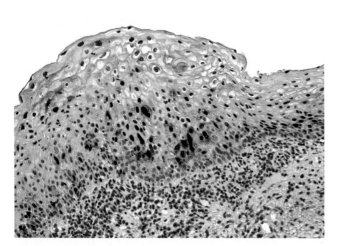

Figure 2.9 Focal p16 reactivity is non-specific and can be seen with reactive squamous metaplasia as well as LSIL (shown).

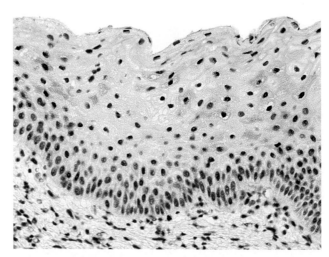

Figure 2.10 Weak or blush p16 reactivity should be interpreted as negative.

(Figure 2.9)[46,47,51]. Variable weak staining or cytoplasmic-only staining is non-specific and should be interpreted as negative (Figure 2.10). While negative p16 supports a benign reactive process, focal, strong p16 is best interpreted as equivocal. Further evaluation with HPV in situ hybridization or HPV polymerase chain reaction may be useful in equivocal cases to determine if high-risk HPV is present.

ProEx C immunohistochemistry

ProEx C is an assay composed of monoclonal antibodies directed against topoisomerase II-alpha and minichromosome maintenance protein-2. It detects aberrant S-phase induction and has been shown to perform similarly to p16[52,53]. Interpretation of ProEx C relies on determining the extent of nuclear reactivity within the vertical layers of the mucosa, since normal ectocervix is characterized by diffuse staining of 1–2 cell layers of the basal layer. The criteria used for defining ProEx C as positive varies from >25% to >33% of the mucosal thickness[53]. Extent of staining loosely correlates with grade of dysplasia; CIN3 typically shows full-thickness or near full-thickness staining of the mucosa.

Ki-67 immunohistochemistry

Several studies have advocated the use of immunohistochemical stain for the proliferation marker Ki-67 as an aid in the diagnosis of cervical dysplasia[47,52,56]. There is general agreement that only strong nuclear staining of cells in the upper two-thirds of the mucosa should be interpreted as positive; some studies specify a requirement for a cluster of two or more positive cells. Accurate interpretation of Ki-67 stain requires well-oriented specimens since tangential sectioning can make it difficult to determine the location of the positive cells. Ki-67 is best used in conjunction with a sensitive marker for high-risk HPV such as p16; false-positive Ki-67 results can occur in the setting of benign reactive or reparative conditions[47,57,59].

Human papillomavirus in situ hybridization

For paraffin-embedded tissue, there are two commercially available slide-based chromogenic in situ hybridization assays for HPV: Ventana Inform (Tucson, AZ) and Dako GenPoint (Carpinteria, CA). The Ventana Inform HPV III Family 16 probe targets multiple high-risk HPV types (6, 11, 16, 18, 31, 33, 35, 39, 45, 51, 52, and 66) but is weighted towards detection of HPV16. Dako GenPoint has both wide spectrum (6, 11, 16, 18, 31, 33, 35, 39, 45, 51, and 52) and type-specific (6/11, 16/18, 31/33) probe sets. The advantage of HPV in situ hybridization is high specificity and the ability to determine viral integration status. Non-integrated virus appears as diffuse nuclear staining, while integrated virus exhibits punctate nuclear staining (Figure 2.11). However, with high viral load, integrated virus may appear as diffuse nuclear staining. The drawback of HPV in situ hybridization is the low sensitivity of the assay in comparison with p16 immunohistochemistry. In a study comparing a Dako high-risk HPV probe (no longer available) and Ventana HPV III probe with p16, the sensitivity of in situ hybridization was 56–69% vs. 82% for diffuse, strong p16[46]. Although less sensitive, HPV in situ

(A)

(B)

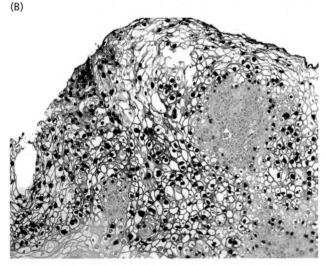

Figure 2.11 Human papillomavirus in situ hybridization. (A) Punctate nuclear staining correlates with viral integration; (B) diffuse nuclear staining correlates with episomal HPV but can also be seen with high concentrations of integrated HPV.

hybridization is more specific than p16 and may be useful for further evaluation of cases with equivocal p16 results.

DIFFERENTIAL DIAGNOSIS

Low-grade squamous intraepithelial lesion

Glycogenation

Glycogen halos can mimic koilocytes, but the nuclei in glycogenation are not enlarged or hyperchromatic (Figure 2.12). Binucleation may be seen, but the nuclei are centrally located and maintain an even distance from the edge of the nucleus to the edge of the halo. The lack of cytologic atypia should preclude a diagnosis of dysplasia (Table 2.3).

Table 2.3 Histologic features of benign squamous mucosa vs. low-grade squamous intraepithelial lesion (LSIL)

	Benign	Low-grade squamous intraepithelial lesion
Nuclear size	Smaller than basal cell nuclei	Enlarged
Binucleation	May be present	May be present
Chromatin	Normal	Hyperchromatic
Nuclear membranes	Smooth	Irregular
Nucleoli	May be present	None
Cytoplasmic halo	Even shape, nucleus located in center of halo	Irregular contours, nucleus located off-center

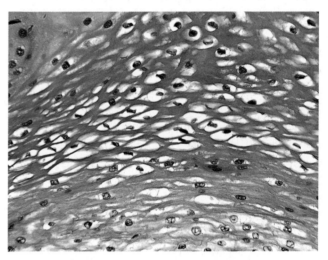

Figure 2.12 Glycogenation of squamous mucosa can mimic koilocytes with the appearance of halos, but note the absence of nuclear atypia in this section of benign esophageal squamous mucosa.

Inflammatory/reactive changes

Inflammatory halos are uniform and round with less-distinct borders between the edge of the halo and the cytoplasm (Figure 2.13). The nuclei may be mildly enlarged with prominent nucleoli, but will be located in the center of the halo with an even distance from the edge of the nucleus to the edge of the halo. The nuclei will also maintain smooth nuclear contours and lack hyperchromasia. Acute and chronic inflammatory cells frequently infiltrate the squamous mucosa, and intercellular edema may also be seen (Table 2.2).

High-grade squamous intraepithelial lesion

Immature squamous metaplasia

Squamous metaplastic cells have increased nuclear-to-cytoplasmic ratios, but the nuclei are uniform with smooth

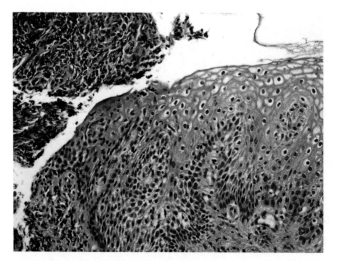

Figure 2.13 Inflammatory halos are even with indistinct edges.

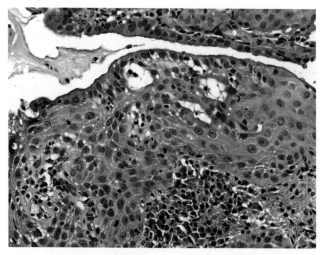

Figure 2.14 Squamous metaplastic cells have increased nuclear-to-cytoplasmic ratios but are evenly spaced; the presence of overlying endocervical glands is a helpful indicator of a benign process.

(A)   (B)

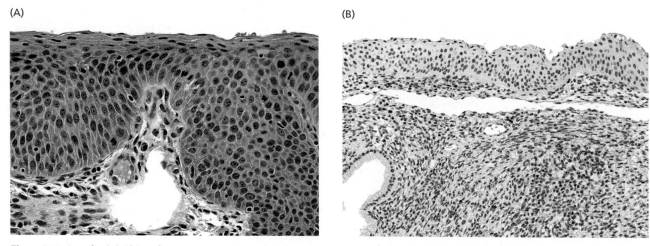

Figure 2.15 Atrophy (A) Thinned squamous mucosa with hyperchromatic nuclei and high nuclear-to-cytoplasmic ratio but smooth nuclear contours; (B) p16 immunohistochemical stain is negative.

nuclear membranes and even chromatin. The cells are not crowded and show retention of polarity (Figure 2.14). Prominent nucleoli and mitotic activity may be seen but there should not be any abnormal mitotic figures. If present, overlying mucinous endocervical epithelium on the surface is a helpful indicator of metaplasia rather than dysplasia (Table 2.3).

Atrophy

Atrophy can be difficult to distinguish from thin high-grade squamous intraepithelial lesion, as both can have cells with high nuclear-to-cytoplasmic ratios and hyperchromatic nuclei. However, with atrophy, the nuclei should be relatively uniform with even chromatin and smooth nuclear contours (Figure 2.15). Mitotic activity should be absent. In cases where the distinction cannot be confidently

made based on histologic features alone, p16 and Ki-67 immunohistochemistry can be helpful (see *Ancillary diagnostic tests*, above).

Squamous cell carcinoma

Displaced epithelium

Prior procedures can displace fragments of benign squamous epithelium into lymphatic-vascular spaces, mimicking lymphatic-vascular invasion (Figure 2.16). The lack of cytologic atypia and presence of degenerative changes are clues to this artifact. With excision specimens, sectioning of the gross specimen can also displace fragments of dysplastic or malignant epithelium into lymphatic-vascular spaces. This can be harder to discern since the fragments

(A)

(B)

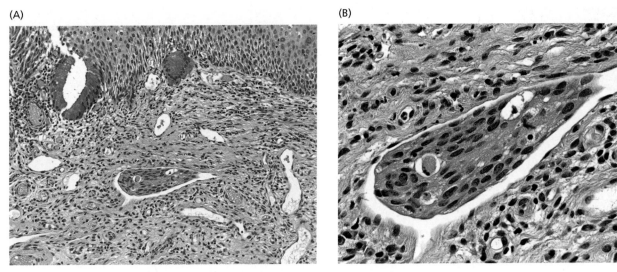

Figure 2.16 (A, B) Benign epithelium can be displaced into a lymphatic-vascular space as a result of a prior biopsy. Note the absence of nuclear atypia and presence of apoptosis, indicating presence of degenerative changes.

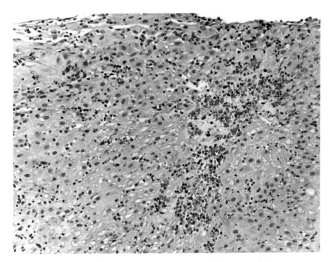

Figure 2.17 Placental site nodules are well circumscribed and composed of intermediate trophoblasts embedded in hyalinized stroma.

will appear abnormal. If the cluster within the space is not attached to the wall and not associated with fibrin, it is best to avoid a definitive diagnosis of lymphatic-vascular invasion.

Squamous intraepithelial lesion

The warty subtype of squamous cell carcinoma resembles a condyloma on the surface, with invasive squamous cell carcinoma apparent at the base of the lesion. Superficial biopsies can lead to an underdiagnosis as low-grade squamous intraepithelial lesion. If condylomatous changes are seen and the junction with the submucosa cannot be evaluated, or if the biopsy represents sampling of a larger mass, consideration should be given to the possibility of a warty squamous cell carcinoma. A deeper sample may be necessary for definitive diagnosis.

Placental site nodule

Placental site nodules are benign remnants of placental implantation sites. While they occur more commonly in the endometrium and myometrium, one-third to two-thirds are found in the lower uterine segment and upper endocervix[60]. Placental site nodules are well circumscribed and composed of intermediate trophoblasts with hyalinized intercellular stroma. The trophoblasts are large cells with hyperchromatic irregular nuclei, prominent nucleoli, and abundant eosinophilic to amphophilic cytoplasm (Figure 2.17)[61]. Mitotic figures are rare. If the trophoblastic nature of the cells is not recognized, the cytologic atypia and eosinophilic cytoplasm can lead to a mistaken diagnosis of squamous cell carcinoma. Immunohistochemical stain for p16 can be helpful, as placental site nodules exhibit no or focal weak staining, while most squamous cell carcinomas are diffusely positive[62]. Placental site nodules are positive for inhibin-α (cytoplasmic), placental alkaline phosphatase, and human placental lactogen (focal), which can also be helpful since these stains are negative in squamous cell carcinoma[61,63].

Epithelioid trophoblastic tumor

Epithelioid trophoblastic tumor represents the neoplastic form of the placental site nodule. They are composed of intermediate trophoblastic cells forming nests and cords of cells with mild to marked nuclear atypia, prominent nucleoli, and moderate to abundant amounts of eosinophilic to clear cytoplasm. The surrounding stroma is hyalinized, and mitotic activity and necrosis are commonly seen. Fibrillary eosinophilic hyaline material in the center of the tumor

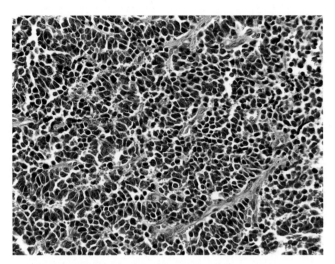

Figure 2.18 Small cell carcinoma has characteristic trabecular growth pattern and tumor cells with stippled chromatin and nuclear molding.

nests can be mistaken for keratin. Similar to placental site nodules, epithelioid trophoblastic tumors occur more commonly in the uterine corpus but can also occur in the cervix where they can mimic invasive squamous cell carcinoma. The neoplastic cells can also replace the overlying normal endocervical mucosa and give the impression of an in situ component (see Chapter 17). However, in contrast to squamous cell carcinoma, the cells of epithelioid trophoblastic tumors tend to be arranged parallel to the basement membrane. Immunohistochemical stain for p16 is typically negative in epithelioid trophoblastic tumors, in contrast with the diffuse positive staining seen in the majority of squamous cell carcinomas[62]. Epithelioid trophoblastic tumors are focally positive for human placental lactogen and hCG[64].

Small cell carcinoma

Poorly differentiated squamous cell carcinoma with small cells can resemble small cell neuroendocrine carcinoma. However, the architectural patterns and nuclear features are distinctive. Small cell neuroendocrine carcinoma grows as sheets, trabeculae, and ribbons of tumor. Rosettes may also be present. In contrast, squamous cell carcinoma invades as irregularly shaped nests. Although both may show single-cell infiltration, the cells of neuroendocrine carcinoma have nuclei with smudgy or stippled chromatin, and lack prominent nucleoli. Nuclear molding and crush artifact are also distinctive (Figure 2.18). Small cell carcinomas are characteristically positive for neuroendocrine markers (e.g., chromogranin, synaptophysin) and negative for p63, while squamous cell carcinomas will exhibit the opposite immunohistochemical profile.

REFERENCES

1. Parkin DM, Bray F, Ferlay J, Pisani P. Global cancer statistics, 2002. *CA Cancer J Clin* 2005;**55**:74–108.
2. Devesa SS, Young JL, Jr., Brinton LA, Fraumeni JF, Jr. Recent trends in cervix uteri cancer. *Cancer* 1989;**64**:2184–90.
3. Devesa SS, Blot WJ, Stone BJ, *et al.* Recent cancer trends in the United States. *J Natl Cancer Inst* 1995;**87**:175–82.
4. US Cancer Statistics Working Group. United States Cancer Statistics: 1999–2007 Incidence and Mortality Data. Centers for Disease Control and Prevention and National Cancer Institute; 2009. (Accessed Oct 18 2011, at www.cdc.gov/uscs.)
5. Walboomers JM, Jacobs MV, Manos MM, *et al.* Human papillomavirus is a necessary cause of invasive cervical cancer worldwide. *J Pathol* 1999;**189**:12–19.
6. Munoz N, Bosch FX, de Sanjose S, *et al.* Epidemiologic classification of human papillomavirus types associated with cervical cancer. *N Engl J Med* 2003;**348**:518–27.
7. Clifford GM, Smith JS, Plummer M, Munoz N, Franceschi S. Human papillomavirus types in invasive cervical cancer worldwide: a meta-analysis. *Br J Cancer* 2003;**88**:63–73.
8. Jancar N, Kocjan BJ, Poljak M, Lunar MM, Bokal EV. Distribution of human papillomavirus genotypes in women with cervical cancer in Slovenia. *Eur J Obstet Gynecol Reprod Biol* 2009;**145**:184–8.
9. FUTURE II Study Group. Quadrivalent vaccine against human papillomavirus to prevent high-grade cervical lesions. *N Engl J Med* 2007;**356**:1915–27.
10. Paavonen J, Naud P, Salmeron J, *et al.* Efficacy of human papillomavirus (HPV)-16/18 AS04-adjuvanted vaccine against cervical infection and precancer caused by oncogenic HPV types (PATRICIA): final analysis of a double-blind, randomised study in young women. *Lancet* 2009;**374**:301–14.
11. Comparison of risk factors for invasive squamous cell carcinoma and adenocarcinoma of the cervix: collaborative reanalysis of individual data on 8,097 women with squamous cell carcinoma and 1,374 women with adenocarcinoma from 12 epidemiological studies. *Int J Cancer* 2007;**120**:885–91.
12. Holmes RS, Hawes SE, Toure P, *et al.* HIV infection as a risk factor for cervical cancer and cervical intraepithelial neoplasia in Senegal. *Cancer Epidemiol Biomarkers Prev* 2009;**18**:2442–6.
13. Vajdic CM, McDonald SP, McCredie MR, *et al.* Cancer incidence before and after kidney transplantation. *JAMA* 2006;**296**:2823–31.
14. Schulz TF. Cancer and viral infections in immunocompromised individuals. *Int J Cancer* 2009;**125**:1755–63.
15. Joseph MG, Cragg F, Wright VC, *et al.* Cyto-histological correlates in a colposcopic clinic: a 1-year prospective study. *Diagn Cytopathol* 1991;**7**:477–81.
16. Stuart GC, McGregor SE, Duggan MA, Nation JG. Review of the screening history of Alberta women with invasive cervical cancer. *CMAJ* 1997;**157**:513–19.
17. Lonky NM, Sadeghi M, Tsadik GW, Petitti D. The clinical significance of the poor correlation of cervical dysplasia and cervical malignancy with referral cytologic results. *Am J Obstet Gynecol* 1999;**181**:560–6.
18. Gullotta G, Margariti PA, Rabitti C, *et al.* Cytology, histology, and colposcopy in the diagnosis of neoplastic non-invasive epithelial lesions of the cervix. *Eur J Gynaecol Oncol* 1997;**18**:36–8.
19. Pretorius RG, Peterson P, Azizi F, Burchette RJ. Subsequent risk and presentation of cervical intraepithelial neoplasia (CIN) 3 or cancer after a colposcopic diagnosis of CIN 1 or less. *Am J Obstet Gynecol* 2006;**195**:1260–5.

20. Holowaty P, Miller AB, Rohan T, To T. Natural history of dysplasia of the uterine cervix. *J Natl Cancer Inst* 1999;**91**:252–8.

21. McCredie MR, Sharples KJ, Paul C, *et al*. Natural history of cervical neoplasia and risk of invasive cancer in women with cervical intraepithelial neoplasia 3: a retrospective cohort study. *Lancet Oncol* 2008;**9**:425–34.

22. Quinn MA, Benedet JL, Odicino F, *et al*. Carcinoma of the cervix uteri. FIGO 26th Annual Report on the Results of Treatment in Gynecological Cancer. *Int J Gynaecol Obstet* 2006;**95**(Suppl 1):S43–103.

23. Delgado G, Bundy B, Zaino R, *et al*. Prospective surgical-pathological study of disease-free interval in patients with stage IB squamous cell carcinoma of the cervix: a Gynecologic Oncology Group study. *Gynecol Oncol* 1990;**38**:352–7.

24. Bean SM, Kurtycz DF, Colgan TJ. Recent developments in defining microinvasive and early invasive carcinoma of the uterine cervix. *J Low Genit Tract Dis* 2011;**15**:146–57.

25. Ostor AG. Pandora's box or Ariadne's thread? Definition and prognostic significance of microinvasion in the uterine cervix. Squamous lesions. *Pathol Annu* 1995;**30**(Pt 2):103–36.

26. Ostor AG, Rome RM. Micro-invasive squamous cell carcinoma of the cervix: a clinico-pathologic study of 200 cases with long-term follow-up. *Int J Gynecol Cancer* 1994;**4**:257–64.

27. Creasman WT, Kohler MF. Is lymph vascular space involvement an independent prognostic factor in early cervical cancer? *Gynecol Oncol* 2004;**92**:525–9.

28. Schwartz LB, Carcangiu ML, Bradham L, Schwartz PE. Rapidly progressive squamous cell carcinoma of the cervix coexisting with human immunodeficiency virus infection: clinical opinion. *Gynecol Oncol* 1991;**41**:255–8.

29. Holcomb K, Maiman M, Dimaio T, Gates J. Rapid progression to invasive cervix cancer in a woman infected with the human immunodeficiency virus. *Obstet Gynecol* 1998;**91**:848–50.

30. Wright TC, Jr., Massad LS, Dunton CJ, *et al*. 2006 Consensus Guidelines for the Management of Women with Cervical Intraepithelial Neoplasia or Adenocarcinoma in Situ. *Am J Obstet Gynecol* 2007;**197**:340–5.

31. Kesic V. Management of cervical cancer. *Eur J Surg Oncol* 2006;**32**:832–7.

32. ACOG Committee on Practice Bulletins—Gynecology. ACOG Practice Bulletin no. 35: Diagnosis and treatment of cervical carcinomas. *Obstet Gynecol* 2002;**99**:855–67.

33. Koliopoulos G, Sotiriadis A, Kyrgiou M, *et al*. Conservative surgical methods for FIGO stage IA2 squamous cervical carcinoma and their role in preserving women's fertility. *Gynecol Oncol* 2004;**93**: 469–73.

34. Landoni F, Maneo A, Colombo A, *et al*. Randomised study of radical surgery versus radiotherapy for stage Ib-IIa cervical cancer. *Lancet* 1997;**350**:535–40.

35. Stoler MH, Schiffman M. Interobserver reproducibility of cervical cytologic and histologic interpretations: realistic estimates from the ASCUS-LSIL Triage Study. *Jama* 2001;**285**:1500–5.

36. Castle PE, Stoler MH, Solomon D, Schiffman M. The relationship of community biopsy-diagnosed cervical intraepithelial neoplasia grade 2 to the quality control pathology-reviewed diagnoses: an ALTS report. *Am J Clin Pathol* 2007;**127**:805–15.

37. Carreon JD, Sherman ME, Guillen D, *et al*. CIN2 is a much less reproducible and less valid diagnosis than CIN3: results from a histological review of population-based cervical samples. *Int J Gynecol Pathol* 2007;**26**:441–6.

38. Tseng CJ, Pao CC, Tseng LH, *et al*. Lymphoepithelioma-like carcinoma of the uterine cervix: association with Epstein-Barr virus and human papillomavirus. *Cancer* 1997;**80**:91–7.

39. Noel J, Lespagnard L, Fayt I, Verhest A, Dargent J. Evidence of human papilloma virus infection but lack of Epstein-Barr virus in lymphoepithelioma-like carcinoma of uterine cervix: report of two cases and review of the literature. *Hum Pathol* 2001;**32**: 135–8.

40. Bais AG, Kooi S, Teune TM, Ewing PC, Ansink AC. Lymphoepithelioma-like carcinoma of the uterine cervix: absence of Epstein-Barr virus, but presence of a multiple human papillomavirus infection. *Gynecol Oncol* 2005;**97**:716–18.

41. Chao A, Tsai CN, Hsueh S, *et al*. Does Epstein-Barr virus play a role in lymphoepithelioma-like carcinoma of the uterine cervix? *Int J Gynecol Pathol* 2009;**28**:279–85.

42. Pecorelli S. Revised FIGO staging for carcinoma of the vulva, cervix, and endometrium. *Int J Gynaecol Obstet* 2009;**105**:103–4.

43. Bader AA, Winter R, Haas J, Tamussino KF. Where to look for the sentinel lymph node in cervical cancer. *Am J Obstet Gynecol* 2007;**197**:678.e1–7.

44. Yuan SH, Xiong Y, Wei M, *et al*. Sentinel lymph node detection using methylene blue in patients with early stage cervical cancer. *Gynecol Oncol* 2007;**106**:147–52.

45. Sakuragi N, Satoh C, Takeda N, *et al*. Incidence and distribution pattern of pelvic and paraaortic lymph node metastasis in patients with Stages IB, IIA, and IIB cervical carcinoma treated with radical hysterectomy. *Cancer* 1999;**85**:1547–54.

46. Kong CS, Balzer BL, Troxell ML, Patterson BK, Longacre TA. p16INK4A immunohistochemistry is superior to HPV in situ hybridization for the detection of high-risk HPV in atypical squamous metaplasia. *Am J Surg Pathol* 2007;**31**:33–43.

47. Keating JT, Cviko A, Riethdorf S, *et al*. Ki-67, cyclin E, and p16INK4 are complimentary surrogate biomarkers for human papilloma virus-related cervical neoplasia. *Am J Surg Pathol* 2001;**25**:884–91.

48. Sano T, Oyama T, Kashiwabara K, Fukuda T, Nakajima T. Expression status of p16 protein is associated with human papillomavirus oncogenic potential in cervical and genital lesions. *Am J Pathol* 1998;**153**:1741–8.

49. Klaes R, Friedrich T, Spitkovsky D, *et al*. Overexpression of p16 (INK4A) as a specific marker for dysplastic and neoplastic epithelial cells of the cervix uteri. *Int J Cancer* 2001;**92**:276–84.

50. Kalof AN, Evans MF, Simmons-Arnold L, Beatty BG, Cooper K. p16INK4A immunoexpression and HPV in situ hybridization signal patterns: potential markers of high-grade cervical intraepithelial neoplasia. *Am J Surg Pathol* 2005;**29**:674–9.

51. Nielsen GP, Stemmer-Rachamimov AO, Shaw J, *et al*. Immunohistochemical survey of p16INK4A expression in normal human adult and infant tissues. *Lab Invest* 1999;**79**:1137–43.

52. Pinto AP, Schlecht NF, Woo TY, Crum CP, Cibas ES. Biomarker (ProEx C, p16(INK4A), and MiB-1) distinction of high-grade squamous intraepithelial lesion from its mimics. *Mod Pathol* 2008;**21**:1067–74.

53. Badr RE, Walts AE, Chung F, Bose S. BD ProEx C: a sensitive and specific marker of HPV-associated squamous lesions of the cervix. *Am J Surg Pathol* 2008;**32**:899–906.

54. Conesa-Zamora P, Domenech-Peris A, Ortiz-Reina S, *et al*. Immunohistochemical evaluation of ProEx C in human papillomavirus-induced lesions of the cervix. *J Clin Pathol* 2009;**62**:159–62.

55. Shi J, Liu H, Wilkerson M, *et al*. Evaluation of p16INK4a, minichromosome maintenance protein 2, DNA topoisomerase IIalpha, ProEX C, and p16INK4a/ProEX C in cervical squamous intraepithelial lesions. *Hum Pathol* 2007;**38**:1335–44.

56. Pirog EC, Baergen RN, Soslow RA, *et al.* Diagnostic accuracy of cervical low-grade squamous intraepithelial lesions is improved with MIB-1 immunostaining. *Am J Surg Pathol* 2002;**26**:70–5.

57. Iaconis L, Hyjek E, Ellenson LH, Pirog EC. p16 and Ki-67 immunostaining in atypical immature squamous metaplasia of the uterine cervix: correlation with human papillomavirus detection. *Arch Pathol Lab Med* 2007;**131**:1343–9.

58. Kruse AJ, Baak JP, de Bruin PC, *et al.* Ki-67 immunoquantitation in cervical intraepithelial neoplasia (CIN): a sensitive marker for grading. *J Pathol* 2001;**193**:48–54.

59. Qiao X, Bhuiya TA, Spitzer M. Differentiating high-grade cervical intraepithelial lesion from atrophy in postmenopausal women using Ki-67, cyclin E, and p16 immunohistochemical analysis. *J Low Genit Tract Dis* 2005;**9**:100–7.

60. Van Dorpe J, Moerman P. Placental site nodule of the uterine cervix. *Histopathology* 1996;**29**:379–82.

61. Young RH, Kurman RJ, Scully RE. Placental site nodules and plaques. A clinicopathologic analysis of 20 cases. *Am J Surg Pathol* 1990;**14**:1001–9.

62. Mao TL, Seidman JD, Kurman RJ, Shih I eM. Cyclin E and p16 immunoreactivity in epithelioid trophoblastic tumor – an aid in differential diagnosis. *Am J Surg Pathol* 2006;**30**:1105–10.

63. Shih IM, Seidman JD, Kurman RJ. Placental site nodule and characterization of distinctive types of intermediate trophoblast. *Hum Pathol* 1999;**30**:687–94.

64. Fadare O, Parkash V, Carcangiu ML, Hui P. Epithelioid trophoblastic tumor: clinicopathological features with an emphasis on uterine cervical involvement. *Mod Pathol* 2006;**19**:75–82.

3 CERVIX: ADENOCARCINOMA AND PRECURSORS, INCLUDING VARIANTS

INTRODUCTION

While the overall age-adjusted incidence of cervical squamous cell carcinoma has declined in countries that have implemented organized cervical Pap smear surveillance programs, the incidence of adenocarcinoma and adenosquamous carcinoma has increased considerably from 1.30 and 0.15 cases per 100 000 women, respectively, in 1970–1972, to 1.83 and 0.41 per 100 000 women in 1994–1996. Moreover, the overall increase in incidence has been observed primarily in women less than 50 years of age. Although initial increases were attributed to increasing prevalence of persistent oncogenic HPV infection (and its cofactors) as well as inherent limitations of cervical cytology in detecting precursor glandular lesions, recent data indicate that cytologic screening, if performed and interpreted properly, can detect these early lesions. In fact, the decrease in glandular lesions of the cervix observed in several countries during the latter part of the 1990s strongly suggests that cytology screening is detecting more preinvasive adenocarcinomas than in previous decades, and further suggests that screening may be starting to have a protective impact on adenocarcinoma.

However, diagnostic issues concerning cervical glandular lesions continue to plague the cytopathologist and surgical pathologist. The key problematic areas revolve around (1) the diagnosis of adenocarcinoma in situ and the exclusion of benign mimics; (2) the presence of early or superficially invasive adenocarcinoma (we do not use the term "microinvasive adenocarcinoma"); (3) identification of the primary site of origin of problematic glandular proliferations in uterine samplings: that is, is it cervical, or endometrial, or metastatic; and (4) special variants. Over the years, a variety of strategies have been proposed for each of these diagnostic problems, some of which have proven to be more useful than others. The more useful strategies are highlighted in this discussion, but it is important to recognize that even these have their limitations, and in some cases a definitive diagnosis simply cannot be made. Since it is just as important to convey this information to the treating clinician as it is to convey more definitive diagnoses, these more "borderline" distinctions are also discussed.

ADENOCARCINOMA IN SITU

With improved screening, pathologists are increasingly faced with biopsy and small cervical cone specimens for evaluation of possible involvement by adenocarcinoma in situ. In some instances the lesions are focal and superficial, requiring serial sectioning before they can be identified, while others are extensive and require serial sectioning in order to exclude a possible invasive focus. Still other lesions are subtle and require ancillary diagnostic tests in order to establish the diagnosis.

Clinical characteristics

Adenocarcinoma in situ is most common during the reproductive years (mean age: 37 years), but women less than 35 as well as women aged 55 years or older may be affected. The risk factors are generally similar to those for squamous intraepithelial neoplasia. Most women are asymptomatic, and the diagnosis is established during the work-up of an abnormal Pap smear, or discovered incidentally after biopsy for squamous intraepithelial neoplasia.

Morphology

Gross pathology
Most adenocarcinoma in situ lesions are not associated with a macroscopic abnormality. Occasional cases may come to clinical attention due to excess mucin production, but colposcopic abnormalities are distinctly less common than with squamous intraepithelial lesions.

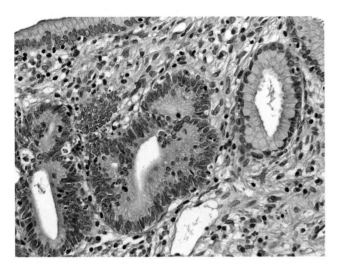

Figure 3.1 Adenocarcinoma in situ. There is nuclear enlargement and nuclear hyperchromasia with mitotic figures.

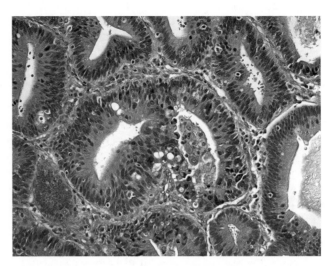

Figure 3.2 Adenocarcinoma in situ. Nuclear stratification is often present.

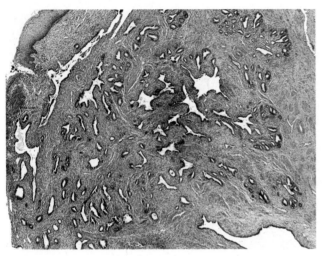

Figure 3.3 Adenocarcinoma in situ. Most adenocarcinoma in situ involves surface epithelium and underlying glands near the transformation zone, but it may be confined entirely to the glands.

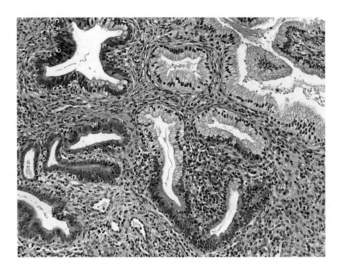

Figure 3.4 Partial gland involvement in adenocarcinoma in situ.

Since adenocarcinoma in situ arises in the glandular region, affected areas may appear on colposcopy as densely white island lesions in the columnar epithelium, but almost one-half of all adenocarcinoma in situ occurs high in the endocervical canal and cannot be visualized on colposcopic examination.

Microscopic pathology

The histologic diagnosis of adenocarcinoma in situ hinges on the identification of unequivocal dysplastic changes, which are typically manifested by low-power basophilia, nuclear enlargement, nuclear hyperchromasia with either fine or coarsely granular chromatin, nuclear apoptotic or karyorrhectic debris, apical mitotic figures, and loss of polarity (which may be subtle) (Figure 3.1). Nuclear stratification with tufting may also be present (Figure 3.2). The involved glands exhibit a lobular architecture that may appear more pronounced than adjacent uninvolved endocervical glands, but irregular infiltration into stroma is absent (Figure 3.3). The cytoplasm of the adenocarcinoma in situ cells may exhibit pale, even abundant intracytoplasmic mucin, but more commonly appears eosinophilic. Partial gland involvement is common, but this may be seen in reactive and even in some metastatic processes, so this feature should not be relied upon as a sole discriminating criterion (Figure 3.4).

Recently, a superficial (early) form of adenocarcinoma in situ has been described in the superficial columnar mucosa, featuring similar cytologic alterations, but less pronounced atypia (Figure 3.5). This lesion is thought to

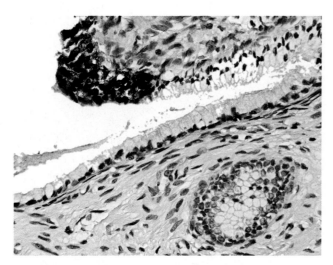

Figure 3.5 p16 highlights focus of superficial ("early") adenocarcinoma in situ.

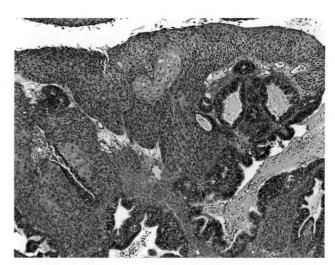

Figure 3.6 Adenocarcinoma in situ with cervical intraepithelial neoplasia.

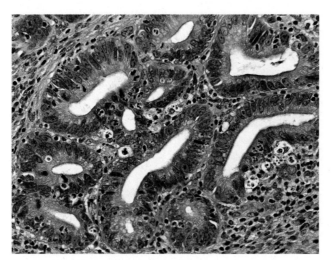

Figure 3.7 Usual adenocarcinoma in situ.

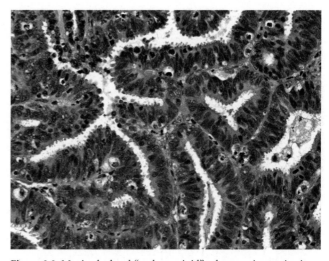

Figure 3.8 Mucin-depleted "endometrioid" adenocarcinoma in situ.

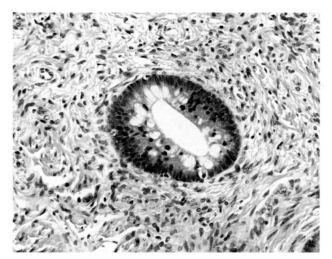

Figure 3.9 Mucinous adenocarcinoma in situ with goblet cells.

occur more commonly in a younger age group (mean: 26 years) and so has been interpreted as an "early" form of adenocarcinoma in situ.

Adenocarcinoma in situ is often associated with squamous intraepithelial lesion (40 to 100% of cases, depending on the series), which can be focal or multifocal (Figure 3.6). Although the literature often emphasizes origin in the columnar epithelium and multifocality, recent studies have suggested that adenocarcinoma in situ likely arises in the transformation zone and extends contiguously, albeit irregularly into the endocervical canal.

Most cases of adenocarcinoma in situ cytologically resemble the cells in invasive usual endocervical adenocarcinoma (mucinous endocervical type) (Figure 3.7), but mucin-depleted "endometrioid" (Figure 3.8), mucinous intestinal (Figure 3.9), and tubal (Figure 3.10) types can

(A)

(B)

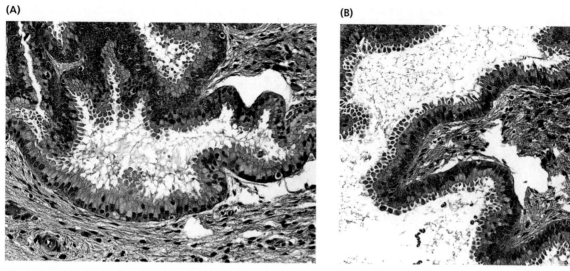

Figure 3.10 (A, B) Adenocarcinoma in situ with tubal features.

(A)

(B)

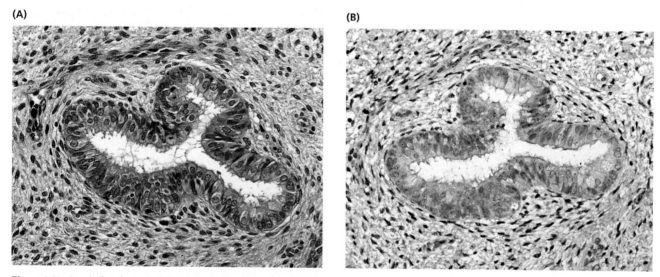

Figure 3.11 Atypical endocervical glands with some features that suggest adenocarcinoma in situ. (A) There is some pseudostratification and nuclear enlargement, but mitotic figures are not prominent. (B) p16 is negative.

also be seen. The tubal type may pose the most significant diagnostic problems, especially on a small biopsy specimen, due to the presence of admixed ciliated cells. The diagnosis hinges on identification of the cytologic features of adenocarcinoma in situ; namely nuclear pseudostratification, nuclear enlargement, coarse chromatin, loss of polarity, and mitotic figures.

Not uncommonly, glandular lesions can be seen in the cervix that exhibit some but not all the features of adenocarcinoma in situ (Figure 3.11). Some, but by no means all of these lesions are associated with adenocarcinoma in situ, high-grade squamous intraepithelial lesion, or invasive adenocarcinoma. Several lines of evidence indicate that

these atypical lesions tend to occur at a younger age and may harbor high-risk HPV; suggesting they may be precursor lesions of adenocarcinoma in situ. The World Health Organization (WHO) has designated these lesions as glandular dysplasia; however, the prevalence, progression rate to adenocarcinoma in situ, diagnostic criteria for this designation, and overall clinical implications are either poorly understood or are not uniformly agreed upon. Moreover, the reproducibility of the diagnosis of *glandular dysplasia*, even with a controlled scoring method, is at best "good" (43%, kappa = 0.6); whereas the reproducibility of the diagnosis of adenocarcinoma in situ using the same scoring system is excellent (95%, kappa = 0.8). In contrast,

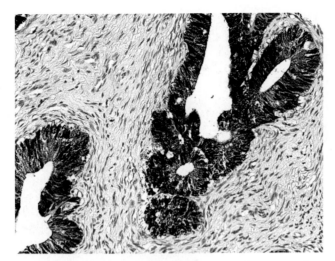

Figure 3.12 p16 in adenocarcinoma in situ is typically strong, nuclear and/or cytoplasmic, and diffuse.

collapsing benign and *glandular dysplasia* into a single benign category using the same scoring method yields a very high concordance (94%) amongst pathologists[1]. For these reasons, while we agree that there is likely an adenocarcinoma in situ precursor lesion, we and others refrain from making the diagnosis of *glandular dysplasia* in the clinical setting.

So, how does a pathologist approach these lesions? Our current strategy is three-fold: (1) additional level sections with intervening unstained slides; (2) immunohistochemistry with p16 and Ki-67; and (3) exclusion of endometrial origin (or metastasis from another site), if indicated. The diagnosis of adenocarcinoma in situ can often be established on the basis of additional sections alone, but when this is not possible, immunohistochemical evaluation of the intervening unstained slides often proves to be useful. The utility of these ancillary studies is discussed in the following sections.

If, after using these adjunct studies, the diagnosis is still unclear, the best course of action is to convey this uncertainty to the treating clinician; a diagnosis of "atypical glandular proliferation, cannot exclude adenocarcinoma" with a recommendation to consider additional sampling and/or imaging studies is perfectly acceptable in this setting.

Ancillary diagnostic tests

The use of biomarkers, particularly a combination of Ki-67 and p16, has been confirmed in a variety of studies to be a highly useful technique in the differential diagnosis of adenocarcinoma in situ. In general, strong, diffuse expression of p16 in conjunction with increased Ki-67 is more commonly associated with adenocarcinoma in situ (Figure 3.12); whereas weak or focal p16 expression with or without increased Ki-67 is more supportive of an adenocarcinoma in situ mimic. Exceptions occur, and so it is important to be thoroughly aware of the variant expression patterns of these markers in the individual lesions in order to prevent misinterpretation on the basis of staining patterns alone[2].

One of the most notable exceptions is minimal deviation adenocarcinoma, which is not usually a high-risk-HPV-associated tumor, and therefore does not overexpress p16[23]. Another exception is mesonephric adenocarcinoma[3]. The differential expression of PAX2 in benign and malignant endocervical glandular lesions has been reported to be a useful adjunctive test in establishing (or excluding) these last two diagnoses. PAX2 is a nuclear transcription protein, involved in urogenital tract differentiation, that is expressed in normal mullerian tissues including endometrium, fallopian tube mucosa, and endocervix, as well as in a spectrum of urologic neoplasms. Since it appears to be expressed in benign endocervical glandular epithelium (Figure 3.13), but not in malignant endocervical glandular cells, it has been suggested that PAX2 may be helpful in evaluating those atypical endocervical glandular lesions that are not associated with high-risk HPV[4]. However, data are limited and we have observed strong expression of PAX2 in mesonephric carcinoma (Figure 3.14). As with p16, interpretation should be conducted with careful consideration of the histology and clinical setting[5].

The characteristic p16/Ki-67 expression profile in the common benign mimics, as well as in the special variants of endocervical carcinoma (in situ and invasive), is discussed more fully in the differential diagnosis and variant sections of this chapter.

Differential diagnosis

A variety of processes mimic adenocarcinoma in situ and, in some instances, invasive adenocarcinoma; these include tubal or tuboendometrioid metaplasia, Arias-Stella reaction, endometriosis, endosalpingiosis, endocervicosis, reactive endocervical cells, radiation atypia, and a variety of endocervical cell alterations that do not necessarily appear to represent a reactive process. These last alterations often pose the most diagnostic difficulty and are classified on the basis of the abnormality present: mitotically active endocervical mucosa; stratified endocervical mucosa; atypical oxyphilic metaplasia, and intestinal metaplasia.

(A)

(B)

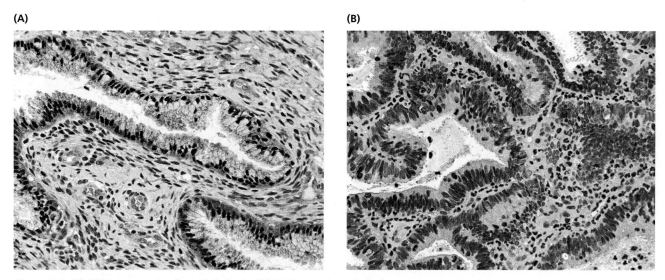

Figure 3.13 (A) PAX2 in normal endocervical glands. (B) PAX2 in endocervical adenocarcinoma.

(A)

(B)

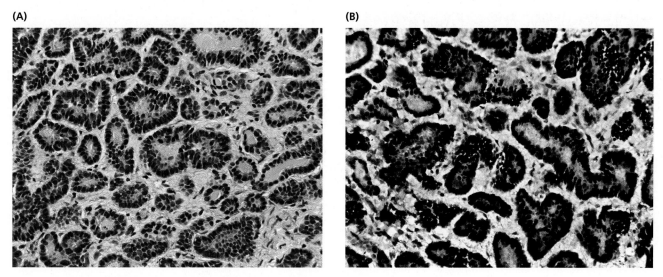

Figure 3.14 (A) Mesonephric carcinoma. (B) PAX2 in mesonephric carcinoma.

Tubal, endometrioid, and tuboendometrioid metaplasia

Tubal or tuboendometrioid metaplasia (TEM), the most common of the adenocarcinoma in situ differential diagnostic entities, is recognized by the presence of cilia and terminal bars along the apical cytoplasm. Nuclear hyperchromasia, elongation, and crowding may be present, but the chromatin is homogeneous and bland as opposed to coarse, and mitotic figures are usually sparse (Figure 3.15). Tuboendometrioid metaplasia may occur deep in the endocervical glands, where it may be associated with periglandular edema. Extensive involvement of the endocervix has been reported in women with in utero exposure to diethylstilbestrol (DES)[6]. The glands are typically small or medium in size, but may vary in size and shape; branching

may be present. In most cases, the constituent cells are heterogeneous, with tall columnar cells alternating with cells exhibiting more optically clear cytoplasm, similar to peg cells in the fallopian tube. Increased expression of Ki-67 (MIB1) in conjunction with diffuse, strong expression of p16 may be useful in the distinction of adenocarcinoma in situ from tuboendometrioid metaplasia, provided the sampling is of sufficient size to be representative (Figure 3.16). The secretory (non-ciliated) columnar cells in tuboendometrioid metaplasia are positive for PAX2[4]; whereas ciliated cells and peg cells are negative. Most tuboendometrioid metaplasia expresses Ki-67 in less than 10% of the constituent cells, while adenocarcinoma in situ may express Ki-67 in over 50% of cells, but overlap exists and we do not use this marker to make the distinction.

(A)

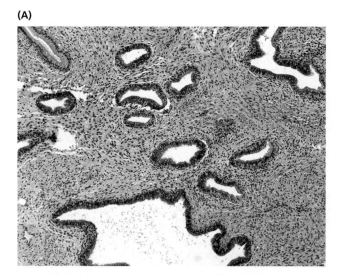

(B)

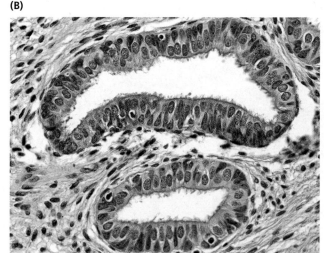

Figure 3.15 (A, B) Tuboendometrioid metaplasia.

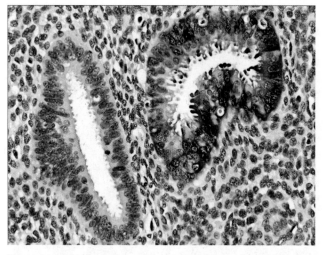

Figure 3.16 p16 may be present in tuboendometrioid metaplasia, but is usually patchy in distribution.

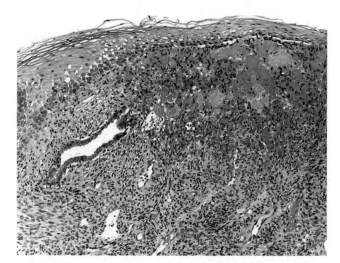

Figure 3.17 Endometriosis.

Tuboendometrioid metaplasia may express carcinoembryonic antigen (CEA), and so this marker is not helpful in this distinction.

Arias-Stella reaction

The histologic features of Arias-Stella reaction are identical to those in the endometrium, and consist of vacuolated cytoplasm, tufting, hobnail cells, clear or oxyphilic cytoplasm, and intranuclear pseudoinclusions[7]. A dense, smudged nuclear chromatin pattern is characteristic (see Figure 18.5).

Arias-Stella reaction is distinguished from adenocarcinoma in situ by the absence or extreme paucity of mitotic figures and apoptotic bodies. The clinical setting and stromal decidual reaction are additional supporting features. The distinction between Arias-Stella reaction and clear cell

carcinoma is more difficult, but the young age, absence of a mass lesion, absence of invasive pattern, and absence of additional patterns of clear cell carcinoma are usually sufficient to exclude carcinoma in this setting.

Endometriosis

Endometriosis may involve the cervix superficially or deep. When superficial, cervical endometriosis may involve the squamocolumnar junction and be confused with adenocarcinoma in situ. When deep, cervical endometriosis may be confused with invasive adenocarcinoma. The individual cells are often pseudostratified and mitotically active, but the nuclei are cytologically bland and similar in appearance to those in the endometrium (Figure 3.17). Endometrial stroma, when present, helps to establish the diagnosis.

(A)

(B)

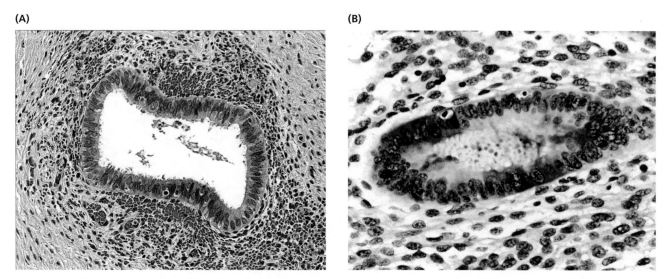

Figure 3.18 (A) Endometriosis. (B) p16 in endometriosis is often present and may be quite strong, although it is usually patchy in distribution.

(A)

(B)

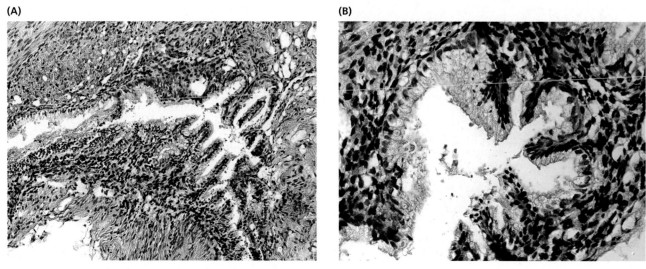

Figure 3.19 (A, B) Endocervicosis.

Caution should be exercised when using biomarkers to help distinguish these two processes, since endometriosis may express high levels of Ki-67, and p16 expression may occur in some cases (Figure 3.18).

Endocervicosis

The outer wall or paracervical tissues may be involved by ectopic endocervical-type glands[8]; this is a rare, but benign process that may mimic a well-differentiated mucinous adenocarcinoma (Figure 3.19). Absence of cervical mucosal involvement essentially excludes a primary cervical adenocarcinoma; although occasional minimal deviation carcinomas appear to arise from the deeper endocervical gland clefts and may not involve mucosa. However,

excluding a cytologically banal metastasis from another site can be more problematic; particularly if there is reactive stroma associated with the endocervicosis. The presence of other mullerian-type glands or endometrial stroma is evidence for endocervicosis. Absence of a mass lesion is additional corroborative support for a benign process.

Endosalpingioisis

Endosalpingiosis may rarely involve the cervical stroma or lower uterine myometrium, occasionally forming a cystic mass-like lesion[9]. The constituent glands have the same appearance of tubal-type glandular epithelium as that seen in more typical sites of involvement.

(A)

(B)

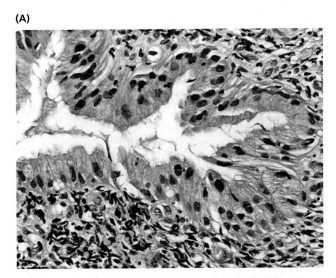
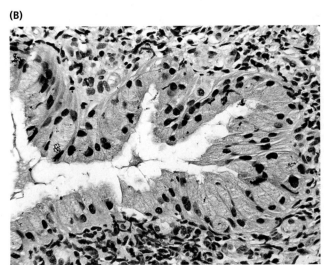

Figure 3.20 (A) Reactive atypia in endocervical glands. (B) p16 is negative.

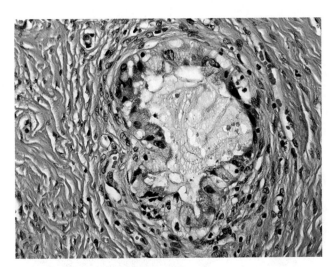

Figure 3.21 Radiation atypia.

Reactive endocervical cell atypia

Inflammatory processes may mimic adenocarcinoma in situ in small biopsies or fragmented curettage specimens. Occasionally, intact biopsy fragments following a prior cervical procedure may demonstrate features of reactive endocervical glands, even though there is little or no associated inflammation. In comparison to adenocarcinoma in situ and invasive adenocarcinoma, reactive endocervical cells exhibit a comparatively low nuclear-to-cytoplasmic ratio and prominent nucleoli (Figure 3.20). Mitotic figures may be numerous and, in these instances, careful attention to the nuclear chromatin pattern (finely stippled as opposed to coarse) and the overall non-infiltrative glandular configuration help to distinguish reactive from neoplastic. Although reactive endocervical cells may exhibit prominent Ki-67 staining,

in most cases, reactive glands should exhibit weak or absent expression of p16.

Radiation changes

Radiation changes may be associated with substantial nuclear atypia, including hyperchromasia, enlargement, pleomorphism, and nucleolar prominence (Figure 3.21). Multinucleated cells may also be present. However, the chromatin is smudged and, unlike adenocarcinoma in situ, mitotic figures are uncommon. The cytoplasm may be eosinophilic or vacuolated[10]. Stromal changes include fibrosis, hyalinization, edema, chronic inflammation, and calcification; the fibroblasts are often atypical. Vascular changes may also be present and are typically manifest by ectasia and intimal thickening. Radiation changes may be focal or diffuse. The differential diagnosis often includes clear cell carcinoma as well as adenocarcinoma in situ. The former is diagnosed on the basis of a mass lesion and gland density (closely packed glands in clear cell carcinoma vs. scattered, irregular glands in radiation). Decreased glands and variation in gland shape and size has also been attributed to long-standing changes secondary to radiation.

Stratified and mitotically active endocervical cells

Cervical glandular epithelium is typically columnar and non-stratified, but, on occasion, normal endocervical cells may take on a more stratified or mitotically active appearance. The stratified "normal variant" features tall columnar cells, but normal gland contours; in most cases, mitotic activity is sparse and the nuclear details

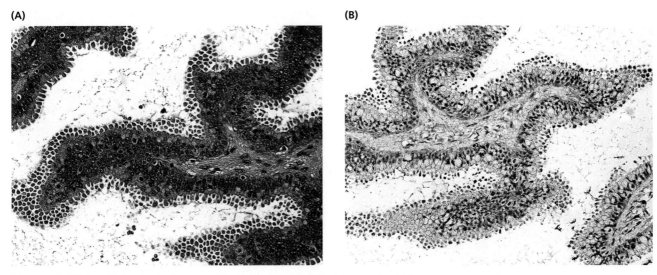

Figure 3.22 (A) Stratified, mitotically active endoecervical glands. (B) p16 expression is absent.

are well preserved and non-dysplastic (Figure 3.22). The mitotically active "normal variant" also features tall, columnar epithelial cells, but there is typically little stratification. Once again, the gland contours are normal; mitotic figures are also normal in this variant. Abnormal division figures or significant nuclear atypia should prompt consideration for adenocarcinoma in situ.

Atypical oxyphilic metaplasia

This is a rare, focal change that may involve the endocervical glandular surface epithelium. The involved cells are cuboidal in contour and have dense eosinophilic cytoplasm and enlarged, hyperchromatic, and irregular nuclei. Cytoplasmic vacuolization with apical snouts may be present, and there may be multinucleated cells. The process is focal, non-stratified, and mitotically inactive. The etiology is unclear, but a secretory-type change has been proposed[11].

Intestinal metaplasia

Very rarely, an otherwise normal-appearing endocervical gland may harbor fully developed goblet cells (intestinal metaplasia)[12]. In the absence of cellular stratification, nuclear atypia, or mitotic activity, this is an innocuous process. However, level sections and/or additional sections should be obtained to exclude an adjacent intestinal-type adenocarcinoma in situ or invasive carcinoma, as the presence of intestinal metaplasia is far more common in these settings.

"EARLY" INVASIVE CERVICAL ADENOCARCINOMA AND THE ASSESSMENT OF INVASION IN THE CERVIX

The diagnosis of invasive cervical adenocarcinoma can be very difficult in early or superficially invasive lesions, as well as in limited (superficial) biopsy specimens. A fundamental problem with assessing depth of invasion in cervical adenocarcinoma is the absence of anatomical planes in the cervix on which a classification of the extent of invasion can logically be based (as can be done in the gastrointestinal tract, for example). The sine qua non of invasive cervical adenocarcinoma is stromal invasion, which is most often manifested by periglandular edema, a chronic inflammatory cell infiltrate, and/or a desmoplastic reaction (Figures 3.23 and 3.24). However, unlike squamous carcinoma of the cervix, invasion may not always be associated with a significant stromal reaction and, in these instances, identification of invasion is based on the presence of marked glandular irregularity, an infiltrative gland pattern, and the presence of enlarged, complex neoplastic glandular structures deep to the normal endocervical crypts. Cribriform, papillary, or solid patterns may be present, but none of these features is pathognomonic[13]. Adenocarcinoma in situ may have irregular glands, a dense periglandular chronic inflammatory infiltrate, and a cribriform or papillary pattern (Figures 3.25 and 3.26). The presence of deep glands in proximity to large vessels may suggest that the process is invasive, but the topographical distribution of normal endocervical glands is often

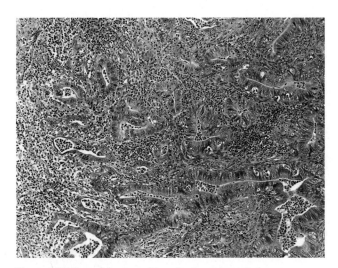

Figure 3.23 Bona fide stromal invasion in endocervical adenocarcinoma.

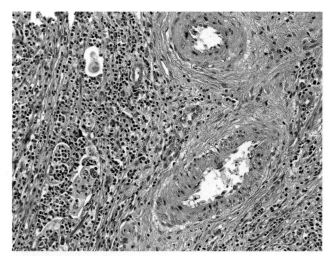

Figure 3.24 Cell clusters near muscular artery in invasive cervical adenocarcinoma.

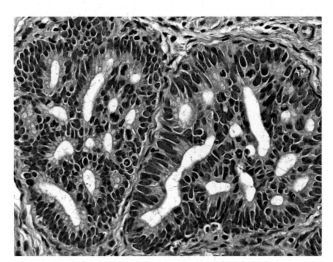

Figure 3.25 Cribriform glands are a feature of invasive adenocarcinoma, but may also be seen in adenocarcinoma in situ.

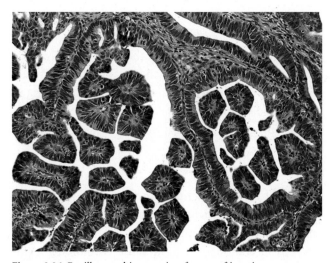

Figure 3.26 Papillary architecture is a feature of invasive adenocarcinoma, but may also be seen in adenocarcinoma in situ.

irregular, and the presence of normal deep-lying glands, often in proximity to large-caliber blood vessels is not uncommon. Moreover, bona fide invasive foci may occur superficial to the deeper-lying endocervical crypts. Therefore, the presence of invasion must be determined on an individual-case basis. The common patterns of invasion that can be seen in invasive cervical adenocarcinoma are presented in Table 3.1 and Figures 3.23–3.28.

Although we do not use the term "microinvasive adenocarcinoma," measurements of the depth of invasion (thickness) and width (diameter) of invasive adenocarcinoma should be determined for all cases deemed to exhibit invasion. The recommended measurements are made from the basement membrane of the epithelium, either surface or glandular, from which the invasive

carcinoma originates, and expressed in millimeters. In practice, it is often more clinically useful to also measure the thickness of the invasive cancer, which is taken from the basement membrane of the surface epithelium (see below). The width is the greatest diameter of the neoplasm measured parallel to the surface. Measurements should be made by calibrated optics. The presence or absence of lymphovascular space involvement should also be reported. Margin status in cone specimens should always be reported, but clear margins are no guarantee that adenocarcinoma in situ and/or invasive adenocarcinoma will not recur, as adenocarcinoma in situ tends to be more commonly multicentric in distribution in comparison to squamous intraepithelial lesions (approximately 25% versus <10%).

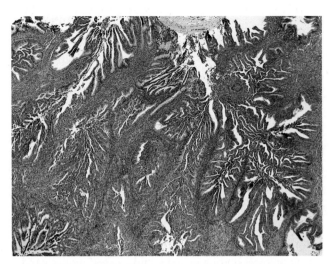

Figure 3.27 Broad invasive front pattern in cervical adenocarcinoma.

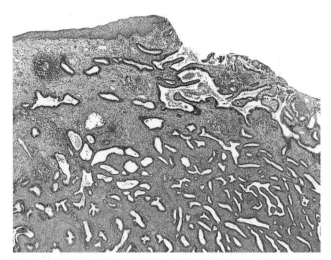

Figure 3.28 Extensive permeative pattern of invasive cervical adenocarcinoma.

Table 3.1 Patterns of invasion in cervical adenocarcinoma[13]

Tiny, finger-like processes

Detached cell clusters

Cytoplasmic eosinophilia – often associated with increased cytoplasm

Claw-like configurations

Prominent intraglandular papillae

Cribriform glands with complex intraglandular bridging

Broad front, often well demarcated from the surrounding cervix – requires exclusion of endocervical lobular hyperplasia

Solid growth – may require mucin stain to confirm glandular differentiation

Superficial mucosal invasion – arises from the surface and thought to represent intramucosal spread

Diffuse permeation by simple glands with minimal or no stromal response – this pattern is subject to significant interobserver disagreement and is best diagnosed only in the hysterectomy specimen in the presence of extensive cervical wall involvement

A maximum depth of invasion of 3 or 5 mm and maximum diameter of 7 mm with negative margins and no lymph vascular invasion[I] is considered by most clinicians as the upper limit for consideration for conservative management, although definitions vary and some authors suggest a maximum depth of 1 or 2 mm of invasion, while others have recommended a tumor volume of less than 500 mm^3. Cone biopsy with or without pelvic lymphadenectomy has been successful in some patients. Recently trachelectomy has also been performed. Women with these findings who wish to preserve fertility are encouraged to complete child-bearing as soon as possible in order to avoid unnecessary risk.

In some cases, a diagnosis of invasion cannot be established with certainty, but is suspected due to a significant deviation from the usual pattern of adenocarcinoma in situ. Abnormal glands with papillary architecture, microglandular architecture (small clusters of glands), or extensive intraglandular bridging are all patterns that, when present, should be regarded as suspicious for invasion. When the specimen is from a hysterectomy and the problematic glands are superficial, they are probably of minimal risk and can probably be regarded as "borderline for invasion" with little clinical consequence; however, when they are encountered in a superficial cone biopsy specimen in a reproductive-aged woman and it is unclear whether the lesion is completely excised, the stakes are considerably higher. In the latter situation, when reproductive conservation is an issue, it is better to convey uncertainty regarding the presence of invasion to the treating clinician rather than make an arbitrary diagnosis of invasion. Level sectioning of the problematic area may provide additional corroborating evidence of invasion; that is, stromal reaction, deeper-lying glands, etc. Alternatively, a repeat superficial cone biopsy and/or imaging studies may help direct further therapy. When reporting these types of cases, the diameter and thickness of the overall lesion should be reported.

In some cases, the lesion is obvious adenocarcinoma, but there is no bona fide cervical stromal invasion; this occurs most commonly with exophytic tumors, but may be seen on occasion in small biopsy specimens. Biopsy or curettage will disclose markedly complex glands with

I The current FIGO definition does not exclude tumors with lymph vascular invasion from the microinvasive category.

sufficient cytologic atypia to warrant diagnosis of adenocarcinoma, but no stromal invasion is seen. In this situation, the pathologist should issue a diagnosis of adenocarcinoma (not adenocarcinoma in situ) with a comment that indicates the lesion is beyond that of an in situ lesion, but invasion per se cannot be determined. When an apparent exophytic adenocarcinoma is identified in the hysterectomy specimen, the tumor should be entirely submitted to exclude small foci of cervical stromal invasion and/or lymphovascular invasion. If no such foci are identified, the tumor dimensions should be reported (i.e., the greatest tumor diameter and tumor thickness) with a comment that no cervical stromal invasion is seen. If minimal or early cervical stromal invasion is present, this too should be reported as depth of invasion in mm. Such tumors are likely to have a better prognosis than a similar grade and size tumor that has invaded the cervical stroma.

Examination of the cone biopsy

Adequate sampling of cone biopsies is critical to the evaluation of the cervix for the presence of adenocarcinoma in situ and invasive adenocarcinoma. Careful orientation is required, and the margins should be inked. At a minimum, the entire cone must be processed, sections should be thin – preferably 2mm – and three levels should be prepared from each block. Additional levels should be obtained if required, especially for determining the state of the margins or for further evaluation of foci suspicious for early invasion. When preparing level sections, it is often useful to obtain alternate unstained sections for possible immunohistochemical studies; if it is determined that routine stain is required in the evaluation of the intervening section, no valuable tissue has been lost. A whole embedding method has also been proposed[13].

Examination of the hysterectomy specimen

As with the cone biopsy, most of the "work" in examining the uterine cervix for adenocarcinoma in situ and adenocarcinoma rests in a careful and thorough macroscopic evaluation. The parametrial tissue should be removed before examining the cervix in order to avoid artifactual parametrial involvement due to contamination by a friable tumor ("floaters"). The parametrium should be carefully examined for all lymph nodes; since the nodes may be quite small, we tend to embed the entire parametrium. For adenocarcinoma in situ or early invasive adenocarcinoma, the

entire cervix should be coned and submitted as described above. For preoperative diagnoses of invasive adenocarcinoma, the examination should focus on identification of the invasive lesion, and sections should be carefully taken to document greatest diameter and thickness of the tumor. The number of sections will vary depending on the size of the uterine cervix and the size of the tumor, but there should be a sufficient number of sections to document the extent of tumor as well as the presence or absence of lymphovascular invasion; we generally submit all of the tumor or, if extremely large, the bulk of the tumor. Keep in mind that multicentric involvement can be seen in up to 25% of cases. Additional sections of the surrounding cervical quadrants, as well as lower uterine segment and corpus, should also be obtained. Coexistent corpus cancer may occur in some instances; in others, the spread pattern to the corpus may prompt additional studies to confirm that the primary lesion is in fact in the cervix.

Examination of the lymph nodes

The macroscopic impression of a positive lymph node is notoriously poor, save for the obvious case of nodal involvement (Figure 3.29). Therefore, all lymph nodes should be entirely submitted; larger nodes should be thinly sectioned to allow sufficient examination. The usual distractors that can be seen in the lymph nodes of the female genital tract – that is, ectopic decidua in pregnancy, endosalpingiosis, endometriosis, psammoma bodies, etc. – should be borne in mind in the microscopic examination (Figure 3.30).

INVASIVE ADENOCARCINOMA, MUCINOUS (USUAL) ENDOCERVICAL TYPE

The discussion that follows pertains to the most common type of endocervical adenocarcinoma: the so-called usual or mucinous, endocervical type. Other specific variants of endocervical carcinoma are discussed separately.

Clinical characteristics

The relative frequency of cervical adenocarcinoma is now approximately 15 to 20% of all invasive cervical carcinomas. While the mean age for women with adenocarcinoma in situ is 37 years, the mean age for early invasive

(A)

(B)

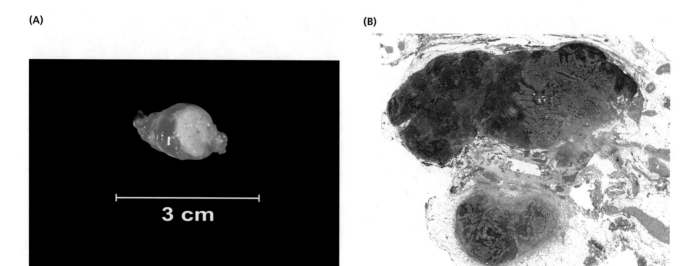

Figure 3.29 (A) Para-aortic lymph node with metastatic endocervical adenocarcinoma. (B) A macroscopically negative lymph node is partially replaced by metastatic adenocarcinoma.

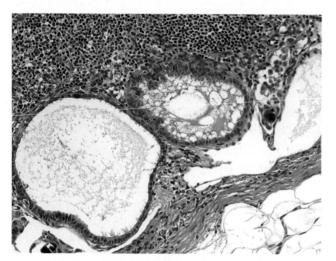

Figure 3.30 Endosalpingiosis in pelvic lymph nodes is common and should not be misinterpreted as metastatic adenocarcinoma.

adenocarcinoma is closer to 40 years (range 39 to 44 years), and the mean age for clinically invasive adenocarcinoma is 46 years (range 44 to 54 years)[13]. However, recent increases in endocervical adenocarcinoma have occurred predominantly in women less than 35 years of age. As with squamous carcinoma, risk factors include number of sexual partners, age at first intercourse, immunosuppression, and history of genital infections, in addition to high-risk HPV infection. Oral contraceptive use has also been suggested to be a risk factor, but it is not clear that this is independent of other risk factors. There is no association between cervical adenocarcinoma and Lynch syndrome[14].

The demographics and presenting symptoms are also similar to cervical squamous cell carcinoma. However,

endocervical adenocarcinoma may demonstrate different patterns of recurrence. For example, metastasis to the ovaries and, possibly, the lungs appears to be more common with adenocarcinoma than with squamous cell carcinoma. Ovarian metastasis may be the presenting sign in some patients.

Morphology

Gross pathology

Adenocarcinoma may present as a flat, ulcerated lesion or be entirely exophytic. In some instances, the only evidence is that of a thickened (barrel-shaped) cervix.

Microscopic pathology

The usual endocervical adenocarcinoma is often not overtly mucinous in appearance. The constituent cells tend to have eosinophilic cytoplasm, occasionally with small intracytoplasmic vacuoles (Figure 3.31). Mitotic figures, which may be concentrated towards the apical portion of the cell, and apoptotic bodies are often numerous. The glands assume irregular branching contours with cribriform, papillary, or villous configurations (Figure 3.32). There are no robust grading schemes for endocervical adenocarcinoma; grading is generally based on a combination of architectural and cytologic features: predominantly glandular lesions with moderate atypia are considered moderately differentiated, while tumors with more solid areas and/or marked cytologic atypia are considered poorly differentiated.

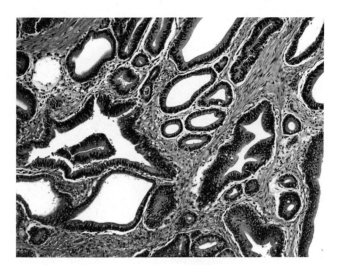

Figure 3.31 Mucinous adenocarcinoma, endocervical type is the most common or "usual" type of endocervical adenocarcinoma. Cytoplasmic mucin may not be particularly prominent.

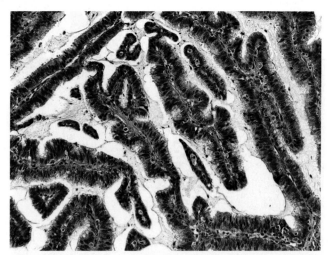

Figure 3.32 Usual endocervical adenocarcinoma typically has a branching pattern.

Well-differentiated endocervical adenocarcinoma of the usual type is rare.

Although invasive adenocarcinoma of the cervix is considered to be a potentially multifocal process, careful sectioning of cervices involved by early adenocarcinoma in situ suggests that multicentricity is seen in only 25% of cases of early invasive adenocarcinoma, and the separation of the invasive foci is usually 3 mm or less[13].

Differential diagnosis

Deep glands
Endocervical glands are often irregularly distributed in the cervix. They may abut blood vessels and extend deep into the outer one-third of the cervical wall[15]. These deep glands may form large cysts (nabothian cysts), creating a mass lesion[16]. Histologically, the glands and cysts are relatively uniform in contour, not overly crowded, and lined by a single layer of cytologically benign epithelium.

Endocervical glandular hyperplasia
There is a large variety of hyperplastic processes that involve endocervical glands; these include microglandular hyperplasia, laminar hyperplasia, tunnel clusters, lobular hyperplasia, mesonephric hyperplasia, and non-specific patterns of hyperplasia. Each of these patterns may exhibit mild cytologic atypia and/or occasional mitotic figures, but in most instances the retention of a low-power lobular architecture, the absence of significant cytologic atypia,

and the well-demarcated arrangement of the glands establishes the diagnosis.

The distinction between hyperplasia and adenoma malignum (minimal deviation adenocarcinoma) is often more problematic, especially in small cervical biopsies. Adenoma malignum should be suspected when the problematic glands are irregular, cystically dilated or "claw-shaped" and appear to infiltrate the stroma with little or no reaction. The constituent cells are notoriously bland, although nuclear enlargement and small nucleoli are typically present. Mitotic figures may also be found, but are often not numerous. Carcinoembryonic antigen expression, if present, may be a helpful differential diagnostic finding, but absence of CEA expression does not exclude the diagnosis. Unlike other adenocarcinomas of the uterine cervix, adenoma malignum does not express p16 (see discussion of *Minimal deviation adenocarcinoma* below).

Microglandular hyperplasia
Microglandular hyperplasia is typically an incidental finding, but may be seen in association with an endocervical polyp or area of cervical erosion[17]. It consists of a tightly packed, back to back, microglandular proliferation lined by low columnar, cuboidal, or flattened epithelium (Figure 3.33). The cytoplasm is often pale, and subnuclear and/or supranuclear vacuoles are typically present (Figure 3.34). Non-keratinizing squamous hyperplasia is common (frequently in a basal distribution). Nuclear atypia is minimal and nucleoli are absent or inconspicuous; mitotic figures are rare. The lumen and stroma are often infiltrated by acute and chronic inflammatory cells.

Occasionally, signet ring cells or a pseudoinfiltrative pattern is present. Initially thought to be associated with pregnancy and oral contraceptive use, it is now recognized that microglandular hyperplasia is often seen in absence of these conditions and can even occur in the postmenopausal setting.

The differential diagnosis is endometrial glandular proliferations with a microglandular pattern: either hyperplasia or carcinoma and clear cell carcinoma. Hyperplastic endometria with a microglandular pattern (with or without atypia) are architecturally similar, but the epithelium is often more attenuated, imparting a mixed microcystic and distended macrocystic appearance with more copious mucin. Endometrial carcinoma with microglandular pattern requires identification of typical endometrial adenocarcinoma merging with the microglandular pattern or the

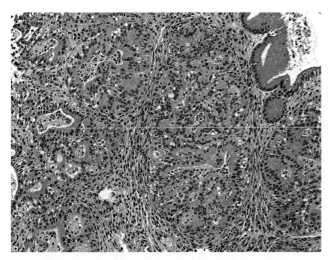

Figure 3.33 Microglandular hyperplasia. Solid microglandular pattern.

presence of significant nuclear atypia. Strategies to identify location are further discussed below. Clear cell carcinoma is recognized on the basis of a mass lesion, more pronounced cytologic atypia, and an infiltrative pattern.

Diffuse laminar endocervical glandular hyperplasia

Diffuse laminar endocervical glandular hyperplasia is typically asymptomatic, but may be associated with a copious watery or mucoid discharge[20]. It tends to occur in premenopausal women. Microscopically, laminar hyperplasia consists of numerous, often closely packed, small-to-medium-sized glands that may be rounded and simple in contour or may exhibit branching and intraglandular papillary tufting (Figure 3.35). Reactive nuclear atypia may also be present, but the absence of marked atypia and the sharp, linear demarcation from underlying cervical stroma provide diagnostic clues in biopsy or excision specimens.

Focal endocervical glandular hyperplasia (tunnel clusters)

According to Fluhmann, the part of the endocervix corresponding to a duct of an exocrine gland is called "the cleft," and the part corresponding to the acinus is the "tunnel." Tunnel clusters, initially described by Fluhmann (also colloquially known as Fluhmann's lumens) consist of two types[21]. The more common type B is composed of closely apposed, simple cystic glands lined by flattened or low cuboidal epithelium arranged in lobules; mitotic activity

(A)

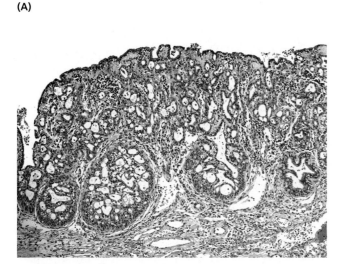

(B)

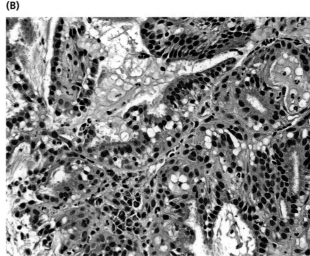

Figure 3.34 (A) Microglandular hyperplasia. (B) Subnuclear vacuoles may suggest clear cell carcinoma, but there is no mass lesion, and other foci of bona fide clear cell carcinoma are absent.

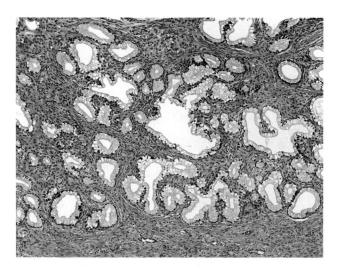

Figure 3.35 Endocervical laminar hyperplasia.

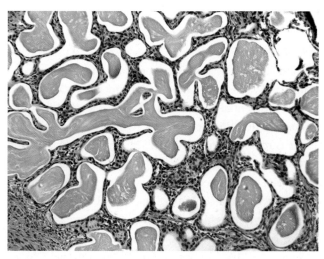

Figure 3.36 Tunnel clusters, type B. Clusters of cystic glands are lined by flattened or low cuboidal mucinous epithelium.

(A)

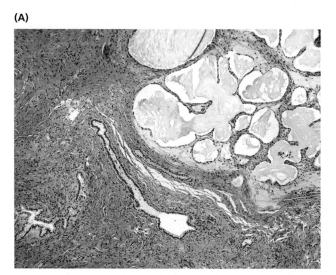

(B)

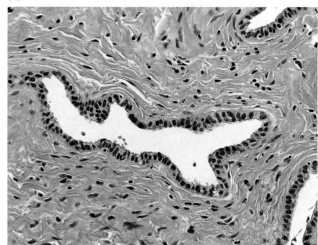

Figure 3.37 (A) Tunnel clusters, type A (lower left) are often admixed with type B tunnel clusters (upper right). (B) The glands in type A tunnel clusters are more elongated and atypical in appearance than in type B.

is minimal (Figure 3.36). The clusters may deeply penetrate the cervical wall, but do not show an infiltrative pattern[22]. The less-recognized type A tunnel clusters are also well circumscribed, but the glands have a more irregular, angular, or pseudoinfiltrative arrangement[23]. The cells in type A are also more prominent, cuboidal or columnar in shape, and may have enlarged nuclei with small nucleoli (Figure 3.37). Type A tunnel clusters are often associated with type B clusters, leading Fluhmann to speculate that type B evolves from type A due to obstruction of the distal endocervical clefts. Recently, type A tunnel clusters have been linked to lobular endocervical glandular hyperplasia on the basis of gastric-type mucin expression and a pyloric gland phenotype[24]. Both types of tunnel clusters tend to

occur in multigravid females, usually over 30 years of age. Affected patients are asymptomatic, but the type B cystic clusters may be macroscopically visible. Multifocal involvement is common.

Tunnel clusters do not exhibit the branching papillary architecture seen in most cases of minimal deviation endometrial carcinoma; the lobular arrangement and absence of cytologic atypia are additional distinguishing features. Tunnel clusters express PAX2[4].

Lobular endocervical glandular hyperplasia

As the name implies, lobular endocervical glandular hyperplasia (Figure 3.38) consists of a multilobular proliferation of rounded small or cystic glands lined by a single layer of

(A)

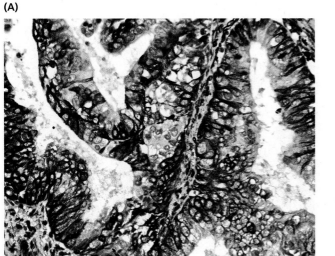

(B)

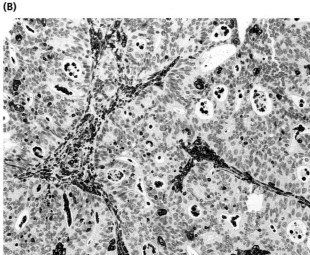

Figure 3.44 Vimentin is often expressed along the basolateral membrane of (A) endometrioid adenocarcinoma; whereas this pattern of expression is not seen in (B) endocervical adenocarcinoma.

characteristic perinuclear or lateral-cell-border pattern in up to 80% of endometrial cancers but in less than 15% of endocervical tumors (Figure 3.44). To circumvent the problems associated with the reliance upon a single antibody, the use of a limited panel of antibodies has been proposed. Using this particular panel, glandular proliferations that are ER positive, vimentin positive, and CEA negative are classified as endometrial in origin; while those that are ER negative, vimentin negative, and CEA positive are classified as endocervical in origin.

However, in practice, most tumors do not conform to these "typical" immunoprofiles for cervical or endometrial adenocarcinoma. For those showing an intermediate and non-specific immunoprofile, the detection of HPV by in situ hybridization or, alternatively, p16 by immunostaining has become the gold standard for distinguishing endocervical from endometrial adenocarcinoma. The detection of HPV by in situ hybridization is more specific, but can be relatively insensitive using current commercially available reagents, and can pose a variety of technical and interpretative challenges. The expression of p16 appears to be highly sensitive but, not surprisingly, suffers from lack of specificity. Overexpression of p16 is highly correlated with the presence of high-risk HPV DNA in cervical intraepithelial lesions and carcinomas, due to the functional inactivation of pRB by viral E7 protein and the resultant overexpression of p16. Because most endocervical adenocarcinomas contain high-risk HPV DNA, while endometrial adenocarcinomas generally do not, the overexpression of p16 can be used as an additional, surrogate marker for the presence of

HPV. Diffuse, strong staining with p16 correlates with an endocervical primary; whereas absent, diffuse weak, or focal strong reactivity correlates with an endometrial primary (Figure 3.45). However, overexpression of p16 can occur in a variety of other carcinomas independent of HPV status, including serous and clear cell carcinoma (Figure 3.46). Moreover, morules in the endometrium are typically strongly positive for p16 (Figure 3.47). Since the distinction between these two sites of origin may be based on whether a strong staining pattern with p16 is focal or diffuse in an individual case, this pattern of reactivity is most useful in whole-tissue sections. In limited samplings, such as are encountered in routine biopsy and curettage specimens, these patterns may be misleading, especially in the presence of glandular variants of uterine serous carcinoma, and should be interpreted with caution and in conjunction with additional markers. Recent studies with ProEx C have shown similar sensitivity, but the specificity is somewhat diminished by the expression of ProEx C in melanoma and in Paget's disease, as well as a variety of reactive glandular processes.

We currently use a panel of three markers that includes ER or PR, p16 or HPV in situ, and vimentin. Addition of other markers does not appear to improve the ability to identify site of origin[2].

It is important to emphasize here that this panel is not useful for differential diagnoses that involve mesonephric adenocarcinoma or classic minimal deviation adenocarcinoma (also the gastric-type mucinous adenocarcinoma: see below), since neither of these tumors are related to high-risk HPV[2,4].

(A)

(B)

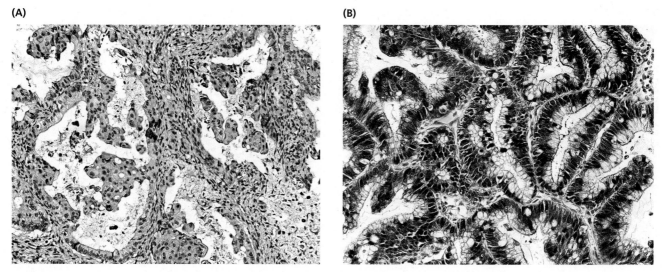

Figure 3.45 p16 expression is absent or patchy in (A) endometrioid adenocarcinoma, but is strongly and diffusely expressed in most types of (B) endocervical adenocarcinoma. Adenoma malignum and mesonephric carcinoma are exceptions.

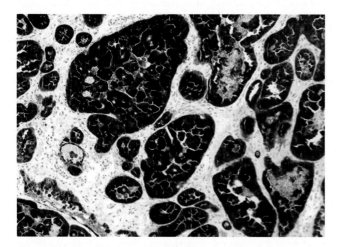

Figure 3.46 Uterine serous carcinoma also expresses p16 in a strong, diffuse pattern. A similar degree of expression may also be seen in clear cell carcinoma.

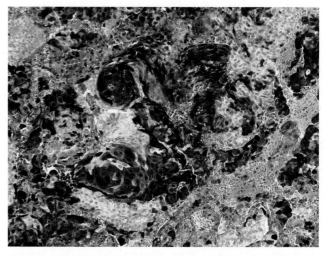

Figure 3.47 Foci of squamous and morular differentiation often express p16 in a strong, diffuse pattern. Morules are also positive for CDX2 (not shown).

METASTATIC GLANDULAR PROLIFERATIONS

The most common sites of origin for metastatic carcinomas presenting in uterine curettings are stomach, ovary, colon, and breast. Most patients have a prior history of carcinoma, and the metastasis is not the first presentation of disease; however, not all treating clinicians and, therefore, not all pathologists may be aware of this history at the time of their evaluation (see Chapter 16). Lymphoma and melanoma, although rare, also continue to pose diagnostic problems when encountered in this location because of their mimicry of undifferentiated carcinoma or sarcoma. Use of a basic panel for undifferentiated tumors and a low threshold for suspecting metastasis will prevent most misclassifications.

OTHER SPECIFIC SUBTYPES OF ENDOCERVICAL ADENOCARCINOMA

Adenocarcinoma of the usual or mucinous endocervical type accounts for 70% of cervical adenocarcinomas. Two variants, adenoma malignum (minimal deviation adenocarcinoma) and villoglandular adenocarcinoma, are very uncommon, but the source of frequent diagnostic problems. Other named types include clear cell, "endometrioid," mesonephric, endocervical intestinal-type, gastric, adenoid basal, adenoid cystic, serous, and neuroendocrine carcinoma. The distinctions between these named subtypes are somewhat arbitrary and are not based on pathogenesis

Table 3.5 Endocervical adenocarcinoma subtypes (WHO Classification)

Mucinous endocervical adenocarcinoma, usual type[a]

  Villoglandular adenocarcinoma (well differentiated)

  Minimal deviation adenocarcinoma (adenoma malignum)

    Mucinous subtype[a]

    Endometrioid subtype

Mucinous adenocarcinoma, intestinal type

  Mucinous (colloid-type) subtype

  Signet ring cell subtype

Endometrioid

Clear cell

Adenoid basal

Adenoid cystic

Mesonephric

Serous

Adenosquamous

  Glassy cell

[a] A subset of mucinous (usual) endocervical adenocarcinomas and mucinous minimal deviation adenocarcinoma are also classified as gastric-type cervical adenocarcinoma, but gastric-type adenocarcinoma is not currently recognized by WHO. See text for more details.

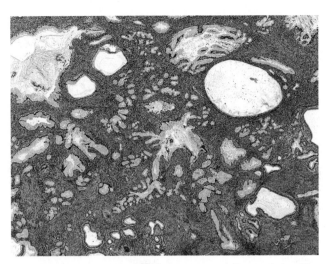

Figure 3.48 Minimal deviation adenocarcinoma. Abnormal claw-like configurations are a characteristic of minimal deviation adenocarcinoma (adenoma malignum).

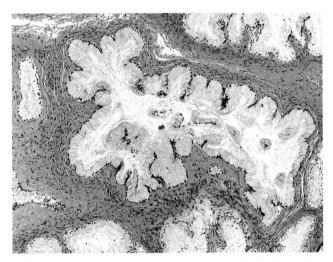

Figure 3.49 Minimal deviation adenocarcinoma. Abnormal glands are lined by abundant, pale, mucinous epithelium.

or immunophenotype; they will likely undergo revision in the next WHO (Table 3.5).

Minimal deviation carcinoma (adenoma malignum)

This tumor, also known as adenoma malignum and characterized by a deceptively benign histologic appearance,

accounts for less than 10% of all cervical adenocarcinomas[33,344]. Patients present with irregular bleeding, diffuse cervical enlargement, and/or vaginal mucus discharge. An association with Peutz–Jeghers syndrome has been reported, and somatic mutations in the *STK11* gene have been identified in these tumors. A wide age range has been reported, but virtually all patients are over 20 years of age. Patients may be biopsied due to abnormal imaging studies that suggest a possible minimal deviation carcinoma, but this is a non-specific radiologic finding; most such patients have a benign condition and carcinoma is not identified, even following diagnostic hysterectomy.

Microscopically, the tumor features cystically dilated, irregular (claw-shaped) glands with minimal cytologic atypia and minimal stromal reaction (Figures 3.48 and 3.49). The diagnosis is most easily established by careful search for foci of cytologic atypia, stromal reaction, or conventional-type adenocarcinoma (Figure 3.50). This tumor can replace normal endocervical and endometrial glandular tissue, mimicking mucinous metaplasia in uterine curettings and biopsy (Figure 3.51). Intracytoplasmic CEA staining may be helpful in some cases, but not all adenoma malignum carcinomas are CEA positive, and normal endocervical glands may express CEA on occasion, although usually only along the surface (glycocalyx)[35]. Expression of ER/PR is often absent[36]. Expression of PAX2 is reported to be lacking, whereas normal endocervical glands are often positive for one or both hormone receptors as well as PAX2.

The more common mucinous variant of minimal deviation adenocarcinoma does not harbor high-risk HPV and does not stain for p16[2]. However, high-risk HPV (and p16

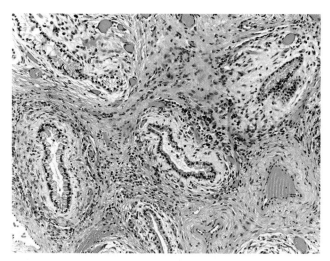

Figure 3.50 Minimal deviation adenocarcinoma. The glands are surrounded by loose, reactive stroma.

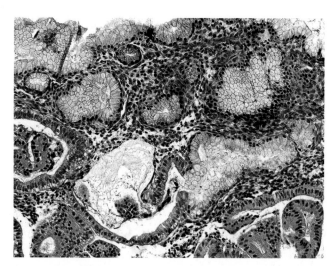

Figure 3.51 Minimal deviation adenocarcinoma may extend into the endometrium, simulating endometrial mucinous metaplasia.

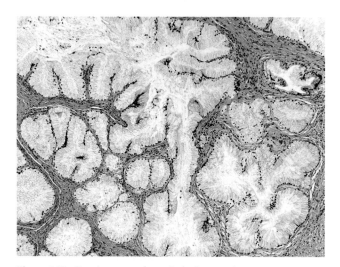

Figure 3.52 Gastric-type endocervical adenocarcinoma.

expression) can be seen in minimal deviation tumors with endometrioid differentiation (see *Endometrioid carcinoma*, below).

The differential diagnosis of minimal deviation adenocarcinoma includes a number of benign endocervical glandular proliferations, most notably lobular endocervical glandular hyperplasia, tunnel clusters, deep glands, and endocervical-type adenomyoma.

Gastric-type adenocarcinoma

The WHO currently classifies mucinous endocervical adenocarcinomas into endocervical and intestinal types, with the endocervical type being the "usual" endocervical adenocarcinoma. In reality, however, many of the mucinous tumors currently classified as endocervical type do not resemble

normal endocervical glandular epithelium. In recent years, a gastric immunophenotype of mucinous endocervical adenocarcinoma has been recognized[37,38]. This "gastric type" exhibits a spectrum of differentiation, with the well-differentiated form corresponding to minimal deviation adenocarcinoma, and the less-differentiated form corresponding to a subset of endocervical-type mucinous adenocarcinomas. Histologically, gastric-type mucinous adenocarcinomas are defined as mucinous carcinomas showing clear and/or pale eosinophilic voluminous cytoplasm, with distinct cell borders (Figure 3.52). These tumors are further characterized by immunopositivity for the gastric marker HIK1083[39]. As with the classic minimal deviation adenocarcinoma, most gastric-type mucinous adenocarcinomas of the uterine cervix are p16 negative and not related to high-risk HPV[40].

Gastric-type mucinous adenocarcinoma is considered to be an aggressive tumor, but it is not clear whether the observed behavior is due to more advanced stage at the time of diagnosis, highly infiltrating pattern of growth as seen in cases of minimal deviation adenocarcinoma, resulting in positive margins, and/or resistance to chemoradiation therapy.

Villoglandular carcinoma

This tumor occurs predominantly in young women and is characterized by villoglandular architectural growth pattern and low nuclear grade (Figure 3.53). The cells may show endometrioid, mucinous, or eosinophilic differentiation, but there appears to be no relationship to adenocarcinomas with similar differentiation arising in the corpus[41,42]. These tumors tend to occur in younger women (mean age: 35 years) and have a good prognosis, but only if

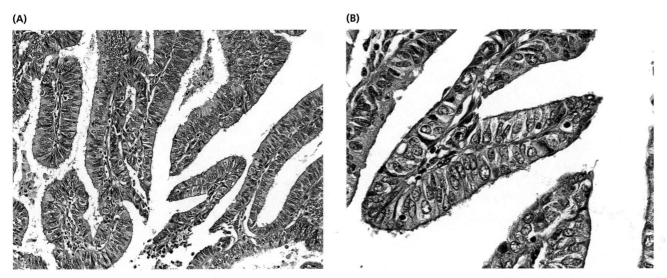

Figure 3.53 (A) Villoglandular endocervical adenocarcinoma. (B) The cells show minimal endocervical mucinous differentiation in this example.

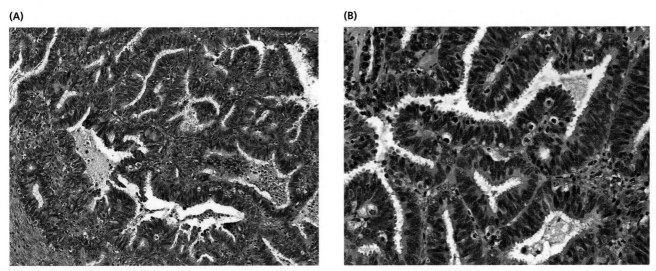

Figure 3.54 (A) Endocervical adenocarcinoma with endometrioid histology. (B) The cells are columnar and contain cilia, similar to endometrioid adenocarcinoma in the uterine corpus.

they are exophytic with minimal or no invasion. These tumors are often associated with high-grade squamous intraepithelial lesion or adenocarcinoma in situ; they are p16 positive and associated with high-risk HPV[43].

Because it is associated with a comparatively good prognosis, a definitive diagnosis of low-grade villoglandular carcinoma should not be made on the basis of a curetting or biopsy specimen; evaluation of the entire lesion is required to exclude a higher-grade component.

"Endometrioid" carcinoma

This is an uncommon tumor type in the cervix, but is so named because it tends to resemble the more common tumor that arises in the endometrium[44]. Some gynecologic pathologists question whether it exists as a separate entity, preferring to classify it with the mucinous, endocervical type (so-called mucin-poor endocervical adenocarcinoma). Despite these classificatory issues, endocervical tumors with this morphology may pose differential diagnostic problems with uterine corpus cancer, and are important to recognize. The constituent cells in this variant are columnar and harbor pseudostratified, ovoid or elongated nuclei, similar to endometrioid tumors arising in the corpus (Figure 3.54). However, unlike corpus endometrioid adenocarcinoma, squamous differentiation (morules, keratinization) is uncommon in "endometrioid" carcinoma arising in the cervix. Included in this variant is the "endometrioid" type of minimal

(A)

(B)

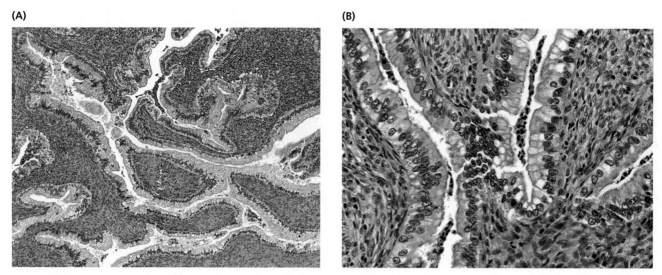

Figure 3.55 (A, B) Minimal deviation adenocarcinoma with "endometrioid" histology elsewhere in the lesion. This type at adenoma malignum is p16-positive and harbors high-risk HPV.

(A)

(B)

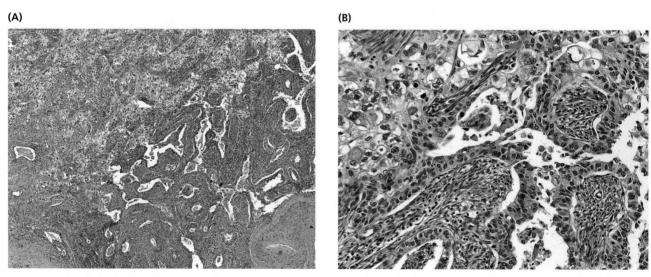

Figure 3.56 (A, B) Adenosquamous carcinoma.

deviation adenocarcinoma[45,46], which consists of very well-differentiated "endometrioid" glands deeply invading the cervical wall, often with only focal nuclear atypia, mitotic activity, or stromal reaction (Figure 3.55).

Unlike its corpus counterpart, significant hormone expression is absent in cervical "endometrioid" adenocarcinoma, and there is an association with high-risk HPV; this association appears to extend to the "endometrioid" type of minimal deviation adenocarcinoma[2].

Intestinal-type adenocarcinoma

This is a rare subtype of endocervical adenocarcinoma characterized by the presence of goblet cells and

occasionally Paneth cells[47]. Argentaffin cells are often present, but these cell types may be seen in other types of carcinomas. Signet ring cells may be seen, but these cells may also occur in poorly differentiated areas of other subtypes of endocervical adenocarcinoma. Some tumors resemble colloid carcinoma[48].

Adenosquamous carcinoma

Adenosquamous carcinoma consists of a mixture of glandular and squamous elements (Figure 3.56). The glandular component typically has usual or mucinous histology, while the squamous component is moderately to poorly differentiated. The better-differentiated tumors feature

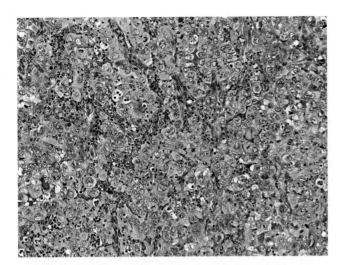

Figure 3.57 Glassy cell carcinoma. The tumor cells are large, eosinophilic, and have distinct cell borders.

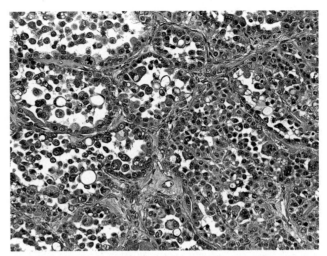

Figure 3.58 Clear cell adenocarcinoma, gland pattern. Clear cell carcinoma of the cervix is similar to clear cell carcinoma in the corpus.

keratin pearls, intracellular keratin, and intercellular bridges. In less-differentiated tumors, the squamous component may feature areas of extensive cytoplasmic clearing due to intracellular glycogen. In the past, these tumors have been associated with a poorer prognosis than squamous cell carcinomas, but when controlled for size and stage, there are no appreciable differences in prognosis with pure squamous cell carcinoma[49].

Glassy cell carcinoma

Glassy cell carcinoma is widely considered a poorly differentiated variant of adenosquamous carcinoma, but the absence of significant amounts of keratin or mucin in tumor cells has led to an alternative suggestion that this subtype is a distinct entity[50]. "Glassy cell carcinoma" should be reserved for those tumors containing an abundance of large, undifferentiated cells with (1) eosinophilic, ground-glass cytoplasm, (2) distinct cell membranes that can be accentuated by PAS (periodic acid-Schiff) stain, and (3) large vesicular nuclei with prominent nucleoli (Figure 3.57)[51]. These tumors often contain a heavy inflammatory infiltrate consisting of eosinophils. Squamous or glandular differentiation may be present but is typically less conspicuous than the glassy cell component. The fraction of glassy cells considered necessary for the diagnosis of a glassy cell carcinoma is under-specified in the pathology literature. Initially considered to have a poor prognosis, recent studies have shown a survival rate closely resembling that for squamous cervical cancer at a similar stage of disease, with multimodal treatment strategies, including surgery and radiation with or without

chemotherapy[52]. The differential diagnosis is that of other large-cell undifferentiated tumors, and includes melanoma, sarcoma, and lymphoma.

Clear cell adenocarcinoma

Clear cell carcinoma may occur in young women (DES exposure in utero) or older women, and may arise in the ectocervix (typically, associated with DES exposure) or endocervix[53,54]. The overall incidence of clear cell carcinoma in daughters exposed to DES is approximately 1/1000. Although the peak affected age is close to 19 years, the increased risk persists, and most affected women have continued follow-up. Diethylstilbestrol-associated clear cell carcinomas typically arise in areas of adenosis in the upper third of the vagina or ectocervix. Currently, most cervicovaginal clear cell carcinomas are not associated with exposure to DES or other synthetic estrogens. These non-DES cancers occur at a wide range of ages, affecting pediatric patients as well as postmenopausal women (mean: 53 years). When they occur in the cervix, they have the same prognosis, stage for stage, as usual cervical carcinoma[54]. Even though clear cell carcinoma often expresses strong p16, neither DES nor non-DES cervical clear cell cancers appear to have a strong association with high-risk HPV[55]. A variety of patterns, including tubulocystic or glandular, solid, and papillary may be seen, often in combination (Figure 3.58). Yolk sac tumor, alveolar soft part sarcoma, Arias-Stella reaction, and microglandular and mesonephric hyperplasia should be excluded. Misclassification as mucinous carcinoma may also occur.

(A)

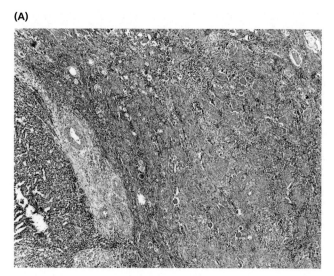

(B)

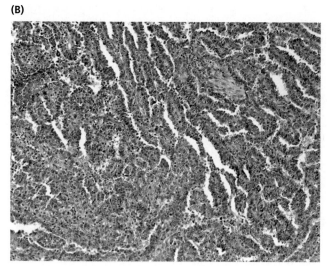

Figure 3.59 (A) Moderately differentiated mesonephric carcinoma (at left) arising in mesonephric hyperplasia (at right). (B) Anastomosing glands are lined by a single layer of cuboidal epithelial cells.

Serous adenocarcinoma

Although described in the cervix[56], in our experience primary endocervical serous carcinoma is extraordinarily rare; most cases we have encountered have been clear cell adenocarcinoma, endocervical adenocarcinoma of usual type with prominent papillary architecture, villoglandular adenocarcinoma with foci or high-grade cytology, or implants from a uterine corpus, fallopian tube, or ovarian primary.

Mesonephric carcinoma

Mesonephric remnants may develop hyperplasia and carcinoma; often a spectrum of these changes is seen in the carcinomas[31,57,58,59]. The carcinomas often pose significant diagnostic difficulty due to their lateral and deep location within the cervix. There may be no surface component. Ductal, retiform, tubular, solid, and spindle patterns may be seen in the carcinomas (Figure 3.59). Most are low to moderate nuclear grade, and some cases may be difficult to distinguish from florid mesonephric hyperplasia. The distinction is often based on loss of lobular architecture and infiltrative pattern in conjunction with the presence of cytologic atypia; mitotic figures are often increased. Diagnosis of higher-grade mesonephric adenocarcinoma is based on identification of residual normal or hyperplastic mesonephric tubules, with their characteristic eosinophilic luminal material. Prognosis is uncertain due to limited numbers of cases, but probably similar to similar-stage usual endocervical adenocarcinoma. Mesonephric carcinomas are often positive for calretinin and CD10 (Figure 3.60),

but negative for CEA, ER, and PR[31,59]. These tumors are not known to be associated with HPV and are usually p16 negative[55,2]. They are reported to be negative for PAX2, but this has not been our experience (Figure 3.14)[5,4]. Mesonephric carcinoma needs to be distinguished from small gland patterns of invasive endometrial cancer (Figure 3.61).

Adenoid basal carcinoma

Adenoid basal cell carcinoma occurs in postmenopausal, elderly women (mean age: 65 years). Most are asymptomatic and the tumor is discovered during evaluation of an abnormal Pap smear. Indeed, it is often associated with high-grade squamous intraepithelial lesion[28,60,61,62]. The cervix is often normal on culposcopic and physical examination. The tumor is cytologically bland (often looking like "bland squamous cell carcinoma") and consists of widely separated clusters of small glands with basaloid and adenoid, as well as squamoid differentiation (Figure 3.62). The adenoid areas consist of small closely packed tubules, occasionally with intraluminal secretions reminiscent of mesonephric tubules. The constituent cells are small, ovoid, and uniform in appearance; nucleoli are absent or inconspicuous (Figure 3.62). Mitotic figures are rare or absent. There is typically no stromal response. The tumor is frequently superficial, although it can extend deeply into the cervical stroma. The small, basaloid nests can also be colonized by severely dysplastic squamous cells. When this occurs, it is important to look for evidence of destructive stromal invasion beyond the

(A)

(B)

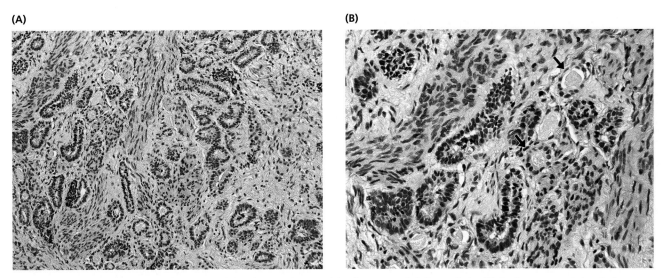

Figure 3.60 (A, B) Well-differentiated mesonephric adenocarcinoma arising in mesonephric hyperplasia. (B) Benign mesonephric tubules (arrows) are admixed with malignant glands.

(A)

(B)

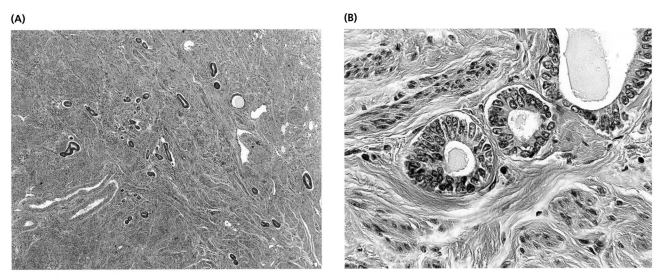

Figure 3.61 (A, B) Sertoliform pattern of invasive endometrial adenocarcinoma may mimic a primary endocervical glandular lesion.

(A)

(B)

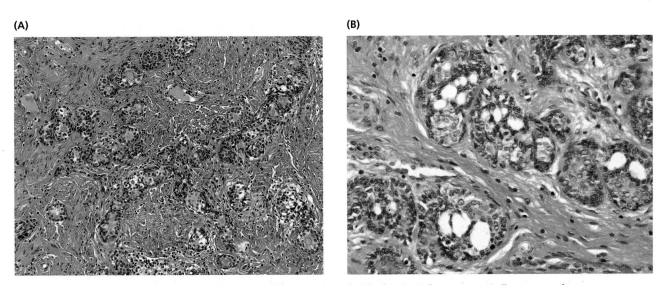

Figure 3.62 (A) Adenoid basal carcinoma. (B) Basaloid cells are cytologically bland; mitotic figures are typically sparse or absent.

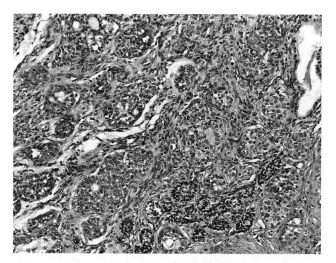

Figure 3.63 Adenoid basal-like adenoid cystic carcinoma.

Table 3.6 Differential diagnosis of uterine cervical "basaloid" proliferations

Adenoid basal hyperplasia (adenoid basal epithelioma)
Adenoid basal carcinoma
Adenoid cystic carcinoma
Usual type
Solid variant
Combined adenoid basal and adenoid cystic carcinoma
Basaloid squamous cell carcinoma
Keratinizing
Non-keratinizing, large cell type
Non-keratinizing, small cell type
Neuroendocrine carcinoma
Small cell neuroendocrine carcinoma
Large cell neuroendocrine carcinoma
Other neoplasms with potential for basaloid morphology
Carcinosarcoma (malignant mixed mullerian tumor: MMMT) with basaloid carcinomatous component(s)
Metastatic carcinoma (basaloid, neuroendocrine, or undifferentiated)
Amelanotic malignant melanoma (primary cervical, or metastatic)

compact nests of the background tumor. Many pathologists diagnosis "adenoid basal epithelioma" when destructive stromal invasion is lacking because metastasis has not been reported in that setting, even when the small, basaloid nests extend deeply into the cervical wall. However, there is a risk of metastatic carcinoma when destructive stromal invasion is present. Similarly, a diagnosis of "adenoid basal carcinoma" is often used when histologically typical invasive squamous or adenosquamous carcinoma arises in a background of adenoid basal epithelioma. The situation is analogous to diagnosing invasive carcinoma in the setting of a low-grade, non-invasive adenofibromatous tumor.

Pure adenoid basal carcinoma has a favorable prognosis and needs to be distinguished from the adenoid cystic pattern of cervical adenocarcinoma, which does not have a favorable prognosis[27]. In most instances, the distinction is straightforward. Adenoid cystic carcinoma features a well-developed cribriform architecture with spherules of basement membrane material. A stromal response is often present. The constituent cells are larger and more mitotically active and pleomorphic than in adenoid basal carcinoma. Moreover, patients with adenoid cystic carcinoma typically present with vaginal bleeding and a mass lesion is detected on examination. However, in some cases, the distinction can be problematic, as adenoid basal-like areas can be seen in adenoid cystic carcinoma (Figure 3.63) and vice versa[63]; when this problem is encountered in a biopsy or curettage specimen it is important to alert the treating physician to the ambiguous histology, so that appropriate management can be implemented. When encountered in a hysterectomy or cone excision specimen, it is important to thoroughly

sample the tumor to exclude adenoid cystic carcinoma or another more aggressive synchronous carcinoma variant (adenosquamous, clear cell, neuroendocrine carcinoma, and, rarely, carcinosarcoma)[64]. Whether all hybrid adenoid cystic/adenoid basal tumors have clinical behavior similar to that of pure adenoid cystic carcinoma, or a more intermediate clinical course, is unknown. The differential diagnosis of basaloid proliferations in the uterine cervix is presented in Table 3.6.

Adenoid cystic carcinoma

Adenoid cystic carcinoma resembles adenoid cystic carcinoma of the salivary gland. Like adenoid basal carcinoma, adenoid cystic carcinoma occurs more frequently in postmenopausal women (mean age: 70 years). Unlike adenoid basal carcinoma, adenoid cystic carcinoma pursues an aggressive clinical course[28,61,63,65]. Patients present with vaginal bleeding, often associated with large, friable and necrotic tumor masses. The glands are arranged in cribriform patterns with intraluminal spherules of basement membrane material (Figure 3.64). Cellular palisading along the periphery is also present, but this may be a focal finding. Trabecular, corded, and nested patterns may also be seen. As in the salivary gland, solid variants occur; they are recognized as adenoid cystic on the basis of the presence of basement membrane material. In addition, there

(A)

(B)

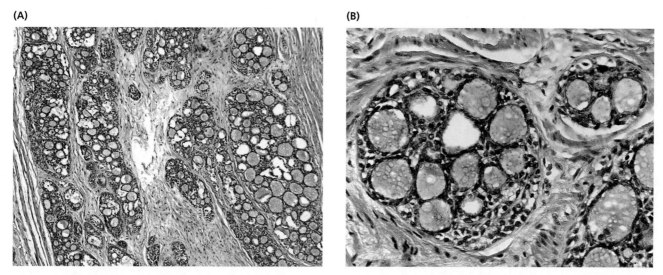

Figure 3.64 (A) Adenoid cystic carcinoma. (B) Solid nests of cells are punctuated by spherical aggregates of basement membrane-like material.

(A)

(B)

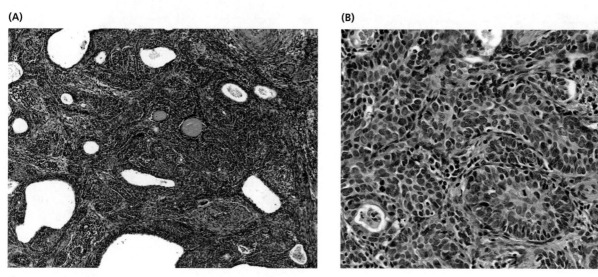

Figure 3.65 (A, B) Squamous cell carcinoma with basaloid features.

may be foci of squamous cell carcinoma. Despite the similarity to the usual salivary gland adenoid cystic carcinoma, myoepithelial cells are inconspicuous or absent. High-risk HPV, in particular type 16, is associated with this uncommon type of primary cervical cancer[66].

The differential diagnosis of adenoid cystic carcinoma includes adenoid basal carcinoma (see above), basaloid squamous cell carcinoma, squamous cell carcinoma with basaloid features (Figure 3.65), neuroendocrine carcinoma, and metastasis. Basaloid squamous cell carcinoma is rare in the cervix, and a well-defined cribriform architecture is lacking. Neuroendocrine carcinoma should express chromogranin or synaptophysin. Metastasis, although unusual, should always be considered if there is a history of a prior

salivary gland tumor, as salivary gland adenoid cystic carcinomas may pursue a prolonged clinical course.

Neuroendocrine carcinoma

Neuroendocrine carcinoma (both small cell and large cell variants) account for less than 5% of all cervical carcinomas. They occur in a wide age range, but most are seen in the fifth decade. These highly aggressive tumors may present as small lesions, but most are large, bulky, and necrotic tumors that are deeply invasive[67]. More than 50% of patients have advanced stage disease (FIGO III/IV). Ectopic hormone production (ACTH, ADH, insulin, etc.) is rare. Cervical small cell neuroendocrine

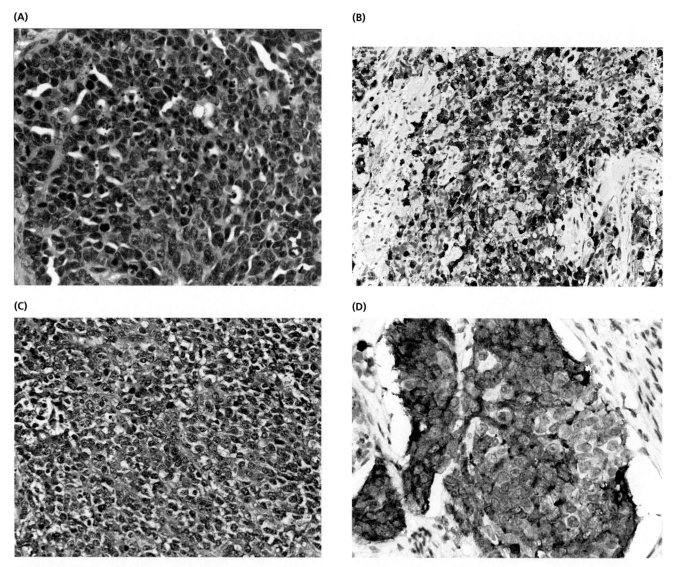

Figure 3.66 (A) Neuroendocrine carcinoma, small cell type. (B) p16 in neuroendocrine carcinoma. (C) Neuroendocrine carcinoma, large cell type. (D) Synaptophysin in large cell neuroendocrine tumor.

carcinoma exhibits the usual features of neuroendocrine carcinoma (e.g., nuclear hyperchromasias, nuclear molding, dispersed chromatin, inconspicuous nucleoli); high mitotic rates, apoptosis, and necrosis are common (Figure 3.66). The large cell variant consists of medium to large cells with moderate to abundant cytoplasm that may contain eosinophilic granules. Neuroendocrine carcinoma is often associated with adenocarcinoma in situ, high-grade squamous intraepithelial lesion, and conventional invasive cervical adenocarcinoma. Most express one or more neuroendocrine markers. Both small and large cell types are p16 positive and harbor high-risk HPV (usually HPV18)[69,71]. First-line systemic chemotherapy with either cisplatin or carboplatin, in combination with etoposide, is recommended for most patients

with metastatic or high-stage disease; however, response durations are often short[72].

Other small blue cell malignancies should be excluded before issuing a diagnosis of small cell carcinoma in the cervix; poorly differentiated small cell non-keratinizing squamous cell carcinoma, basaloid squamous cell carcinoma, rhabdomyosarcoma, lymphoma, and melanoma are the chief mimics. Metastasis should always be excluded.

Well-differentiated neuroendocrine tumors

Rarely, well-differentiated neuroendocrine tumors (so-called "carcinoid" and "atypical carcinoid") may occur in the cervix, and the prognosis for this tumor may be

(A)

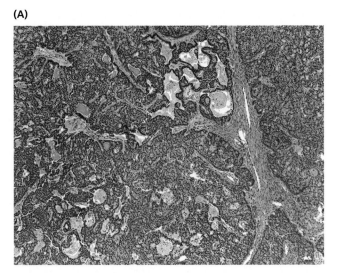

(B)

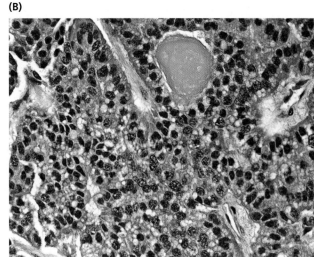

Figure 3.67 (A, B) Carcinoid tumor in the cervix. These tumors tend to behave more aggressively than their gastrointestinal counterparts.

somewhat better (Figure 3.67). Mitotic index and Ki-67 are useful in confirming low-grade histology, and may be useful in predicting prognosis in these better-differentiated examples. Well-differentiated neuroendocrine tumors arising in the cervix should be managed similarly to gastroenteropancreatic neuroendocrine tumors[73].

REFERENCES

1. Ioffe OB, Sagae S, Moritani S, *et al.* Proposal of a new scoring scheme for the diagnosis of noninvasive endocervical glandular lesions. *Am J Surg Pathol* 2003;**27**:452–60.

2. Kong C, Beck A, Longacre T. A panel of three markers including p16, ProEx C, or HPV ISH is optimal for distinguishing between primary endometrial and endocervical adenocarcinomas *Am J Surg Pathol* 2010;**34**:915–26.

3. Park KJ, Kiyokawa T, Soslow RA, *et al.* Unusual endocervical adenocarcinomas: an immunohistochemical analysis with molecular detection of human papillomavirus. *Am J Surg Pathol* 2011; **35**:633–46.

4. Rabban JT, McAlhany S, Lerwill MF, *et al.* PAX2 distinguishes benign mesonephric and mullerian glandular lesions of the cervix from endocervical adenocarcinoma, including minimal deviation adenocarcinoma. *Am J Surg Pathol* 2010;**34**:137–46.

5. DiMaio M, Beck A, Montgomery K, *et al.* PAX8 and WT1 are superior to PAX2 and BRST2 in distinguishing mullerian tract tumors from breast carcinomas. *Mod Pathol* 2011;**24**:243A.

6. Vang R, Vinh TN, Burks RT, *et al.* Pseudoinfiltrative tubal metaplasia of the endocervix: a potential form of in utero diethylstilbestrol exposure-related adenosis simulating minimal deviation adenocarcinoma. *Int J Gynecol Pathol* 2005;**24**:391–8.

7. Nucci MR, Young RH. Arias-Stella reaction of the endocervix: a report of 18 cases with emphasis on its varied histology and differential diagnosis. *Am J Surg Pathol* 2004;**28**:608–12.

8. Young RH, Clement PB. Endocervicosis involving the uterine cervix: a report of four cases of a benign process that may be confused with deeply invasive endocervical adenocarcinoma. *Int J Gynecol Pathol* 2000;**19**:322–8.

9. Clement PB, Young RH. Florid cystic endosalpingiosis with tumor-like manifestations: a report of four cases including the first reported cases of transmural endosalpingiosis of the uterus. *Am J Surg Pathol* 1999;**23**:166–75.

10. Lesack D, Wahab I, Gilks CB. Radiation-induced atypia of endocervical epithelium: a histological, immunohistochemical and cytometric study. *Int J Gynecol Pathol* 1996;**15**:242–7.

11. Jones MA, Young RH. Atypical oxyphilic metaplasia of the endocervical epithelium: a report of six cases. *Int J Gynecol Pathol* 1997;**16**:99–102.

12. Trowell JE. Intestinal metaplasia with argentaffin cells in the uterine cervix. *Histopathology* 1985;**9**:551–9.

13. Ostor AG. Early invasive adenocarcinoma of the uterine cervix. *Int J Gynecol Pathol* 2000;**19**:29–38.

14. Mills AM, Liou S, Kong CS, *et al.* Are women with endocervical adenocarcinoma at risk for Lynch syndrome? Evaluation of 101 cases including unusual subtypes and lower uterine segment tumors. *Int J Gyn Pathol* 2012; in press.

15. Daya D, Young RH. Florid deep glands of the uterine cervix. Another mimic of adenoma malignum. *Am J Clin Pathol* 1995;**103**:614–17.

16. Clement PB, Young RH. Deep nabothian cysts of the uterine cervix. A possible source of confusion with minimal-deviation adenocarcinoma (adenoma malignum). *Int J Gynecol Pathol* 1989; **8**:340–8.

17. Greeley C, Schroeder S, Silverberg SG. Microglandular hyperplasia of the cervix: a true "pill" lesion? *Int J Gynecol Pathol* 1995;**14**:50–4.

18. Nichols TM, Fidler HK. Microglandular hyperplasia in cervical cone biopsies taken for suspicious and positive cytology. *Am J Clin Pathol* 1971;**56**:424–9.

19. Young RH, Scully RE. Atypical forms of microglandular hyperplasia of the cervix simulating carcinoma. A report of five cases and review of the literature. *Am J Surg Pathol* 1989;**13**:50–6.

20. Jones MA, Young RH, Scully RE. Diffuse laminar endocervical glandular hyperplasia. A benign lesion often confused with adenoma malignum (minimal deviation adenocarcinoma). *Am J Surg Pathol* 1991;**15**:1123–9.

21. Fluhmann CF. Focal hyperplasis (tunnel clusters) of the cervix uteri. *Obstet Gynecol* 1961;**17**:206–14.

22. Segal GH, Hart WR. Cystic endocervical tunnel clusters. A clinicopathologic study of 29 cases of so-called adenomatous hyperplasia. *Am J Surg Pathol* 1990;**14**:895–903.

23. Jones MA, Young RH. Endocervical type A (noncystic) tunnel clusters with cytologic atypia. A report of 14 cases. *Am J Surg Pathol* 1996;**20**:1312–18.

24. Kondo T, Hashi A, Murata SI, et al. Gastric mucin is expressed in a subset of endocervical tunnel clusters: type A tunnel clusters of gastric phenotype. *Histopathology* 2007;**50**:843–50.

25. Nucci MR, Clement PB, Young RH. Lobular endocervical glandular hyperplasia, not otherwise specified: a clinicopathologic analysis of thirteen cases of a distinctive pseudoneoplastic lesion and comparison with fourteen cases of adenoma malignum. *Am J Surg Pathol* 1999;**23**:886–91.

26. Kawauchi S, Kusuda T, Liu XP, et al. Is lobular endocervical glandular hyperplasia a cancerous precursor of minimal deviation adenocarcinoma? A comparative molecular-genetic and immunohistochemical study. *Am J Surg Pathol* 2008;**32**:1807–15.

27. Brainard JA, Hart WR. Adenoid basal epitheliomas of the uterine cervix: a reevaluation of distinctive cervical basaloid lesions currently classified as adenoid basal carcinoma and adenoid basal hyperplasia. *Am J Surg Pathol* 1998;**22**:965–75.

28. Grayson W, Cooper K. A reappraisal of "basaloid carcinoma" of the cervix, and the differential diagnosis of basaloid cervical neoplasms. *Adv Anat Pathol* 2002;**9**:290–300.

29. Ferry JA, Scully RE. Mesonephric remnants, hyperplasia, and neoplasia in the uterine cervix. A study of 49 cases. *Am J Surg Pathol* 1990;**14**:1100–11.

30. Seidman JD, Tavassoli FA. Mesonephric hyperplasia of the uterine cervix: a clinicopathologic study of 51 cases. *Int J Gynecol Pathol* 1995;**14**:293–9.

31. McCluggage WG, Oliva E, Herrington CS, et al. CD10 and calretinin staining of endocervical glandular lesions, endocervical stroma and endometrioid adenocarcinomas of the uterine corpus: CD10 positivity is characteristic of, but not specific for, mesonephric lesions and is not specific for endometrial stroma. *Histopathology* 2003;**43**:144–50.

32. Longacre TA, Atkins KA, Kempson RL, et al. The uterine corpus. In: Sternberg S, Mills S, eds. *Diagnostic Surgical Pathology*. New York: Raven Press; 2009:2184–277.

33. Gilks CB, Young RH, Aguirre P, et al. Adenoma malignum (minimal deviation adenocarcinoma) of the uterine cervix. A clinicopathological and immunohistochemical analysis of 26 cases. *Am J Surg Pathol* 1989;**13**:717–29.

34. Kaminski PF, Norris HJ. Minimal deviation carcinoma (adenoma malignum) of the cervix. *Int J Gynecol Pathol* 1983;**2**:141–52.

35. Michael H, Grawe L, Kraus FT. Minimal deviation endocervical adenocarcinoma: clinical and histologic features, immunohistochemical staining for carcinoembryonic antigen, and differentiation from confusing benign lesions. *Int J Gynecol Pathol* 1984;**3**:261–76.

36. Toki T, Shiozawa T, Hosaka N, et al. Minimal deviation adenocarcinoma of the uterine cervix has abnormal expression of sex steroid receptors, CA125 and gastric mucin. *Int J Gyn Pathol* 1999;**18**:215–19.

37. Kawakami F, Mikami Y, Kojima A, et al. Diagnostic reproducibility in gastric-type mucinous adenocarcinoma of the uterine cervix: validation of novel diagnostic criteria. *Histopathology* 2010;**56**:551–3.

38. Mikami Y, Kiyokawa T, Hata S, et al. Gastrointestinal immunophenotype in adenocarcinomas of the uterine cervix and related glandular lesions: a possible link between lobular endocervical glandular hyperplasia/pyloric gland metaplasia and 'adenoma malignum'. *Mod Pathol* 2004;**17**:962–72.

39. Kojima A, Mikami Y, Sudo T, et al. Gastric morphology and immunophenotype predict poor outcome in mucinous adenocarcinoma of the uterine cervix. *Am J Surg Pathol* 2007;**31**:664–72.

40. Kusanagi Y, Kojima A, Mikami Y, et al. Absence of high-risk human papillomavirus (HPV) detection in endocervical adenocarcinoma with gastric morphology and phenotype. *Am J Pathol* 2010;**177**:2169–75.

41. Jones MW, Silverberg SG, Kurman RJ. Well-differentiated villoglandular adenocarcinoma of the uterine cervix: a clinicopathological study of 24 cases. *Int J Gynecol Pathol* 1993;**12**:1–7.

42. Young RH, Scully RE. Villoglandular papillary adenocarcinoma of the uterine cervix. A clinicopathologic analysis of 13 cases. *Cancer* 1989;**63**:1773–9.

43. Jones MW, Kounelis S, Papadaki H, et al. Well-differentiated villoglandular adenocarcinoma of the uterine cervix: oncogene/tumor suppressor gene alterations and human papillomavirus genotyping. *Int J Gynecol Pathol* 2000;**19**:110–17.

44. Alfsen GC, Thoresen SO, Kristensen GB, et al. Histopathologic subtyping of cervical adenocarcinoma reveals increasing incidence rates of endometrioid tumors in all age groups: a population based study with review of all nonsquamous cervical carcinomas in Norway from 1966 to 1970, 1976 to 1980, and 1986 to 1990. *Cancer* 2000;**89**:1291–9.

45. Rahilly MA, Williams AR, al-Nafussi A. Minimal deviation endometrioid adenocarcinoma of cervix: a clinicopathological and immunohistochemical study of two cases. *Histopathology* 1992;**20**:351–4.

46. Young RH, Scully RE. Minimal-deviation endometrioid adenocarcinoma of the uterine cervix. A report of five cases of a distinctive neoplasm that may be misinterpreted as benign. *Am J Surg Pathol* 1993;**17**:660–5.

47. Lee KR, Trainer TD. Adenocarcinoma of the uterine cervix of small intestinal type containing numerous Paneth cells. *Arch Pathol Lab Med* 1990;**114**:731–3.

48. Lewis TL. Colloid (mucus secreting) carcinoma of the cervix. *J Obstet Gynaecol Br Commonw* 1971;**78**:1128–32.

49. Shingleton HM, Bell MC, Fremgen A, et al. Is there really a difference in survival of women with squamous cell carcinoma, adenocarcinoma, and adenosquamous cell carcinoma of the cervix? *Cancer* 1995;**76**:1948–55.

50. Kato N, Katayama Y, Kaimori M, et al. Glassy cell carcinoma of the uterine cervix: histochemical, immunohistochemical, and molecular genetic observations. *Int J Gynecol Pathol* 2002;**21**:134–40.

51. Littman P, Clement PB, Henriksen B, et al. Glassy cell carcinoma of the cervix. *Cancer* 1976;**37**:2238–46.

52. Gray HJ, Garcia R, Tamimi HK, et al. Glassy cell carcinoma of the cervix revisited. *Gynecol Oncol* 2002;**85**:274–7.

53. Kaminski PF, Maier RC. Clear cell adenocarcinoma of the cervix unrelated to diethylstilbestrol exposure. *Obstet Gynecol* 1983;**62**:720–7.

54. Thomas MB, Wright JD, Leiser AL, et al. Clear cell carcinoma of the cervix: a multi-institutional review in the post-DES era. *Gynecol Oncol* 2008;**109**:335–9.

55. Houghton O, Jamison J, Wilson R, et al. p16 immunoreactivity in unusual types of cervical adenocarcinoma does not reflect human papillomavirus infection. *Histopathology* 2010;**57**:342–50.

56. Zhou C, Gilks CB, Hayes M, *et al.* Papillary serous carcinoma of the uterine cervix: a clinicopathologic study of 17 cases. *Am J Surg Pathol* 1998;**22**:113–20.

57. Bague S, Rodriguez IM, Prat J. Malignant mesonephric tumors of the female genital tract: a clinicopathologic study of 9 cases. *Am J Surg Pathol* 2004;**28**:601–7.

58. Clement PB, Young RH, Keh P, *et al.* Malignant mesonephric neoplasms of the uterine cervix. A report of eight cases, including four with a malignant spindle cell component. *Am J Surg Pathol* 1995;**19**:1158–71.

59. Silver SA, Devouassoux-Shisheboran M, Mezzetti TP, *et al.* Mesonephric adenocarcinomas of the uterine cervix: a study of 11 cases with immunohistochemical findings. *Am J Surg Pathol* 2001;**25**:379–87.

60. Ferry JA. Adenoid basal carcinoma of the uterine cervix: evolution of a distinctive clinicopathologic entity. *Int J Gynecol Pathol* 1997;**16**:299–300.

61. Ferry JA, Scully RE. "Adenoid cystic" carcinoma and adenoid basal carcinoma of the uterine cervix. A study of 28 cases. *Am J Surg Pathol* 1988;**12**:134–44.

62. Hart WR. Symposium part II: special types of adenocarcinoma of the uterine cervix. *Int J Gynecol Pathol* 2002;**21**:327–46.

63. Grayson W, Taylor LF, Cooper K. Adenoid cystic and adenoid basal carcinoma of the uterine cervix: comparative morphologic, mucin, and immunohistochemical profile of two rare neoplasms of putative 'reserve cell' origin. *Am J Surg Pathol* 1999; **23**:448–58.

64. Parwani AV, Smith Sehdev AE, Kurman RJ, *et al.* Cervical adenoid basal tumors comprised of adenoid basal epithelioma associated with various types of invasive carcinoma: clinicopathologic features, human papillomavirus DNA detection, and p16 expression. *Hum Pathol* 2005;**36**:82–90.

65. Albores-Saavedra J, Manivel C, Mora A, *et al.* The solid variant of adenoid cystic carcinoma of the cervix. *Int J Gynecol Pathol* 1992;**11**:2–10.

66. Grayson W, Taylor L, Cooper K. Detection of integrated high risk human papillomavirus in adenoid cystic carcinoma of the uterine cervix. *J Clin Pathol* 1996;**49**:805–9.

67. Gersell DJ, Mazoujian G, Mutch DG, *et al.* Small-cell undifferentiated carcinoma of the cervix. A clinicopathologic, ultrastructural, and immunocytochemical study of 15 cases. *Am J Surg Pathol* 1988;**12**:684–98.

68. Gilks CB, Young RH, Gersell DJ, *et al.* Large cell neuroendocrine [corrected] carcinoma of the uterine cervix: a clinicopathologic study of 12 cases. *Am J Surg Pathol* 1997;**21**:905–14.

69. Ishida GM, Kato N, Hayasaka T, *et al.* Small cell neuroendocrine carcinomas of the uterine cervix: a histological, immunohistochemical, and molecular genetic study. *Int J Gynecol Pathol* 2004;**23**:366–72.

70. Sato Y, Shimamoto T, Amada S, *et al.* Large cell neuroendocrine carcinoma of the uterine cervix: a clinicopathological study of six cases. *Int J Gynecol Pathol* 2003;**22**:226–30.

71. Grayson W, Rhemtula HA, Taylor LF, *et al.* Detection of human papillomavirus in large cell neuroendocrine carcinoma of the uterine cervix: a study of 12 cases. *J Clin Pathol* 2002;**55**:108–14.

72. Strosberg JR, Coppola D, Klimstra DS, *et al.* The NANETS consensus guidelines for the diagnosis and management of poorly differentiated (high-grade) extrapulmonary neuroendocrine carcinomas. *Pancreas;***39**:799–800.

73. Gardner GJ, Reidy-Lagunes D, Gehrig PA. Neuroendocrine tumors of the gynecologic tract: a Society of Gynecologic Oncology (SGO) clinical document. *Gynecol Oncol* 2011;**122**:190–8.

4 MISCELLANEOUS CERVICAL ABNORMALITIES

ARIAS-STELLA REACTION

Up to 10% of gravid hysterectomy specimens contain foci of Arias-Stella reaction in endocervical glands. Patients range in age from 19 to 44 years; almost all are pregnant, but a history of oral contraceptive use has also been reported[1]. The histologic features are identical to those in the endometrium, and consist of vacuolated cytoplasm, tufting, hobnail cells, clear or oxyphilic cytoplasm, and intranuclear pseudoinclusions. A dense, smudged nuclear chromatin pattern is characteristic (see Figure 18.5).

DECIDUAL REACTION

Decidual stromal reaction can occur anywhere in the female genital tract and peritoneum. Although it is typically associated with pregnancy, it may also be seen in the setting of progestin treatment (so-called pseudodecidual reaction; see Chapter 5). It is usually an incidental finding, but may present as cervical erosion or bleeding during pregnancy (Figure 4.1). Distinction from squamous cell

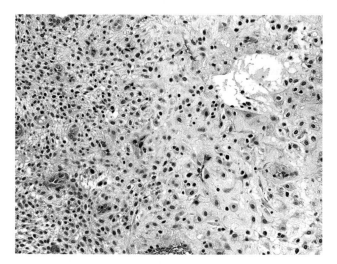

Figure 4.1 Decidua in cervix can be quite extensive and simulate a neoplastic process.

carcinoma is based on bland nuclear features and absence of mitotic figures; decidual stromal reaction does not express cytokeratin.

ENDOCERVICAL POLYP

Endocervical polyps are common. They are usually small and lined by a mix of squamous and endocervical mucinous epithelium (Figure 4.2). The surfaces are often eroded and there is usually a component of acute and chronic inflammation – which may consist of numerous plasma cells. Foci of microglandular hyperplasia may also be present. The constituent glands can be small, or large and cystic; in the presence of cystic, or elongated and compressed glands, adenosarcoma should be excluded (see Chapter 11). Most endocervical polyps occur in reproductive-aged women.

Rarely, a tubulosquamous polyp may present in the cervix. This polyp, which typically occurs in the upper vagina of postmenopausal women, consists of cytologically benign, well-circumscribed nests of glycogenated or non-glycogenated squamous epithelium, with admixed small tubules at the periphery of some of the nests. The tubules may be positive for prostatic acid phosphatase and prostate-specific antigen; derivation from paraurethral Skene glands, the female equivalent of prostatic glands in the male, has been proposed[2].

POLYPOID ADENOMYOMA

Although polypoid adenomyoma is more common in the corpus, similar polyps may arise in the cervix (Figure 4.3). The constituent glands are small, rounded or slightly compressed, and exhibit endocervical glandular differentiation. The surrounding stroma is fibromuscular. Most cervical polypoid adenomyomas are small (<5 mm), but larger

(A)

(B)

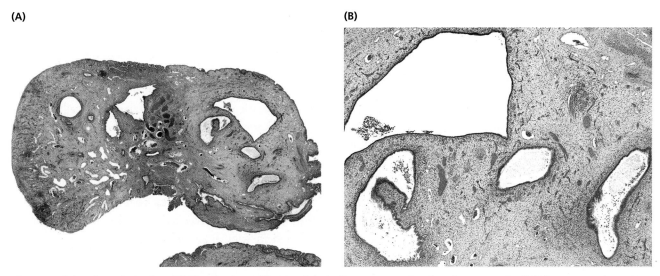

Figure 4.2 (A) Endocervical polyp. (B) The glands are dilated and set in fibrous stroma, but there is no stromal cellularity or stromal cell atypia.

(A)

(B)

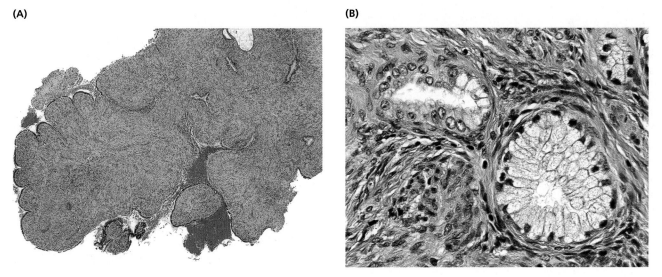

Figure 4.3 (A) Polypoid adenomyoma arising in cervix. (B) The constituent endocervical glands are small with banal cytology.

polyps may raise the differential diagnosis of a smooth muscle tumor. They are benign.

MULLERIAN PAPILLOMA

This lesion occurs in children, usually between the ages of two and five years, and is often associated with vaginal bleeding or discharge[3]. A distinct papillary or polypoid mass is almost always present, which may extend to 2 cm in size. Microscopically, the polyp is composed of branching papillary structures lined by a single layer of bland epithelium that is flattened, cuboidal, or low columnar; squamous metaplasia may be present. The papillary

connective tissue cores are usually composed of dense cervical stromal tissue, but edema, inflammation, and calcifications may also be seen.

INVERTED TRANSITIONAL CELL PAPILLOMA

Rare cervical polyps show histologic features similar to those of urinary tract inverted papilloma[4]. Like the inverted papilloma elsewhere, this polyp features inverted anastomosing epithelial nests divided by fibrovascular septa. The epithelial nests show peripheral palisading and uniform, oval nuclei with longitudinal grooves. There is no significant atypia, and mitotic activity is absent. Inside the nests, foci of intraepithelial glandular metaplasia resembling glandular cystitis of the urinary bladder may be seen. Most occur in adult, reproductive-aged women, but they have also been reported in older women.

CERVICITIS

Inflammation of the cervix is common. Most cervices show variable degrees of lymphocytic and plasmacytic inflammation, but occasional cases show a predominance of plasma cells replete with Russell bodies (plasma cell cervicitis), eosinophils (eosinophilic cervicitis), histiocytes (xanthogranulomatous cervicitis), or non-infectious necrobiotic granulomas[5–9]. The last two processes may be

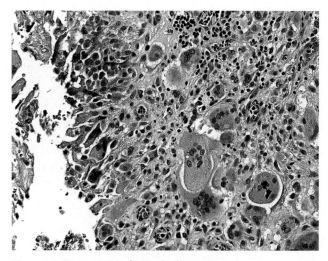

Figure 4.4 Post-curettage foreign body reaction.

due to prior procedure, particularly electrocautery. Foreign body giant cells, pigment, and the presence of elongated and flattened surface epithelium with nuclear hyperchromasia and smudged chromatin may also be seen in postcautery change (Figure 4.4). The presence of a marked tissue eosinophilic infiltrate is typically secondary to a prior biopsy procedure, but carcinoma (glassy cell type, or other) with marked eosinophilic stromal infiltration should always be excluded.

Occasionally, the lymphoid infiltrate is associated with exophytic papillary structures (papillary endocervicitis; Figure 4.5) or pronounced subepithelial and periglandular lymphoid follicles, often with germinal centers (follicular cervicitis). Both processes are benign, although the latter may be confused with lymphoma (see below).

Chlamydia infection has been associated with florid follicular cervicitis[10]. Other infectious etiologies are listed in Table 4.1.

LYMPHOMA-LIKE LESION (PSEUDOLYMPHOMA)

Lymphoma-like lesions of the female genital tract are florid reactive inflammatory processes that mainly occur in women in their reproductive years. They are characterized by a dense lymphoid infiltrate with admixed large cells that is often suspicious for lymphoma. Occasional cases have been associated with CMV, herpes simplex virus (HSV), or EBV infection (Figure 4.6)[21]. Often superficial erosion of the cervical mucosa is present, but, in contrast to

(A)

(B)

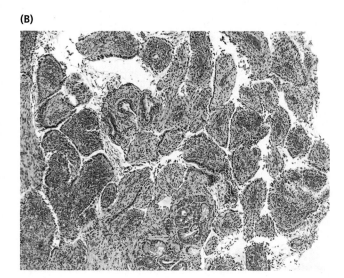

Figure 4.5 (A, B) Papillary endocervicitis.

Table 4.1 Infectious lesions of the cervix

Agent	Pathology and key features
Viral	
Human papillomavirus (HPV)	See Chapter 2
Cytomegalovirus (CMV)[11,12]	Dense acute and chronic inflammation; may have lymphoid follicles. Intracytoplasmic inclusions in endocervical cells; cytoplasmic and/or intranuclear inclusions in endothelial cells and stromal cells. Note: CMV may be an incidental finding in patients not known to be immunocompromised
Herpes[10]	Necrotic ulcer with predominant lymphocytic inflammation with admixed neutrophils and histiocytes. Inclusions may not be present, so diagnosis often requires cultures
Bacterial	
Chlamydia[10]	Follicular cervicitis. Diagnosis requires cultures or molecular studies
Tuberculosis[13,14]	Necrotizing granulomatous inflammation; often disease elsewhere. May form a mass lesion
Syphilis[15]	Ulcer or erosion with prominent lymphocytic and plasmacytic infiltration; swollen endothelial cells with or without vasculitis. Diagnosis made by serology, cultures, or molecular studies
Actinomycosis[16]	Non-specific acute and chronic inflammation. Distinctive sulfur granules – not to be confused with pseudoactinomycotic radiate granules (PAMRAGs). Actinomycotic granules are positive on gram and silver stains; PAMRAGs are not. History of intrauterine device (IUD)
Parasitic	
Schistosomiasis[17,18]	Granulomatous inflammation, but may be sparse depending on immune response. Diagnosis based on identification of eggs. Calcifications may indicate old infection. History of travel in endemic area – typically *Schistosoma haematobium*
Entamoeba histolytica[19]	Ulcers or erosions with exudate. May be associated with verrucoid epithelial hyperplasia, mimicking squamous cell carcinoma. Diagnosis made on wet mounts, serology
Trypanosoma cruzi (Chaga's disease)[20]	Acute and chronic inflammation. Multinucleated giant cells containing amastigotes. History of immunodeficiency

lymphoma, there is no evidence of a mass, deep cervical stromal invasion, or prominent sclerosis[22]. Immunohistochemical studies often show a mixture of B and T cells without immunoglobulin light chain restriction, but recently clonal *IGH* gene rearrangements have been detected by polymerase chain reaction methods in some lymphoma-like lesions; as the latter cases all had a benign clinical course, caution should be exercised, and careful correlation of clinical, histologic, immunophenotypic, and genetic features is required to prevent misdiagnosis[23].

PSAMMOMATOUS CALCIFICATIONS

Psammoma bodies within the stroma may occasionally be seen in the cervix and uterine corpus. They are often an incidental finding, but may be associated with psammomatous calcifications in a Pap smear[24]. Careful evaluation of the surrounding glandular tissue to exclude a subtle serous carcinoma is warranted, particularly if there are suspicious clinical findings[25], but in most cases stromal psammoma bodies have no clinical significance.

MULTINUCLEATED STROMAL GIANT CELLS

Multinucleated stromal giant cells, identical to those that occur in fibroepithelial polyps and, occasionally, in benign endometrial polyps, are common in the cervical stroma (Figure 4.7). They appear to be rare in women under 30 years of age, but increase with age[26,27]. Depending on the assiduity of the pathologist, up to 80% of cervices contain scattered multinucleated stromal cells in the sixth decade[27]. They are generally confined to the loose subepithelial connective tissue stroma in the ectocervix. They are negative for cytokeratin and muscle markers.

FIBROEPITHELIAL POLYP

Fibroepithelial polyps may rarely occur in the cervix[28]. They exhibit similar features to those seen in the more common vulvovaginal fibroepithelial polyp. Cell types range from small spindle cells to enlarged, bizarre angulated and multinucleated forms. The absence of a clear demarcation between the lesional cells and the stromal–epithelial interface, and the presence of characteristic stellate multinucleate stromal cells, facilitate the correct diagnosis (Figure 4.8). The multinucleated atypical cells are often enriched along the stromal–epithelial interface.

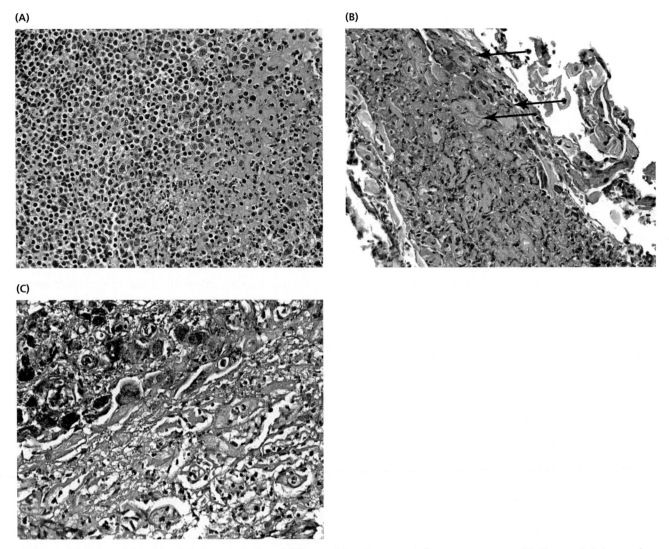

Figure 4.6 (A) Herpes simplex virus infection may incite a striking pseudolymphomatous inflammatory response. (B) Characteristic intranuclear inclusions (arrows) may be difficult to detect amidst the atypical lymphoid infiltrate. (C) Immunhistochemical detection of the HSV virus facilitates the diagnosis.

ARTERITIS

Giant cell arteritis or polyarteritis nodosa can involve the entire female genital tract, although the cervix is most commonly involved by polyarteritis nodosa (Figure 4.9). Giant cell arteritis tends to occur in post-menopausal women (Figure 4.10), while polyarteritis nodosa can occur in a wide age range[29–31]. Almost all affected patients are asymptomatic; most are isolated, microscopic findings, but rare cases are reported to be associated with a systemic disease. In these last cases, the systemic disease may be pre-existing, or the arteritis is the initial manifestation. When such cases are encountered, it is important to emphasize that, while most cases are isolated, the possibility of systemic disease should be considered, especially if there are other supportive clinical findings.

LIGNEOUS CERVICITIS

Ligneous cervicitis is rare, but almost always associated with ligneous conjunctivitis. The cervix is the most common site of female genital tract involvement. Patients may have vaginal discharge or an apparent cervical lesion on clinical examination. The histologic features of ligneous cervicitis are extensive deposition of hyaline or amorphous, eosinophilic fibrinous material (Figure 4.11), some of which is necrotic[32]. Ligneous cervicitis has been linked to a deficiency in plasminogen[33].

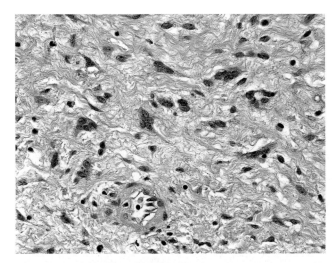

Figure 4.7 Multinucleated stromal cells are common in the cervical stroma. In absence of stromal cellularity, this is a benign finding.

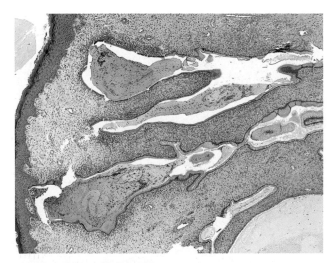

Figure 4.8 Fibroepithelial polyp.

(A)

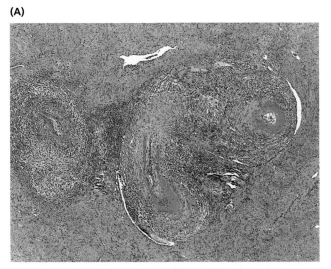

(B)

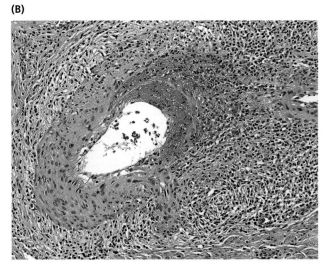

Figure 4.9 (A, B) Polyarteritis nodosum.

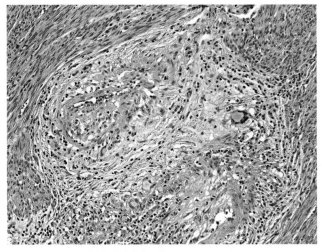

Figure 4.10 Localized giant cell arteritis.

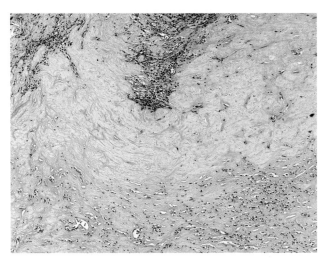

Figure 4.11 Ligneous cervicitis.

(A)

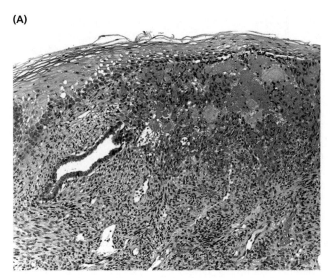

(B)

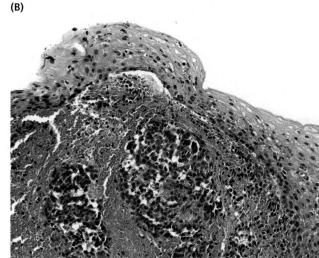

Figure 4.12 Endometriosis. (A) The endometrial stroma may be masked by hemorrhage and inflammation. (B) Disintegrating stroma in cervical endometriosis may simulate a neoplasm.

AMYLOIDOSIS

Localized amyloidosis may rarely occur in the uterine cervix[34,35]. Several reported cases have been related to cervical squamous cell carcinoma[36]. Other reports have been associated with systemic involvement or myeloma[37].

OTHER ECTOPIAS

In addition to the more common gland-forming ectopias (endometriosis, endocervicosis, endosalpingiosis), a variety of other ectopic tissues can be seen in the cervix (Figure 4.12). These include prostate[38], sebaceous glands[39], fat[40], bone[41], and adnexal (hair follicles) structures[42]. Ectopic prostate tissue resembles typical prostatic glandular tissue, including basal cells that are positive for high molecular weight keratin and glandular cells that are immunoreactive for prostatic acid phosphatase and/or prostate-specific antigen[43]. Squamous metaplasia may be prominent, and it is possible that the entire process represents a metaplastic lesion as opposed to a true ectopia. The presence of sebaceous glands, hair follicles, bone, and cartilage may represent retained fetal parts. The presence of bone may also represent a metaplastic process, secondary to abortion, chronic endometritis, metabolic disorders, and loop electrosurgical excision[44]. Recent data indicate that the presence of mature adipose tissue is likely to be a normal constituent of the cervical stroma and not a true ectopia[40]. Extramedullary hematopoiesis can also occur in the cervix[45].

MELANOTIC LESIONS

These are discussed under ***Miscellaneous uterine mesenchymal tumors*** in Chapter 14.

REFERENCES

1. Nucci MR, Young RH. Arias-Stella reaction of the endocervix: a report of 18 cases with emphasis on its varied histology and differential diagnosis. *Am J Surg Pathol* 2004;**28**:608–12.
2. McCluggage WG, Young RH. Tubulo-squamous polyp: a report of ten cases of a distinctive hitherto uncharacterized vaginal polyp. *Am J Surg Pathol* 2007;**31**:1013–19.
3. Smith YR, Quint EH, Hinton EL. Recurrent benign mullerian papilloma of the cervix. *J Pediatr Adolesc Gynecol* 1998;**11**:29–31.
4. Albores-Saavedra J, Young RH. Transitional cell neoplasms (carcinomas and inverted papillomas) of the uterine cervix. A report of five cases. *Am J Surg Pathol* 1995;**19**:1138–45.
5. Chen KT, Hendricks EJ. Malakoplakia of the female genital tract. *Obstet Gynecol* 1985;**65**:84S–7S.
6. Evans CS, Goldman RL, Klein HZ, *et al.* Necrobiotic granulomas of the uterine cervix. A probable postoperative reaction. *Am J Surg Pathol* 1984;**8**:841–4.
7. Ladefoged C, Lorentzen M. Xanthogranulomatous inflammation of the female genital tract. *Histopathology* 1988;**13**:541–51.
8. Pikarsky E, Maly B, Maly A. Ceroid granuloma of the uterine cervix. *Int J Gynecol Pathol* 2002;**21**:191–3.
9. Stewart CJ, Leake R. Reactive plasmacytic infiltration with numerous Russell bodies involving the uterine cervix: 'Russell body cervicitis'. *Pathology* 2006;**38**:177–9.
10. Kiviat NB, Paavonen JA, Wolner-Hanssen P, *et al.* Histopathology of endocervical infection caused by Chlamydia trachomatis, herpes simplex virus, Trichomonas vaginalis, and Neisseria gonorrhoeae. *Hum Pathol* 1990;**21**:831–7.

11. Byard RW, Mikhael NZ, Orlando G, *et al.* The clinicopathological significance of cytomegalovirus inclusions demonstrated by endo-cervical biopsy. *Pathology* 1991;**23**:318–21.

12. McGalie CE, McBride HA, McCluggage WG. Cytomegalovirus infection of the cervix: morphological observations in five cases of a possibly under-recognised condition. *J Clin Pathol* 2004; **57**:691–4.

13. Shobin D, Sall Pellman C. Genitourinary tuberculosis simulating cervical carcinoma. *J Reprod Med* 1976;**17**:305–8.

14. Vuong PN, Houissa-Vuong S, Bleuse B, *et al.* Pseudotumoral tuberculosis of the uterine cervix. Cytologic presentation. *Acta Cytol* 1989;**33**:305–8.

15. Gutmann EJ. Syphilitic cervicitis simulating stage II cervical cancer. Report of two cases with cytologic findings. *Am J Clin Pathol* 1995;**104**:643–7.

16. Snowman BA, Malviya VK, Brown W, *et al.* Actinomycosis mimicking pelvic malignancy. *Int J Gynaecol Obstet* 1989;**30**:283–6.

17. Adeniran A, Dimashkieh H, Nikiforov Y. Schistosomiasis of the cervix. *Arch Pathol Lab Med* 2003;**127**:1637–8.

18. Sharma S, Boyle D, Wansbrough-Jones MH, *et al.* Cervical schisto-somiasis. *Int J Gynecol Cancer* 2001;**11**:491–2.

19. Nopdonrattakoon L. Amoebiasis of the female genital tract: a case report. *J Obstet Gynaecol Res* 1996;**22**:235–8.

20. Concetti H, Retegui M, Perez G, *et al.* Chagas' disease of the cervix uteri in a patient with acquired immunodeficiency syndrome. *Hum Pathol* 2000;**31**:120–2.

21. Hachisuga T, Ookuma Y, Fukuda K, *et al.* Detection of Epstein-Barr virus DNA from a lymphoma-like lesion of the uterine cervix. *Gynecol Oncol* 1992;**46**:69–73.

22. Ma J, Shi QL, Zhou XJ, *et al.* Lymphoma-like lesion of the uterine cervix: report of 12 cases of a rare entity. *Int J Gynecol Pathol* 2007;**26**:194–8.

23. Geyer JT, Ferry JA, Harris NL, *et al.* Florid reactive lymphoid hyperplasia of the lower female genital tract (lymphoma-like lesion): a benign condition that frequently harbors clonal immunoglobulin heavy chain gene rearrangements. *Am J Surg Pathol* 2010;**34**:161–8.

24. Misdraji J, Vaidya A, Tambouret RH, *et al.* Psammoma bodies in cervicovaginal cytology specimens: a clinicopathological analysis of 31 cases. *Gynecol Oncol* 2006;**103**:238–46.

25. Fadare O, Chacho MS, Parkash V. Psammoma bodies in cervicova-ginal smears: significance and practical implications for diagnostic cytopathology. *Adv Anat Pathol* 2004;**11**:250–61.

26. Clement PB. Multinucleated stromal giant cells of the uterine cervix. *Arch Pathol Lab Med* 1985;**109**:200–2.

27. Hariri J, Ingemanssen JL. Multinucleated stromal giant cells of the uterine cervix. *Int J Gynecol Pathol* 1993;**12**:228–34.

28. Nucci MR, Young RH, Fletcher CD. Cellular pseudosarcomatous fibroepithelial stromal polyps of the lower female genital tract: an underrecognized lesion often misdiagnosed as sarcoma. *Am J Surg Pathol* 2000;**24**:231–40.

29. Bell DA, Mondschein M, Scully RE. Giant cell arteritis of the female genital tract. A report of three cases. *Am J Surg Pathol* 1986;**10**:696–701.

30. Ganesan R, Ferryman SR, Meier L, *et al.* Vasculitis of the female genital tract with clinicopathologic correlation: a study of 46 cases with follow-up. *Int J Gynecol Pathol* 2000;**19**:258–65.

31. Hoppe E, de Ybarlucea LR, Collet J, *et al.* Isolated vasculitis of the female genital tract: a case series and review of literature. *Virchows Arch* 2007;**451**:1083–9.

32. Deen S, Duncan TJ, Hammond RH. Ligneous cervicitis; is it the emperor's new clothes? Case report and different analysis of aeti-ology. *Histopathology* 2006;**49**:198–9.

33. Biswas J, Billingham K, Biswas S, *et al.* Ligneous cervicitis: an unusual cause of post-coital bleeding in a postmenopausal woman. *J Obstet Gynaecol* 2009;**29**:163–5.

34. Gibbons D, Lindberg GM, Ashfaq R, *et al.* Localized amyloidosis of the uterine cervix. *Int J Gynecol Pathol* 1998;**17**:368–71.

35. Harry VN, Lyall M, Cruickshank ME, *et al.* Cervical amyloidosis: a rare cause of cervical ectopy in a postmenopausal woman. *Eur J Obstet Gynecol Reprod Biol* 2008;**137**:252–3.

36. Tsang WY, Chan JK. Amyloid-producing squamous cell carcinoma of the uterine cervix. *Arch Pathol Lab Med* 1993;**117**:199–201.

37. Taylor E, Gilks B, Lanvin D. Amyloidosis of the uterine cervix pre-senting as postmenopausal bleeding. *Obstet Gynecol* 2001;**98**:966–8.

38. Nucci MR, Ferry JA, Young RH. Ectopic prostatic tissue in the uterine cervix: a report of four cases and review of ectopic prostatic tissue. *Am J Surg Pathol* 2000;**24**:1224–30.

39. Kazakov DV, Hejda V, Kacerovska D, *et al.* Hyperplasia of ectopic sebaceous glands in the uterine cervix: case report. *Int J Gynecol Pathol*;**29**:605–8.

40. Doldan A, Otis CN, Pantanowitz L. Adipose tissue: a normal constituent of the uterine cervical stroma. *Int J Gynecol Pathol* 2009;**28**:396–400.

41. Sabatini L, Rainey AJ, Tenuwara W, *et al.* Osseous metaplasia of cervical epithelium. *BJOG* 2001;**108**:333–4.

42. Robledo MC, Vazquez JJ, Contreras-Mejuto F, *et al.* Sebaceous glands and hair follicles in the cervix uteri. *Histopathology* 1992;**21**:278–80.

43. McCluggage WG, Ganesan R, Hirschowitz L, *et al.* Ectopic pro-static tissue in the uterine cervix and vagina: report of a series with a detailed immunohistochemical analysis. *Am J Surg Pathol* 2006;**30**:209–15.

44. Bedaiwy MA, Goldberg JM, Biscotti CV. Recurrent osseous meta-plasia of the cervix after loop electrosurgical excision. *Obstet Gyne-col* 2001;**98**:968–70.

45. Pandey U, Aluwihare N, Light A, *et al.* Extramedullary haemopoi-esis in the cervix. *Histopathology* 1999;**34**:556–7.

5 NON-NEOPLASTIC ENDOMETRIUM

INTRODUCTION

A variety of normal physiologic, abnormal but non-neoplastic, and artifactual changes in endometrial specimens can pose diagnostic problems for the pathologist (Tables 5.1 and 5.2). These changes may occur in isolation or superimposed on another underlying benign or malignant process. An understanding of these alterations and their differential diagnosis is essential to evaluation of the endometrium, whether it is in a biopsy, curettage, polypectomy, or hysterectomy specimen (Tables 5.1 and 5.2). This chapter will emphasize the key problem areas, pitfalls, and differential diagnostic decisions that need to be made in the evaluation of the non-neoplastic endometrium. A series of tables and figures supplement the discussion in order to provide a cogent, practical approach for the surgical pathologist (see Table 5.3).

PHYSIOLOGIC CYCLING ENDOMETRIUM

Normal endometrium varies in appearance depending on the site within the uterus and the prevailing hormonal milieu. Fully developed, normal, physiologic cycling endometrial tissue is most representative in the superficial layer within the uterine fundus (stratum functionalis); while the lower layer within the fundus (stratum basalis) and the entire endometrium (strata functionalis and basalis) in the lower uterine segment are less hormonally responsive. Full sections of lower uterine segment often show the basalis of the fundus merging imperceptibly with lower uterine segment endometrium, such that there is no clear demarcation between functionalis and basalis. As a result, it can be difficult to determine whether a biopsy specimen is from the lower uterine segment or the basalis endometrium.

The cyto-architectural features of normal cycling endometria have been well described[1] and are not further

Table 5.1 Artifacts in the endometrial biopsy/curettage specimen

Artifact	Description	Differential diagnosis
Excessive fragmentation	Strips of endometrium with scant attached stroma form discrete, but dense tissue fragments simulating stromal breakdown	Menstrual endometrium, stromal breakdown
Pseudopapillary change	Atrophic surface endometrium coils in on itself, imparting a papillary appearance	Endometrial hyperplasia, metaplasia, or carcinoma
Excessive crowding	Strips of detached surface endometrium with minimal stroma align together to impart an apparent increased gland-to-stroma ratio	Endometrial hyperplasia
Telescoping	Apparent gland-within-gland pattern due to intussusception of the glands during the curettage procedure	Endometrial hyperplasia
Stratum basalis	Artifactual crowding of glands due to tangential sectioning of stratum basalis or lower uterine segment	Endometrial hyperplasia
Cervical tissue contaminant	Squamous or mucinous glandular epithelium, mucin pools, pseudo-signet ring cells, metaplastic or dysplastic squamous epithelium, microglandular hyperplasia, endocervical adenocarcinoma	Endometrial hyperplasia, endometrial carcinoma
Intracavitary histiocytes	Sheet-like aggregates of histiocytes or inflammatory cells, due to hydrometra, mucometra, pyometra	Endometrial stromal neoplasm
Uterine perforation	Adipose tissue (rarely, colonic mucosa)	Ectopic adipose tissue, lipoleiomyoma or lipoma – requires direct connection with cervical/ endometrial stroma

Table 5.2 Artifacts in the hysterectomy specimen

Artifact	Description	Differential diagnosis
Intravascular menstrual endometrium	Vascular spaces in myometrium contain disaggregated menstrual stroma and/or glands – usually focal with degenerative changes	Lymphovascular space invasion
Intravascular adenomyosis	Similar to intravascular menstrual endometrium	Intravascular leiomyomatosis
Gland-poor adenomyosis	Nodules of dense, but atrophic endometrial stroma within myometrium, but no mass lesion – often has glands elsewhere; typically occurs in postmenopausal patient	Endometrial stromal sarcoma
Post-curettage atypia	Surface cells are eosinophilic with papillary syncytial change, may have smudged and/or hyperchromatic nuclei with mitotic figures	Serous intraepithelial carcinoma
Intravascular carcinoma	Plugs of tumor in ectatic vascular spaces secondary to artifactual displacement (either during or after laparoscopic or robotic surgery)	Lymphovascular space invasion
Cornual fallopian tube	Intramyometrial tube – may have simple or slightly more convoluted architecture	Adenomyosis, possibly carcinoma if carcinoma is present elsewhere in the uterus

Table 5.3 Common diagnostic problems encountered in the non-neoplastic uterus in clinical practice[a]

Problem	Description
Proliferative vs. secretory endometrium	Focal or patchy subnuclear vacuolization can occur in proliferative endometria, especially in the setting of chronic anovulation. However, the cytoplasmic vacuoles are less well developed in extent and uniformity than is seen in physiologic early secretory endometrium
Proliferative vs. disordered proliferative endometrium	Mild irregularity in gland size, contour, and distribution can be seen in normal proliferative endometrium. The diagnosis of disordered proliferative endometrium should be reserved for specimens with intact surface endometrium; the glands should exhibit clearly disordered architecture (focally or in a multifocal distribution) interspersed with more normal-appearing proliferative or, in some cases, weakly proliferative endometrial glands
Secretory endometrium vs. gestational endometrium	In comparison to late secretory endometrium, early gestational endometrium exhibits prominent stromal deciduation with more pronounced glandular secretions, prominent cytoplasmic vacuolation, and gland distension with marked stromal edema and thick spiral arteries. Arias-Stella reaction may also be present
Normal cycling endometrium vs. pill effect	Oral contraceptive use may impart a subtle spindled cell appearance to the endometrial stroma; often the glands are not as well developed
Normal cycling endometrium vs. progestin effect	The secretory changes in progestin effect are muted: glands are small with minimal vacuolation, and the stroma has a spindled appearance with minimal predecidual change
Polypoid secretory endometrium vs. endometrial polyp	Florid secretory endometrium may form pseudopolypoid configurations on gross or hysteroscopic examination, distinguished from true polyps by the absence of central thick-walled blood vessels
Benign endometrial polyp vs. endometrial polyp with hyperplasia	Benign endometrial polyps may have irregular, clustered glands with a variety of superimposed metaplastic changes, but the process is focal, and adjacent fragments of endometrium do not show features of hyperplasia, whereas hyperplasia should be a more diffuse process
Endometrial polyp with increased cellularity or stromal atypia vs. sarcoma	The stromal cellularity or stromal atypia is limited to the polyp and unassociated with the typical glandular changes seen in adenosarcoma, and there is no condensation of stroma around the glands. The atypia appears degenerative, with nuclear hyperchromasia and smudged chromatin
Atrophy vs. insufficient sampling	It is important to be able to distinguish atrophy from an inadequate or insufficient endometrial sampling. Atrophy is a very common cause of postmenopausal bleeding (approximately 25% of cases). If the patient is postmenopausal and the treating clinician reports scant tissue despite a good sampling, a diagnosis of an atrophic pattern is appropriate. However, if there is concern by the treating clinician or the pathologist that the sampling may not be representative

continued on next page

Table 5.3 (continued)

Problem	Description
	(uterine enlargement, thickened endometrial stripe, young age with no clinical history to support endometrial atrophy, etc.), a descriptive diagnosis of "scant inactive endometrial tissue," with a comment indicating that further evaluation and correlation with clinical and/or imaging studies is required to exclude other processes, is appropriate
Endometrial tissue vs. cervical tissue	When the glands are lined by columnar epithelium with ovoid, pseudostratified nuclei, recognition of endometrial tissue is straightforward, but mucinous metaplasia can mimic endocervix; in these cases, attention to the stroma and adjacent tissue may provide a clue to the location. The immunopanel used for distinguishing malignant cervical and endometrial glandular lesions is less useful in this differential diagnosis, since benign endocervical glands may express hormone receptors
Florid stromal breakdown vs. menstrual endometrium	Extensive breakdown may obscure underlying tissue and prevent a definitive diagnosis; in this situation, the distinction between breakdown due to dysfunctional uterine bleeding (or other cause) and menstrual endometrium may be impossible. In absence of strong clinical and histologic evidence for physiologic, menstrual-related bleeding, florid stromal and glandular breakdown should not be diagnosed as menstrual endometrium
Menstrual endometrium vs. stromal neoplasm	Stromal breakdown in menstrual endometrium may result in condensed aggregates of gland-poor stroma, simulating a stromal neoplasm, but apoptotic bodies, fibrin, and other degenerative features are also present
Menstrual endometrium vs. endometrial carcinoma	Glandular breakdown in menstrual endometrium may result in crowded epithelium with hyperchromasia, simulating adenocarcinoma, but degenerative changes with other features of breakdown are almost always present
Hobnail cells vs. clear cell or serous carcinoma	The nuclei in benign endometrial cells with hobnail change are small, round, and often have dense chromatin; while the nuclei in clear cell or serous carcinoma are pleomorphic, often with prominent nucleoli
Arias-Stella reaction vs. clear cell carcinoma	Arias-Stella is focal, mitotically inactive, and associated with decidua; clear cell carcinoma is more diffuse, occurs in older patients, and not associated with decidua
Late secretory or early gestational endometrium vs. clear cell carcinoma	Secretory and, particularly, early gestational endometrium may have prominent cytoplasmic vacuolation, but there is no significant nuclear atypia; mitotic figures are absent and there is no associated decidua
Intermediate trophoblast vs. squamous cell carcinoma	Intermediate trophoblast or decidua can mimic squamous cell carcinoma in pregnancy; this is generally not a problem unless it is an unsuspected pregnancy. The presence of edema and stromal granulocytes and the absence of intercellular bridges, keratinization, and mitotic figures are key distinguishing features of pregnancy changes
Syncytiotrophoblast vs. anaplastic or giant cell carcinoma	This is a problem only when there is scant tissue; distinction is based on patient demographics and histology in adjacent endometrial tissue
Atypical polypoid adenomyoma (APA) vs. endometrioid carcinoma	Atypical polypoid adenomyoma is focal, associated with a non-inflamed fibromuscular stroma, and often admixed with fragments of proliferative or secretory endometrium (see Chapter 7)
Hydropic abortus vs. molar pregnancy	See Chapter 17

[a] Also see Chapter 6.

discussed in this chapter (Table 5.4). Accurate dating requires intact fragments from the corpus functionalis (not the corpus basalis or lower uterine segment), with intact surface endometrium. Dating cannot be conducted in polyps, endometrial tissue involved by chronic endometritis, endometrial hyperplasia, endometrial carcinoma, atrophy, or disordered proliferation (anovulation). Endometrial tissue is also undatable in patients with a persistent corpus luteum or exogenous hormone treatment.

PHYSIOLOGIC PREMENARCHAL AND POSTMENOPAUSAL ENDOMETRIUM

Atrophy is a normal, physiologic pattern in the premenarchal and late postmenopausal years[1]. The endometrial glands in atrophy are either small and tubular (Figure 5.1) or cystically dilated (so-called "cystic atrophy"; Figure 5.2). The hallmark of atrophy is the low columnar, cuboidal, or, in some instances, flattened glandular epithelium with small, mitotically inactive nuclei (Figure 5.2). The stroma is typically

Table 5.4 Physiologic cycling endometrial tissue

What type of gland is present?

Proliferative gland (early proliferative, midproliferative, late proliferative, interval)

   Is the gland straight or coiled?

      Straight: early proliferative

      Coiled: midproliferative, late proliferative, interval

   Is there stromal edema?

      Yes: midproliferative

      No: late proliferative, interval

   Are there scattered subnuclear vacuoles present (less than 50% of the glands exhibiting uniform subnuclear vacuolization)?

      No: late proliferative

      Yes: interval, consistent with but not diagnostic of POD 1

Secretory gland, vacuolated (early secretory)

   POD 2: subnuclear vacuolization uniformly present, leading to exaggerated nuclear pseudostratification; mitotic figures frequent (over 50% of the glands exhibit uniform subnuclear vacuolization)

   POD 3: subnuclear vacuoles and nuclei uniformity aligned; scattered mitotic figures

   POD 4: vacuoles assume luminal position; mitotic figures rare

   POD 5: vacuoles infrequent; secretion in lumen of gland, non-vacuolated cells with non-vacuolated secretory appearance

Secretory gland, non-vacuolated (midsecretory, late secretory, menstrual)

   Is there normal stromal predecidualization?

      No: midsecretory

         POD 6: secretion prominent

         POD 7: beginning stromal edema

         POD 8: maximal stromal edema

      Yes: late secretory, menstrual

   Is there crumbling of the stroma?

      No: late secretory

         POD 9: spiral arteries first prominent

         POD 10: thick periarterial cuffs of predecidua

         POD 11: islands of predecidua in superficial compactum

         POD 12: beginning coalescence of islands of predecidua

         POD 13: confluence of surface islands; stromal granulocytes prominent

         POD 14: extravasation of red cells in stroma; prominence of stromal granulocytes

      Yes: menstrual

   Late menstrual: regenerative changes prominent

Abbreviation: POD, postovulatory day.

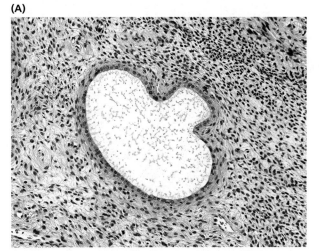

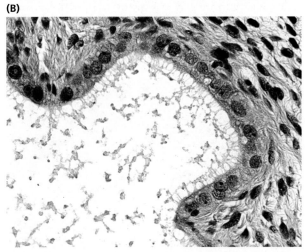

Figure 5.1 (A) Endometrial atrophy. Atrophic endometrial glands are round or only mildly irregular in contour, but may vary in size. The surrounding stroma is paucicellular and often more fibrous in comparison to proliferative phase stroma. (B) The epithelium is low columnar to cuboidal.

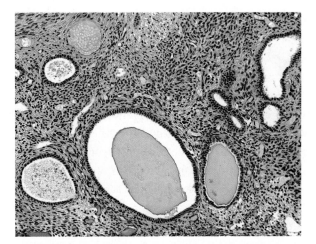

Figure 5.2 Cystic atrophy. The constituent cells are cuboidal to low columnar and mitotically inactive. Often, there is a prominence of ciliated cells.

dense and collagenized or slightly spindled, but mitotically inactive. Eosinophilic tubal-type and/or ciliated metaplasia (change) are often present in atrophic endometria. The gland-to-stroma ratio is decreased (typically ≤1). Often,

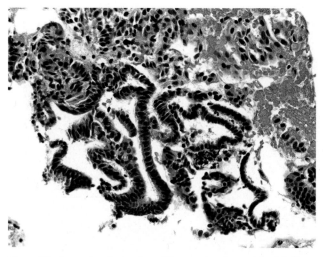

Figure 5.3 Scant, detached strips of disrupted endometrial epithelium and irregular fragments of crushed stroma are characteristic of atrophic endometrium in endometrial curettage specimens.

Table 5.5 Differential diagnosis of atrophic/weakly proliferative pattern

Atrophy	Premenarchal or postmenopausal?
Stratum basalis only	Is surface endometrium (stratum functionalis) present?
Lower uterine segment	Are there hybrid endocervical-endometrial glands present?
Thin mucosa overlying leiomyoma	Are there fragments of smooth muscle beneath endometrium?
Fragments of endometrial polyp	Are there thick-walled vessels in the atrophic fragments? Other fragments showing normal cycling endometria?
Progestin effect	Are there predecidual changes present?

(A)

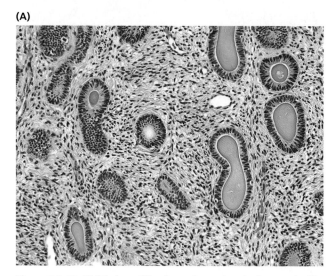

(B)

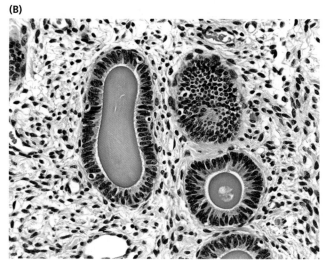

Figure 5.4 (A, B) Weak proliferative endometrium is characterized by pseudostratified columnar epithelium with rare mitotic figures.

all that is present in curettage specimens obtained from atrophic endometria is scant, detached strips of endometrial glandular epithelium with minimal supporting, partially crushed stroma (Figure 5.3). Weakly proliferative endometria differ from those that are atrophic; the cells in weakly proliferative endometrium are pseudostratified and elongated rather than cuboidal or flattened; the nuclei are more basophilic and may contain occasional mitotic figures (Figure 5.4).

Atrophic endometria are a common cause of postmenopausal bleeding, and although there is a paucity of tissue in an atrophic endometrial biopsy or curettage specimen, it is not insufficient or inadequate. In the appropriate clinical setting, the scant tissue is likely to be the only tissue present and is therefore representative of the endometrium. Often, the treating clinician will convey the clinical suspicion of

atrophy (e.g., "good scrape, but scant tissue"). By doing so, it is expected that the pathologist will interpret scant, inactive tissue as compatible with atrophy, and not as insufficient with a recommendation for re-biopsy.

However, the presence of atrophic and weakly proliferative-appearing endometrium is distinctly abnormal during the reproductive years, unless there is a history of hormonal medication or premature ovarian failure. If the pathologist is unable to assign an etiology for a scant and/or atrophic specimen in this setting, it is appropriate to make a diagnosis of "insufficient for evaluation." The differential diagnosis for endometrial tissue with an apparent atrophic or weakly proliferative pattern is provided in Table 5.5. In our experience the most common source of confusion is the presence of fragments of lower uterine segment in scant curettage specimens (Figure 5.5).

(A)

(B)

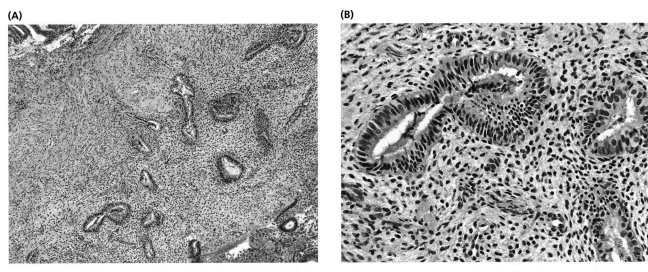

Figure 5.5 (A) Lower uterine segment may be mistaken for a possible atrophic, weakly proliferative, or disordered-proliferative endometrium. (B) Lower uterine segment is recognized by the presence of often irregular, but inactive glands set in fibrous endometrial stroma.

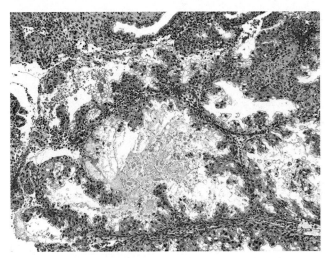

Figure 5.6 Early gestational endometrium is characterized by hypersecretory glands with cytoplasmic vacuolization and prominent intraluminal secretions.

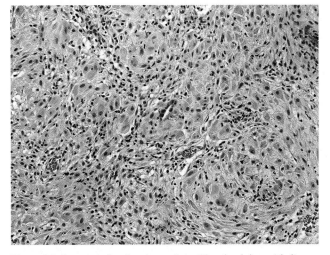

Figure 5.7 Late gestational endometrium. The glandular epithelium is less prominent and the decidua predominates.

PHYSIOLOGIC GESTATIONAL ENDOMETRIUM

The appearance of gestational endometrium varies depending on the duration of gestation. Early gestational endometria show hypersecretory glands with prominent cytoplasmic vacuolization, prominent intraluminal secretions, and prominent stromal edema (Figure 5.6). Arias-Stella change may be present (see below). The stromal cells undergo deciduation, forming large, polyhedral cells with well-defined cell membranes and central round-to-oval nuclei with inconspicuous nucleoli. Stromal granulocytes are common. In the fully developed gestational endometrium, the glandular epithelium becomes less

prominent and the decidua dominates. Sheets of decidua surround glands lined by relatively low cuboidal or flattened, indistinct epithelium (Figure 5.7). The glands may be dilated and gaping, rather than coiled. Glandular cells with inclusion-like cleared chromatin can be seen; although they resemble nuclei infected with herpesvirus, eosinophilic inclusions and nuclear molding are absent and there is no evidence that virus is present in such cells (Figure 5.8). This change may be related to intranuclear accumulation of biotin[2,3].

The changes that occur in the endometrium during gestation can also be seen in patients harboring an ectopic pregnancy, as well as in patients receiving progestogen therapy. The presence of chorionic villi, fetal parts, and/or unambiguous trophoblastic cells is required to confirm the presence of an intrauterine pregnancy.

Arias-Stella reaction

Arias-Stella reaction is characterized by the presence of hypersecretory glands lined by large cells with abundant clear-to-amphophilic and vacuolated cytoplasm and enlarged hyperchromatic nuclei with smudged chromatin (Figure 5.9)[4]. Mitotic figures are very rare. The Arias-Stella reaction may be focal; in some cases, the remainder of the endometrium may or may not exhibit a secretory reaction.

The Arias-Stella reaction may also be seen in gestational trophoblastic disease, ectopic gestation, and in association with the administration of exogenous hormones[7,8]. Rarely, there is no apparent history of endogenous or exogenous progestin. Extraendometrial sites of involvement include the cervix, fallopian tubes, and foci of endometriosis.

PHYSIOLOGIC PERIMENARCHAL AND PERIMENOPAUSAL ENDOMETRIUM

The endometrium during the perimenarchal and perimenopausal years has a characteristic disordered proliferative pattern. Disordered proliferative endometria consist of glands lined by bland, pseudostratified, mitotically active epithelium (Figure 5.10). The gland-to-stroma ratio is roughly normal, but,

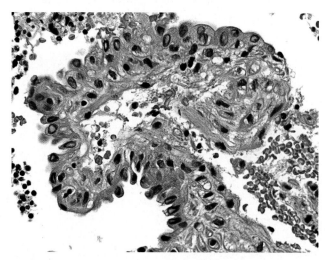

Figure 5.8 Nuclear inclusions in gestational endometrium may mimic a viral process.

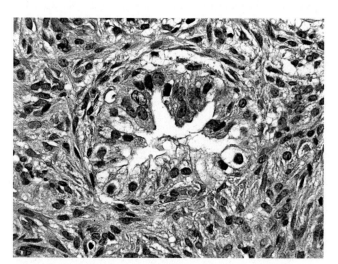

Figure 5.9 Arias-Stella reaction in endometrial polyp removed during pregnancy.

(A)

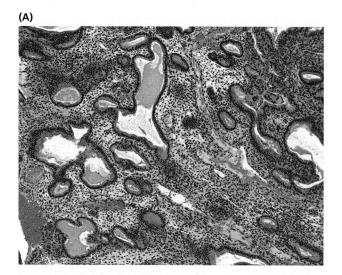

(B)

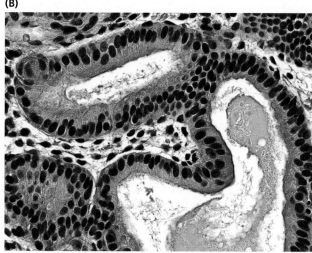

Figure 5.10 Disordered proliferative endometrium. (A) The glands assume irregular contours and are abnormally distributed, but the overall gland-to-stroma ratio is only minimally increased and does not approach the level seen in endometrial hyperplasia (gland-to-stroma ratio ≥ 3 : 1). (B) The cells are often mitotically active and pseudostratified.

endometria (Figure 5.15). Chronic breakdown may result in foci of nodular stromal hyperplasia (Figure 5.16), fibrosis or hyalinization, hemosiderin deposits, or xanthoma cells, and may feature foci of secondary chronic endometritis.

When pronounced, the glands may be artifactually crowded, simulating hyperplasia; alternatively, the stroma may be artifactually cellular, simulating stromal sarcoma (Figure 5.17). Attention to the nuclear debris, fibrin thrombi, and other features of breakdown often provides the correct diagnosis, but there are occasional cases in which the changes are so pronounced that a neoplastic process cannot be confidently excluded. In these cases, correlation with clinical and imaging studies and a request for additional sampling is in order.

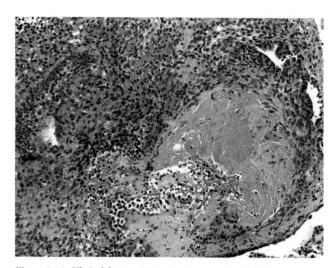

Figure 5.15 Fibrin lakes are common in estrogen-related dysfunctional uterine bleeding and stromal breakdown.

(A) (B)

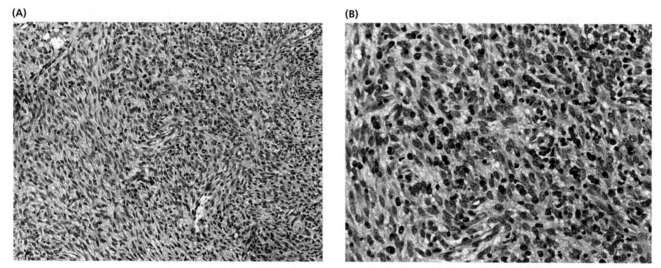

Figure 5.16 (A, B) Prominent stromal cellularity in this example of chronic endometritis is secondary to intrauterine device.

(A) (B)

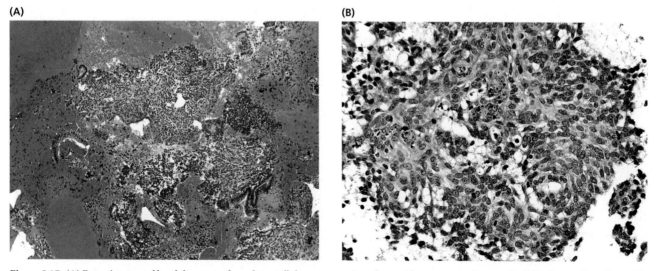

Figure 5.17 (A) Extensive stromal breakdown may form dense cellular aggregates in endometrial curettage specimens, mimicking low-grade endometrial stromal sarcoma. (B) Careful attention to the presence of apoptotic debris and other evidence of breakdown resolves most diagnostic problems.

Extensive stromal breakdown is not limited to dysfunctional uterine bleeding; it occurs in a variety of conditions and may well mask a variety of specific benign conditions (polyp, leiomyoma, endometritis). However, it does not appear to pose a significant risk for concealing a malignant condition.

MISCELLANEOUS PATTERNS

Stromal decidual reaction

A stromal decidual reaction is typically encountered during pregnancy or exogenous hormonal therapy, but can be seen in women with no apparent (at least to the pathologist) history of pregnancy or hormonal exposure. It is also encountered in women with dysfunctional uterine bleeding who have been treated with a trial (or two) of progestin prior to evaluation.

Stromal decidual reaction may be associated with stromal and glandular breakdown; the glands may be secretory (gestational type), inactive, or atrophic. In the atrophic pattern, the decidua assumes a more compact, cellular appearance with plump, ovoid cells and indistinct cell borders, which if gland-poor may simulate an endometrial stromal neoplasm (Figure 5.18). The latter is excluded on the basis of clinical correlation – absence of a mass lesion, history of hormonal exposure, etc. – or if necessary, additional evaluation.

In other instances, the tissue may be abundant, forming large polypoid structures, and the constituent glands may be dilated and inactive or exhibit only mild secretory activity (Figure 5.19). When stromal mitotic figures are

also present, the overall appearance may suggest a possible adenofibroma or adenosarcoma. The absence of multiple epithelial types and the history of progestin therapy are important clues to the correct diagnosis.

Decidua can take on a number of other secondary alterations, including signet ring-type change, coalescent granulomatous-type change, edematous or myxoid change, and endometritis-type change (Figure 5.20).

Exogenous hormone effects

Most endometria exhibiting signs of exogenous hormone effect are secondary to oral contraceptive use or one form or another of progestin therapy. The specific morphologic effects depend on the baseline status of the underlying

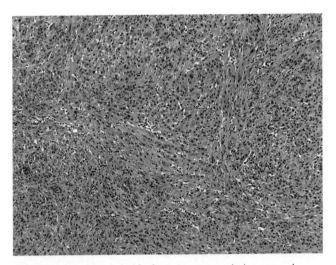

Figure 5.19 Exuberant decidual response may mimic a stromal neoplasm.

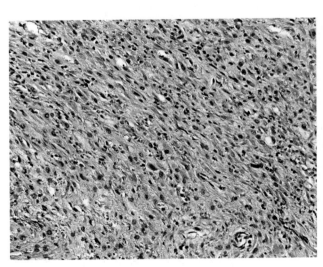

Figure 5.18 Atrophic pattern of decidual response.

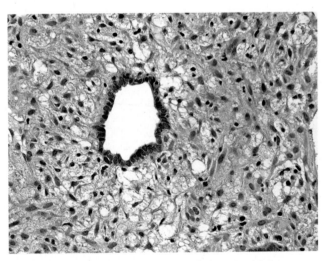

Figure 5.20 Decidua may undergo a spindled or myxoid change, which may mimic a mesenchymal neoplasm.

endometrium, the type and dose of exogenous hormone, and the duration of exposure. They range from the predominantly decidual pattern previously described, to abnormal secretory or even atrophic gland patterns. The abnormal secretory pattern typically consists of poorly developed secretory-type glands set in predeciduated stroma (dyssynchrony between glands and stroma) (Figure 5.21). While the more atrophic gland pattern consists of small, inactive glands with small cytoplasmic vacuoles surrounded by abundant spindled cell stroma; areas of edematous or myxoid stromal change may also be seen in this pattern (Figure 5.22).

Combined estrogen and progestin replacement therapy usually shows atrophic or weak proliferative endometrium; a superimposed weak progestin effect may also be present in the constituent glands. Effects of specific hormonal agents on endometrial tissue are summarized in Table 5.11.

Tamoxifen is a selective estrogen receptor modulator (SERM) with anti-estrogenic effects on breast epithelia but partial estrogenic effects on endometrial epithelia. A variety of uterine effects have been attributed to tamoxifen exposure, and most women who are on long-term tamoxifen therapy are evaluated periodically to detect possible abnormal endometrial proliferation(s). The relative risk of developing endometrial carcinoma in this setting is still poorly defined. However, in contrast to unopposed estrogen therapy, a relative increased risk of developing high-grade carcinomas and sarcomas has been observed with tamoxifen therapy. In general, any patient on tamoxifen with abnormal bleeding or an abnormal endometrial stripe on ultrasound is evaluated by biopsy or curettage. The most common finding in our experience is atrophy, followed by mucinous metaplasia, and/or polyps featuring mucinous or secretory-type metaplastic change (Figure 5.23).

Focal gland atypia

In some cases of exogenous hormone therapy, an Arias-Stella-type reaction can be seen. A less recognized pattern of glandular atypia consists of a peculiar, more focal reaction, characterized by nuclear enlargement with nuclear hyperchromasia, which in some cases may even harbor rare mitotic figures (Figure 5.24). The constituent cells in this latter reaction typically have eosinophilic or amphophilic cytoplasm with or without small cytoplasmic vacuoles; hobnail cells may also be seen. The clue to their correct

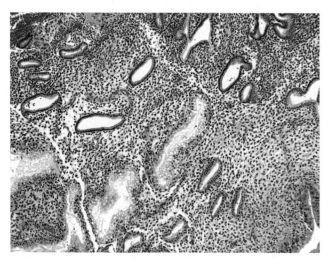

Figure 5.21 Abnormal secretory pattern is characterized by poorly developed secretory glands set in a predeciduated stroma.

(A)

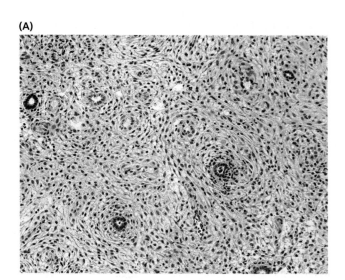

(B)

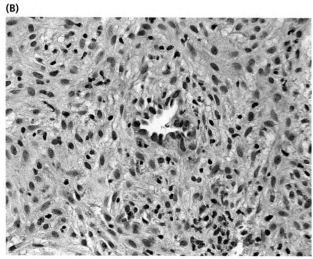

Figure 5.22 (A, B) Atrophic secretory pattern. Atrophic glands are scattered throughout a prominent predeciduated stroma.

Table 5.11 Exogenous hormonal effects on endometrial tissue

Hormonal agent	Mode of action	Major use(s)	Major morphologic effect on endometrium
Estrogen	Proliferation	Control menopausal symptoms	Proliferative or disordered proliferative endometrium, with or without breakdown; hyperplasia; metaplasia; carcinoma (two to three years unopposed estrogen)
Progestin	Suppress ovulation and endometrial proliferation; secretory maturation	Dysfunctional uterine bleeding; contraception; medical treatment of hyperplasia and low-grade carcinoma	Stromal decidual pattern with or without breakdown (see text for full description)
Combined estrogen–progestin	Proliferation and secretory maturation	Oral contraception; hormone replacement therapy	Under-developed proliferative or secretory pattern, depending on phase of cycle if sequential; atrophic endometrium if combined
Tamoxifen	Selective estrogen receptor modulator (antagonist in breast; weak agonist in endometrium)	Breast cancer	Mucinous metaplasia; mucinous polyps; other metaplasia; hyperplasia; carcinoma; sarcoma
Raloxifene	Selective estrogen receptor modulator (antagonist in breast; no agonist effect in endometrium)	Breast cancer	Atrophy
Clomifene	Anti-estrogen	Infertility	Variable: secretory phase may be normal or appear diminished in number and caliber of glands, secretory activity, and stromal predeciduation
Danazol	Weak progestin effect	Endometriosis; hyperplasia	Atrophic glands with vacuolated cells
Gonadotropins	LH and FSH effects	Infertility	Variable: normal glandular development or glandular and stromal dyssynchrony
Gonadotropin-releasing hormone agonists	Gonadotropin-releasing hormone effects	Oocyte retrieval and in vitro fertilization; suppression of endometrium before ablation; decrease leiomyomas before surgical resection	Weak proliferative, inactive, or atrophic endometrium
Progesterone receptor modulators	Progesterone receptor antagonist	Contraception; treatment of endometriosis and leiomyomas	Atrophic or inactive endometrium; glandular secretions; glandular and stroma dyssynchrony; cystic glands; ciliated cells

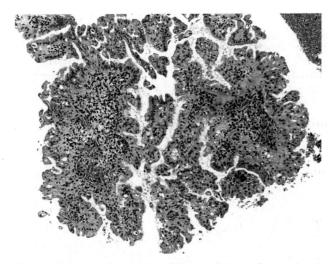

Figure 5.23 Mucinous and eosinophilic metaplasia may be prominent following tamoxifen treatment.

diagnosis is the focal nature of the process; the atypical glands are typically set amidst benign inactive glands. The presence of a decidual stromal reaction provides additional evidence of a hormone-mediated effect, but this may not always be present.

ENDOMETRIAL METAPLASIA

Endometrial metaplasia denotes the presence of epithelial cell differentiation not ordinarily identified in endometrial cells, or ordinarily identified in only a minority of normal endometrial cells (e.g., ciliated cells) (Table 5.12). The term metaplasia is used because it is thought that the etiology of many of these cellular alterations is due to metaplasia,

Table 5.12 Classification of endometrial metaplasia

Type	Description
Ciliated (tubal)	Low columnar, cuboidal, or pear-shaped cells with cilia; cytoplasm often eosinophilic, but may be basophilic; nuclei are round with small nucleoli
Clear cell	Cytoplasmic clearing (not due to glycogen or mucin); cytoplasm may be foamy
Eosinophilic	Columnar or cuboidal epithelium with abundant eosinophilic cytoplasm, round nuclei, and fine chromatin; may have nucleoli
Hobnail	Non-stratified, low columnar epithelium with hobnail pattern; round nuclei, fine chromatin
Mucinous	Intracellular mucin; may be endocervical like or microglandular hyperplasia like
Oxyphilic	Abundant, granular eosinophilic cytoplasm; nuclei are uniform, round, and regular
Papillary syncytial	Syncytia of eosinophilic cells forming small papillae; nuclei often dark and pyknotic; apoptosis; common pattern in stromal breakdown (may be reparative or degenerative)
Squamous (morular) metaplasia	Keratinizing or non-keratinizing; sheets of elongate or rounded (morular pattern) spindled cells; may have central necrosis

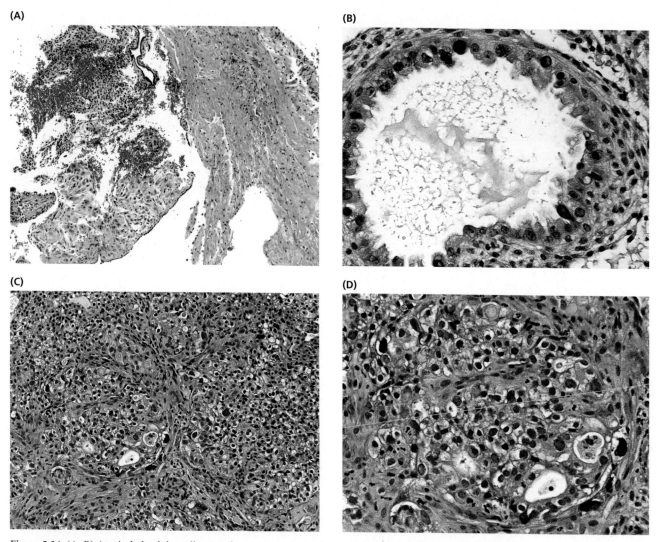

Figure 5.24 (A, B) Atypical glandular cells secondary to exogenous hormonal therapy may also be seen in association with intrauterine devices. (C, D) Mirena intrauterine device with focal Arias-Stella reaction.

but some changes may be hormone induced, reactive, or degenerative[10]. This may lead to differences in terminology (i.e., "metaplasia" versus "change" versus "differentiation"). In clinical practice, the nomenclature is not important; instead, it is most important to be able to distinguish whether the alterations represent a benign or malignant process[11].

Squamous metaplasia (Figures 5.25–5.27) and ciliated cell (tubal) metaplasia or change (Figure 5.28) are seen most commonly, although eosinophilic and oxyphilic

(Figure 5.29), papillary syncytial (Figure 5.30), papillary (Figure 5.31), mucinous (Figure 5.32), and clear cell or hobnail cell (Figure 5.33) changes also occur. Although each of these cellular types is individually identified, mixed patterns of metaplasia are very common (Figure 5.34).

Metaplasia can be seen in non-hyperplastic, hyperplastic, and malignant endometrial glands. Polyps often harbor metaplastic cells, particularly ciliated and mucinous types. Classification of the underlying glandular process is based on gland density, gland architecture, and the presence/degree of cytologic atypia; not on the presence/type of cellular metaplasia. In some instances, metaplastic cells may normally exhibit mild atypia (e.g., ciliated cells may

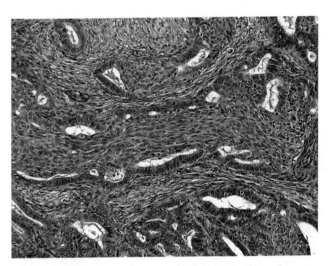

Figure 5.25 Squamous metaplasia typically takes the form of a spindled morular proliferation within the lumen of the endometrial glands. It can be seen (rarely) in atrophic endometrium, in disordered proliferative endometrium, in endometrial hyperplasia, and in carcinoma. It can be confused with squamous proliferations of the uterine cervix; this confusion is compounded by expression of p16 in endometrial squamous epithelium (see Figure 3.47).

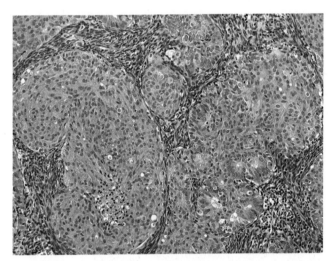

Figure 5.26 Extensive morular metaplasia fills the glands to the extent that their outer contours are essentially obliterated, imparting the appearance of infiltration into the adjacent stroma.

(A)

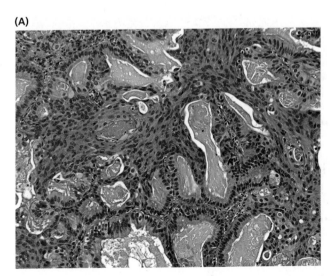

(B)

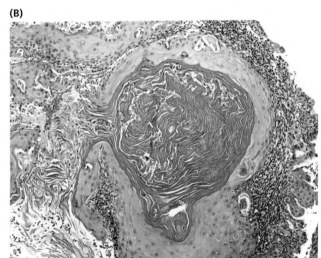

Figure 5.27 Squamous metaplasia may exhibit (A) focal or (B) prominent keratinization.

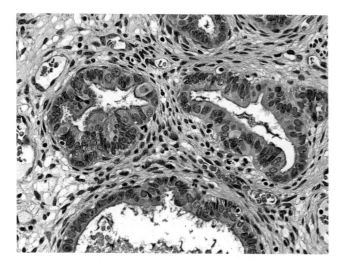

Figure 5.28 Ciliated cells are present in normal endometrium, but increase under estrogenic stimulation. The terms "ciliated cell change" or "ciliated cell prominence" have been proposed, since their presence does not strictly qualify as a metaplastic process.

have nucleoli), and this must be taken into account when making an assessment of the overall glandular process.

Squamous metaplasia can form immature morules or fully keratinizing and glycogenated squamous cells (Figures 5.25–5.27). The morular form may exhibit a spindled appearance that can be mistaken for a malignant process if not properly recognized. Squamous metaplasia can be seen in disordered proliferative and other non-hyperplastic endometrial proliferations, and should not be considered "hyperplastic" or "atypical" in absence of the glandular and cytologic changes required for these diagnoses.

Ciliated cells normally occur in the endometrium, but are considered "metaplastic" when present in more pronounced numbers; alternative designations are ciliated prominence and ciliated (tubal) cell change. Most ciliated metaplasia is non-stratified, but some ciliated metaplasia

(A)   **(B)**

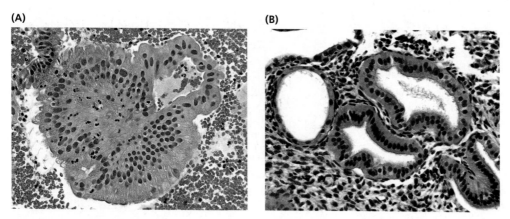

Figure 5.29 (A) Eosinophilic cell metaplasia. (B) Eosinophilic "oxyphilic" metaplasia. Note slightly enlarged nuclei and small nucleoli, and granular cytoplasm.

(A)   **(B)**

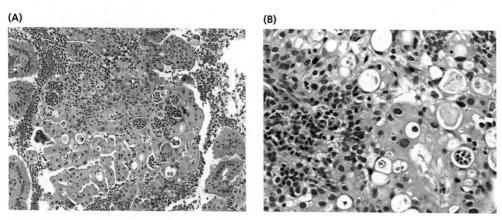

Figure 5.30 (A) Papillary syncytial metaplasia. (B) The nuclei may be hyperchromatic, but the chromatin is smudged.

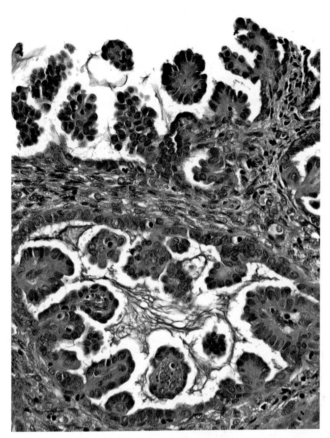

Figure 5.31 Prominent papillary change can mimic hyperplasia and, on occasion, carcinoma. The cytoplasm in papillary change is often eosinophilic, and the cytologic features are bland.

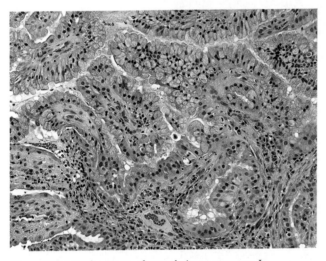

Figure 5.34 Mixed patterns of metaplasia are common. In this example, mucinous, ciliated cell, and eosinophilic cell changes are present. Here, the metaplastic gland exhibits complex architecture, but the overall gland-to-stroma ratio is not increased.

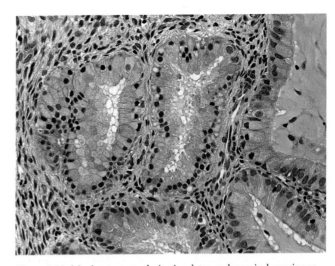

Figure 5.32 Mucinous metaplasia simulates endocervical mucinous epithelial cells and can be mistaken for an endocervical process (and vice versa). A key that the lesion may be endometrial is the presence of other types of metaplasia: typically eosinophilic cell metaplasia (not depicted here).

(A)

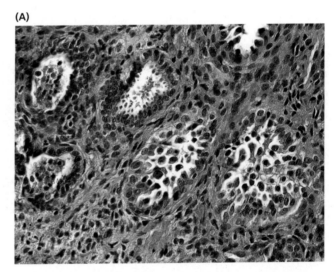

(B)

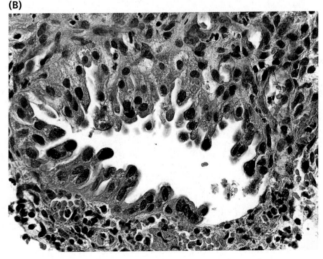

Figure 5.33 (A, B) Hobnail change in benign endometrium.

may appear more complex with a stratified, cribriform, or pseudopapillary pattern (Figure 5.28). Nucleoli are often present in ciliated cells, and this does not signify cytologic atypia. In absence of changes required for a diagnosis of hyperplasia, the pathologist should simply diagnose the lesion as ciliated metaplasia or ciliated change.

Eosinophilic (pink cell) metaplasia often merges with ciliated and/or mucinous metaplasia (Figure 5.29). When the cytoplasm is granular, eosinophilic metaplasia is considered oncocytic[12]. The nuclei may be enlarged, but the chromatin is fine in eosinophilic metaplasia.

Papillary syncytial metaplasia is common (Figure 5.30). When it is seen in association with stromal and glandular breakdown, it has been referred to as syncytial papillary change[10], but it can also be seen in association with hyperplasia and carcinoma (usually FIGO grade 1 or 2). In the latter two settings, the metaplastic epithelium is usually most pronounced along the surface endometrium, but may also involve deep glands. It is common for the metaplastic cells in papillary syncytial metaplasia to merge with mucinous and squamous cells.

True papillary metaplasia (Figure 5.31) is less common, but often raises concern for serous carcinoma. However, the papillae are small and are lined by cells with minimal atypia. The chromatin may appear dark, since most cases of papillary metaplasia appear to be mitotically inactive. Also, the disheveled appearance of many examples of serous carcinoma is absent in papillary metaplasia.

Mucinous metaplasia can be simple or complex (Figure 5.32). Papillary and microglandular patterns are commonly seen in polyps and hyperplastic endometrium. The individual cells are usually columnar with basal nuclei and pale, endocervical-type mucinous cytoplasm. Goblet cells may also be seen in mucinous metaplasia, but are far less common. Mucinous metaplasia is often seen in association with eosinophilic metaplasia (Figure 5.34).

Hobnail change is uncommon, but can be disconcerting when present in benign endometrial tissue (Figure 5.33). The nuclei in benign hobnail change are small, but often hyperchromatic, imparting a smudged appearance. Mitotic figures may be present, but marked atypia is absent. Hobnail change is distinguished from clear cell carcinoma and serous carcinoma with hobnail cells on the basis of focality (hobnail change is often discrete and focal or multifocal, but not diffuse) and absence of significant cytologic atypia or other features of clear cell carcinoma. Other forms of metaplasia are listed in Table 5.12.

POLYPS

Although polyps are included in the discussion of this chapter, they are considered benign neoplasms. Clonal abnormalities have been identified in the mesenchyme of usual endometrial polyps, as well as several karyotypic abnormalities involving chromosomes 6 and 12. Usual endometrial polyps vary considerably in size, are often single, but may be multiple, and occur over a wide age range. They are recognized microscopically on the basis of their polypoid shape, dense stroma, and presence of thick-walled arteries and disordered glands (Figure 5.35). Larger polyp fragments exhibit surface epithelium over three sides, which may be eroded or overlay collections of small, ectatic thin-walled veins. Surface infarction or complete hemorrhagic infarction secondary to torsion may

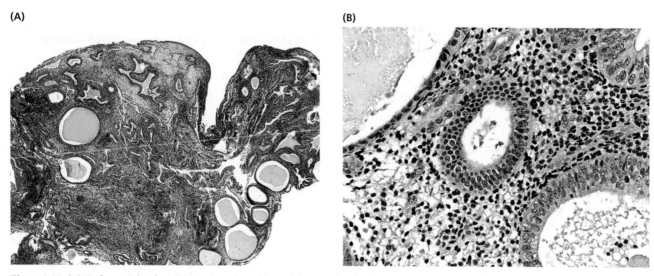

(A) **(B)**

Figure 5.35 (A) Endometrial polyp. (B) Cystic and weakly proliferative glands often harbor ciliated cells in endometrial polyps.

(A)

(B)

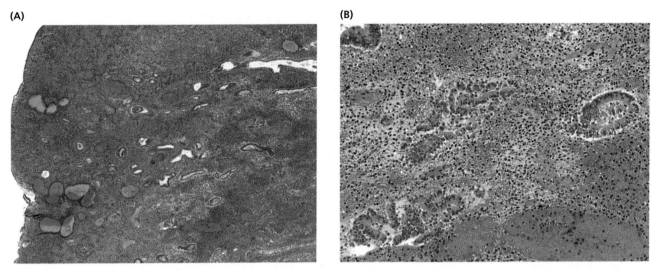

Figure 5.36 (A) Endometrial polyp with extensive hemorrhage secondary to torsion. (B) Disintegrating glands may exhibit cytologic and/or cytoplasmic changes that may pose concern for a neoplastic process.

(A)

(B)

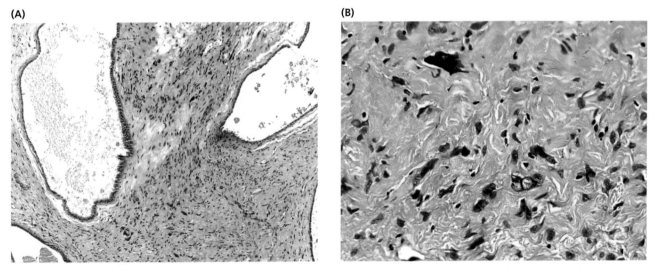

Figure 5.37 (A, B) Endometrial polyps may contain atypical stromal cells similar to those seen in fibroepithelial polyps.

also be present (Figure 5.36). The glands are typically irregular in contour, resembling disordered proliferative glands; ciliated cells or eosinophilic cell change may be present. Atrophic (endometrial glands and stroma are atrophic), functional (secretory or proliferative glands), mixed (endometrial and endocervical glands), and adenomyomatous (see *Polypoid adenomyoma* and *Atypical polypoid adenomyoma* below) variants can be seen. Occasionally, the glands are dilated, but large and irregular cystic structures with polypoid intrusions are uncommon and should prompt consideration for adenofibroma or adenosarcoma (see Chapter 11).

Most endometrial polyps are easily recognized, but a variety of alterations may occur in otherwise benign polyps that can pose diagnostic problems. The most common alterations

include (1) increased mitotic figures (up to 5 mitotic figures per 10 high-power fields [5 MF/10 HPF]); (2) atrophic and/or degenerative changes; (3) hobnail, eosinophilic, or clear cell metaplastic changes; (4) prominent stromal cellularity or stromal atrophy; (5) a non-specific plasmacellular infiltrate; and (6) bizarre stromal cell atypia (Figure 5.37).

On occasion, atrophic or degenerative changes in postmenopausal endometrial polyps can masquerade as endometrial intraepithelial carcinoma; absence of strong p53 expression and, typically, a paucity of mitotic figures may aid in this distinction; but in some instances uncertainty remains after full evaluation of one of these problematic endometrial samplings (Figure 5.38). Often, re-sampling resolves the problem, avoiding an unnecessary surgical procedure.

(A)

(B)

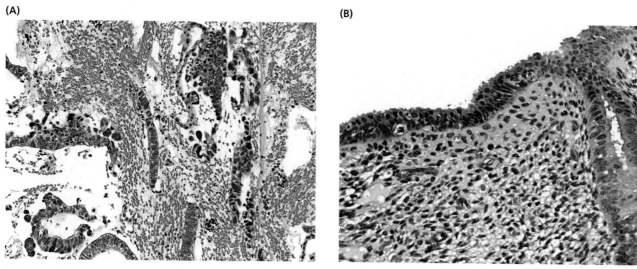

Figure 5.38 (A) Endometrial polyps may undergo degenerative changes, which may result in (B) abnormal epithelium in curettage specimens.

(A)

(B)

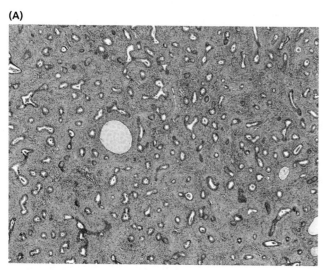
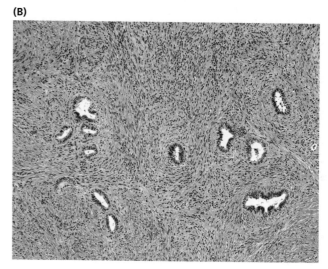

Figure 5.39 (A, B) Polypoid adenomyoma.

All polyps should be submitted in their entirety for microscopic examination, since approximately 1–2% may harbor a malignancy.

POLYPOID ADENOMYOMA

Polypoid adenomyomas or adenomyo*fibro*mas (PAs) are circumscribed aggregates of fibromuscular tissue containing small, architecturally simple glands without branching or budding[13]. The constituent cells are cytologically bland (Figure 5.39). Morules may be present, but they are usually not prominent, and endometrial stroma may be present. Polypoid adenomyomas uncommonly present as an exophytic polypoid growth and are thought to represent endometrial polyps or submucosal leiomyomas until they are examined

histologically. These lesions are benign. They usually do not pose a significant diagnostic problem unless they are confused with the atypical polypoid adenomyoma.

ATYPICAL POLYPOID ADENOMYOMA[1]

Atypical polypoid adenomyomas or adenomyo*fibro*mas (APAs) are distinctive endometrial lesions that closely mimic hyperplasia or adenocarcinoma[14]. They are characterized by a localized, polypoid endometrial proliferation

---

[1] Although APA is included in the non-neoplastic chapter, it is probably a benign neoplastic process. Certainly, the APA-LMP (atypical polypoid adenomyoma of low malignant potential) appears to represent a low-grade neoplasm.

(A)

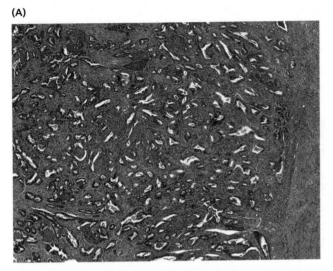

(B)

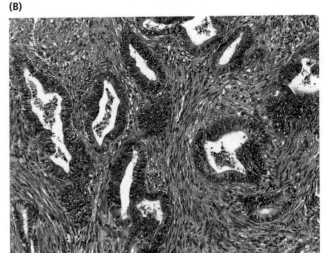

Figure 5.40 (A, B) Atypical polypoid adenomyoma.

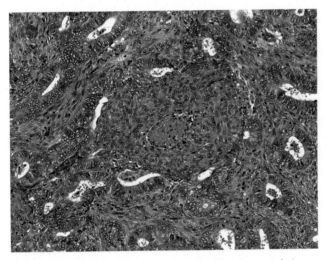

Figure 5.41 Atypical polypoid adenomyoma. Morular metaplasia is typically prominent and may serve as a clue to the diagnosis in a curettage specimen.

with architecturally complex glands set in a stroma composed of smooth muscle or, more commonly, smooth muscle and fibrous tissue (Figure 5.40). Trichrome stain often confirms the impression of a mixture of spindled smooth muscle cells and collagen. In most cases stromal mitotic figures do not exceed 2 per 10 HPF, but focal increased stromal mitotic figures (3–5 MF/10 HPF) may occasionally be present. Morular and/or squamous metaplasia are present in most cases and are often florid (Figure 5.41). Keratinization and necrosis within the areas of squamous metaplasia are common. The endometrial samplings typically consist of large fragments or chunks of tissue. Most of the samplings also contain smaller admixed, but separate fragments of normal proliferative phase or secretory phase endometrium imparting a low-power dimorphic appearance.

Most atypical polypoid adenomyomas occur in premenopausal or perimenopausal women, with a mean age of about 40 years. Many of the patients are nulliparous, and a clinical history of infertility is not uncommon. Atypical polypoid adenomyomas may occur in women with Turner syndrome. The hysteroscopic appearance is usually that of a polypoid mass within the uterine fundus or lower uterine segment. Occasionally, more than one polyp is present. These lesions can recur locally, but do not have metastatic potential. Approximately one-third of patients managed with local excision develop recurrent disease, often over the course of several years[15]. Some patients experience multiple recurrences. The histology of the recurrent or persistent atypical polypoid adenomyoma usually resembles that of the initial atypical polypoid adenomyoma; however some recurrences develop increasingly complex glandular architecture. Reproductive conservation utilizing procedures short of hysterectomy is warranted for the conventional atypical polypoid adenomyoma, since affected patients may have successful pregnancies even with recurrent lesions[15]. Such patients require clinical follow-up because of the risk for recurrence and, in some cases, progression.

A subset of atypical polypoid adenomyomas contain glands that are sufficiently complex to satisfy the criteria for well-differentiated carcinoma (Figure 5.42), and we have designated them as APA-LMP inasmuch as they appear to be capable of locally aggressive, infiltrative behavior and rarely demonstrate evidence of malignant behavior (i.e., extrauterine disease or metastasis)[15]. Such tumors have been reported in the literature as invasive, well-differentiated adenocarcinoma arising in atypical polypoid adenomyoma,

(A)

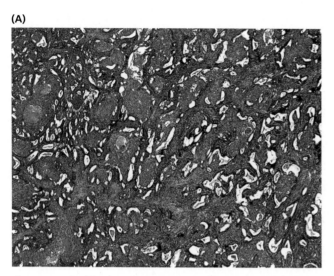

(B)

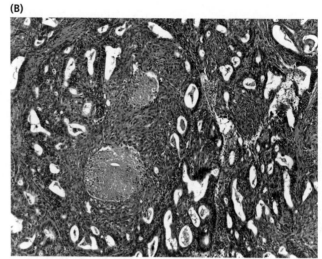

Figure 5.42 (A, B) Atypical polypoid adenomyoma may contain marked glandular complexity similar to that which occurs in low-grade endometrioid adenocarcinoma. When this occurs, the lesion is designated as atypical polypoid adenomyoma with low malignant potential (APA-LMP), as these polyps may occasionally invade the myometrium. Some gynecologic pathologists classify these polyps as carcinoma arising in an atypical polypoid adenomyoma, but since there have never been any reports of spread beyond the uterus, we think this diagnosis is inaccurate.

but we are aware of only one case where disease progression occurred beyond the uterus. In contrast, no atypical polypoid adenomyoma without marked architectural complexity has demonstrated convincing myoinvasion. The incidence of recurrence after local excision of the atypical polypoid adenomyoma of low malignant potential is higher than that for the atypical polypoid adenomyoma (60% versus 33%), but these lesions do not otherwise significantly differ with respect to clinical, histologic or immunohistologic features.

The distinction between atypical polypoid adenomyoma and myoinvasive carcinoma in an endometrial sampling is best accomplished on the basis of a cluster of clinicopathologic features that include patient age, hysteroscopic or microscopic evidence of a focal process, the presence of a biphasic glandular and fibromuscular stromal proliferation, absence of severe cytologic atypia, and a low architectural complexity[15]. Whereas most atypical polypoid adenomyomas and atypical polypoid adenomyomas of low malignant potential contain separate fragments of benign proliferative or secretory endometrium elsewhere in the endometrial sampling, most myoinvasive adenocarcinomas contain separate fragments of adenocarcinoma that are unassociated with the myoinvasive fragments elsewhere in the endometrial sampling.

ADENOMYOSIS

Endometrial tissue (glands and stroma) is considered ectopic in the uterus if it is present on the uterine serosa

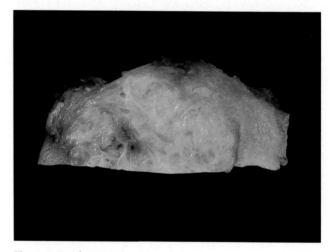

Figure 5.43 Adenomyosis.

(endometriosis) or if it is located "excessively" deep in the myometrium. In well-developed cases, the uterus is grossly abnormal. When it is focal, adenomyosis mimics a leiomyoma in being a roughly spheric, intramural lesion, but it differs from leiomyoma in that the mass cannot be shelled out easily from the surrounding uninvolved myometrium; an important point for infertility surgeons. When involvement is diffuse, the uterus is enlarged in a "globoid" fashion. The cut surface is coarsely trabecular, often with visible microcysts (Figure 5.43). At the microscopic level, foci of basalis-type endometrial glands and stroma are delimited by hypertrophied bands of smooth muscle (Figure 5.44).

The glands in adenomyosis may undergo the same alterations that the glands in the overlying endometrium

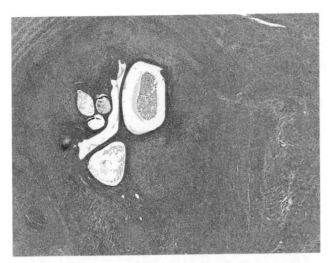

Figure 5.44 Adenomyosis. Well-circumscribed glands set in stroma are surrounded by concentric smooth muscle in the myometrium.

(A)

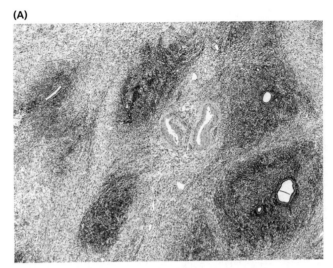

(B)

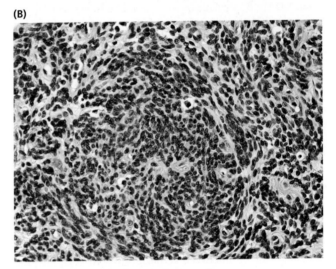

Figure 5.45 (A, B) Gland-poor adenomyosis.

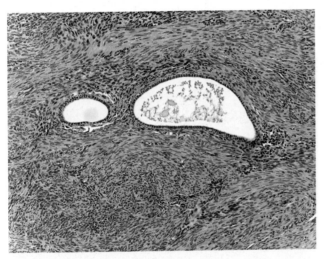

Figure 5.46 Stroma-poor adenomyosis.

undergo, including atrophy, metaplasia, hyperplasia, and carcinoma. Atrophic changes may result in gland-poor adenomyosis (Figure 5.45), or stroma-poor adenomyosis (Figure 5.46).

Gland-poor adenomyosis (adenomyosis with sparse glands) has the characteristic zonal phenomenon of usual adenomyosis, with an atrophic or attenuated cuff of smooth muscle hypertrophy surrounding a focus of endo-metrial stroma depleted of glands. The nuclei in this context are small and atrophic (Figure 5.45). In contrast, stroma-poor adenomyosis features naked glands set within the myometrium, with minimal surrounding stroma (Figure 5.46). The finding of areas of preserved stroma and more-typical areas of adenomyosis aids in the distinction from an invasive, very well-differentiated adenocarcinoma.

ENDOMETRITIS

Endometritis may be acute or chronic. Most endometritis is chronic, but acute, suppurative endometritis can be seen in the postpartum or postabortion period due to secondary infection[9].

Acute endometritis

Acute endometritis is infrequent, but has a striking micro-scopic appearance. It is almost always limited to the post-partum or postabortion setting (peurperal sepsis), but could conceivably occur post-instrumentation. The endo-metrial stromal and glandular tissue is extensively replaced by neutrophils, often with necrosis and microabscess for-mation; in the endometrial biopsy or curettage specimen,

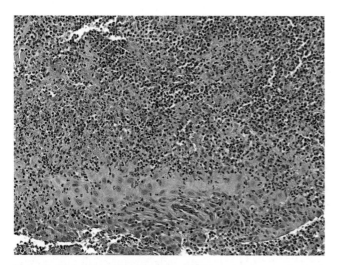

Figure 5.47 Acute suppurative endometritis.

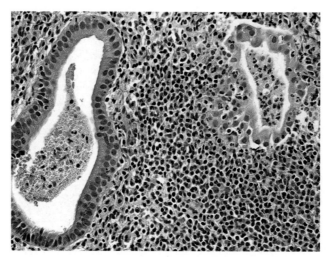

Figure 5.48 Chronic endometritis. Plasma cells are numerous.

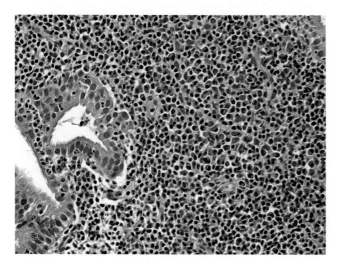

Figure 5.49 Chronic endometritis.

there is also extensive stromal and glandular breakdown (Figure 5.47). Granulation tissue may be present in severe cases. Distinction from menstrual endometrium or stromal breakdown secondary to dysfunctional uterine bleeding is based on the pronounced acute, suppurative inflammatory cell process, and the clinical setting.

Chronic endometritis

The definition and histologic diagnostic criteria for chronic endometritis have undergone a series of revisions in the last decade. While the identification of even a single plasma cell was once considered sufficient evidence to diagnose chronic endometritis, current standard of practice mandates the presence of more numerous and easily identifiable plasma cells before rendering a diagnosis of chronic endometritis (Figure 5.48). This rule is especially true in

absence of other clinical or pathologic features associated with the inflammatory process[18]. Although the plasma cell continues to be the sine qua non of chronic endometritis, most cases of bona fide chronic endometritis also show (1) increased numbers of lymphocytes with lymphoid follicles, and (2) variable numbers of histocytes, eosinophils and neutrophils (Figure 5.49). In addition: (3) the stroma is reactive with elongated spindle cells, (4) neutrophils often sprinkle the surface epithelium, and there is (5) altered gland development, with (6) stromal and glandular breakdown[9]. Plasma cells may be focal and scattered, or diffusely permeate the endometrial stroma. They tend to aggregate in the subepithelial and periglandular regions and may also be detected in the vicinity of lymphoid follicles. The intensity of plasma cell infiltrate does not necessarily correlate with severity of inflammation. In addition to stromal atypia, the glandular epithelium is also atypical. These reactive changes include: cytoplasmic eosinophilia, cellular stratification, nuclear enlargement, chromatin clearing, nucleoli, and mitotic figures.

The presence of prominent lymphoid aggregates may simulate lymphoma (so-called lymphoma-like lesion), but the absence of a mass lesion and the presence of reactive germinal centers within the aggregates, and a mixed inflammatory cell infiltrate with plasma cells elsewhere in the endometrium, distinguish lymphoma-like lesion from true lymphoma. Because monoclonal *IGH* gene rearrangements have been detected by polymerase chain reaction methods in some lymphoma-like lesions, caution should be exercised in the evaluation of these specimens. Correlation of all clinical, histologic, and ancillary studies is required to prevent misdiagnosis[19,20].

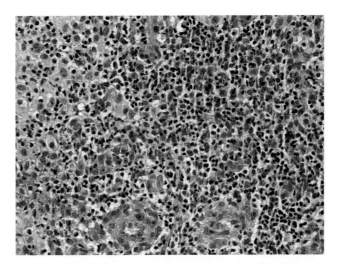

Figure 5.50 Deciduated tissue in dysfunctional uterine bleeding with focal plasma cell aggregates. The significance of this finding is uncertain in this setting, but it likely represents breakdown-associated changes.

Disordered proliferative endometria, persistent proliferative endometria with breakdown, and a variety of endometria from women with dysfunctional uterine bleeding and focal stromal breakdown may contain occasional plasma cells in absence of any evidence of clinical infection (Figure 5.50)[18]. Whether these patients harbor a subclinical and undetected infection is currently pure conjecture; therefore, in absence of additional clinical or histologic evidence of infection, a definitive diagnosis of endometritis should be avoided in these cases. A comment in the body of the report noting the presence of occasional plasma cells, the significance of which is uncertain (given the absence of other findings), is sufficient. Sometimes it can be difficult to discriminate between extensive stromal breakdown with low levels of plasma cells, and chronic endometritis with stromal breakdown; in those instances a diagnosis of "extensive stromal breakdown" with a comment suggesting the possibility of chronic endometritis is warranted. Because of the difficulty in distinguishing endometrial stromal cells from bona fide plasma cells, use of CD138 (syndecan-1) has been advocated by some authors, but we do not routinely use this marker for that purpose.

Specific infections

Most infections do not have a specific histologic correlate. However, in some cases the etiology is apparent (i.e., retained products of conception). In others, the pattern of inflammation may suggest one or another diagnosis.

Chlamydia trachomatis has been associated with a diffuse, often marked inflammatory infiltrate consisting of plasma cells, lymphocytes with prominent reactive lymphoid follicles, and macrophages. However, this pattern of inflammation is not specific, and milder degrees of inflammation can be seen in polymerase chain reaction-proven cases of chlamydial endometritis.

Actinomyces israeli endometritis occurs in association with the use of an intrauterine device. The inflammation is a dense mix of plasma cells, lymphocytes, and neutrophils. Characteristic sulfur granules need to be distinguished from pseudoactinomycotic radiate granules. Actinomycotic granules are positive on gram and silver stains; while pseudoactinomycotic radiate granules are not.

Mycoplasma has been associated with a predominantly lymphocytic and histiocytic inflammatory infiltrate; plasma cells tend to be rare in this infection. The lymphocytes form loose aggregates beneath the surface epithelium and around glands and vessels, and can be difficult to distinguish from normal lymphoid infiltrates.

The cervix is a more common site for viral infection, but severe cervical infections may extend to involve the endometrium. Cytomegalovirus forms characteristic intranuclear and intracytoplasmic inclusions in endothelial cells and in the glandular epithelium. Herpes virus also exhibits characteristic ground-glass inclusions; however, non-viral nuclear-inclusion-like changes can also be seen in a variety of non-infectious endometrial processes, including trophoblasts, Arias-Stella reaction, squamous metaplastic cells, and exogenous hormone therapy.

Granulomatous inflammation is seen in *Mycobacterium tuberculosis* and fungal infections. Both are rare in the United States, but *Mycobacterium tuberculosis* endometritis is a significant contributor to endometritis in regions where there is a higher rate of infection. Well-formed granulomas may not be present if the endometrium is evaluated during the proliferative or early secretory phase of the menstrual cycle (Figure 5.51). Acid fast and/or Fite stains are rarely positive; tissue culture is required. In the United States, prior ablation therapy or other possible iatrogenic causes should be considered, as these are more common causes for granulomatous inflammation of the endometrium. Rarely, sarcoid may involve the uterus.

The differential diagnosis of endometritis includes: (1) stromal granular lymphocytes in secretory or gestational endometrium; (2) collections of neutrophils in stroma secondary to tissue necrosis; (3) neutrophils in gland lumens secondary to entrapment of cellular debris; (4) luminal histiocytes secondary to mucin secretions or cervical stenosis; and (5) tissue eosinophils in leiomyomas or secondary to curettage or other procedure; (6) mast cells in polyps, leiomyomas, and endometrial hyperplasia; and (7) histiocytes in normal myometrium and leiomyomas. Finally (8) inflamed cervical tissue often contains a marked plasmacellular infiltrate; this finding does not indicate the presence of chronic endometritis.

Xanthogranulomatous endometritis

This condition typically occurs in postmenopausal women as a result of cervical stenosis (Figure 5.52). A prior history of radiation therapy may be present[21]. The endometrium is replaced by numerous histiocytes with abundant foamy

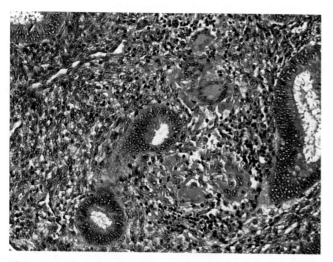

Figure 5.51 Tuberculous endometritis. Endometrial granulomas in tuberculosis are poorly formed and may not show characteristic necrosis.

or eosinophilic, granular cytoplasm; admixed neutrophils, plasma cells, lymphocytes, and hemosiderin-laden histiocytes are also present[22]. There may be necrosis, cholesterol clefts, and dystrophic calcification. Extension to involve the myometrium may be seen. The inflammatory process is typically sterile, but secondary bacterial infection can occur. The differential diagnosis includes malakoplakia, and changes secondary to ablation therapy. Malokoplakia is diagnosed on the basis of identification of the characteristic Michaelis–Gutmann bodies and intracellular bacilli[23].

POST-CURETTAGE CHANGES

The surface and superficial glandular epithelium may show marked atypia following a curettage procedure. The involved cells typically take on a more pronounced cytoplasmic eosinophilia, with hobnail contour. The nuclei are enlarged and hyperchromatic, and nucleoli are often prominent. Mitotic figures and apoptosis may also be present. The clinical history of a prior procedure and the presence of edema and inflammation (which may be neutrophilic, histiocytic, and/or eosinophilic) in the adjacent stroma are helpful diagnostic cues. Stromal hemosiderin or hemosiderin-laden stromal cells and/or histiocytes are additional clues, if present. Also, there is typically a discontinuous involvement of the endometrium by this repair process (Figure 5.53). Although this last feature is best appreciated in a hysterectomy specimen, focal involvement may also be detected in an endometrial sampling specimen.

(A)

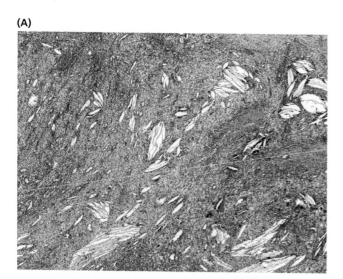

(B)

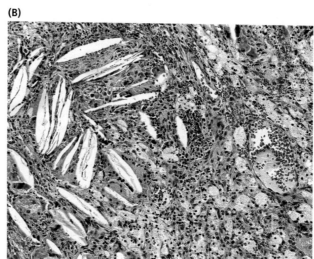

Figure 5.52 (A, B) Xanthogranulomatous endometritis.

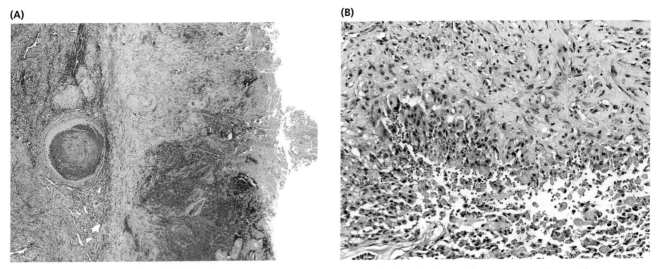

Figure 5.53 Post-curettage changes. (A) Florid endometrial hemorrhage and vascular thrombosis secondary to recent endometrial curettage. (B) Organizing fibrosis and foreign-body-type reaction due to endometrial curettage.

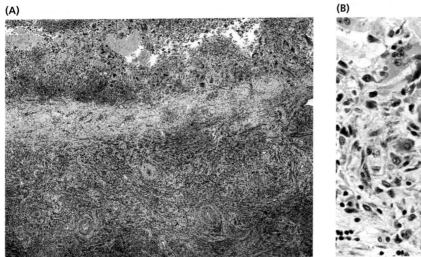

Figure 5.54 (A, B) Endometrial ablation secondary to roller ball.

ABLATION

Depending on the type of ablation procedure and the post-ablation interval, a variety of changes may be seen in the endometrium and superficial myometrium[24]. In the initial month, there is full-thickness endometrial necrosis, followed by a chronic repair–regeneration phase. Foreign body giant cells and other remnants of the ablation may persist for several years (Figure 5.54). Intracavitary balloon thermal ablation may show loss of nuclei and increased cytoplasmic eosinophilia early; later changes may consist of gland-poor, fibrous-appearing endometrial stroma (Figure 5.55). Other forms of thermal ablation therapy may result in a necrotizing granulomatous inflammatory response, often associated

with a foreign body giant cell reaction[25]. Refractile hematoidin pigment or black carbon pigment is also seen.

RADIATION

Radiation changes in the uterus may be visible grossly (Figure 5.56A) or only on microscopic examination (Figure 5.56B). Grossly, the uterus may be small and fibrotic or large, globoid, and fibrotic (Figure 5.56A). Microscopic changes in the endometrial surface and glandular epithelium consist of low-power cytoplasmic eosinophilia and nuclear hyperchromasia[26]. The nuclei vary in size and shape, and hobnail cells can be seen (Figure 5.56B). However, the nuclear chromatin has

(A)

(B)

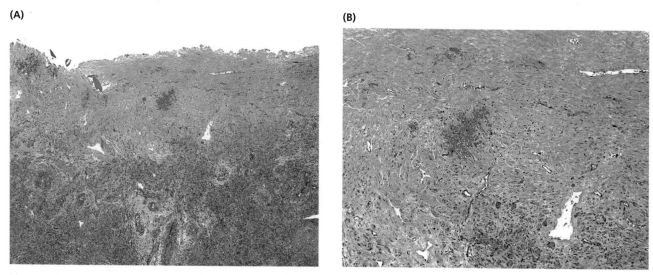

Figure 5.55 (A, B) Endometrial ablation secondary to thermal balloon procedure.

(B)

(A)

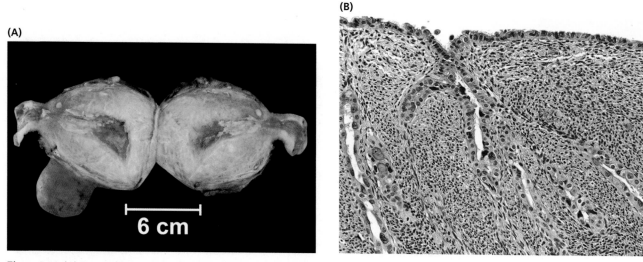

Figure 5.56 (A) Post-radiation uterus is markedly fibrotic. (B) Gland atypia in the post-radiated uterus.

a smudged appearance, and mitotic figures are typically absent. Cytoplasmic vacuolization may be seen, but is neither required nor diagnostic of radiation change. The affected glands are not crowded, but are rather widely spaced and set in a more fibrous-appearing stroma. Stromal fibroblast atypia is often also present. The vasculature may also show ectasia and thickening. In some instances, a xanthogranulomatous reaction may be seen, but, in our experience, this change is more commonly seen in association with chemotherapy.

MYOMETRIAL XANTHOMATOSIS

This recently described condition is characterized by extensive infiltration of the myometrium by foamy histiocytes, in absence of other inflammatory cells (Figure 5.57)[27].

Endometritis is absent. Myometrial xanthomatosis is an incidental finding in reproductive-aged women. A documented history of cesarean section in two cases points to a possible inciting event for this phenomenon, but suture material or refractile foreign body material is absent, and there is no granulomatous component to the foam cell infiltrate.

HETEROTOPIAS

Ectopic bone, fat, cartilage, and glia can be seen in the uterus (Figure 5.58)[28]. The most common site of involvement is the endometrium, followed by the cervix and myometrium. Possible etiologies include implantation of fetal tissue during spontaneous or therapeutic abortion, metaplasia, dystrophy, or true heterotopia. The presence

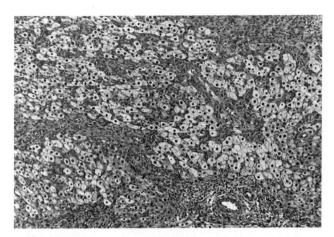

Figure 5.57 Myometrial xanthomatosis.

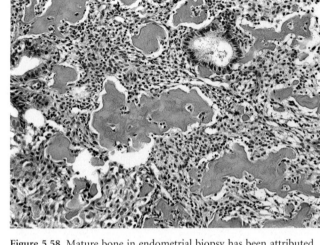

Figure 5.58 Mature bone in endometrial biopsy has been attributed to retained fetal parts as well as osseous metaplasia, perhaps due to inflammation.

(A)

(B)

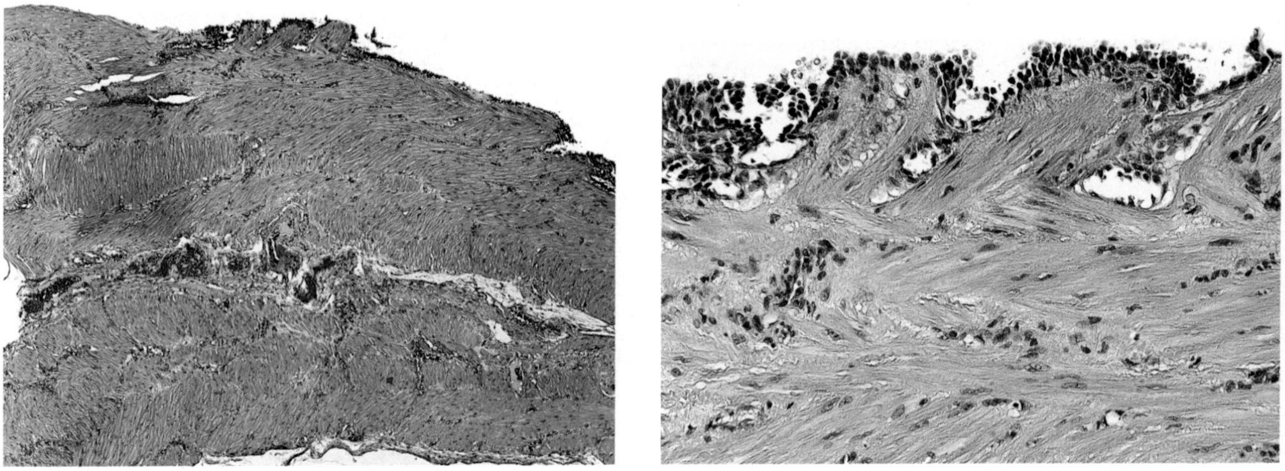

Figure 5.59 (A, B) Mullerian cyst in uterine corpus.

of fat in an endometrial sampling should also prompt consideration for possible uterine perforation.

EXTRAMEDULLARY HEMATOPOIESIS

Extramedullary hematopoiesis is rarely encountered in the endometrium or myometrium[31]. Some, but not all cases have had an associated hematologic disorder. Recent pregnancy with retained products of conception has also been attributed to this finding.

CONGENITAL ABNORMALITIES

A variety of congenital abnormalities occur in the uterus, including atresia, aplasia, and mullerian duct fusion defects. Most patients present with obstetric difficulties. Rarely, patients present with a uterine or pelvic mass lesion due to congenital myometrial cyst[32]. The congenital myometrial cyst may be mullerian or mesonephric. The more common mullerian cyst is located within the midline anterior or posterior wall, and is lined by a single layer of endometrioid, ciliated or mucinous (endocervical-type) columnar cells (Figure 5.59), while the mesonephric cyst is lateral and lined by non-ciliated, non-mucinous columnar or cuboidal epithelium. The cysts are unilocular and surrounded by myometrium; they vary in size, but can be quite large, measuring up to 12 cm. By definition, no communication with the endocervix or endometrium should be present. The differential diagnosis is adenomyosis with a prominent cystic component (presence of stromal elements) or hydrosalpinx of intramural tube (characteristic location and predominant tubal-type epithelium).

REFERENCES

1. Longacre TA, Atkins KA, Kempson RL, *et al.* The uterine corpus. In: Sternberg S, Mills S, eds. *Diagnostic Surgical Pathology.* New York: Raven Press; 2009:2184–277.

2. Mazur MT, Hendrickson MR, Kempson RL. Optically clear nuclei. An alteration of endometrial epithelium in the presence of trophoblast. *Am J Surg Pathol* 1983;**7**:415–23.

3. Yokoyama S, Kashima K, Inoue S, *et al.* Biotin-containing intranuclear inclusions in endometrial glands during gestation and puerperium. *Am J Clin Pathol* 1993;**99**:13–17.

4. Arias-Stella J. Gestational endometrium. In: Hertig A, Norris H, Abell M, eds. *The Uterus.* Baltimore: Williams & Wilkins; 1973: 185–212.

5. Arias-Stella J. The Arias-Stella reaction: facts and fancies four decades after. *Adv Anat Pathol* 2002;**9**:12–23.

6. Arias-Stella J, Jr., Arias-Velasquez A, Arias-Stella J. Normal and abnormal mitoses in the atypical endometrial change associated with chorionic tissue effect [corrected]. *Am J Surg Pathol* 1994;**18**: 694–701.

7. Clement PB, Young RH, Scully RE. Nontrophoblastic pathology of the female genital tract and peritoneum associated with pregnancy. *Semin Diagn Pathol* 1989;**6**:372–406.

8. Huettner PC, Gersell DJ. Arias-Stella reaction in nonpregnant women: a clinicopathologic study of nine cases. *Int J Gynecol Pathol* 1994;**13**:241–7.

9. Mazur MT, Kurman RJ. *Diagnosis of Endometrial Biopsies and Curettings: A Practical Approach.* New York: Springer-Verlag; 2005.

10. Zaman SS, Mazur MT. Endometrial papillary syncytial change. A nonspecific alteration associated with active breakdown. *Am J Clin Pathol* 1993;**99**:741–5.

11. Hendrickson MR, Kempson RL. Endometrial epithelial metaplasias: proliferations frequently misdiagnosed as adenocarcinoma. Report of 89 cases and proposed classification. *Am J Surg Pathol* 1980;**4**:525–42.

12. Silver SA, Cheung AN, Tavassoli FA. Oncocytic metaplasia and carcinoma of the endometrium: an immunohistochemical and ultrastructural study. *Int J Gynecol Pathol* 1999;**18**:12–19.

13. Gilks CB, Clement PB, Hart WR, *et al.* Uterine adenomyomas excluding atypical polypoid adenomyomas and adenomyomas of endocervical type: a clinicopathologic study of 30 cases of an underemphasized lesion that may cause diagnostic problems with brief consideration of adenomyomas of other female genital tract sites. *Int J Gynecol Pathol* 2000;**19**:195–205.

14. Clement P, Young R. Atypical polypoid adenomyoma of the uterus associated with Turner's syndrome. A report of three cases, including a review of "estrogen-associated" endometrial neoplasms and neoplasms associated with Turner's syndrome. *Int J Gynecol Pathol* 1987;**6**:104–13.

15. Longacre TA, Chung MH, Rouse RV, *et al.* Atypical polypoid adenomyofibromas (atypical polypoid adenomyomas) of the uterus. A clinicopathologic study of 55 cases. *Am J Surg Pathol* 1996; **20**:1–20.

16. Mazur M. Atypical polypoid adenomyomas of the endometrium. *Am J Surg Pathol* 1981;**5**:473–82.

17. Young R, Treger T, Scully R. Atypical polypoid adenomyoma of the uterus. A report of 27 cases. *Am J Clin Pathol* 1986;**86**:139–45.

18. Gilmore H, Fleischhacker D, Hecht JL. Diagnosis of chronic endometritis in biopsies with stromal breakdown. *Hum Pathol* 2007;**38**:581–4.

19. Geyer JT, Ferry JA, Harris NL, *et al.* Florid reactive lymphoid hyperplasia of the lower female genital tract (lymphoma-like lesion): a benign condition that frequently harbors clonal immunoglobulin heavy chain gene rearrangements. *Am J Surg Pathol* 2010; **34**:161–8.

20. Young R, Harris N, Scully R. Lymphoma-like lesions of the lower female genital tract: a report of 16 cases. *Int J Gynecol Pathol* 1985;**4**:289–99.

21. Russack V, Lammers R. Xanthogranulomatous endometritis. Report of six cases and a proposed mechanism of development. *Arch Pathol Lab Med* 1990;**114**:929–32.

22. Ladefoged C, Lorentzen M. Xanthogranulomatous inflammation of the female genital tract. *Histopathology* 1988;**13**:541–51.

23. Kawai K, Fukuda K, Tsuchiyama H. Malacoplakia of the endometrium. An unusual case studied by electron microscopy and a review of the literature. *Acta Pathol Jpn* 1988;**38**:531–40.

24. Davis JR, Maynard KK, Brainard CP, *et al.* Effects of thermal endometrial ablation. Clinicopathologic correlations. *Am J Clin Pathol* 1998;**109**:96–100.

25. Colgan TJ, Shah R, Leyland N. Post-hysteroscopic ablation reaction: a histopathologic study of the effects of electrosurgical ablation. *Int J Gynecol Pathol* 1999;**18**:325–31.

26. Silverberg SG, DeGiorgi LS. Histopathologic analysis of preoperative radiation therapy in endometrial carcinoma. *Am J Obstet Gynecol* 1974;**119**:698–704.

27. DiMaio M, Longacre TA. Myometrial xanthomatosis: possible relationship to prior pregnancy procedure. *Int J Gynecol Path* 2012; in press.

28. Nogales FF, Pavcovich M, Medina MT, *et al.* Fatty change in the endometrium. *Histopathology* 1992;**20**:362–3.

29. Roca A, Guajardo M, Estrada W. Glial polyp of the cervix and endometrium. Report of a case and review of the literature. *Am J Clin Pathol* 1980;**73**:718–20.

30. Tyagi SP, Saxena K, Rizvi R, *et al.* Foetal remnants in the uterus and their relation to other uterine heterotopia. *Histopathology* 1979; **3**:339–45.

31. Valeri RM, Ibrahim N, Sheaff MT. Extramedullary hematopoiesis in the endometrium. *Int J Gynecol Pathol* 2002;**21**:178–81.

32. Sherrick J, Vega J. Congenital intramural cysts of the uterus. *Obstet Gynecol* 1962;**19**:486–93.

6 ENDOMETRIAL CARCINOMA PRECURSORS: HYPERPLASIA AND ENDOMETRIAL INTRAEPITHELIAL NEOPLASIA

INTRODUCTION

There are currently three major classification systems for low-grade endometrial carcinoma precursor lesions, each of which tend to overlap at the more complex end of the spectrum (Diagram 6.1). While the endometrial intra-epithelial neoplasia (EIN) classification is based on a series of molecular genetic alterations (which may or may not translate into biologically or clinically relevant risk lesions), each classification scheme ultimately utilizes a series of histologic features, usually a combination of architecture and cytology to establish a diagnosis. Obviously, different pathologists may apply different histologic criteria to diagnose an endometrial cancer precursor lesion, depending on the classification system used, and this may result in different thresholds for diagnosing these risk lesions; that is, some proliferations may be deemed to be at risk for progression to carcinoma in one scheme, but not in another. Fortunately, these discrepant cases are a minority and most "at risk" endometrial glandular proliferations are similarly classified by all three classification schemes. The similarities and discordance are highlighted in Diagram 6.1.

The most commonly utilized classification system for endometrial hyperplasia was outlined by the WHO in 1994 (Table 6.1). The classification criteria for this system are based on the 1985 study by Kurman and colleagues[1]. This study, which demonstrated a 23% risk of progression to carcinoma for atypical endometrial hyperplasia compared to only 2% for non-atypical hyperplasia, informs the rationale for separating atypical hyperplasia from non-atypical hyperplasia. In this system, hyperplasia is further subdivided into "simple" and "complex" based on architectural features; although this has less bearing on prognosis than the presence or absence of atypia, most atypical endometrial hyperplasias are also complex. Subsequent reports have buttressed the findings of Kurman et al., with some suggesting an even higher progression rate of 20–30%[2]. The four categories of endometrial hyperplasia recognized by the WHO classification schema are: (1) simple hyperplasia without atypia; (2) complex hyperplasia without atypia; (3) simple atypical hyperplasia; and (4) complex atypical hyperplasia. The WHO classification system has proven clinically useful and is the most widely used endometrial precancer scheme in the United States. However, it is imprecise and suffers from significant inter-observer variability due to its reliance on cytology, which is notoriously subjective[3].

An alternative precancer classification scheme is the EIN system[4,5]. The molecular foundation of this system rests on a series of meticulous studies characterizing the expression of phosphatase and tensin homolog (PTEN) in endometrial glands[6,7]. Loss of phosphatase and tensin homolog expression initially appeared to be closely correlated with future development of endometrioid adenocarcinoma;

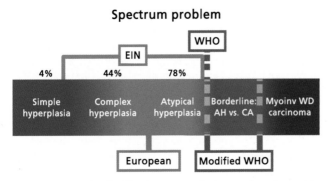

Diagram 6.1 Major classification systems for low-grade endometrial carcinoma precursor lesions. Abbreviations: myoinv WD carcinoma, myoinvasive well-differentiated carcinoma; AH, atypical hyperplasia; CA, carcinoma.

Table 6.1 Low-grade endometrial cancer precursor lesions: World Health Organization classification system

Simple hyperplasia without atypia
Complex hyperplasia without atypia
Simple hyperplasia with atypia
Complex hyperplasia with atypia

Table 6.2 Low-grade endometrial cancer precursor lesions: endometrial intraepithelial neoplasia (EIN) classification system

Benign hyperplasia
Endometrial intraepithelial neoplasia

Table 6.3 Low-grade endometrial cancer precursor lesions: European classification system

Endometrial hyperplasia
Endometrial neoplasia

however subsequent studies have shown a less direct correlation with progression to malignancy[8,9]. In practice, the criteria for diagnosis of endometrial intraepithelial neoplasia are not entirely dissimilar from those used in the WHO system, and center primarily around the relative proportions of tissue occupied by glands and stroma (Table 6.2). In the EIN system this is quantified as a "volume percentage stroma" (VPS) score, and a cutoff of <55% is used for the diagnosis of a precancer lesion (designated as endometrial intraepithelial neoplasia as opposed to endometrial hyperplasia with atypia). Such foci must measure over 1 mm[4,5].

Although the WHO and EIN systems both recognize the importance of glandular density in predicting progression, the EIN system is less reliant on cytologic atypia. This leads to a slight discordance between the types of cases labeled as high risk by these two classification systems. Approximately 4% of glandular proliferations classified as simple hyperplasia without atypia and 44% of glandular proliferations classified as complex hyperplasia without atypia are classified as endometrial intraepithelial neoplasia, while 78% of glandular proliferations classified as atypical hyperplasia are classified as endometrial intraepithelial neoplasia, with most of the remaining atypical hyperplasia classified as carcinoma using the EIN system[4,5,10]. However, when compared head to head, the two classification systems show similar diagnostic reproducibility and a similar ability to predict the development of carcinoma[11,12]. Thus, while the PTEN story provides insight into the molecular pathway(s) associated with low-grade endometrial adenocarcinoma, a more precise identification of precursor lesions in the clinical setting remains elusive.

To improve on diagnostic reproducibility of the WHO classification, Bergeron and colleagues suggested a simplified classification of hyperplasia and endometrial neoplasia, whereby hyperplasia consisted of simple and complex hyperplastic glandular proliferations, and neoplasia consisted of atypical hyperplasia and well-differentiated adenocarcinoma[13]. Using this scheme, glandular crowding is the chief criterion for diagnosing

hyperplasia, and nuclear pleomorphism is the chief criterion for endometrioid neoplasia, although nuclear enlargement, vesicular chromatin, and nucleoli are additional features. Although preliminary studies suggested that the diagnoses of hyperplasia and endometrioid neoplasia were highly reproducible when this classification scheme was employed, this system has not been widely adopted (Table 6.3).

In our practice, the WHO system is used in the evaluation of endometrial precancer lesions; this system is preferred because (1) there is more experience with this system, both for the pathologists as well as the treating physicians in our centers; and (2) some of the lesions classified as endometrial intraepithelial neoplasia do not, in our experience, pose the same level of risk as do other endometrial intraepithelial neoplasia and atypical hyperplastic lesions. However, in the spirit of full disclosure, both systems are presented in the following discussion.

CLINICAL CHARACTERISTICS

Morphology

Gross pathology

The endometrial curettage may be voluminous. In addition, the uterine cavity may be expanded by the hyperplastic endometria. Pseudopolyps are not uncommon, and occasionally true polyps are also present. Hemorrhage and, rarely, necrosis may be present; the necrosis is generally secondary to polypoid areas of hyperplastic tissue that become torsed or overgrow their blood supply. However, extensive necrosis in a biopsy sample should be viewed with caution, and a full curettage should be considered to exclude a more severe lesion.

Although hyperplasia is considered a diffuse process, focal endometrial hyperplasia may be seen in some hysterectomy specimens (Figure 6.1). This may translate into an apparent focal hyperplastic process in an endometrial sampling. Provided the sampling is adequate and contains sufficient intact tissue to make an assessment of the overall gland-to-stroma ratio, "focal endometrial hyperplasia" is

(A)

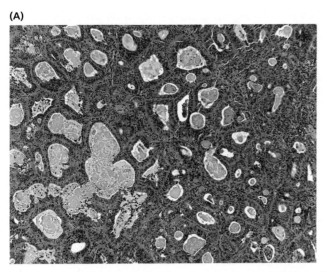

(B)

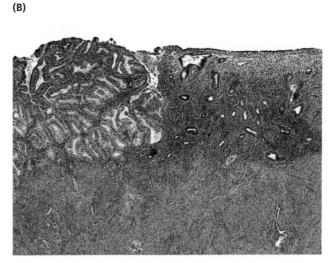

Figure 6.1 (A) Endometrial hyperplasia most commonly exhibits gland crowding, with a resultant gland-to-stroma ratio of 3 : 1 or more. This feature of hyperplasia is best detected on low magnification. In this example, the hyperplastic glands exhibit extensive mucinous metaplasia. (B) Although it is generally considered to be a diffuse process, hyperplasia may be a discrete focal lesion.

a reasonable diagnosis. The significance of focal hyperplasia (as opposed to the more common diffuse process) has not been well studied.

Microscopic pathology

ENDOMETRIAL HYPERPLASIA

Endometrial hyperplasia is typically a response to estrogen stimulation unchecked by progesterone. It is important to emphasize that endometrial hyperplasia is not considered to be a precursor lesion for all histologic subtypes of endometrial carcinoma; high-grade serous carcinoma appears to be largely estrogen independent. Given its association with hormonal imbalance, it is not surprising that endometrial hyperplasia is most often encountered around or following menopause, although premenopausal women with sclerocystic ovaries and/or obesity are also at increased risk. In the perimenopausal setting, estrogen excess may be due to either exogenous hormone replacement therapy or endogenous factors, such as anovulation. Obesity contributes to estrogen excess through conversion of androgens into estrogen within adipose tissue. Tamoxifen therapy may also contribute to increased risk of hyperplasia. Most women with endometrial hyperplasia present with abnormal uterine bleeding. Endometrial hyperplasia forms a continuum of morphologic appearances, with the earliest proliferation represented by crowded glands with simple tubular architecture composed of cells resembling proliferative endometrium; while advanced proliferations in this continuum are characterized by crowded glands with complex architecture,

often containing cells with nuclear atypia resembling low-grade endometrioid adenocarcinoma.

While it is generally accepted that endometrial hyperplasia represents a risk factor for the development of adenocarcinoma, the degree of perceived risk and the preferred treatment varies depending on the clinical setting. In postmenopausal women, hysterectomy is often appropriate even for low-risk lesions; while in younger women who wish to maintain fertility, less invasive therapies are often initially employed, even when the diagnostic considerations also include low-grade endometrioid adenocarcinoma.

Endometrial hyperplasia may be grossly unremarkable, but typically manifests as an increased endometrial stripe on transvaginal ultrasound, and increased volume of endometrial tissue on hysteroscopy and/or curettage. Although hyperplasia may be associated with high endometrial tissue volume, the increase in bulk is typically no more impressive than is observed in normal secretory phase endometrium; the appearance is that of the diffuse, somewhat polypoid, tan, velvety tissue that is characteristic of normal, secretory endometrium. In some instances, localized hyperplasia may mimic a polyp or in fact arise in a polyp. Hyperplasia may also involve adenomyosis, including deep (outer one-half of myometrium) foci.

Endometrial hyperplasia is morphologically defined as proliferating endometrium with architectural abnormalities. These architectural changes range from cystic dilatation to more complex configurations, including glandular budding and branching, papillary infoldings, exophytic villous and villoglandular growths, and cribriform structures. In addition to abnormal architecture, a diagnosis of hyperplasia usually requires an increased glandular density with a gland-to-stroma ratio of ~3 : 1 (Figure 6.1)[14]. Some authors propose a lower gland-to-stroma ratio (>2 : 1), but there is often overlap with artifactual compression of glands in curettage specimens at this level. Luminal spaces and villoglandular structures are both included in the glandular component for this calculation. If the gland-to-stroma ratio fails to meet the required

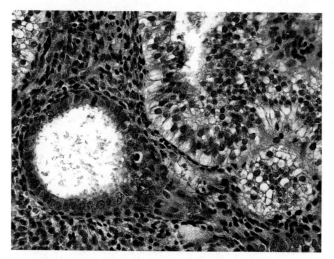

Figure 6.2 Endometrial hyperplastic proliferations generally feature enlarged cells (relative to the uninvolved normal endometrium, if present) with enlarged nuclei and nuclear pseudostratification. Mitotic figures are typically present, although not depicted in this image. Benign mimics (e.g., florid secretory or gestational endometrium) can be excluded by evaluating suspected hyperplastic proliferations on higher magnification.

cutoff, a lesion is probably best classified as disordered proliferative endometrium rather than hyperplasia. In most instances, the constituent cells are larger than those of normal endometrium and exhibit proliferative features including nuclear pseudostratification and increased mitotic figures (Figure 6.2); in the absence of these latter features, an endometrial metaplastic process should be considered.

While hyperplastic endometria may have cytologic atypia, this criterion is neither required nor sufficient for the diagnosis. The assessment of atypia is poorly reproducible, but the various criteria include nuclear rounding and enlargement, nuclear pleomorphism, loss of polarity, increased nuclear-to-cytoplasm ratios, prominent nucleoli, irregular nuclear borders, vesicular chromatin, and clumped chromatin. Atypical cells may show tufting and focal stratification, although extensive nuclear stratification merits a diagnosis of malignancy. Hyperplastic endometria with cytologic atypia are considered to pose a more significant risk for endometrial adenocarcinoma than hyperplastic endometria without atypia[1,12].

Although the morphologic features of hyperplasia usually occur in concert with increased overall volume when compared to the background endometrial tissue, in rare instances the architectural criteria for hyperplasia are satisfied in the absence of any increased tissue volume. Isolated foci of hyperplasia may also be identified in a background of otherwise unremarkable endometrium; this has been referred to as "focal hyperplasia," and while the significance of this is uncertain there is evidence to suggest that the risk of coincident myoinvasive carcincoma is very low[15].

Hyperplasic endometria often contain areas of metaplasia and a variety of secondary changes (Figure 6.1A, 6.3, 6.4).

(A)

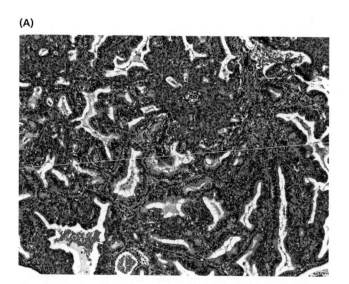

(B)

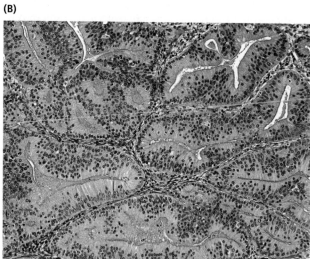

Figure 6.3 (A) Endometrial hyperplasia with morular metaplasia. (B) Endometrial hyperplasia with ciliated (pink cell) metaplasia.

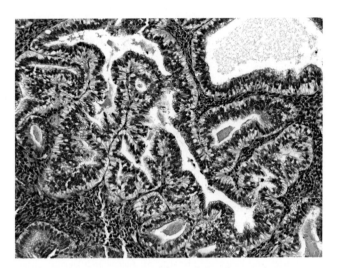

Figure 6.4 Secretory endometrial hyperplasia. The constituent glands exhibit diffuse subnuclear vacuolization.

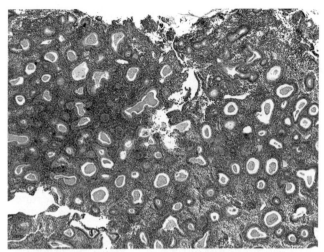

Figure 6.5 Simple hyperplasia consists of minimally branched, closely packed glands with gland-to-stroma ratio of 3 : 1.

Squamous metaplasia, in particular, can be extensive, filling and expanding hyperplastic glands (Figure 6.3). This feature can emphasize the crowded appearance of the lesion. Importantly, the presence and extent of metaplasia has no bearing on prognosis of endometrial hyperplasia and should be ignored when assessing for associated carcinoma.

Simple hyperplasia without atypia

Simple hyperplasia is characterized by densely packed, cystically dilated glands of variable size, separated by normal intervening stroma (Figure 6.5). While the glandular patterns in simple hyperplasia may be similar to what is observed in disordered proliferative endometria, the latter fails to meet the 3 : 1 gland-to-stroma ratio. Ciliated cells are often quite prominent in simple hyperplasia; squamous morular metaplasia may also occur.

Simple hyperplasia is distinguished from cystic atrophy and clusters of normally occurring weakly proliferative or inactive glands based on cytologic features: the cells in hyperplasia are columnar, pseudostratified, and mitotically active; whereas the cells in atrophic/inactive glands are flattened or cuboidal, form a single layer, and are mitotically inactive.

Complex hyperplasia without atypia

Complex hyperplasia without atypia is defined as glands with abnormal, irregular architecture set in a background of scant intervening stroma. The background stroma is generally less prominent than in simple hyperplasia. Some

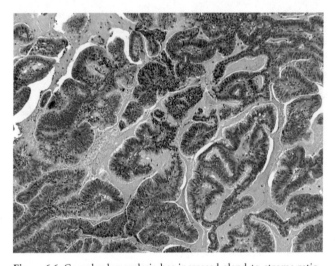

Figure 6.6 Complex hyperplasia has increased gland-to-stroma ratio (≥3 : 1), and gland complexity – due to either branching, outward budding, internal papillary infoldings, or internal bridges.

stroma must be present, however, and even in cases where glands are apparently back to back, close examination reveals basement membrane lining individual glands and a rim of intervening stroma between them.

In addition to back-to-back, cribriform-like arrangements, other glandular architectural abnormalities warranting designation as complex hyperplasia include outpouchings, infoldings, and budding (Figure 6.6). Although these abnormal glands may be lined by only a single layer of cells, up to four cell layers may be present, and focal tufting into the lumen can be seen. Squamous or morular metaplasia, as well as eosinophilic and ciliated cell change, is frequently encountered in glands exhibiting features of complex hyperplasia. Complex hyperplasia may be

(A)

(B)

(C)

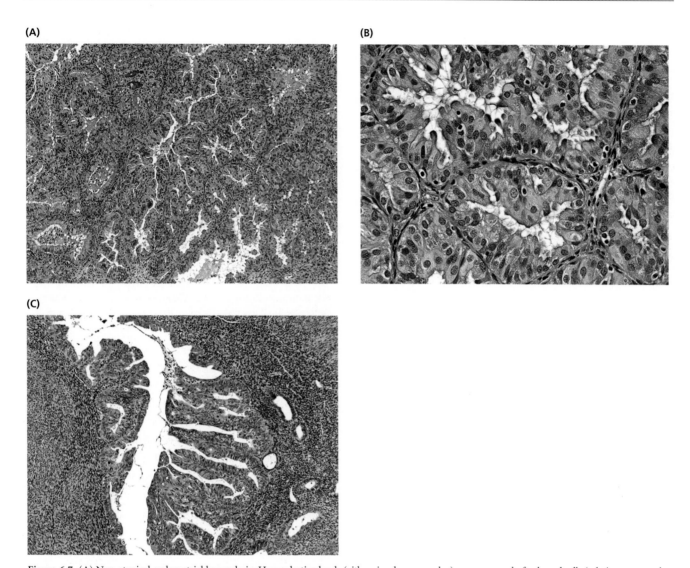

Figure 6.7 (A) Non-atypical endometrial hyperplasia. Hyperplastic glands (either simple or complex) are composed of enlarged cells (relative to normal endometrial cells) with enlarged nuclei, and nuclear pseudostratification. (B) However, the nuclear membranes are smooth and the chromatin is evenly dispersed. Nucleoli may be present, but they are small and rather indistinct. (C) Involvement of foci of adenomyosis is common in endometrial hyperplasia.

associated with simple hyperplasia; the distinction between simple and complex architecture in these cases may be subjective.

Cytologically, epithelial cells are identical to those seen in simple hyperplasia and are characterized by pseudostratification, smooth oval nuclei with evenly dispersed chromatin, inconspicuous nucleoli, and variable mitoses (Figure 6.7). These features are reminiscent of those seen in normal proliferative endometrial cells, although nuclei are often larger in hyperplasia.

Simple atypical hyperplasia

The nuclear criteria for atypia mirror those required for complex atypical hyperplasia and are described below. Cytologic atypia in the absence of architectural complexity is rare.

Complex atypical hyperplasia

Most cases of atypical endometrial hyperplasia fall into this category. This lesion is differentiated from complex non-atypical hyperplasia solely on the basis of cytologic abnormalities. Unlike the smooth, oval nuclei seen in non-atypical hyperplasia, atypical nuclei are rounder and may have irregular membranes (Figure 6.8). Chromatin is often irregularly dispersed and clumpy, imparting a vesicular appearance. True stratification with loss of polarity in relation to the basement membrane is common, and differs from the pseudostratification seen with non-atypical hyperplasia. Apoptotic bodies may be seen. Perhaps the most reproducible criterion for atypical endometrial hyperplasia is the presence of enlarged nucleoli.

Neither the degree nor the extent to which the atypia must be present to diagnose atypical hyperplasia is well

(A)

(B)

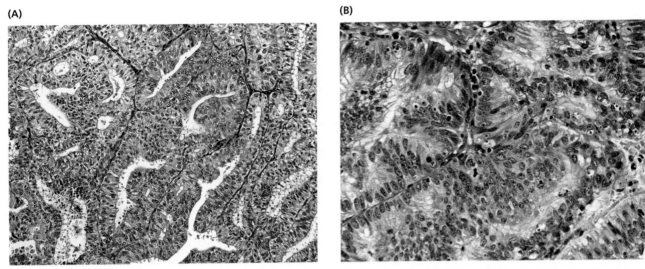

Figure 6.8 (A, B) Atypical endometrial hyperplasia is recognized by the presence of distinct nucleoli, nuclear pleomorphism, irregular nuclear membranes and dispersed or clumpy chromatin. The extent of atypia in this proliferation qualifies this as atypical hyperplasia. The significance of small foci of atypia set in a hyperplasic process that is otherwise banal is uncertain.

specified, but in general, atypia should involve a significant proportion of the hyperplastic proliferation, rather than an isolated focus, to warrant a definitive diagnosis of atypical hyperplasia (Figure 6.8). However, occasional curettage specimens may contain glandular tissue with marked complexity, but only focal cytologic atypia. In these instances, we classify the architecture (e.g., complex hyperplasia, borderline, or carcinoma – see below) and note the degree and extent of atypia. The surrounding stroma is typically compressed, but may appear more fibrous, or exhibit features of stromal breakdown (the breakdown may artifactually increase the apparent gland-to-stroma ratio). Stromal foam cells may also be seen; this feature helps to localize the proliferation to the endometrium in those cases in which the morphologic features are ambiguous[14].

Although the criteria appear straightforward, application of this system can be difficult in clinical practice. The determination of atypia is particularly troublesome and accounts for considerable lack of reproducibility in the classification of endometrial hyperplasia (interobserver variability in the classification of simple versus complex hyperplasia also exists, but this distinction does not appear to carry the same clinical import)[12]. An additional confounding factor in the practical application of these criteria is the observation that occasional low-grade endometrial adenocarcinomas (and presumably their precursor lesions) exhibit very little cytologic atypia; this is particularly a problem with complex mucinous endometrial proliferations (see Chapter 9).

ENDOMETRIAL INTRAEPITHELIAL NEOPLASIA CLASSIFICATION SYSTEM

In contrast to the WHO criteria, the EIN criteria are informed not only by clinical outcome data, but also by molecular data. As such, endometrial intraepithelial neoplasia is essentially a monoclonal proliferation of architecturally and cytologically altered endometrial glands having a high likelihood of concurrent occult carcinoma, as well as an increased risk for progression to adenocarcinoma over time. Like endometrial hyperplasia, endometrial intraepithelial neoplasia arises in a background of increased estrogen, but it is thought that the development of somatically acquired mutations is more closely correlated to the endometrial intraepithelial neoplasia lesion than estrogen excess per se. The level of risk is reported to be higher in endometrial intraepithelial neoplasia than in atypical hyperplasia (14-fold versus 45-fold), but a head-to-head comparison with equivalent follow-up times has not been conducted (the one study that did compare the two systems found no significant differences in predictive value or diagnostic reproducibility with relatively short-term follow-up). The diagnosis of endometrial intraepithelial neoplasia requires the presence of five criteria within a single tissue fragment (Table 6.4).

Many of the admonitions mentioned in the evaluation of the non-neoplastic endometrium (e.g., benign polyps, normal basalis, and secretory endometrium may mimic hyperplasia) are also applicable to endometrial intraepithelial neoplasia; therefore careful morphologic assessment is

Table 6.4 Criteria for endometrial intraepithelial neoplasia[a]

Criterion	Comments
Architecture	Area of glands exceeds area of stroma
Size	Focus of crowded and cytologically altered glands ≥1 mm
Cytology	Cytology in area of gland crowding differs from background endometrium
Exclude benign mimics	Disordered proliferative endometrium, benign endometrial hyperplasia, polyps, secretory endometrium, artifacts, etc.
Exclude malignant mimics	Low-grade endometrioid carcinoma

[a] All five criteria must be met in a single tissue fragment to diagnose endometrial intraepithelial neoplasia. Note that loss of PTEN expression is not a criterion for endometrial intraepithelial neoplasia.

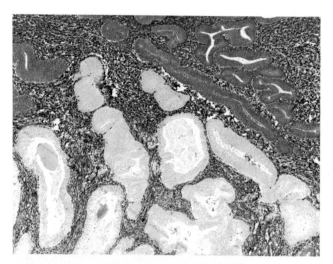

Figure 6.9 Loss of PTEN expression is seen in this disordered proliferative endometrium. Although loss of PTEN is associated with endometrial neoplasia, it is not specific for neoplasia and is not recommended for use in routine diagnosis or in risk stratification.

required. Although loss of PTEN has been proposed as a useful marker for endometrial intraepithelial neoplasia, loss of PTEN is not specific for endometrial intraepithelial neoplasia and may be seen in histologically normal secretory glands as well as in disordered proliferative glands (Figure 6.9). Endometrial intraepithelial neoplasia is not to be confused with endometrial intraepithelial carcinoma, which is a high-grade putative precursor to serous carcinoma (see Chapter 8).

DOES FOCAL HYPERPLASIA (OR ENDOMETRIAL INTRAEPITHELIAL NEOPLASIA) EXIST?

Although endometrial hyperplasia is generally taken to imply a diffuse process, it is clear that, in some instances (non-atypical or atypical), hyperplasia or endometrial intraepithelial neoplasia may only focally involve the endometrium. This is best confirmed in the intact hysterectomy specimen (Figure 6.1), but this pattern can occasionally be encountered in a uterine curetting; in the latter setting, the sampling consists of a dimorphic pattern of abnormal endometrium with separate fragments of normal cycling endometrium in the premenopausal patient, and inactive or weakly proliferative endometrium in the postmenopausal patient. Apparent isolated involvement of a polyp may also be present. While there are some data regarding the rarity of associated myoinvasive carcinoma after a diagnosis of

focal atypical hyperplasia[15]. It would seem that curettage followed by a trial of progestin therapy may be warranted in this situation.

A PRACTICAL APPROACH TO DIAGNOSING PRECANCER IN THE ENDOMETRIUM

In practice, the key distinctions to be made in endometrial hyperplasia or endometrial intraepithelial neoplasia are: (1) the presence or absence of cytologic alterations (defined either by set criteria in the WHO system or by difference from background endometrium in the EIN system); (2) exclusion of benign mimics that pose no risk for progression to endometrial carcinoma; and (3) exclusion of low-grade endometrial carcinoma. Most at-risk endometria feature a complex glandular architecture and exhibit diffuse atypia. Focal cytologic alterations may be present in some hyperplastic endometria, but the significance of such focal alterations is uncertain. If the architecture is sufficiently complex, these lesions may be diagnosed as "hyperplasia with focal atypia" or "complex lesion, bordering on endometrial intraepithelial neoplasia"; the degree and extent of cytologic alteration should be mentioned in a comment section of the report, and a follow-up sampling should be considered. If the hyperplastic process is otherwise banal and the sampling appears to be representative, we diagnose these lesions as "hyperplasia" and indicate the presence of focal atypia in the comment section, with the note that the degree and extent of atypia is insufficient to warrant a definitive diagnosis of atypia (or EIN, if that is the system being used). At the other end of the spectrum are markedly complex endometrial glandular proliferations that appear to fall short of that typically seen in low-grade adenocarcinoma, but are nevertheless worrisome for well-differentiated adenocarcinoma (Diagram 6.2). Since the endometrial sampling is essentially a screening

procedure, these cases are best diagnosed as "borderline" or "at least complex atypical hyperplasia (or endometrial intraepithelial neoplasia), cannot exclude well-differentiated adenocarcinoma" (Table 6.5)[14,16]. The exclusion of benign mimics that pose no risk for progression is discussed below.

ANCILLARY DIAGNOSTIC TESTS

Over the years, a variety of ancillary tests have been evaluated for aiding in the distinction from carcinoma, as well as accurate diagnosis of significant cancer precursor lesions. However, in our opinion, none have proven to be sufficiently sensitive or specific to justify their use in routine clinical practice.

DIFFERENTIAL DIAGNOSIS

Hyperplasia without atypia (benign hyperplasia)

Artifactual changes are among the chief mimickers of benign (non-atypical) endometrial hyperplasia (see Chapter 5). Stromal breakdown in actively bleeding endometria can lead to an apparent elevation of the gland-to-stroma ratio. Telescoping of glands within one another can impart a low-power appearance of complexity (Figure 6.10), and surface epithelium can become so tightly coiled in a curettage

Competing "precancer" criteria

Kurman	WHO	EIN	European
Hyperplasia	SH without atypia	Hyperplasia	Hyperplasia
	CH without atypia		
Atypical hyperplasia	SH with atypia	EIN	Endometrial neoplasia
	CH with atypia		
Carcinoma	Carcinoma	Carcinoma	

Diagram 6.2 The degree of relatedness between the various classifications for endometrial hyperplasia and carcinoma is depicted in this figure. Endometrial precancer classification schemes are not equivalent, particularly with respect to the WHO and EIN schemes. The degree of overlap (and non-overlap) between WHO and EIN classification schemes is an approximation based on extrapolation of the published data. Abbreviations: SH, simple hyperplasia; CH, complex hyperplasia; EIN, endometrial intraepithelial neoplasia; WHO, World Health Organization.

Table 6.5 Classification systems for low-grade endometrial precancer lesions[a]

WHO	EIN	European	WHO (modified)[b]
Simple hyperplasia without atypia	Hyperplasia	Hyperplasia	Hyperplasia without atypia
Complex hyperplasia without atypia	Hyperplasia	Hyperplasia	Hyperplasia without atypia
Simple hyperplasia with atypia[c]	Endometrial intraepithelial neoplasia	Endometrial neoplasia	Hyperplasia with atypia/borderline
Complex hyperplasia with atypia	Endometrial intraepithelial neoplasia	Endometrial neoplasia	Hyperplasia with atypia/borderline
Carcinoma	Carcinoma		Carcinoma

Abbreviations: WHO, World Health Organization; EIN, endometrial intraepithelial neoplasia.

[a] Note that the classification schemes are not equivalent, particularly with respect to the WHO and Endometrial neoplasm schemes. The degree of overlap (and non-overlap) between WHO and EIN classification schemes is based on extrapolation of the published data. Approximately 4% of glandular proliferations classified as simple hyperplasia without atypia and 44% of glandular proliferations classified as complex hyperplasia without atypia are classified as endometrial intraepithelial neoplasia, while 78% of atypical hyperplasia is classified as endometrial intraepithelial neoplasia, with most of the remaining atypical hyperplasia classified as carcinoma using the EIN system. Some of these discrepancies may be due to the lack of nuclear atypia in many complex metaplastic lesions.

[b] The introduction of the "borderline" category captures both the uncertainty and poor interobserver reproducibility of diagnoses for glandular proliferations that lie within the morphologic transition zone of the hyperplasia–carcinoma spectrum, and can be applied to EIN as well as WHO.

[c] Simple hyperplasia with atypia is rare. Most atypical hyperplasia is complex.

(A)

(B)

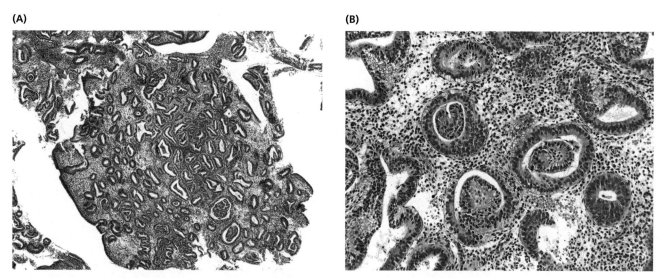

Figure 6.10 (A, B) Telescoping of endometrial glands can be misinterpreted as disordered proliferative endometrium or hyperplasia on low magnification. However, the cells are bland, without the usual features of hyperplasia (nuclear enlargement, increased mitotic figures, nuclear pseudostratification, etc).

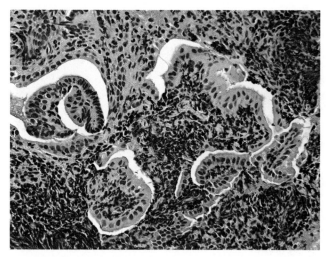

Figure 6.11 Pseudopapillary pattern due to curettage. The endometrium is folded or coiled into itself, creating the impression of papillae.

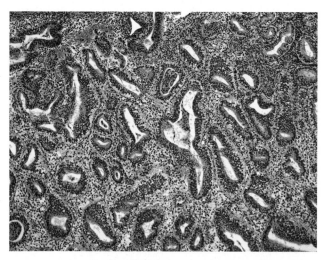

Figure 6.12 Disordered proliferative endometrium may show focal gland crowding, but the overall gland-to-stroma ratio is less than 3 : 1 (often, less than 2 : 1). The constituent cells may exhibit various degrees of metaplasia, but cytologic atypia is absent.

specimen that it simulates a papillary architectural pattern (Figure 6.11). The basalis may be over-represented in a biopsy specimen. All of these artifacts are particularly common in fragmented curettage specimens, where areas of non-crowded glands may or may not be present. If, after thoroughly evaluating a fragmented uterine sampling, a determination cannot be made about the process (i.e., hyperplasia versus benign, non-hyperplasia), it is reasonable to suggest consideration for repeat biopsy or curettage.

Disordered proliferative endometrium can closely resemble hyperplasia, although the stroma is more abundant than is permitted for a hyperplasia or endometrial intraepithelial neoplasia diagnosis. Disordered proliferative

endometrial glands often exhibit irregular contours, cystic expansion, and focal crowding, but the gland-to-stroma ratio does not reach 3 : 1, and the cytology is not dissimilar to uninvolved endometrial glands (Figure 6.12).

Polyps should also be in the differential for non-atypical hyperplasia or endometrial intraepithelial neoplasia, particularly in limited samples (Figure 6.13). Polyps can have architectural complexity reminiscent of hyperplasia and may show significant ciliated or squamous metaplasia – both common features in endometrial hyperplasia and endometrial intraepithelial neoplasia. While they may represent a focal hyperplasia of the uterine basalis,

(A)

(B)

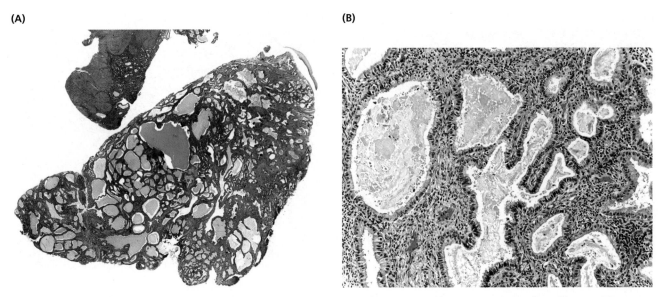

Figure 6.13 (A, B) Endometrial polyp. The glands in endometrial polyps are often crowded and irregular in contour, typically resembling disordered proliferative endometrium; recognition of the fibrous stroma, thick-walled blood vessels, and overall polypoid configuration will prevent overdiagnosis of hyperplasia.

(A)

(B)

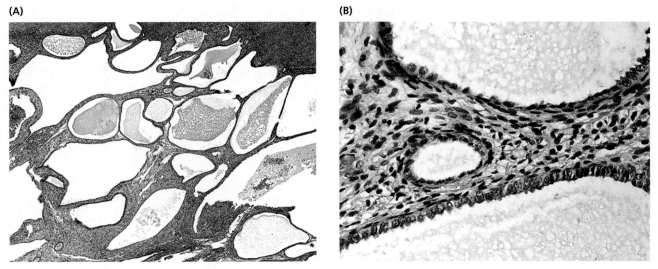

Figure 6.14 (A, B) Cystic atrophy consists of dilated glands lined by atrophic endometrial cells. Mitotic figures are absent.

endometrial polyps do not appear to be estrogen related and do not carry the risks associated with true endometrial hyperplasia. The presence of dense stroma, thick-walled vessels, and normal adjacent endometrium helps solidify a polyp diagnosis and avoid an overdiagnosis of hyperplasia or endometrial intraepithelial neoplasia. However, since polyps may contain foci of hyperplasia/endometrial intraepithelial neoplasia or even carcinoma (both low grade and high grade), the glands contained within endometrial polyps should always be carefully evaluated. When evaluating the cytologic characteristics of suspicious glands in endometrial polyps, it is important to base any

comparisons on the background glandular epithelium of the polyp and not on the glands outside the polyp.

Cystic atrophy is encountered in endometria from postmenopausal women; it is distinguished from cystic hyperplasia and endometrial intraepithelial neoplasia by the presence of attenuated and non-stratified, atrophic epithelium, often with prominent ciliated cells set in an eosinophilic, fibrous stroma (Figures 6.14 and 6.15). Mitotic figures are absent. Since the underlying process reflects a low estrogenic state, the volume of involved endometrial tissue is typically less than that encountered in hyperplasia.

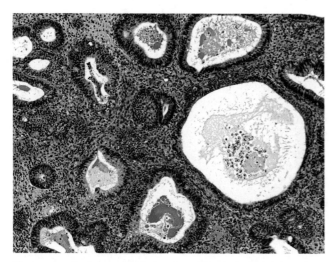

Figure 6.15 Cystic hyperplasia consists of closely spaced, enlarged, proliferative glands. Mitotic figures are typically present. Most cases exhibit additional hyperplastic foci with marked (>3:1) gland crowding.

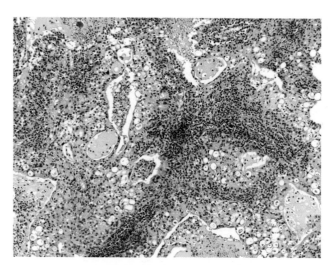

Figure 6.16 Papillary syncytial change consists of a sheet-like proliferation of eosinophilic cells with indistinct cell borders.

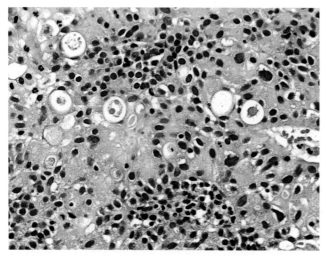

Figure 6.17 Nuclear atypia may be present in papillary syncytial change, but usually consists of small nucleoli or a smudged chromatin pattern. Mitotic figures may be present but are typically sparse.

Hyperplasia with atypia

Despite the efforts to develop clinically relevant and diagnostically reproducible criteria for risk prediction, the distinction between hyperplasia and atypical hyperplasia or endometrial intraepithelial neoplasia continues to be one of the more problematic areas in surgical pathology. A misdiagnosis of atypical hyperplasia or endometrial intraepithelial neoplasia has a higher penalty than a misdiagnosis of non-atypical (benign) hyperplasia, since the former carries a greater risk of progression to cancer and is therefore more likely to trigger definitive clinical action. As with non-atypical hyperplasia, however, multiple artifactual and benign changes can complicate accurate diagnosis of atypical hyperplasia or endometrial intraepithelial

neoplasia. Unsettling artifacts include nuclear changes such as stratification and hobnail-like morphology. Similarly, normal proliferative endometrium can have rounded cells with coarse chromatin, reminiscent of those sometimes seen in atypical hyperplasia or endometrial intraepithelial neoplasia. In all of these cases, it is the absence of abnormal architecture that excludes atypical hyperplasia or endometrial intraepithelial neoplasia.

Endometrial metaplasia

Metaplasias can be particularly problematic when assessing an endometrial proliferation; in part because these changes are more commonly seen under estrogenic stimulation and often occur in concert with hyperplasia and, in part, because the metaplastic epithelium may exhibit cytologic changes that begin to overlap with those in atypical hyperplasia or endometrial intraepithelial neoplasia. However, in isolation metaplasia has no neoplastic potential, and its presence alone should not be taken as synonymous with increased risk. Papillary syncytial change (also referred to as surface syncytial change and papillary syncytial metaplasia) is among the most eye-catching of these alterations (Figures 6.16 and 6.17); characterized by a sheet-like proliferation of eosinophilic cells with indistinct cell borders, this change is often observed in the setting of bleeding and breakdown, and is thought to represent a degenerative or reparative process rather than a true metaplasia. Reactive cytologic atypia may be present. Another form of eosinophilic metaplasia consists of cuboidal to columnar cells with pale to dark pink cytoplasm, resembling tubal metaplasia, but without cilia (Figure 5.29). The nuclei in eosinophilic

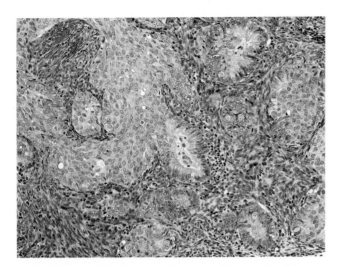

Figure 6.18 Morules fill the gland lumens in this example of squamous metaplasia.

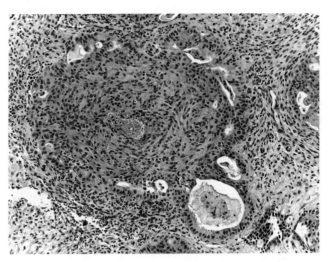

Figure 6.19 Squamous or morular metaplasia may contain foci of punctate necrosis, but this finding has no bearing on risk for progression, and should not be misinterpreted as evidence of atypia or malignancy.

metaplasia may exhibit hyperchromasia, posing concern for a cytologically atypical process, but the chromatin is smudged. Ciliated cells typically exhibit small nucleoli and on occasion are mistaken for atypical hyperplasia.

Squamous metaplasia can also be problematic, particularly when it is extensive. Squamous metaplastic cells are typically non-keratinizing and contain moderate amounts of eosinophilic cytoplasm; they can form sheets and morules and often fill glandular lumens (Figure 6.18), creating the impression of a significant solid component (although this should not be included in overall assessment of the lesional architecture). Central necrosis is frequently encountered within morules, and should not be misinterpreted as evidence of atypia or malignancy (Figure 6.19). It is not uncommon for extensive morular metaplasia to be misdiagnosed as complex atypical hyperplasia or even carcinoma due to the sheet-like growth pattern and the presence of small nucleoli in the squamous metaplastic cells[17]. In order to prevent these overdiagnoses, classification should be made on the basis of an assessment of the architecture and cytology of the glandular components.

The distinction between benign mucinous metaplasia, atypical hyperplasia or endometrial intraepithelial neoplasia with mucinous metaplasia, and well-differentiated mucinous carcinoma can be difficult[14]. In these instances, careful assessment of the glandular architecture is critical. Since mucinous carcinomas may be deceptively bland and may not differ significantly from background endometrium, whenever the glandular configuration of a mucinous proliferation is indeterminate between hyperplasia and carcinoma, the term "complex mucinous proliferation"

should be employed to convey uncertainty (Figure 6.20). Evaluation for a possible cervical source is also prudent in these cases[18,19].

When interpreted without the relevant clinical history, the architectural and nuclear changes seen in florid secretory or gestational endometria can also raise the possibility of atypical hyperplasia or endometrial intraepithelial neoplasia. Secretory changes include the accumulation of luminal secretions and vacuolated cytoplasm, which may be associated with stromal breakdown. Nuclear hobnailing reminiscent of Arias-Stella reaction can also be seen[20]. These changes may also occur focally or diffusely within hyperplasic glands (Figure 6.21). Identification of cytologic alterations can be difficult in this setting because secretory features can mask nuclear changes. If atypia cannot be excluded, recommendation for possible re-biopsy is warranted. Endometritis can show features concerning for atypia, such as nuclear enlargement and stratification; however, the presence of abundant spindled, reactive stroma and plasma cells provides reassurance. In some cases, examination of the sample may offer clues to the etiology behind endometritis (such as retained implantation site or placental site nodule), although more often than not this information is derived from the clinical history.

Benign endometrial polyp

Fragmented benign endometrial polyps are also common mimickers of atypical hyperplasia or endometrial intra-epithelial neoplasia, particularly in curetting specimens.

(A)

(B)

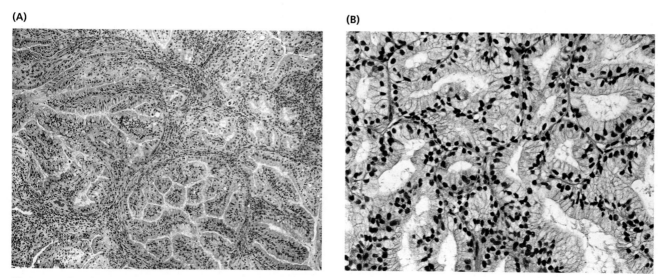

Figure 6.20 (A, B) Mucinous metaplasia can exhibit a variety of appearances, but the most common form mimics endocervical mucinous epithelium. In this example, the architecture is complex, but the cytology is banal. Mucinous proliferations that are indeterminate between hyperplasia and carcinoma should be diagnosed as "complex mucinous proliferation."

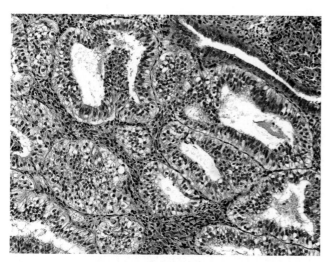

Figure 6.21 Secretory hyperplasia consists of hyperplastic endometrial glands with prominent subnuclear or, occasionally, supranuclear cytoplasmic vacuoles, similar to secretory endometrium. When the gland architecture meets criteria for adenocarcinoma, such superimposed secretory changes have been referred to as secretory carcinoma.

Many polyps contain irregular, basalis-type glands that can bear nuclear atypia. While a diagnosis of polyp is easily rendered when their polypoid shape, dense stroma, and thick-walled blood vessels are readily apparent, in fragmented samples these features are not always obvious. In these cases additional sampling may be considered.

Atypical polypoid adenomyoma

Since atypical polypoid adenomyomas (APAs) contain complex, irregular glands with altered cytology, misdiagnoses of

atypical hyperplasia, endometrial intraepithelial neoplasia, or endometrial carcinoma may occur (Figure 6.22). However, these localized, polypoid proliferations can be safely treated by polypectomy and/or hormonal therapy without significant risk for progression to carcinoma provided there is careful clinical follow-up. Since atypical polypoid adenomyomas typically occur in young women (often under 40 years of age), reproductive conservation is particularly desirable with this lesion. A clue that the lesion is focal is the presence in curettage or biopsy specimens of additional fragments of normal proliferative or secretory pattern endometrium admixed with the atypical polypoid adenomyoma fragments[21].

Adenocarcinoma

Perhaps the most important and problematic entity in the differential diagnosis of atypical hyperplasia (or endometrial intraepithelial neoplasia) is well-differentiated carcinoma. This distinction remains a focus of debate as well as a source of confusion in gynecologic pathology[25–27]. Despite the difficulties that arise in their application, pathologists generally agree on three criteria for the diagnosis of well-differentiated carcinoma. They are: (1) the presence of large macroglands with complex cribriform or papillary internal structure; (2) a confluent, haphazard pattern of branching glands with interconnecting gland lumina without intervening stroma; and (3) extensive or confluent papillary formations[16,28]. The presence of any one of these three features merits a diagnosis of well-differentiated adenocarcinoma. However, it is often not possible to securely

(A)

(B)

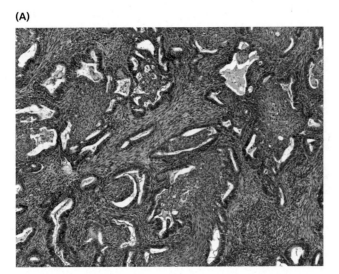

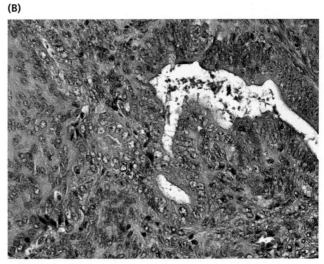

Figure 6.22 (A) Atypical polypoid adenomyoma is recognized by the presence of irregular glands set in a prominent fibromuscular stroma. Morular metaplasia is common. (B) The irregular glands may exhibit cytologic atypia, but these lesions can be managed by curettage and hormonal therapy.

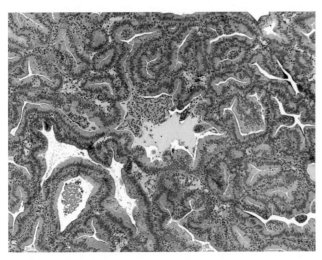

Figure 6.23 Complex glandular proliferation with atypia borders on low-grade endometrioid adenocarcinoma at right. In absence of more definitive features, the small volume in this case could be diagnosed as "borderline" or "at least complex atypical hyperplasia, cannot exclude adenocarcinoma."

place a proliferation in the malignant category based on small, fragmented samples. Cases in which the distinction between the two processes cannot be made with confidence are best diagnosed as "borderline" or "at least complex atypical hyperplasia (endometrial intraepithelial neoplasia), cannot exclude well-differentiated adenocarcinoma" (Figure 6.23)[14,16]. It is important to emphasize that some endometrial adenocarcinomas may exhibit less cytologic atypia than atypical hyperplasia or endometrial intraepithelial neoplasia; this is especially true with some of the mucinous adenocarcinomas.

Other difficulties that may be encountered in endometrial sampling specimens include: extensive fragmentation, extensive squamous or morular metaplasia, and desmoplastic stroma unassociated with a glandular proliferation. In many of these cases, a definitive diagnosis may not be possible, and consideration should be given for further evaluation, including repeat sampling[14,16]. Rarely, gland forming serous carcinoma may be misinterpreted as atypical hyperplasia (Figure 7.43). The presence of severe nuclear atypia is a feature that suggests the correct diagnosis.

EVALUATION OF PROGESTIN TREATMENT IN ENDOMETRIAL HYPERPLASIA (OR ENDOMETRIAL INTRAEPITHELIAL NEOPLASIA)

Patients with complex endometrial hyperplasia (or endometrial intraepithelial neoplasia) and well-differentiated endometrial adenocarcinoma are often treated with oral progestin or with a progesterone-releasing intrauterine device in order to induce a hormonal ablation[29]. Such therapy is useful both in young women wishing to preserve fertility and in postmenopausal patients who are poor surgical candidates or otherwise wish to avoid a surgical hysterectomy procedure. The response rate varies from <40 to 100% of patients so treated, but tends to be more successful for hyperplasia with lesser degrees of atypia; postmenopausal women appear to demonstrate a better

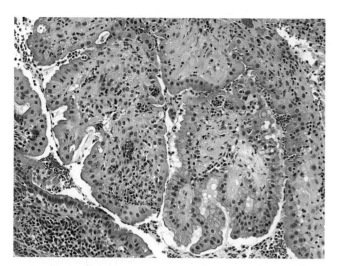

Figure 6.24 Progestin effects on endometrial tissue show stromal pseudodecidual reaction and atrophic, inactive, or weakly proliferative glandular epithelium.

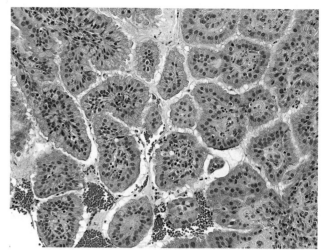

Figure 6.25 Mucinous metaplasia is a frequent effect of progestin therapy. Since hyperplasia and carcinoma may also feature prominent mucinous metaplasia, the prior, pre-treatment curettage should be evaluated in conjunction with the post-treatment sampling in order to determine whether or not there is a persistent lesion.

response than premenopausal women, presumably due to the effects of circulating estrogens. However, atypical hyperplasia and even well-differentiated endometrial carcinoma can respond to progestin therapy, and this is often the initial trial of therapy in premenopausal patients who wish to preserve their fertility. Pathologists are often asked to evaluate the follow-up biopsy or curettage in these patients to assess overall response. This is best accomplished by comparison with the prior, pre-treatment sampling.

A variety of changes may occur secondary to the progestin therapy; these include predecidual change, decreased gland confluence and complexity, increased metaplasia (squamous, eosinophilic, and mucinous), decreased nuclear size, and decreased cytologic atypia (Figures 6.24 and 6.25)[32]. The nuclei may be rounder than in the pre-treated lesion, and the chromatin tends to be finer and more homogenized. Mitotic figures are rare or absent altogether. A papillary or cystic architecture may also be seen. Since persistence of significant cytologic atypia or complex architecture may be present only focally in the post-treated endometrium, these samplings should be carefully screened in order to alert the treating physician to the possibility of persistent and/or possibly recurrent atypical hyperplasia (or endometrial intraepithelial neoplasia). Although the clinical significance of focal hyperplasia is undetermined (see the subsection *Does focal hyperplasia (or endometrial intraepithelial neoplasia) exist?*, above), the presence of focal hyperplasia in this setting implies incomplete response to medical management or inadequate therapy (too low a dose, or too short an interval, or both). Hormonal therapy should not be discontinued if

there is any evidence of residual disease. The presence of cytologic atypia after six months of adequate progestin therapy indicates poor response to medical therapy.

REFERENCES

1. Kurman R, Kaminski P, Norris H. The behavior of endometrial hyperplasia. A long-term study of "untreated" hyperplasia in 170 patients. *Cancer* 1985;**56**:403–12.
2. Huang S, Amparo E, Fu Y. Endometrial hyperplasia: histologic classification and behavior. *Surg Pathol* 1988;**1**:215–29.
3. Kendall BS, Ronnett BM, Isacson C, *et al.* Reproducibility of the diagnosis of endometrial hyperplasia, atypical hyperplasia, and well-differentiated carcinoma. *Am J Surg Pathol* 1998;**22**:1012–19.
4. Mutter GL. Histopathology of genetically defined endometrial precancers. *Int J Gynecol Pathol* 2000;**19**:301–9.
5. Mutter GL, Baak JP, Crum CP, *et al.* Endometrial precancer diagnosis by histopathology, clonal analysis, and computerized morphometry. *J Pathol* 2000;**190**:462–9.
6. Mutter GL, Ince TA, Baak JP, *et al.* Molecular identification of latent precancers in histologically normal endometrium. *Cancer Res* 2001;**61**:4311–14.
7. Mutter GL, Lin MC, Fitzgerald JT, *et al.* Altered PTEN expression as a diagnostic marker for the earliest endometrial precancers. *J Natl Cancer Inst* 2000;**92**:924–30.
8. Lacey JV, Jr., Mutter GL, Ronnett BM, *et al.* PTEN expression in endometrial biopsies as a marker of progression to endometrial carcinoma. *Cancer Res* 2008;**68**:6014–20.
9. Mutter GL, Lin MC, Fitzgerald JT, *et al.* Changes in endometrial PTEN expression throughout the human menstrual cycle. *J Clin Endocrinol Metab* 2000;**85**:2334–8.
10. Mutter GL. Endometrial intraepithelial neoplasia (EIN): will it bring order to chaos? The Endometrial Collaborative Group. *Gynecol Oncol* 2000;**76**:287–90.

11. Baak JP, Mutter GL, Robboy S, *et al.* The molecular genetics and morphometry-based endometrial intraepithelial neoplasia classification system predicts disease progression in endometrial hyperplasia more accurately than the 1994 World Health Organization classification system. *Cancer* 2005;**103**:2304–12.

12. Lacey JV, Jr., Mutter GL, Nucci MR, *et al.* Risk of subsequent endometrial carcinoma associated with endometrial intraepithelial neoplasia classification of endometrial biopsies. *Cancer* 2008;**113**:2073–81.

13. Bergeron C, Nogales FF, Masseroli M, *et al.* A multicentric European study testing the reproducibility of the WHO classification of endometrial hyperplasia with a proposal of a simplified working classification for biopsy and curettage specimens. *Am J Surg Pathol* 1999;**23**:1102–8.

14. Longacre TA, Atkins KA, Kempson RL, *et al.* The uterine corpus. In: Sternberg S, Mills S, eds. *Diagnostic Surgical Pathology.* New York: Raven Press; 2009:2184–277.

15. Leitao MM Jr, Han G, Lee LX, *et al.* Complex atypical hyperplasia of the uterus: characteristics and prediction of underlying carcinoma risk. *Am J Obstet Gynecol* 2010;**203:349**.e1–6. Epub **2010** Jun 23.

16. Longacre TA, Chung MH, Jensen DN, *et al.* Proposed criteria for the diagnosis of well-differentiated endometrial carcinoma. A diagnostic test for myoinvasion. *Am J Surg Pathol* 1995;**19**: 371–406.

17. Blaustein A. Morular metaplasia misdiagnosed as adenoacanthoma in young women with polycystic ovarian disease. *Am J Surg Pathol* 1982;**6**:223–8.

18. Kong CS, Beck AH, Longacre TA. A panel of three markers including p16, ProEx C, or HPV ISH is optimal for distinguishing between primary endometrial and endocervical adenocarcinomas. *Am J Surg Pathol* 2010;**34**:915–26.

19. Mills AM, Longacre TA. Endometrial hyperplasia. *Semin Diagn Pathol* 2010;**27**:199–214.

20. Arias-Stella J. Gestational endometrium. In: Hertig A, Norris H, Abell M, eds. *The Uterus.* Baltimore: Williams & Wilkins; 1973:185–212.

21. Clement P, Young R. Atypical polypoid adenomyoma of the uterus associated with Turner's syndrome. A report of three cases, including a review of "estrogen-associated" endometrial neoplasms and neoplasms associated with Turner's syndrome. *Int J Gynecol Pathol* 1987;**6**:104–13.

22. Longacre TA, Chung MH, Rouse RV, *et al.* Atypical polypoid adenomyofibromas (atypical polypoid adenomyomas) of the uterus. A clinicopathologic study of 55 cases. *Am J Surg Pathol* 1996;**20**:1–20.

23. Mazur M. Atypical polypoid adenomyomas of the endometrium. *Am J Surg Pathol* 1981;**5**:473–82.

24. Young R, Treger T, Scully R. Atypical polypoid adenomyoma of the uterus. A report of 27 cases. *Am J Clin Pathol* 1986; **86**:139–45.

25. Soslow RA. Problems with the current diagnostic approach to complex atypical endometrial hyperplasia. *Cancer* 2006;**106**:729–31.

26. Trimble CL, Kauderer J, Zaino R, *et al.* Concurrent endometrial carcinoma in women with a biopsy diagnosis of atypical endometrial hyperplasia: a Gynecologic Oncology Group study. *Cancer* 2006;**106**:812–19.

27. Zaino RJ, Kauderer J, Trimble CL, *et al.* Reproducibility of the diagnosis of atypical endometrial hyperplasia: a Gynecologic Oncology Group study. *Cancer* 2006;**106**:804–11.

28. Kurman R, Norris H. Evaluation of criteria for distinguishing atypical endometrial hyperplasia from well-differentiated carcinoma. *Cancer* 1982;**49**:2547–59.

29. Kaku T, Yoshikawa H, Tsuda H, *et al.* Conservative therapy for adenocarcinoma and atypical endometrial hyperplasia of the endometrium in young women: central pathologic review and treatment outcome. *Cancer Lett* 2001;**167**:39–48.

30. Randall TC, Kurman RJ. Progestin treatment of atypical hyperplasia and well-differentiated carcinoma of the endometrium in women under age 40. *Obstet Gynecol* 1997;**90**:434–40.

31. Reed SD, Newton KM, Garcia RL, *et al.* Complex hyperplasia with and without atypia: clinical outcomes and implications of progestin therapy. *Obstet Gynecol*;**116**:365–73.

32. Wheeler DT, Bristow RE, Kurman RJ. Histologic alterations in endometrial hyperplasia and well-differentiated carcinoma treated with progestins. *Am J Surg Pathol* 2007;**31**:988–98.

7 ENDOMETRIOID ADENOCARCINOMA

INTRODUCTION

Endometrioid adenocarcinomas, which comprise approximately 85% of all endometrial cancers, are the most common type of endometrial carcinoma and the most commonly diagnosed gynecologic cancer in North America. Despite the high prevalence of this tumor type, the vast majority of affected patients can be cured without chemotherapy. Endometrioid adenocarcinomas are considered type I endometrial cancers according to the Bokhman classification[1] because of their epidemiologic association with estrogen. The current model of estrogen-dependent endometrial carcinogenesis involves progression from hyperplasia, with increasing degrees of architectural and cytologic atypia (complex atypical hyperplasia). The development of an invasive neoplasm heralds the emergence of "adenocarcinoma" in this context. These generalities pertain mostly to differentiated endometrioid adenocarcinomas, grades 1 and 2 in the FIGO system.

In practice, endometrioid adenocarcinoma is often a default diagnosis for carcinomas of the endometrium. As these tumors occur rather frequently, the default leads to correct diagnosis in most cases. The shotgun approach is, in fact, fairly accurate when the tumor is differentiated and exhibits low nuclear grade; however, this approach is often inaccurate in tumors with high nuclear grade and those demonstrating solid architecture. Tricky diagnostic challenges exist at both ends of the differentiation spectrum. Meaningful criteria that separate hyperplasia and adenocarcinoma are still being debated, as are those that distinguish gland-forming endometrioid adenocarcinoma and serous carcinoma, and clear cell carcinoma in some cases. Last, insufficient attention has been paid to the characteristics that divide poorly differentiated endometrioid adenocarcinomas (FIGO grade 3) from serous carcinomas with solid architecture, undifferentiated and neuroendocrine carcinomas, and primitive neuroectodermal tumors.

CLINICAL CHARACTERISTICS

The clinical characteristics of patients with low-grade endometrioid adenocarcinomas are those of Bokhman type I carcinomas (Table 7.1)[1]. Most patients with differentiated endometrioid adenocarcinomas are obese, diabetic, or hypertensive, and are exposed to high levels of unopposed estrogen, whether from endogenous sources such as polycystic ovarian syndrome, estrogen-secreting tumors, or excess adipose tissue, or exogenous sources such as tamoxifen or unopposed estrogen therapy. The typical patient is postmenopausal, but up to 25% of patients are premenopausal.

Published details regarding the clinical characteristics of patients with poorly differentiated endometrioid adenocarcinoma are few. Some of these tumors may arise in a background of hyperestrinism, whereas others probably do not. Only about 20% of these patients have coincident hyperplasia on hysterectomy[2]. The typical patient with FIGO grade 3 endometrioid adenocarcinoma is older than one with grade 1 or 2 carcinoma (Table 7.2). About one-half of patients are older than 65 years, and approximately one-half have extrauterine disease at presentation (Table 7.3).

Most endometrioid adenocarcinomas occur sporadically, but approximately 2–5% of these tumors arise in the setting of a hereditary syndrome. Chief among these syndromes is Lynch syndrome, the hereditary non-polyposis

Table 7.1 Bokhman type I and type II endometrial carcinoma

Feature	Type I	Type II
Estrogen excess	Present	Absent
Patient age	Younger	Older
Endometrial hyperplasia	Present	Absent
Prototypic diagnosis	Endometrioid (FIGO grades 1 and 2)	Serous

Table 7.2 International Federation of Gynecology and Obstetrics (FIGO) grading for endometrioid adenocarcinoma

Architectural features	Nuclear features	FIGO grade
Well-formed glands or papillae	Mild to moderate pleomorphism	1
Well-formed glands or papillae	Severe pleomorphism[a]	2
Glands or papillae with 6–50% solid, non-squamous growth	Mild to moderate pleomorphism	2
Glands or papillae with 6–50% solid, non-squamous growth	Severe pleomorphism[a]	3
More than 50% solid, non-squamous growth	Any	3

[a] Should be fairly diffuse or multifocal. Consider a diagnosis of serous or clear cell carcinoma instead of endometrioid adenocarcinoma. Do NOT use FIGO when there is uncertainty regarding classification as endometrioid adenocarcinoma.

Table 7.3 2009 FIGO staging[3]

Stage I	Tumor confined to the corpus uteri
IA	No or less than half myometrial invasion
IB	Invasion equal to or more than half of the myometrium
Stage II	Tumor invades cervical stroma, but is confined to the uterus
Stage III	Local and/or regional spread of tumor
IIIA	Tumor invades the uterine serous or adnexal structures[a]
IIIB	Vaginal and/or parametrial involvement
IIIC	Metastases to pelvic and/or para-aortic lymph nodes
IIIC1	Positive pelvic nodes, but not para-aortic nodes
IIIC2	Positive para-aortic nodes
Stage IV	Tumor invades bladder and/or bowel mucosa, and/or distant metastases
IVA	Tumor invasion of bladder and/or bowel mucosa
IVB	Distant metastases, including intra-abdominal metastases and/or inguinal lymph nodes

[a] Positive cytology (i.e., pelvic washing) should be reported separately.

colorectal carcinoma syndrome (HNPCC)[4,5]. Endometrioid cancers can also arise in a setting of Muir–Torre syndrome (a variant of Lynch syndrome) and Cowden syndrome.

Preoperative assessment

A diagnosis of endometrial cancer rendered on review of biopsy or curettage material allows planning for definitive treatment. In most centers, a diagnosis of nonendometrioid adenocarcinoma (i.e., serous carcinoma) or FIGO grade 2 or 3 endometrioid adenocarcinoma prompts hysterectomy, salpingo-oophorectomy, pelvic and para-aortic lymph node dissection, and staging. Treatment planning for patients with a preoperative diagnosis of FIGO grade 1 endometrioid adenocarcinoma is not as straightforward. If reflexive lymph node dissection and staging were to be performed in all patients, as many as 80% of patients will have undergone an unnecessary procedure, while omitting lymph node dissection would leave approximately 20% of FIGO grade 1 carcinoma patients in need of a second surgery for staging and/or adjuvant therapy. A detailed understanding of the accuracy of preoperative assessment is therefore necessary. In up to 15% of cases[6], a diagnosis of FIGO grade 1 endometrioid adenocarcinoma on biopsy or curettage is upgraded to FIGO grade 2 or 3 endometrioid carcinoma in the follow-up hysterectomy. Moreover, approximately 1% have pure nonendometrioid carcinoma or mixed endometrioid and nonendometrioid carcinoma at hysterectomy. A diagnosis based on evaluation of a dilatation and curettage specimen rather than an endometrial biopsy allows a more accurate preoperative diagnosis of FIGO grade 1 adenocarcinoma[6], as does a preoperative diagnosis of adenocarcinoma when associated with complex atypical hyperplasia[7], especially in patients 55 years of age or younger.

Frozen section evaluation

Because of the possible upgrade of a biopsy/curettage diagnosis at hysterectomy, and to evaluate the extent of uterine myometrial involvement, intraoperative examination of endometrial carcinomas is commonly used to estimate the risk of lymph node metastasis. A historical general rule of thumb is that lymph node dissection can be omitted in patients with FIGO grade 1 carcinomas that invade less than 50% of the myometrium. However, a small proportion of patients whose tumors meet these criteria will be suboptimally staged or require adjuvant therapy; it is estimated that approximately 3% of patients with well-differentiated, superficially invasive tumors will have lymph node metastases (most of these tumors have lymphovascular invasion or measure more than 2 cm)[8]. In addition, the intraoperative assessment of the uterus can be inaccurate. According to a recent study[6], criteria for lymph node dissection or adjuvant therapy were ultimately met in approximately 20% of patients with FIGO grade 1 carcinoma who underwent frozen section evaluation. Only approximately 5% of patients without myometrial invasion on frozen section were found to have deep invasion or grade 2–3 carcinoma in permanent sections, whereas approximately 20% of patients with myometrial invasion of less than 50% on frozen section had similar high-risk features on permanent sections. More than 90% of patients with deep myometrial invasion on frozen section had high-risk features on review of permanent sections. Discrepancies in frozen section diagnosis and permanent section diagnosis are generally due to sampling errors; interpretive errors account for a minority of cases.

Sentinel lymph node mapping

Sentinel lymph node mapping has been studied in an effort to provide a more accurate estimate of the risk of lymph node metastasis. A recent pilot study evaluating the feasibility of sentinel lymph node mapping for FIGO grade 1 endometrioid adenocarcinoma[9] reported that sentinel lymph nodes were visualized intraoperatively in 86% of patients who underwent cervical and/or fundal injections of radioactive technetium and blue dye. Advanced age, obesity, and surgical inexperience with sentinel node mapping were recognized as factors that limited the ability to detect sentinel lymph nodes. It is also well known that bulky lymph node metastases may lead to failed mapping. In this study, 89% of the sentinel nodes were external or internal iliac or obturator nodes, whereas only 8% were common iliac and 3% para-aortic. A median of three sentinel lymph nodes was identified. The pathology protocol used in this study involved the preparation of two sets of two 5 μm sections separated by 50 μm. A hematoxylin and eosin stain and an AE1/AE3 cytokeratin immunohistochemical stain were performed on each set. Eleven percent of patients (four patients in total) had positive lymph nodes. Three metastases were recognizable on the original hematoxylin and eosin stained sections, and one was reported as having isolated cytokeratin-positive cells detectable with AE1/AE3 cytokeratin immunohistochemical stains. All node-positive cases were picked up by sentinel lymph node mapping, and there were no false-negative cases. Despite the potential efficacy of this procedure, the optimal injection medium, site of injection, pathology protocol, and cost–benefit ratio have not been rigorously studied. Sentinel lymph node mapping remains of theoretical interest because it obviates the need to perform frozen sections for assessing myometrial invasion. More important is its potential to spare low-risk patients full lymphadenectomy and the development of resulting debilitating lower extremity edema.

Prognosis

Clinical outcomes for patients with endometrioid adenocarcinomas are linked to grade (Table 7.2), stage (Table 7.3), patient age, and the presence of medical co-morbidities. Most FIGO grade 1 and 2 carcinomas are organ confined at presentation. Tumors that demonstrate deep myometrial invasion and obvious lymphovascular invasion are at highest risk for occult pelvic and para-aortic lymph node metastasis. These patients may also present with pelvic visceral and soft tissue metastasis, including ovarian, tubal, and serosal disease. Peritoneal dissemination from a low-grade endometrioid adenocarcinoma of endometrium, however, is extraordinary in this setting; it tends to be seen in patients with clinically obvious, locally advanced tumor, usually in those patients who have experienced symptoms for long periods of time. Patients with organ-confined disease have superior outcomes, with survival rates in the 90–100% range after hysterectomy. Patients with only superficially invasive FIGO grade 3 carcinoma probably also experience good outcomes, but great care should be exercised to ensure that serous, neuroendocrine, and undifferentiated carcinomas are excluded. These latter patients should also be offered comprehensive surgical staging. Regardless of tumor grade, patients with extrauterine disease such as pelvic soft tissue and regional lymph node metastasis have significantly diminished survival rates; perhaps approaching 50–60%. Patients older than 65 years experience worse outcomes than younger patients[2]. The clinical significance of isolated positive pelvic washings in low-grade, organ-confined disease is uncertain, although tumors with these characteristics have been historically considered to be FIGO stage IIIA. The 2009 revision of the FIGO staging system has eliminated pelvic wash status as a staging criterion.

Nomograms have been developed to provide individualized and accurate estimates of overall survival following primary therapy. A nomogram is a chart representing numerical relationships, or a graphic calculation tool. According to a recent proposal[10], an individual endometrial carcinoma patient's prognosis can be estimated using a nomogram that incorporates numerous data points, including age at diagnosis, adequacy of lymph node dissection, lymph node status, FIGO stage, FIGO grade, and histologic subtype. Each data element is assigned a point value, and adding the points together yields an estimate of three-year and five-year overall survival rate. More points are awarded for higher age, inadequate lymph node evaluation, more positive lymph nodes, higher FIGO stage, grade, and nonendometrioid histology, with carcinosarcoma (malignant mixed mullerian tumor), being the most aggressive tumor type. A typical, 65-year-old patient with FIGO grade 1 endometrioid carcinoma, invading less than 50% of the myometrium, but without lymph node dissection, has a 90–95% three-year and 80–90% five-year probability of survival. Note that the survival rates are not disease specific, such that many of the deaths may be attributable to co-morbidities such as heart disease.

Treatment

The standard therapy for endometrial carcinoma is total hysterectomy with salpingo-oophorectomy. Patients who are poor surgical risks, such as the elderly and debilitated, are sometimes offered radiation or hormonal therapy instead. Hormonal therapy may include progestational agents and/or aromatase inhibitors. These agents are usually delivered systemically, but progestin-coated intrauterine devices have also been used. Strategies that encourage weight loss may also be beneficial.

The treatment of reproductive-age endometrial cancer patients is tailored to their desire and ability to become pregnant. Patients who desire a fertility-sparing therapeutic approach are enrolled in a program that ultimately results in months, if not years, of high-dose progestational therapy along with close surveillance. It is appropriate to offer this option to patients with a diagnosis of complex atypical hyperplasia or FIGO grade 1 endometrioid carcinoma (preferably confirmed on second opinion by a gynecologic pathologist) and no evidence of myometrial invasion or extrauterine spread on clinical and radiologic evaluation. The ideal candidate should be able to tolerate high-dose progestin therapy, is motivated to undergo close surveillance, and thoroughly understands and accepts the risks involved in this treatment option. Patients probably need to be treated for at least six to nine months, as pathologic features present in biopsies taken during this time period are most predictive of ultimate response. One study[11] reports that 67% of complex atypical hyperplasia patients and 42% of adenocarcinoma patients experience complete resolution of their neoplasm. Despite these rather encouraging results, some patients' tumors progress during

Table 7.4 Criteria for adjuvant chemotherapy in FIGO stage I–IIA endometrial carcinoma (according to GOG 249)

Age greater than or equal to 70 years with one risk factor
Age greater than or equal to 50 years with two risk factors
Any age with three risk factors
Risk factors: FIGO grade 2 or 3; lymphovascular invasion; outer-half myometrial invasion.

therapy, and some patients experience recurrence after having been treated successfully initially. Some young endometrial cancer patients will elect hysterectomy without salpingo-oophorectomy. As young patients are at higher risk than older patients of having synchronous or metachronous endometrioid carcinomas of the ovary, these patients should undergo surveillance for the emergence of such an ovarian tumor.

The typical patient with FIGO grade 1, non-invasive or minimally invasive endometrial cancer may not be offered adjuvant therapy. The more deeply invasive the tumor, the more likely it is that a radiation oncologist will recommend vaginal brachytherapy in hopes of decreasing the risk of local recurrence. The use of whole pelvic and whole abdominal radiation has become far less common in recent years because of the increasing performance of lymphadenectomy and the recognition of high rates of debilitating side effects. Most of the high-stage patients and almost all patients with nonendometrioid carcinomas are now treated with combination chemotherapy with or without radiation therapy. The presence of significant, life-threatening, coexisting medical problems, such as morbid obesity, hypertension, and diabetes, complicates delivery of adjuvant therapy in some cases. Patients who require adjuvant therapy, but not chemotherapy, may be offered progestins or aromatase inhibitors. Selected patients with low-stage, but histologically "high–intermediate risk" endometrioid carcinomas are currently randomized to a trial by the Gynecologic Oncology Group (GOG 249), one arm of which includes cytotoxic chemotherapy (Table 7.4).

MORPHOLOGY

Gross pathology

The typical endometrioid adenocarcinoma forms a grossly appreciable, dominant tumor mass, or causes a diffuse thickening of the endometrial stripe (Figure 7.1). Most tumors arise in the fundus, but they can be found less

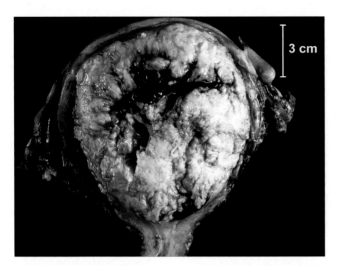

Figure 7.1 Endometrioid adenocarcinoma typically expands the uterus, filling the uterine cavity.

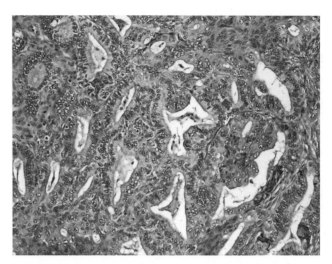

Figure 7.2 Endometrioid adenocarcinoma composed of back-to-back, well-formed tubular glands. Individual glands and constituent cells are reminiscent of the appearance of proliferative endometrium.

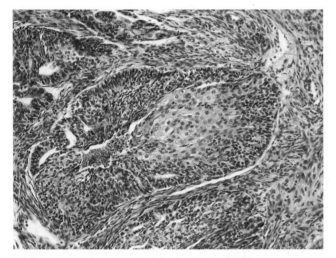

Figure 7.3 Endometrioid adenocarcinoma showing squamous differentiation.

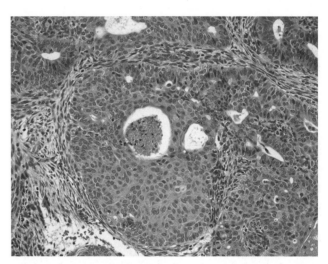

Figure 7.4 Endometrioid adenocarcinoma containing morules (rounded aggregates of non-keratinizing squamous metaplastic cells).

commonly in one of the cornua or in the lower uterine segment. In some cases, the lesion is centered in an endometrial polyp. Endometrioid adenocarcinomas are usually tan in color and soft in consistency. A good gross description will include the size of the tumor, a measurement of the depth of invasion into the myometrium, and document involvement of endocervix, uterine serosa, fallopian tubes, or ovaries, if present. These tissues may be involved by direct extension or metastasis.

Microscopic pathology

Differentiated endometrioid adenocarcinomas should resemble, at least focally, proliferative-type endometrium, with tubular glands, smooth luminal surfaces, and mitotically active columnar cells (Figure 7.2). Histologic features considered typical of endometrioid carcinoma include keratinizing squamous metaplasia (Figure 7.3) or morular metaplasia (non-keratinizing squamous metaplasia) (Figure 7.4), which may show clear cytoplasm and punctate necrosis. Additional features commonly encountered in both non-neoplastic and neoplastic endometrium include tubal metaplasia (Figure 7.5), mucinous metaplasia (Figure 7.6), and secretory (Figure 7.7A), hobnail (Figure 7.8), papillary (Figure 7.9), and clear cell change (Figure 7.7B), with subnuclear or supranuclear cytoplasmic vacuoles.

As mentioned above, endometrioid adenocarcinomas can demonstrate mucinous differentiation and can contain ciliated cells and cells with secretory features. When mucinous differentiation predominates (intracytoplasmic but

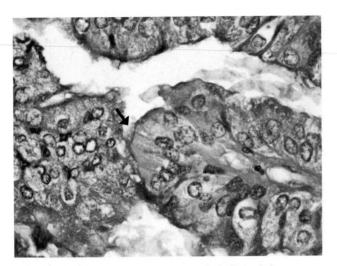

Figure 7.5 Endometrioid adenocarcinoma including tubal metaplastic cells exhibiting a prominent, eosinophilic terminal bar (arrow).

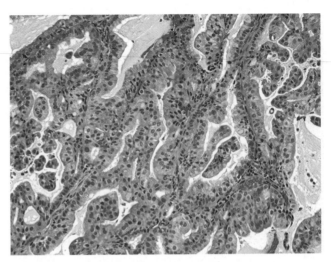

Figure 7.6 Endometrioid adenocarcinoma with mucinous differentiation. Note apical mucin in tumor cells.

(A)

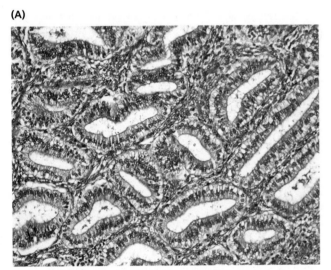

(B)

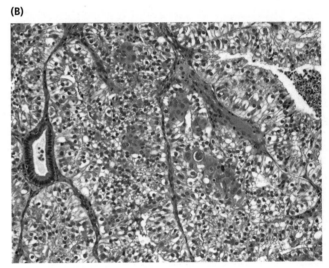

Figure 7.7 (A) Endometrioid adenocarcinoma with subnuclear vacuoles, simulating the appearance of secretory endometrium. (B) Endometrioid adenocarcinoma with extensive clear cell change.

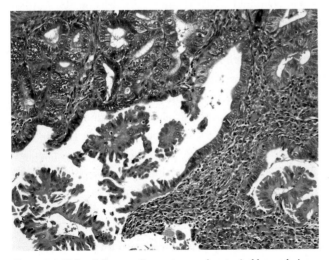

Figure 7.8 Hobnail change adjacent to complex atypical hyperplasia.

not luminal mucin; present in over 50% of cells), the tumor is referred to as "mucinous carcinoma." Likewise, "ciliated carcinoma" and "secretory carcinoma" have been described but are rare. The presence of any secondary component should be noted in the report. Endometrioid adenocarcinomas may also feature papillary architecture. The tumor is referred to as "villoglandular carcinoma" when the papillae are long, slender with delicate fibrovascular cores, and are lined by cytologically low-grade, pseudostratified columnar cells arranged perpendicular to the basement membrane (Figure 7.10). Endometrioid adenocarcinomas with non-villous papillae have also been described. Other findings that can be seen in endometrioid adenocarcinomas include psammomatous calcifications,

(A)

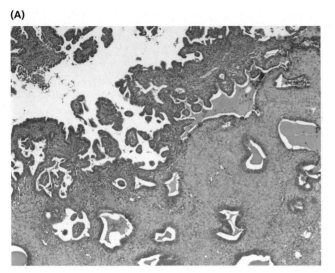

(B)

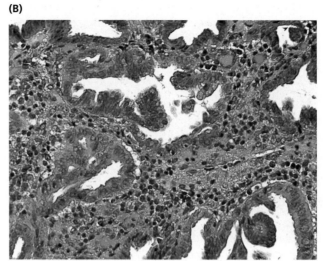

Figure 7.9 (A, B) Papillary change. Bland nuclear features, absent mitotic activity, and well-formed papillae with fibrovascular cores all favor papillary change instead of hyperplasia or carcinoma.

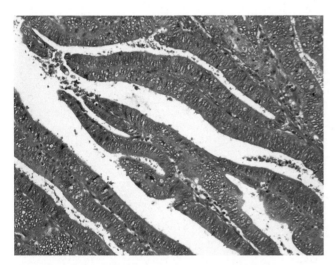

Figure 7.10 Endometrioid adenocarcinoma with long, thin, finger-like papillae. Such carcinomas are diagnosed as villoglandular adenocarcinoma when the nuclear grade is low throughout the tumor.

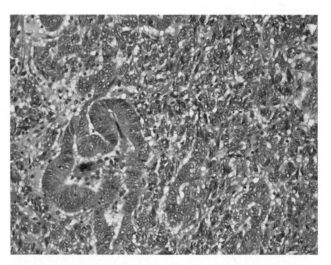

Figure 7.11 Endometrioid adenocarcinoma with spindle cells. The spindle cell component merges with the gland-forming component and is histologically low grade.

cells with clear cytoplasm, spindled cells (Figure 7.11), tubules and trabeculae resembling sex cord ovarian tumors (Figure 7.12), hyalinized and myxoid stroma (Figure 7.13), and, exceptionally, heterologous elements such as osteoid (Figure 7.14) and lobules of cartilage. Finally, differentiated endometrioid adenocarcinomas can undergo dedifferentiation, which results in a tumor showing both gland formation and sheets of undifferentiated tumor. This will be discussed in more detail subsequently.

Therapy-related changes

Endocrine therapy, particularly treatment with the progestin, Megace (megestrol acetate), has been suggested as an alternative to hysterectomy for patients with well-differentiated endometrioid adenocarcinomas who desire fertility preservation. Complete response to Megace results in stromal pseudodecidualization with atrophic glands that sometimes display a variety of metaplastic changes[11]. Incomplete responses usually result in residual foci of back-to-back glands in a background of pseudo-decidua (Figure 7.15). Residual adenocarcinoma retains cytologic atypia and glandular architectural complexity, and frequently demonstrates cytoplasmic eosinophilia. Biopsies taken to detect response to progestational therapy should be reviewed in concert with pre-treatment biopsies.

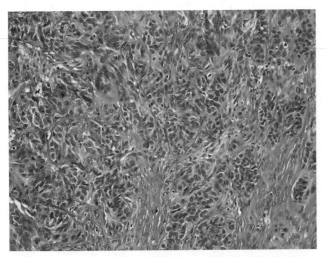

Figure 7.12 Endometrioid adenocarcinoma with sex cord–like features. This example recalls the appearance of adult granulosa cell tumor or Sertoli cell tumor.

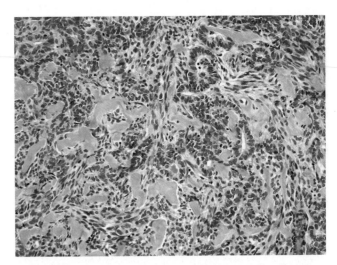

Figure 7.13 Endometrioid adenocarcinoma with spindle cells and hyalinized stroma.

(A)

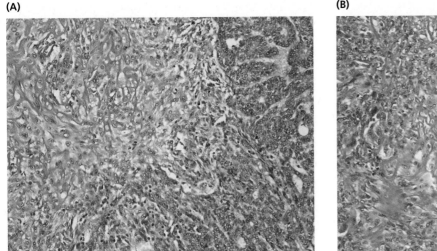

(B)

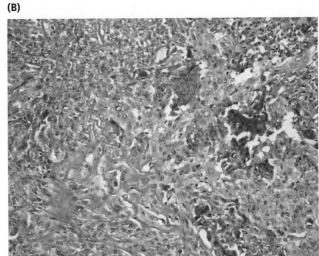

Figure 7.14 Endometrioid adenocarcinoma with hyalinized stroma resembling metaplastic osteoid (A, B), associated with osteoclast-like giant cells (B). Metaplastic bone and cartilage in this context does not necessarily signify the presence of malignant mixed mullerian tumor.

Changes attributable to radiation may be seen in endometrial samples following radiation therapy for cervical or rectal carcinomas. Radiation therapy is also rarely used for primary treatment of endometrial carcinoma when patients are suboptimal candidates for surgery. Radiation changes to neoplastic and non-neoplastic endometrium resemble those commonly encountered in other organs: cellular enlargement with retention of nuclear-to-cytoplasmic ratios, vacuolated cytoplasm, and enlarged, hyperchromatic nuclei (Figure 7.16). Attention to the architectural features of gland crowding and complexity, rather than cytologic atypia alone, should allow the distinction of radiated adenocarcinoma and non-neoplastic

endometrium with radiation atypia. Stromal changes include hyalinization and the presence of sclerotic blood vessels. Immunohistochemistry with p53 and MIB1 can also be used if the differential diagnosis includes serous carcinoma.

Tumor grading

Current practice standards indicate that endometrioid adenocarcinomas should be assigned a FIGO grade by assessing the degree of glandular differentiation (Figures 7.17–7.19) (Table 7.2): grade 1 shows ≤ 5% of solid non-glandular, non-squamous growth; grade 2 is defined by finding between 6 and 50% of solid non-glandular, non-squamous

(A)

(B)

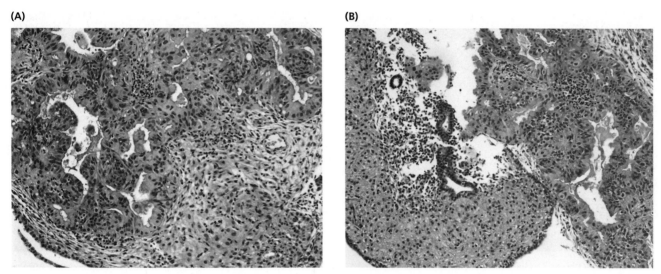

Figure 7.15 Residual endometrioid adenocarcinoma following treatment with progestins (A, B). Glandular complexity is retained, but the cytoplasm is more abundant and eosinophilic as compared to untreated tumor. Note background stromal decidualization (A, B) and residual, non-neoplastic atrophic endometrium (B).

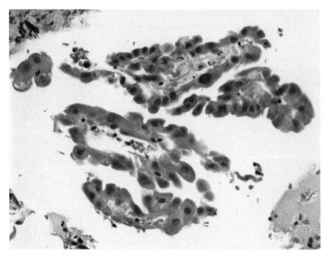

Figure 7.16 Radiation atypia in an endometrial curettage from a patient treated for rectal carcinoma. Note cyto- and nucleomegaly. The nuclei have a smudged, degenerative appearance.

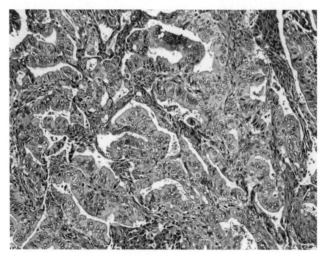

Figure 7.17 International Federation of Gynecology and Obstetrics (FIGO) grade 1 endometrioid adenocarcinoma. The tumor is gland-forming and lacks solid growth. The nuclear grade is 2 on a 3-point scale.

growth; and grade 3 by containing over 50% of solid non-glandular, non-squamous growth. The presence of marked cytologic atypia increases the grade by one[3]. Since many pathologists consider mucinous adenocarcinomas of the endometrium to be closely related to endometrioid adenocarcinomas, it is reasonable to use FIGO grades for those carcinomas as well. However, FIGO grading should not be used when endometrioid or mucinous differentiation is in doubt or cannot be established. All of the other endometrial tumor types carry an intrinsic tumor grade (i.e., serous and clear cell carcinomas are high grade). Gilks' grading scheme can be used if the tumor type is

uncertain (see **Hybrid tumors** in Chapter 8). Strategies for grading mixed epithelial tumors are unresolved, but it is our practice to grade these based on the most aggressive component.

FIGO grades are not always clearly separable in practice. Many pathologists consider tight, small microacini with barely visible lumens as solid growth (Figure 7.20), which means that a significant amount of this in an endometrioid tumor usually leads to classification as FIGO grade 2 or 3. As stated in the FIGO criteria, squamous differentiation should be discounted as evidence of solid growth, but there are inevitable problems with grading

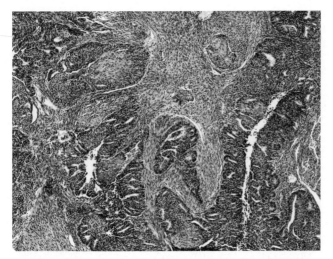

Figure 7.18 FIGO grade 2 endometrioid adenocarcinoma. The tumor features glands, solid, non-squamous components, and focal squamous differentiation. The nuclear grade is 2 on a 3-point scale.

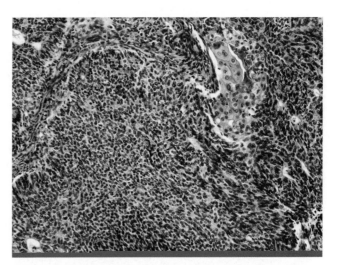

Figure 7.19 FIGO grade 3 endometrioid adenocarcinoma. The tumor has a predominant solid, non-squamous component and minor components of glands and squamous differentiation. The nuclear grade is 2 on a 3-point scale. The carcinoma can be recognized as endometrioid because of a focal glandular component and the presence of mature squamous differentiation. The solid component features nests of cohesive cells that resemble non-keratinizing, poorly differentiated squamous cell carcinoma.

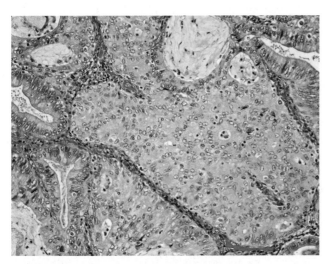

Figure 7.20 FIGO grade 2 endometrioid adenocarcinoma. This tumor is composed mostly of well-formed glands, but the presence of tiny microacini usually prompts a diagnosis of grade 2 adenocarcinoma.

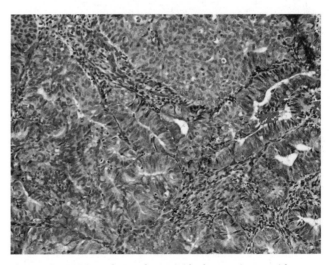

Figure 7.21 FIGO grade 1 endometrioid adenocarcinoma with morules. The presence of solid areas composed of morules or squamous metaplasia does not affect FIGO grade.

tumors with solid growth that resembles immature squamous metaplasia, and tumors that feature fusions between non-keratinizing squamous metaplasia and spindle cell change. It is reasonable to adjudicate these types of cases by paying attention to the nuclear grade, first in the glandular component and then, if that is not informative, in the solid component (Figure 7.21). We usually assign a tumor FIGO grade 3 if the solid areas resemble poorly differentiated non-keratinizing squamous cell carcinoma (Figure 7.19).

Another common problem concerns the degree and extent of nuclear atypia that is sufficient to upgrade a tumor from one FIGO category to another. The philosophy underlying our approach to this problem is that discordance between architectural grade and nuclear grade should be uncommon in endometrioid adenocarcinomas. The first step is to assure oneself that the nuclear features are sufficiently atypical. An easy guideline is to ask, "Is this focus easily appreciated on scanning or intermediate power examination?" and "Is the atypia so bad that I would consider it grade 3 on a 3-point scale?" (Figure 7.22)[3]. If the answers are "yes," sample the tumor extensively to

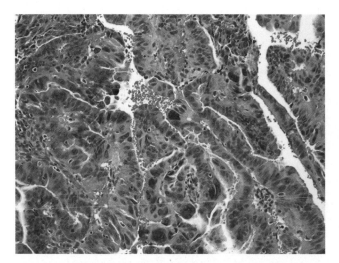

Figure 7.22 This endometrioid adenocarcinoma demonstrates a focus with obvious nuclear enlargement and pleomorphism. This degree of nuclear atypia is sufficient to upgrade an endometrioid adenocarcinoma from one grade to the next. If the component with high nuclear grade constitutes more than 10% of the tumor and demonstrates features that suggest a nonendometrioid component, consider a diagnosis of mixed epithelial carcinoma.

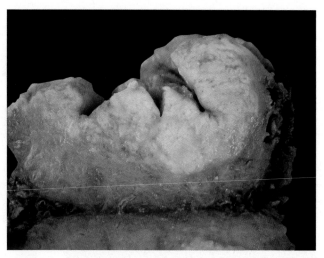

Figure 7.23 Myoinvasion in the uterus may be subtle, but can often be recognized by the presence of slightly firmer, gray-white tissue irregularly extending into the pink myometrium.

determine whether the finding is limited to only a few glands. If the change is diffuse, it is advisable to at least question whether part or all of the tumor could be a serous carcinoma or a clear cell carcinoma, instead of an endometrioid carcinoma (see pages 168–169). It is acceptable to move such a tumor from one FIGO grade to another only after assuring that the tumor is indeed endometrioid throughout. A mixed epithelial carcinoma with an endometrioid component should be diagnosed when the cytologically atypical area is determined to be serous or clear cell on further study (see pages 171–172). One should hesitate to upgrade endometrioid adenocarcinomas containing only a few glands with atypical nuclei; especially if it took a prolonged search at high power magnification to recognize them.

Tumor staging

The current FIGO system for staging endometrial cancers accounts for the depth of myometrial invasion, cervical involvement, extrauterine pelvic disease, and extrauterine extrapelvic disease (Table 7.3). The most difficult issues for practicing pathologists involve diagnosing myometrial invasion, measuring the depth of myometrial invasion, determining cervical involvement and the difference between endocervical mucosal and stromal invasion, and whether tumors involving ovaries, fallopian tubes, or endometriosis represent metastatic

endometrial carcinoma or synchronous carcinoma. Pathologists are also facing emerging problems that have arisen as a result of the increasing performance of lymph node dissections; these problems involve the recognition of micrometastases and isolated tumor cells and the techniques used to detect them. The 2009 changes to the FIGO staging system may alleviate some of the problems concerning measurement of the depth of myometrial invasion and determination of cervical involvement[12].

Myometrial invasion

A variety of non-invasive patterns may be misinterpreted as myometrial invasion, on both macroscopic and microscopic examination. The most common are exophytic tumors, irregular endomyometrial junction, and adenomyosis[13]. Macroscopic examination of the uterus can be especially difficult in the presence of adenomyosis during the intraoperative evaluation. Serial sections through the myometrium at 5 mm intervals to include cornua and lower uterine segment, with selected frozen sections of the most suspicious areas for invasion, are required to accurately provide an intraoperative assessment (Figure 7.23). Microscopically, the endomyometrial–myometrial interface in these situations should show surrounding or interglandular endometrial stroma, benign marker glands at the periphery, absence of surrounding desmoplasia, absence of an inflammatory infiltrate, and smooth, rounded contours (Figure 7.24). The criteria for invasion when faced with an irregular endomyometrial junction are the same as those that distinguish

(A)

(B)

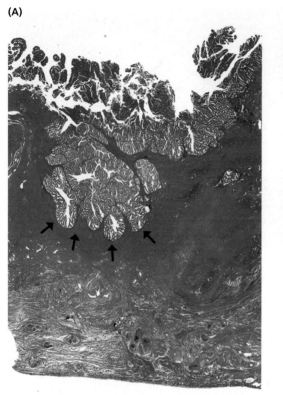

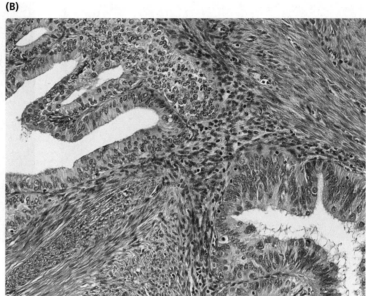

Figure 7.24 Irregular endomyometrial junction (A, B). Rounded contours, focally condensed endometrial stroma at the junction (B), and the absence of desmoplasia are against the presence of myometrial invasion.

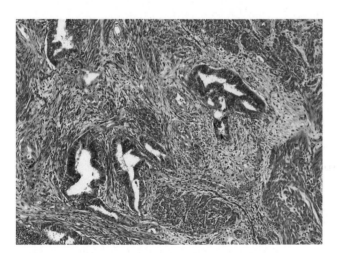

Figure 7.25 Myoinvasive endometrioid adenocarcinoma. Haphazardly arranged and angulated glands with surrounding stromal desmoplasia are evident.

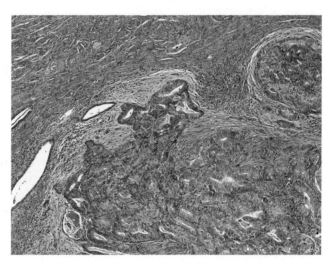

Figure 7.26 Myoinvasive endometrioid adenocarcinoma. Desmoplasia is obvious at the invasive front of this endometrioid adenocarcinoma in the lower uterine segment.

invasive carcinoma and carcinoma involving adenomyosis. Myometrial invasion should be diagnosed when neoplastic epithelial cells are surrounded by myometrium without intervening endometrial stroma. The presence of both a jagged, infiltrative contour and an associated desmoplastic stromal reaction is usually encountered, but invasion can still be diagnosed when either is present, as long as the epithelial elements are not surrounded by endometrial stroma (Figures 7.25 and 7.26). It should be noted that endometrial stroma frequently loses its dense, blue appearance, and thereby mimics the appearance of myometrium; the problem is particularly difficult when the remaining stroma at the myometrial interface is attenuated. In these cases, the stroma usually exhibits poorly formed fascicles of eosinophilic, vaguely fibrillar spindle cells without organized, thick muscle bundles, similar to what is commonly seen in endometrial polyps with pink, fibrillary stroma (Figure 7.27). This pattern should be distinguished from myometrium, in which well-formed fascicles and thick muscle bundles are apparent. These thick muscle bundles are particularly obvious in myometrium surrounding foci of adenomyosis, which can serve as a low-power clue to the presence of adenomyosis, especially when endometrial stroma is sparse and/or eosinophilic.

The depth of myometrial invasion cannot always be reported with complete certainty. When confronted with an exophytic endometrial carcinoma, identifying the adjacent endomyometrial junction can assist in measuring the depth of myometrial invasion (Diagram 7.1). The macroscopic characteristics are also frequently contributory. If one

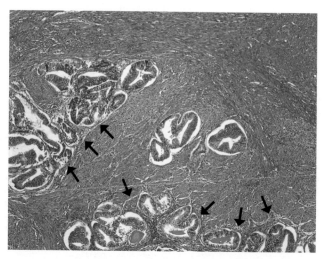

Figure 7.27 Complex atypical hyperplasia colonizing adenomyosis. The endometrial stroma is attenuated, eosinophilic, and fibrillary (arrows), mimicking the appearance of myometrium. Note rounded bands of surrounding hypertrophic myometrium. This finding can be used to support a diagnosis of adenomyosis when endometrial stroma is sparse or altered.

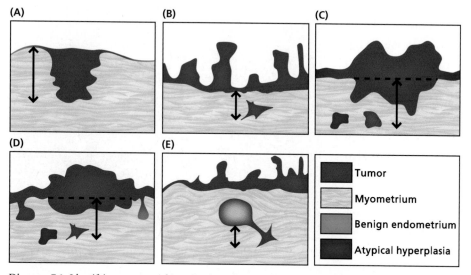

Diagram 7.1 Identifying myometrial invasion in endometrial cancer is based on the presence of irregular permeation into the myometrium. (A) Direct invasion from the endometrium is the most recognizable and reproducible form of invasion, particularly when the advancing front is jagged and associated with a stromal response. In this situation, the depth of invasion is measured from the nearest adjacent uninvolved endometrial–myometrial junction to the deepest focus of invasion. The thickness of the myometrium is measured similarly (i.e., from the nearest junction of the endometrium and myometrium to the serosa). (B) Discontinuous myometrial invasion; ensure discontinuous focus is invasive (illustrated as having spiculated contours), not adenomyosis colonized by carcinoma (illustrated as having rounded contours; see panels C-E). (C and D) Depth of invasion in these cases is measured from a virtual plane whose location is estimated from the adjacent endomyometrial junction. In C, the invasive focus is represented by a broad, pushing front, a pattern that is difficult to evaluate. It can often be recognized by the presence of a more fibrous stroma in response to the invasive glands. In D, the invasive focus is mostly discontinuous; the discontinuous focus of myometrial invasion can be distinguished from adenomyosis because of its spiculated shape. Histologically, the lack of endometrial stroma and presence of surrounding desmoplasia are the two most helpful features that indicate myometrial invasion is present. (E) Rarely, carcinoma may arise in adenomyosis or invade from a deep focus of adenomyosis. In this situation, the depth of invasion should be measured from the junction of the adenomyosis and myometrium to the deepest area of invasive carcinoma.

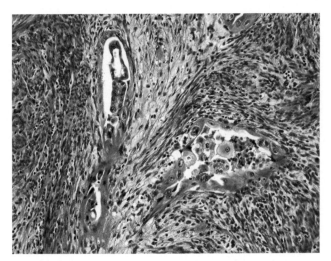

Figure 7.28 Myoinvasive endometrioid adenocarcinoma with a microcystic, elongated and fragmented pattern (MELF). Note histiocyte-like tumor cells, attenuated and squamous metaplastic tumor cells, periglandular stromal pallor, and aggregates of neutrophils.

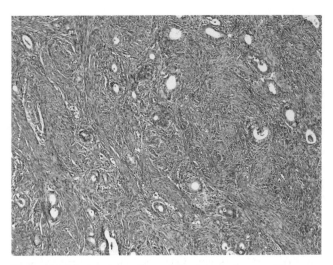

Figure 7.29 Myoinvasive endometrioid adenocarcinoma with an "adenoma malignum–like" pattern. Well-differentiated endometrioid glands are dispersed throughout the myometrium and are unassociated with a desmoplastic host response.

cannot reliably distinguish an irregular endomyometrial junction from true superficial myometrial invasion, it is best to discuss the uncertainty with the gynecologist. We are not aware of guidelines for staging endometrial cancers in which invasion is only found deep in the myometrium adjacent to foci of adenomyosis. It has been our practice to describe the morphologic findings in the pathology report and emphasize that, while the clinical significance is not known with certainty, we think the behavior of such tumors is more akin to superficially invasive carcinoma than to deeply invasive carcinoma.

Certain patterns of myoinvasive endometrial carcinomas may pose diagnostic problems. Patterns that can conceptually present difficulties with measurements of the depth of myometrial invasion are the microcystic, elongated, and fragmented (MELF) pattern (Figure 7.28)[14], the adenoma malignum pattern (Figure 7.29)[15], and the pushing pattern. The MELF pattern is characterized by attenuated neoplastic cells with a squamoid or vacuolated appearance lining small, elongated glands containing neutrophils and denuded neoplastic cells. Foci of MELF invasion are commonly surrounded by pale and inflamed reactive tissue. The reaction to invasion is frequently much more obvious, particularly at low-power examination, than are the invasive epithelial cells. The MELF pattern is treacherous because the invasive epithelial cells may be inapparent, leading to a diagnosis of non-invasive adenocarcinoma. Other common problems include similarities between the appearance of MELF invasion and lymphovascular

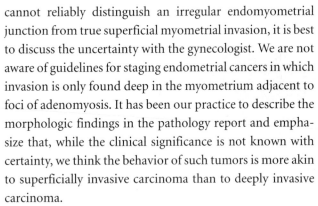

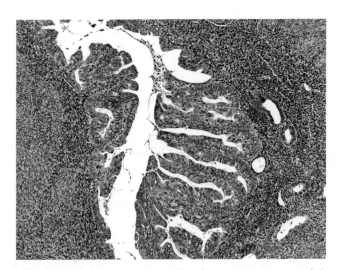

Figure 7.30 Adenomyosis colonized by adenocarcinoma, surrounded by myometrial hypertrophy.

invasion, and finding MELF invasion foci deep in myometrium, apparently discontinuous with the endomyometrial junction, and in some cases adjacent to foci of deeply placed adenomyosis colonized by adenocarcinoma (Figure 7.30). Microcystic, elongated, and fragmented invasion is also thought to be associated with high rates of lymphovascular invasion. The adenoma malignum pattern of invasion[10] describes well-differentiated, neoplastic, tubular endometrioid glands that invade myometrium without an obvious stromal response. Recognition of invasion is facilitated by the abnormal density of glands, a jagged invasive front, and the absence of endometrial stroma – eosinophilic, fibrillary, or otherwise – surrounding glands. The differential diagnosis usually includes a very deeply placed and irregular endomyometrial junction, and extensive stroma-poor adenomyosis. In the pushing pattern, the tumor invades the myometrium in a broad front. It may be difficult to diagnose these carcinomas as invasive unless there is a desmoplastic reaction at the advancing edge. Mimics of this pattern include very irregular endomyometrial junctions, and tumor involvement of adenomyosis, neither of which shows a desmoplastic reaction at its periphery.

Lymphovascular invasion

Lymphovascular invasion is an important determinant of lymph node metastasis and is currently considered part of the risk stratification scheme used to determine which patients with low-stage endometrial cancer should be treated with chemotherapy. Although assessment of lymphovascular invasion is not required for stage assignment, a surgical pathology report lacking this information is generally considered incomplete. Evaluation for the presence of lymphovascular invasion should be undertaken at the advancing edge of an invasive endometrial carcinoma and deeper within the myometrium. The significance of lymphovascular invasion within the main tumor mass is uncertain, especially when the tumor is well differentiated and only minimally myoinvasive. Lymphovascular invasion can sometimes be associated with perivascular lymphoid aggregates, which can serve as a low-power clue to its presence. Lymphovascular invasion should be diagnosed when neoplastic cells are present within an endothelial-cell-lined space and contamination can be excluded with reasonable certainty (see below). In most cases, neoplastic cells within the lymphovascular spaces resemble the predominant cell type found within the tumor (Figure 7.31A); however, in some cases, tumor cells within lymphovascular spaces have more abundant cytoplasm and/or different nuclear features (Figure 7.31B). This is particularly true of lymphovascular invasion associated with MELF invasion.

Distinguishing true lymphovascular invasion from artifactual displacement of tumor cells within vascular lumens can be challenging. Recent work has indicated that certain types of laparoscopic assisted hysterectomies[16,17] and robot assisted hysterectomies lead to disruption of otherwise intact tumors, which results in artifactual displacement of tumor cells (Figure 7.31C). Intravascular adenomyosis is another mimic of lymphovascular invasion (Figure 7.31D). Features that favor contamination are listed in Table 7.5.

Immunohistochemical markers of endothelial differentiation, CD34 and CD31, and the lymphatic endothelial marker podoplanin (D2-40) can be used to verify the presence of a vascular space containing a tumor embolus. The contribution of these tests regarding their association with lymph node metastases and prognosis has not been extensively studied in endometrial cancer.

Cervical involvement

Clinically and grossly obvious cervical involvement by an endometrial carcinoma is easy to appreciate, but detecting microscopic involvement can be challenging (Diagram 7.2)[18,19]. The most common problem concerns the lack of anatomic boundaries that separate corpus and cervix. Cervical involvement can be reported when there is endocervical epithelium proximal to a focus of carcinoma (Figure 7.32). It may therefore be difficult to assess cervical involvement if normal-appearing endocervical-type glands are sparse, such as when there is extensive tubal or tuboendometrioid metaplasia in the upper endocervix. In this case, re-examine the specimen and submit additional tissue that is grossly suspicious for cervical involvement. It would be impossible to make a confident diagnosis of cervical involvement if this was unsuccessful. That being said, there are no convincing clinical reasons that should influence a pathologist to establish a diagnosis of cervical involvement when that diagnosis is in doubt (i.e., there aren't compelling reasons to err on the side of calling cervical involvement when it is not obvious). Furthermore, interobserver variability in diagnosing cervical involvement and distinguishing mucosal from stromal invasion is far from optimal[20]. Revisions to the FIGO staging system have eliminated the need to distinguish involvement of endometrium and endocervical mucosa[12].

The next challenge concerns the distinction of endocervical mucosal and cervical stromal invasion[19], as the boundary between these compartments is neither well demarcated nor anatomically well defined. Surface tumor deposits, tumor colonizing pre-existing endocervical glands, and lobulated aggregates of tumor that could be construed as having expanded and distorted endocervical glands can be confidently diagnosed as endocervical mucosal involvement if the contour at the base of the proliferation is rounded and not jaggedly infiltrative (Figure 7.33). Tumors that replace glands with attenuation of intervening stroma in the superficial zones of the endocervix are usually called "mucosal involvement" (and not stromal invasion) when the tumor is well differentiated and the base of the proliferation is rounded and smooth. Jagged invasion of stroma between glands is sometimes diagnosed as mucosal invasion and sometimes as stromal invasion. Any irregular interface with stroma beneath endocervical glands usually results in a diagnosis of cervical stromal invasion (Figure 7.34).

Table 7.5 Characteristics of artifactual displacement of intravascular tumor cells[a]

The number of affected vessels is disproportionate given the tumor grade and depth of myometrial invasion

Both superficial and deep vessels are involved

Vessels both adjacent to and distant from the main tumor mass are involved

Capillaries, veins, and arterioles are all involved

Intravascular tumor cells are admixed with non-neoplastic elements, including benign epithelium and stroma

[a] Not considered true lymphovascular invasion.

It should be noted that the same range of invasion patterns described in myometrium can be encountered in cervical stroma. Of particular relevance here is the adenoma malignum pattern of endometrioid adenocarcinoma, as discussed above (Figure 7.35). As this pattern features extremely well-differentiated glands without an associated stromal response, correct diagnosis rests on perceiving the abnormal clustering (arrangement) and depth of glands. When neoplastic glands are small and contain eosinophilic secretions, this pattern may resemble benign and hyperplastic mesonephric rests, and, when the neoplastic glands contain ciliated cells, tubal metaplasia becomes an obvious diagnostic trap[21]. Strategies for sorting out these problems are detailed elsewhere in the text (see Chapter 5). Be aware that, in some cases, cervical stromal invasion predominates over myometrial invasion, and that some endometrial

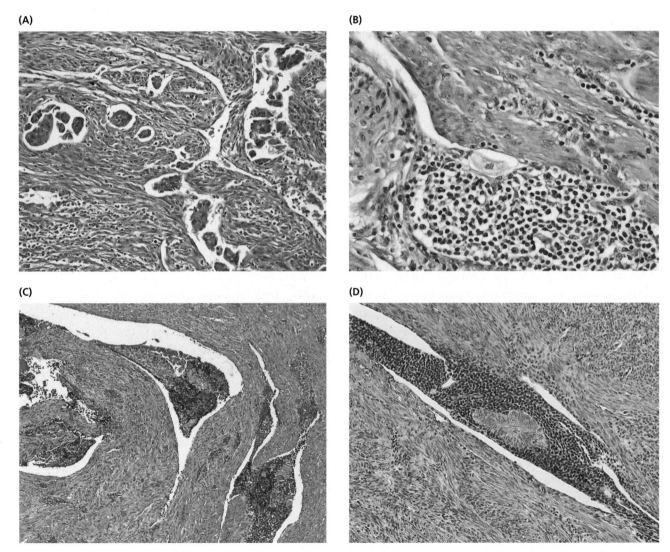

(A)

(B)

(C)

(D)

Figure 7.31 The appearance of lymphovascular invasion (A, B) contrasts with artifactual displacement of tumor and non-neoplastic elements (C) and intravascular adenomyosis (D). Panel B shows an intravascular histiocyte-like tumor cell, which can be seen in the presence of MELF invasion (Figure 7.28).

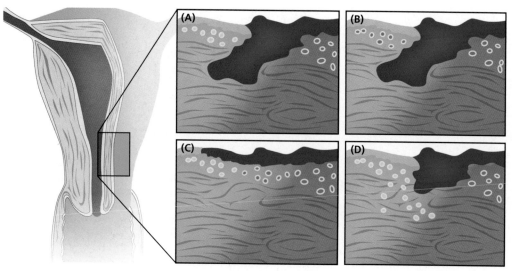

Diagram 7.2 Cervical stromal invasion by endometrial carcinoma. Endometrial glands, unlike endocervical glands, are depicted with blue centers. (A) Cervical stromal invasion must clearly involve endocervical stroma and not lower uterine segment. This is best depicted by the identification of carcinoma (not hyperplasia) within cervical stroma well below endocervical glands. (B) In this panel, endometrial carcinoma invades the lower uterine segment, but not the cervix. Note endometrial glands bordering either side of the invasive front. Because the myometrium in the lower uterine segment is often more fibrous in appearance than in the fundus, the distinction between cervical stroma and lower uterine segment can be difficult without glandular landmarks. (C) In this panel, the endometrial cancer involves the cervix, but does not extend beyond the superficial normal endocervical glands and so does not represent stromal invasion. We would consider this mucosal involvement, which is no longer featured in the current FIGO staging scheme. (D) In this panel, the adenocarcinoma extends beyond the level of the superficial cervical glands, but not beyond the deeper endocervical glands. Whether this pattern constitutes cervical stromal invasion is subject to interobserver disagreement. In the presence of substantial tumor involvement of cervical stroma at the depth depicted in this panel, we would classify this as stromal invasion.

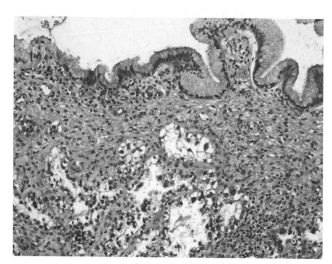

Figure 7.32 Clear cell carcinoma of endometrium involving cervix.

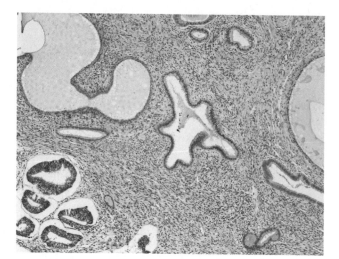

Figure 7.33 Endometrioid adenocarcinoma involving cervix without stromal invasion.

carcinomas that invade cervical stroma show only minimal evidence of tumor in the endometrium. The latter tumors are considered endometrial and not endocervical if an endometrial curettage was diagnostic of endometrioid adenocarcinoma and the histologic appearance and immunophenotype of the tumor in question were incompatible with endocervical adenocarcinoma.

It has been suggested that there are no significant differences in clinical outcome when comparing survival rates for patients with endometrioid adenocarcinoma

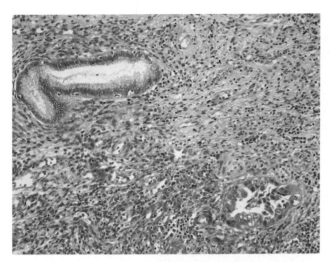

Figure 7.34 Endometrioid adenocarcinoma invading cervical stroma.

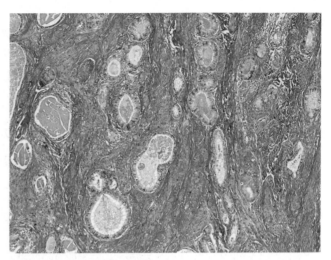

Figure 7.35 Endometrioid adenocarcinoma invading cervical stroma with a focal "adenoma malignum–like" pattern of invasion at center.

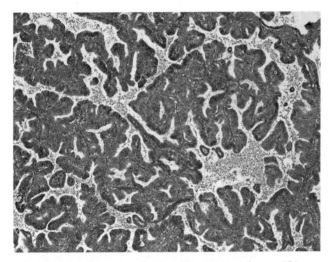

Figure 7.36 Synchronous endometrioid carcinoma of ovary. This primary endometrioid carcinoma of ovary shows expansile invasion without destructive stromal invasion.

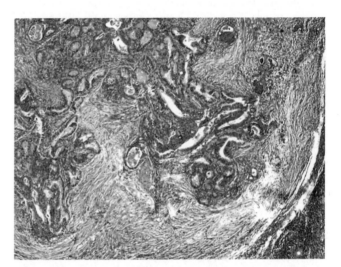

Figure 7.37 Metastatic endometrioid adenocarcinoma to ovary. Features favoring metastasis include deep myometrial invasion, ovarian surface involvement, and a nodular growth pattern with surrounding desmoplasia, illustrated here.

involving mucosa versus stroma[19]. When cervical involvement is present, survival rates are probably driven by tumor type, presence of lymphovascular invasion and depth of myometrial invasion. Many gynecologists will perform radical hysterectomy instead of simple hysterectomy if the cervix is known to be involved preoperatively.

Synchronous and metastatic carcinomas

The younger the endometrial cancer patient, the more likely it is that she harbors a synchronous ovarian carcinoma. In some series, up to one-quarter of endometrial cancer patients less than 40 years of age have synchronous ovarian endometrioid adenocarcinomas[22,23]. At least two categories of tumors can be confidently interpreted as synchronous. The first is a non-invasive or minimally invasive, well-differentiated endometrioid carcinoma of endometrium with coincident complex atypical hyperplasia and a well-differentiated endometrioid carcinoma of ovary with coincident endometriosis or endometrioid adenofibromatous tumor, but without ovarian surface involvement (Figure 7.36). The second concerns endometrial and ovarian tumors of clearly different grades and histologic types. At the other end of the spectrum are the obviously metastatic tumors: deeply invasive, high-grade endometrial carcinomas with multiple ovarian tumor nodules, including ovarian surface deposits (endometrial primary with metastasis to ovary) (Figure 7.37); the occasional, massive ovarian, tubal, or peritoneal carcinoma with small "drop metastases" to the endometrium (ovarian

(A)

(B)

(C)

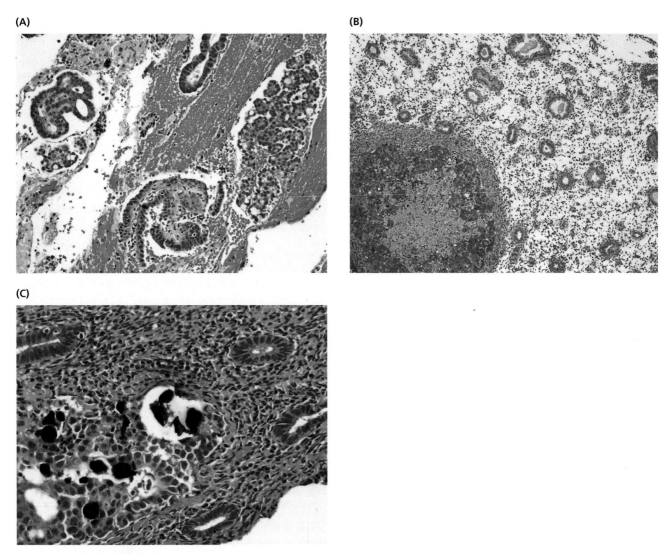

Figure 7.38 Drop metastasis from ovarian serous carcinoma to endometrium. This endometrial curettage (A) contains glandular and papillary fragments of tumor in a background of atrophic endometrium. Hysterectomy failed to reveal carcinoma in the endometrium; salpingo-oophorectomy disclosed large, bilateral, high-grade ovarian serous carcinomas with tubal involvement. Secretory endometrium with a drop metastasis is seen in B, and low-grade serous carcinoma metastatic to atrophic endometrium is illustrated in C.

primary with metastasis to endometrium) (Figure 7.38); and an endometrial serous carcinoma, arising in an endometrial polyp with a serous carcinoma involving ovary, fallopian tube, and peritoneum (favor endometrial primary with metastasis to ovary). Details concerning the latter are provided in Chapter 8.

Scenarios other than the ones described above are common, and this is unfortunate because it can be difficult or impossible to determine whether the tumors are synchronous. In these situations, it is recommended to provide the clinicians with a list of features for and against metastasis (Tables 7.6, 7.7, and 7.8), a comment regarding which features predominate, and, based on that, an indication of whether one possibility is favored over the other.

Table 7.6 Characteristics of synchronous primary tumors of uterus and ovary or fallopian tube

Endometrial tumor is well differentiated and either non-invasive or minimally invasive

No lymphovascular invasion is present

No serous tubal intraepithelial carcinoma is present

Ovarian tumor is associated with endometriosis or endometrioid adenofibromatous tumor

Endometrial and ovarian tumors may be histologically similar or dissimilar[a]

[a] Many synchronous tumors are endometrioid and well differentiated in both organs. These are not interpreted as metastatic if the endometrial tumor is either non-invasive or minimally invasive, the ovarian tumor is associated with an endometrioid adenofibromatous tumor, and/or the ovarian carcinoma is not present on the ovarian surface.

Features in favor of metastasis from uterus to ovary include: poor differentiation in the endometrial tumor; deep myometrial invasion; prominent lymphovascular invasion in uterus and ovarian hilum; ovarian tumor multinodularity and multifocality; absence of endometriosis and endometrioid adenofibroma; presence of destructive stromal invasion in ovary; presence of ovarian surface involvement. Consider an ovarian, peritoneal, or tubal primary when the volume of disease involving ovary or peritoneum greatly exceeds that in endometrium, or when tubal intraepithelial carcinoma is obvious.

Keratin deposition on peritoneal surfaces, usually involving a granulomatous reaction (Figure 7.39) can be misinterpreted as metastatic carcinoma, but neoplastic tumor cells are not identified.

Table 7.7 Characteristics of metastatic endometrial carcinoma to ovary or fallopian tube

Endometrial tumor is moderately or poorly differentiated and more than minimally invasive

Lymphovascular invasion is present

Ovarian tumor is unassociated with endometriosis or endometrioid adenofibromatous tumor and involves the ovarian surface

Endometrial and ovarian tumors are histologically similar[a]

[a] Many endometrioid carcinomas of endometrium metastasize to the ovaries. These must be distinguished from synchronous, well-differentiated endometrioid carcinomas of endometrium and ovary as outlined in Table 7.6.

Lymph nodes

Carcinomas demonstrating the microcystic, elongated, and fragmented pattern (MELF) of myometrial invasion are frequently associated with lymphovascular invasion and tiny deposits of carcinoma in lymph nodes that resemble histiocytes[24] – this is an obvious application of the use of keratin stains to confirm epithelial differentiation and the presence of rare, single tumor cells in lymph node sinuses (Figure 7.40). Keratin stains have also been studied in the setting of sentinel lymph node evaluation, but this does not currently constitute the standard of care. Additional details were presented earlier in the chapter under **Sentinel lymph node mapping**.

Table 7.8 Characteristics of metastatic ovarian or tubal carcinoma[a]

Endometrial tumor is present in the setting of cycling endometrium

Endometrial tumor deposits are small and multifocal and unassociated with an endometrial polyp

Serous tubal intraepithelial carcinoma is present

[a] Pertains mostly to serous carcinoma.

ANCILLARY DIAGNOSTIC TESTS

The immunophenotype of endometrioid carcinoma varies with degrees and types of differentiation (Table 7.9). Endometrioid adenocarcinomas coexpress pan-cytokeratins and vimentin and only rarely show diffuse cytoplasmic staining with carcinoembryonic antigen. Almost all endometrioid neoplasms express CK7 and are largely negative for CK20.

(A)

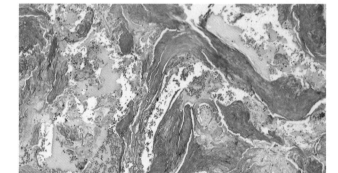

(B)

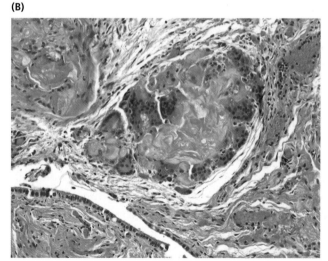

Figure 7.39 Keratin deposition on peritoneal surfaces (A, B) is frequently associated with a granulomatous reaction (B). This should not be misinterpreted as metastatic carcinoma when tumor cells are not present.

(A)

(B)

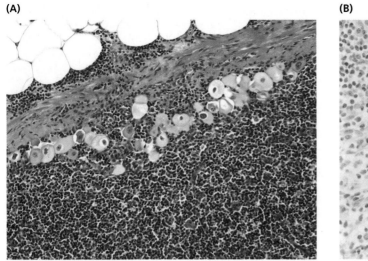
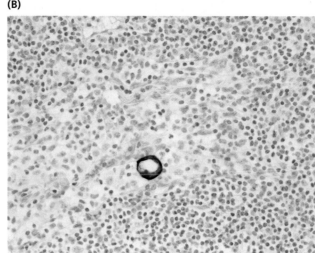

Figure 7.40 Histiocyte-like metastatic endometrioid adenocarcinoma to pelvic lymph node (A, B). In contrast to sinus histiocytes, tumor cells are larger, have more abundant cytoplasm, feature a surrounding halo or clear space, and are keratin positive (B).

Table 7.9 Immunophenotype of endometrioid adenocarcinoma (selected markers)

	Progesterone receptor (PR)	p53	p16
FIGO 1 and 2	+++	+	+
FIGO 3	+	++	++
Serous	−	+++	+++
Clear cell	−	++	++

Symbols: −, negative; +, low level expression/rare cases positive; ++, moderate expression/rare cases show diffuse positivity/overexpression; +++, diffuse positivity/overexpression.

Other commonly expressed antigens include CA125, Ber-EP4, and B72.3. The expression of estrogen and progesterone receptors is almost constant among FIGO grade 1 adenocarcinomas, but this feature is present in a minority of FIGO grade 3 tumors. Overexpression of p53 (expression in greater than 50–75% of nuclei) is seen in a minority of FIGO grade 3 adenocarcinomas, but almost never in FIGO grade 1 tumors[25,26]. The expression of p16 also tends to accumulate with increasing histologic grade[27]. High-molecular-weight cytokeratins, p63, and nuclear β-catenin are preferentially expressed in areas demonstrating squamous differentiation.

DIFFERENTIAL DIAGNOSIS

The differential diagnosis of uterine endometrioid adenocarcinoma includes other uterine carcinomas such as serous and clear cell carcinomas. Immunohistochemical

Table 7.10 Differential diagnosis of endometrioid adenocarcinoma

Complex atypical hyperplasia

Atypical polypoid adenomyoma

Serous carcinoma (both primary and metastatic)

Clear cell carcinoma

Microglandular hyperplasia of cervix

Undifferentiated carcinoma

Transitional cell carcinoma

Squamous cell carcinoma

Small cell neuroendocrine carcinoma

Carcinosarcoma (malignant mixed mullerian tumor)

Uterine tumor resembling ovarian sex cord tumor (UTROSCT)

Mesonephric adenocarcinoma

Metastatic colorectal adenocarcinoma

Alveolar soft part sarcoma

Epithelioid leiomyosarcoma

Endocervical adenocarcinoma

Primitive neuroectodermal tumor

strategies for distinguishing between these entities are summarized in Table 7.9. Other common problems in diagnosis involve the distinction of complex atypical hyperplasia from endometrioid adenocarcinoma, endocervical from endometrial adenocarcinoma, and carcinosarcoma from endometrioid adenocarcinoma (Table 7.10).

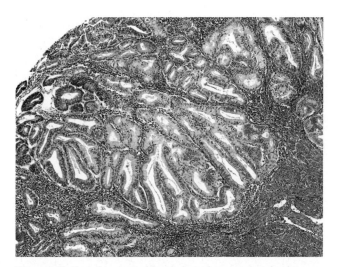

Figure 7.41 Complex atypical hyperplasia demonstrates closely spaced glands with retained interglandular stroma. Extensively fused glands are not present. This pattern is similar to that seen in Gleason pattern 3 prostatic adenocarcinoma.

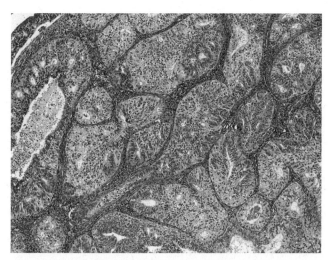

Figure 7.42 Endometrioid adenocarcinoma. Despite the presence of interglandular stroma, the glands are large and have substantial internal complexity (so-called macroglands). This pattern is similar to that seen in Gleason pattern 4 prostatic adenocarcinoma. Compare with Figure 7.41.

(A)

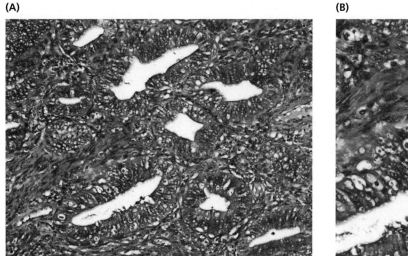

(B)

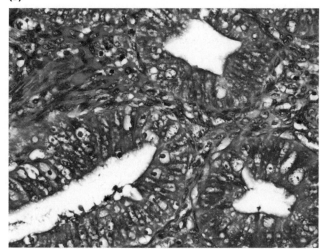

Figure 7.43 (A, B) Endometrial adenocarcinoma. Despite the presence of interglandular stroma, the neoplastic epithelium here demonstrates severely atypical nuclear features that are incompatible with a diagnosis of complex atypical hyperplasia. This degree of atypia should raise concern for serous carcinoma.

Complex atypical hyperplasia

Complex atypical hyperplasia and well-differentiated (FIGO grade 1) endometrial endometrioid carcinoma are both differentiated neoplasms, so endometrioid tubular glands generally predominate in both (Figure 7.41) (Table 7.11). Conceptually, adenocarcinoma is separated from hyperplasia by finding evidence of endometrial stromal invasion[28]. Since the morphologic features of a reaction to invasion in the endometrial stroma are non-specific, the presence of exuberant epithelial growth that excludes endometrial stroma is sufficient to categorize a lesion as

adenocarcinoma in practice. Examples of exuberant epithelial growth (Figure 7.42) include: extensive confluent papillae; so-called macroglands; and cribriform gland formations[28,29]. Marked cytologic atypia also disqualifies a diagnosis of hyperplasia (Figure 7.43)[29]. Some tumors that resemble complex atypical hyperplasia with marked cytologic atypia are found to be endometrioid adenocarcinomas on hysterectomy, whereas others are serous carcinomas, and yet others are endocervical adenocarcinomas.

Hyperplastic lesions with superimposed metaplasia can be diagnostically challenging. Hyperplasia with extensive

Table 7.11 Distinguishing characteristics of low-grade endometrioid adenocarcinoma (versus atypical hyperplasia) – see Diagram 7.3

Epithelial proliferations that obliterate endometrial stroma[a]

- Cribriform structures involving large glands
- Confluent glands with a cribriform-like pattern (fused glands)
- Confluent glands with a maze-like pattern
- Complex papillary growth (papillae [primary papillae] supporting branched papillae [secondary or tertiary papillae])

Severe nuclear atypia, even focal[b]

[a] The risk of coincident adenocarcinoma in a follow-up hysterectomy specimen is higher when these epithelial proliferations are prominent. Most pathologists diagnose "adenocarcinoma" when more than 30% of the lesion is an epithelial proliferation that obliterates endometrial stroma or when these epithelial proliferations measure over 2 mm.

[b] Diffuse nuclear atypia should trigger consideration for endocervical adenocarcinoma when the patient is pre- or perimenopausal, and serous or clear cell carcinoma when the patient is postmenopausal.

morular metaplasia can be difficult to distinguish from adenocarcinoma because the morules commonly efface the underlying glandular architecture. We favor a diagnosis of complex atypical hyperplasia when glands lacking morules are not fused and when the nuclear grade of the glandular component is 1 on a 3-point scale. Pure mucinous carcinomas and endometrioid adenocarcinoma with extensive mucinous differentiation usually appear highly differentiated, leading to confusion with microglandular hyperplasia of the endocervix, discussed subsequently, and complex atypical hyperplasia with mucinous metaplasia (see Chapter 9). Significant nuclear atypia (beyond that of atypical endometrial hyperplasia – which is admittedly highly subjective), or cribriform and extensive papillary growth patterns favor adenocarcinoma.

Two types of lesions exhibit features that fall just short of an unqualified diagnosis of adenocarcinoma: small lesions with well-developed architectural complexity (i.e., tiny carcinomas; Figure 7.44) and lesions that display some architectural complexity (i.e., lesions with some features of hyperplasia and some of carcinoma). Both the Kurman and Norris[28] and Stanford criteria[29] for well-differentiated endometrial carcinoma specify a quantitative limit (1.9 mm and 30%, respectively) below which adenocarcinoma is not diagnosed. The reason behind this is that tiny carcinomas diagnosed in biopsy or curettage material are much less likely than larger carcinomas to manifest either residual carcinoma or, more importantly, deep myometrial invasive carcinoma on hysterectomy. Despite this, there is a

small risk of myometrial invasive carcinoma on follow-up. Some pathologists diagnose these cases as "small foci of endometrioid adenocarcinoma in a background of complex atypical hyperplasia," but we tend to use the terminology "complex atypical hyperplasia bordering on carcinoma." Other pathologists subclassify complex atypical hyperplasia into subtypes or use the term, "adenocarcinoma in situ," to denote that these lesions are at higher risk of residual carcinoma on follow-up as compared to typical examples of complex atypical hyperplasia. Lesions showing some, but not all, of the features of carcinoma are also at higher risk of residual carcinoma on follow-up as compared to cases of straightforward complex atypical hyperplasia. We use the term "complex atypical hyperplasia bordering on carcinoma" for these as well.

Atypical polypoid adenomyoma

Atypical polypoid adenomyoma is a polypoid lesion with muscular or fibromuscular stroma that harbors a proliferation resembling complex atypical hyperplasia, frequently with morular metaplasia (Figure 7.45)[30]. Most lesions are exophytic, but occasional lesions are endophytic. Both exophytic and endophytic lesions sometimes appear concerning for myometrial-invasive carcinoma, especially to those unfamiliar with the entity. One should avoid suggesting the presence of myometrial-invasive carcinoma in biopsy and curettage material since these specimens almost never yield sufficient myometrium for evaluation; furthermore, both adenocarcinoma involving a polyp and atypical polypoid adenomyoma can mimic the appearance of myometrial invasion in a biopsy specimen. In curettage specimens this is most often manifest by admixed fragments of normal cycling endometrium (e.g., proliferative or secretory pattern endometrium) in addition to the fragmented polypoid lesion. The profile at the periphery of the endophytic tumors is usually obvious and distinct from surrounding myometrium, facilitating distinction of myometrial invasive carcinoma from endophytic atypical polypoid adenomyoma. Strategies for distinguishing atypical polypoid adenomyoma and adenocarcinoma are the same as those separating complex atypical hyperplasia and adenocarcinoma. Small foci with well-developed architectural complexity (i.e., tiny carcinomas) in this context have been referred to in the literature as "atypical polypoid adenomyofibromas of low malignant potential"[31] (APA-LMP) (see Chapter 5).

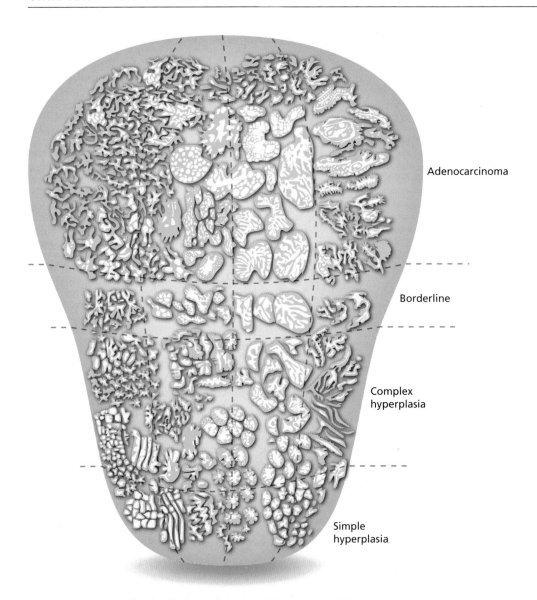

Adenocarcinoma

Borderline

Complex
hyperplasia

Simple
hyperplasia

Diagram 7.3 Diagram for classification of endometrial hyperplasia and low-grade endometrial adenocarcinoma. A subset of gland patterns exhibit architecture that is intermediate between hyperplasia and carcinoma; this subset is depicted in the middle of the diagram and is classified as borderline. The vertical lines depict the main glandular patterns that are seen in the endometrium (commencing from left): budding and/or branching glands; macroglands with internal (cribriform-type) budding; macroglands with internal villi; and exophytic villous and/or papillary glands. Risk of myometrial invasion in the hysterectomy specimen is highest with high-risk architecture (= carcinoma: approximately 20% risk of myoinvasion) and lowest with low-risk architecture (= hyperplasia: <0.05% risk of myoinvasion). This diagram is based only on gland architecture; evaluation of the cytology is also important, as some endometrial carcinomas may be formed by simple glands, but have high-grade cytology and are diagnosed on the basis of their high-grade cytologic atypia (e.g., serous, clear cell, and some cases of endometrioid carcinomas). (Modified from Longacre TA, Chung MH, Jensen DN, *et al.* Proposed criteria for the diagnosis of well-differentiated endometrial carcinoma. A diagnostic test for myoinvasion. *Am J Surg Pathol* 1995;**19**:371–406.)

Serous carcinoma

Carcinomas should be categorized as serous when the background is atrophic, the nuclear grade is high, cellular dyshesion and tufting are present, and cytoplasmic changes associated with endometrioid differentiation are absent (i.e., squamous, morular, or mucinous metaplasia, and the presence of cilia are lacking) (Figure 7.46). Caution is advised when a diagnosis of mixed serous and endometrioid adenocarcinoma is considered (Table 7.12; also see ***Mixed epithelial carcinomas*** and ***Hybrid tumors*** in Chapter 8).

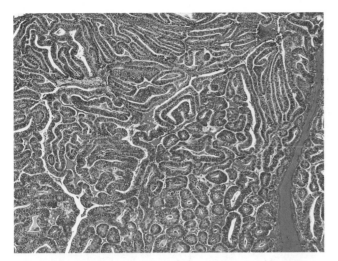

Figure 7.44 The presence of labyrinthine architecture (upper left) signifies the presence of adenocarcinoma, provided more than 30% of the atypical proliferation demonstrates either the architectural or cytologic features of adenocarcinoma.

Clear cell carcinoma

Carcinomas containing cells with clear cytoplasm should be categorized as clear cell carcinomas when a typical papillary or tubulocystic architecture is present and the nuclei are highly atypical (Figure 7.47; Table 7.13). As endometrioid carcinomas may exhibit a variety of patterns of cytoplasmic clearing, one should hesitate to make a diagnosis of clear cell carcinoma if the tumor is predominantly solid, the tumor cells are high columnar instead of cuboidal, and secretory change and/or glycogenated squamous metaplasia cannot be excluded[32]. It is currently unsettled whether tumors with solid architecture and highly atypical clear cells can be accurately subclassified; it is likely that some are clear cell carcinomas, while others are endometrioid, and yet others may well be serous. As with serous carcinomas, a clear cell carcinoma diagnosis

(A)

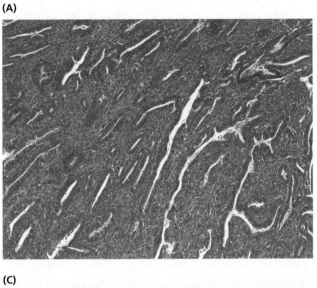

(B)

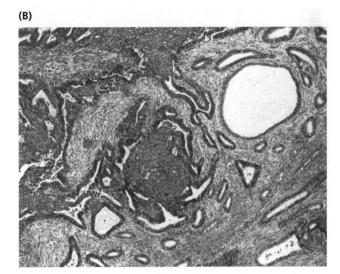

(C)

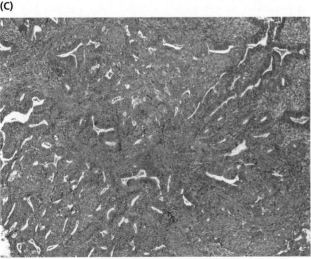

Figure 7.45 Atypical polypoid adenomyoma. The glandular proliferation resembles complex hyperplasia, but it is present within a polyp with muscular stroma (A). Squamous morules are commonly seen (B). The proliferation may be sufficiently architecturally complex to consider a diagnosis of adenocarcinoma (C), but follow-up hysterectomy only rarely demonstrates myometrial invasion.

Table 7.12 Characteristics of serous carcinoma

Presence of endometrial atrophy

Absence of endometrial hyperplasia

Presence of an endometrial polyp

Irregular, serrated, luminal contours due to the presence of micropapillae, tumor cell budding, dyshesion, and detachment

Diffuse, severe nuclear atypia

Architectural and cytologic dyssynchrony

Intraepithelial carcinoma

Gaping gland pattern of myometrial invasion

Table 7.13 Characteristics of clear cell carcinoma

Absence of endometrial hyperplasia

Combinations of solid, tubulocystic, and papillary architecture

Round papillae; lining epithelium is generally less than three cells thick

Hobnail cells

Cuboidal or low-columnar cell shape

Large, round nuclei with prominent nucleoli

Absence of squamous differentiation and intracytoplasmic mucin

No admixture of columnar cells with subnuclear vacuoles

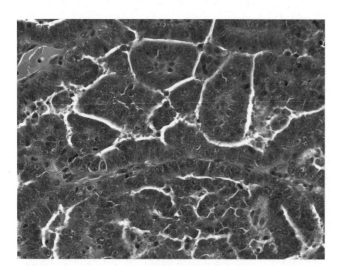

Figure 7.46 Serous carcinoma of endometrium.

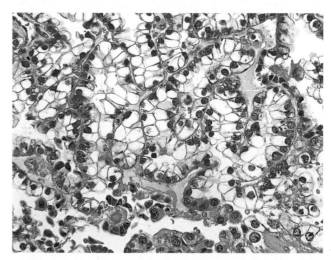

Figure 7.47 Clear cell carcinoma of the endometrium.

should only be rendered when cytoplasmic changes associated with endometrioid differentiation are absent. Caution is advised when a diagnosis of mixed clear cell and endometrioid adenocarcinoma is considered (see Chapter 9).

Microglandular hyperplasia of the cervix

Microglandular hyperplasia of the cervix occurs mostly in premenopausal and perimenopausal women exposed to estrogen and/or progesterone stimulation, such as during pregnancy or while taking oral contraceptives; however it may be seen in postmenopausal women (see Chapter 3). This endocervical lesion is composed of small acini, frequently lined by basaloid cells at the periphery and cuboidal or columnar cells surrounding the lumen (Figure 7.48). The basaloid cells sometimes demonstrate squamous metaplasia, and the luminal cells typically show cytoplasmic clearing, reminiscent of secretory change. Despite the admixture of inflammatory cells, mitotic figures are scarce and nuclear atypia is lacking. On biopsy or curettage, the endometrial

carcinomas for which this lesion is most frequently mistaken are highly differentiated endometrioid adenocarcinoma with mucinous metaplasia and pure, highly differentiated mucinous adenocarcinoma. Endometrial carcinomas may rarely exhibit an extensive microglandular pattern, but the squamous component in these tumors is generally inconspicuous, at least in the microglandular areas. A diagnosis of endometrial carcinoma is favored when the patient is postmenopausal and the lesion shows any appreciable mitotic activity or nuclear atypia.

Undifferentiated carcinoma

A FIGO grade 3 endometrioid adenocarcinoma should be diagnosed only when the tumor is obviously endometrioid in character; so this diagnosis should not be applied to every tumor that exhibits solid growth patterns. Confirmatory endometrioid features in this context include glandular architecture, squamous metaplasia, or trabecular and nested growth patterns. There are likely different types

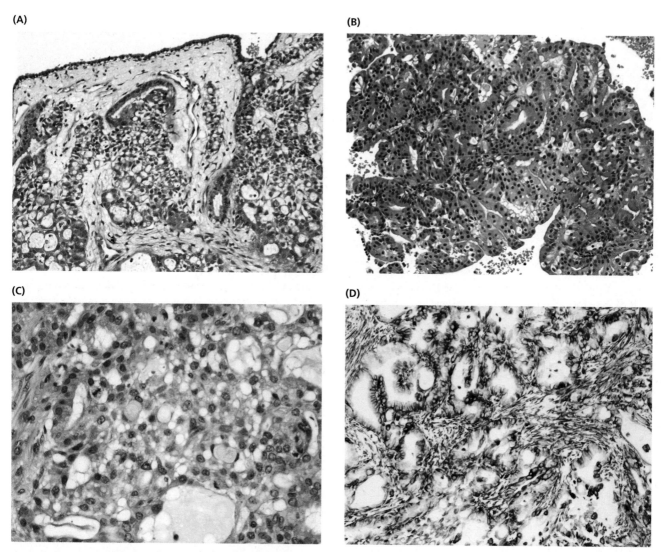

Figure 7.48 Microglandular hyperplasia of endocervix (A). This lesion may be mistaken for mucinous and endometrioid adenocarcinoma of endometrium in biopsy and curettage material. Postmenopausal patients are much more likely to have endometrial carcinoma (B; mucinous carcinoma) rather than microglandular hyperplasia. Microglandular hyperplasia-like endometrial carcinoma has also been described (C). Compared to microglandular hyperplasia, it shows more nuclear atypia, mitotic activity and vimentin expression (D).

of undifferentiated carcinoma. The type that is best described in the literature[33,34] lacks these confirmatory endometrioid features, although it is frequently associated with well-differentiated endometrioid adenocarcinoma, in which case the tumor is classified as "dedifferentiated"[35]. Undifferentiated carcinoma grows in sheets, with irregular myometrial permeation at the periphery (Figure 7.49; Table 7.14). Tumor cells are dyshesive and resemble lymphoma, plasmacytoma or rhabdoid tumor cells. These features, specifically, can be used to separate undifferentiated carcinoma and FIGO grades 2 and 3 endometrioid carcinomas, tumors that more often show solid, trabecular, and nested growth patterns with cohesive tumor cells. Immunohistochemically, rare cells express epithelial membrane

antigen (EMA) or CK18 strongly, but most cells lack an obviously epithelial phenotype, unlike FIGO grades 2 and 3 endometrioid carcinomas. Stains for lymphoid, plasmacytoid, rhabdomyoblastic, and rhabdoid neoplasms are negative, although patchy and weak CD138 staining is sometimes seen (see Chapter 9).

Transitional cell carcinoma

Occasional endometrioid adenocarcinomas demonstrate exophytic, broad papillae lined by multiple layers of stratified cells with squamotransitional features (Figure 7.50). These tumors should be classified as endometrioid if they retain some evidence of glandular differentiation, but they

(A)

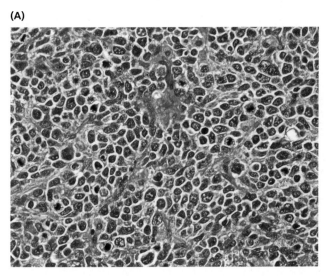

(B)

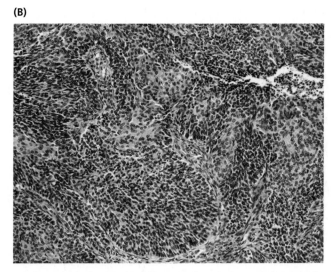

Figure 7.49 Undifferentiated carcinoma (A) and FIGO grade 3 endometrioid adenocarcinoma (B). Undifferentiated carcinomas are formed of poorly cohesive cells, and frequently resemble lymphoma. Poorly differentiated endometrioid adenocarcinoma, in contrast, has cohesive cells that form nests.

Table 7.14 Characteristics of undifferentiated carcinoma

Solid, sheet-like, patternless architecture
No glandular, papillary, trabecular, or nested formations
Cellular dyshesion
Lymphoma-like appearance
Uniform, ovoid cells with vesicular chromatin and nucleoli
Presence of rhabdoid cells in myxoid matrix
Only minimal expression of EMA, keratins, ER and PR[a]

[a] Overt neuroendocrine differentiation should be lacking. At least focal EMA or keratin expression should be present, although evidence of epithelial differentiation is usually scant.

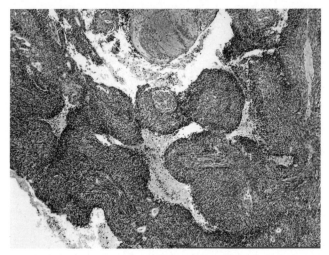

Figure 7.50 Endometrioid adenocarcinoma with a transitional cell–like growth pattern. Although this tumor displays broad papillae, focal glandular differentiation is evident.

can be classified as transitional cell if those features are lacking or only very subtle. In our opinion, almost all endometrial carcinomas so classified are probably endometrioid in differentiation. Rare transitional cell carcinomas of the urinary tract secondarily involve the uterine corpus, but most of these show vaginal and cervical involvement as well.

Squamous cell carcinoma

Strategies for distinguishing between squamous cell carcinoma and endometrioid adenocarcinoma are similar to those that separate transitional cell carcinoma and endometrioid adenocarcinoma. That is, squamous cell carcinoma of the endometrium cannot be diagnosed unless endometrioid glands are lacking. Extension from

a contiguous squamous carcinoma of the cervix should also be excluded (see Chapter 9).

Small cell neuroendocrine carcinoma

Rare endometrioid adenocarcinomas harbor neuroendocrine components. Pure neuroendocrine carcinomas of the endometrium are extraordinary. Tumors with a large cell neuroendocrine carcinoma component are probably more commonly encountered than those with a small cell neuroendocrine component. The diagnostic criteria for these tumors are the same as those used in other organs.

(A)

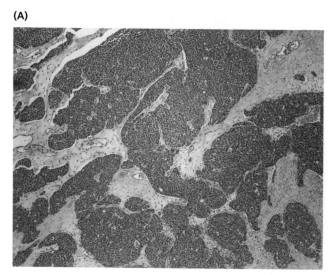

(B)

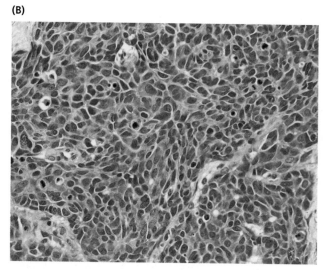

Figure 7.51 Small cell carcinoma (A, B).

Small cell carcinomas should be composed of small cells, with a high nucleus-to-cytoplasm ratio and nuclear molding, but no nucleoli, with an extremely high proliferative rate and numerous apoptotic bodies (Figure 7.51). Large cell neuroendocrine carcinomas are highly proliferative, nested, or trabecular with large cells containing nuclei with nucleoli. Although many pathologists do not require immunohistochemical stains to establish neuroendocrine differentiation for the small cell tumors, many rely on immunohistochemistry for the large cell tumors (see Chapter 9). These latter tumors should show convincing expression of chromogranin and/or synaptophysin and/or CD56 in more than approximately 20% of tumor cells. Note that many endometrioid adenocarcinomas contain a significant percentage of tumor cells that stain positively for neuroendocrine markers, but, in general, these tumors neither resemble neuroendocrine carcinomas nor exhibit widespread immunohistochemical evidence of neuroendocrine differentiation.

Carcinosarcoma (malignant mixed mullerian tumor)

Uterine carcinosarcoma (malignant mixed mullerian tumor) should not be diagnosed when the epithelial and mesenchymal elements are not obviously histologically high grade[36] (see Chapter 10). Examples of high-grade epithelial elements are FIGO grade 3 endometrioid, serous, clear cell, or undifferentiated carcinoma. High-grade mesenchymal elements display cellularity greater than that seen in typical ovarian fibroma, easily found

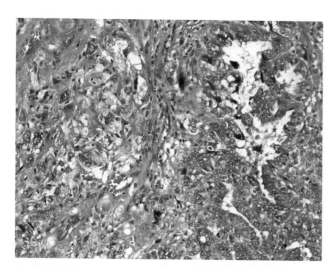

Figure 7.52 Carcinosarcoma (malignant mixed mullerian tumor) is a biphasic neoplasm with distinct epithelial and mesenchymal components that are histologically high grade. Endometrioid adenocarcinomas with spindle cell features are histologically low grade and display seamless transitions from epithelioid to spindle cell components.

mitotic figures in three to five fields at intermediate magnification, any atypical mitotic figures, nuclear hyperchromasia, nuclear pleomorphism recognizable at scanning magnification, and nuclear enlargement three-times that of non-neoplastic myometrial muscle fibers or non-neoplastic endometrial stroma (Figure 7.52; Table 7.15).

Endometrioid adenocarcinoma with spindle cell elements is diagnosed when the epithelial and mesenchymal elements are low grade in appearance[37]. In this tumor, the endometrioid elements, frequently showing squamous metaplasia, fuse imperceptibly with spindle cell elements

Table 7.15 Characteristics of carcinosarcoma[a]

Biphasic appearance

Epithelial and mesenchymal components are distinct

Epithelial component is serous, FIGO grade 3 endometrioid, or too poorly differentiated to subclassify in most cases

Mesenchymal component is spindled, pleomorphic, and mitotically active

Presence of rhabdomyoblasts in the context of a biphasic tumor with high-grade epithelial and mesenchymal components

[a] Occasional endometrioid carcinomas imperceptibly blend with histologically low-grade spindle cell proliferations that may contain metaplastic bone or cartilage. A diagnosis of carcinosarcoma should be avoided when the spindle cell component lacks pleomorphism.

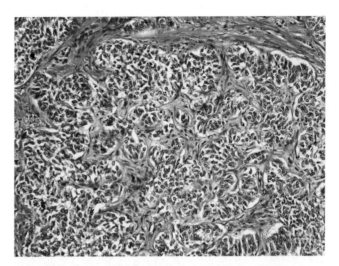

Figure 7.53 Uterine tumor resembling ovarian sex cord tumor (UTROSCT). This tumor exhibits retiform and Sertoli-like patterns, which can be misinterpreted as evidence of glandular differentiation and endometrioid adenocarcinoma.

that are never histologically high grade. In most cases, the endometrioid component is no more than FIGO grade 2, and the spindle cell component is cellular and sometimes mitotically active, but not markedly atypical. Carcinosarcoma contains easily separable, high-grade epithelial and mesenchymal elements, whereas this type of endometrioid adenocarcinoma shows seamless fusion of the two (i.e., element fusion). Although the presence of squamous metaplasia is often a useful clue that a given spindle cell proliferation may represent a low-grade endometrioid process, occasional carcinosarcomas may contain prominent endometrioid differentiation with squamous elements. In these instances, the tumor grade, the presence or absence of "element fusion," and careful evaluation of the mitotic index in the spindle cell component can be used to inform the decision. Endometrioid adenocarcinomas can contain chondroid and osteoid elements[37]. Heterologous elements by themselves do not signify carcinosarcoma, although finding rhabdomyosarcoma along with adenocarcinoma almost always signifies carcinosarcoma.

Uterine tumor resembling ovarian sex cord tumor

Uterine tumors that resemble ovarian sex cord tumors (UTROSCTs) are uncommon uterine tumors, typically myometrial based with pushing, well-demarcated borders (Figure 7.53). Microscopically, the tumors display trabecular, corded, and nested patterns that recall ovarian Sertoli and granulosa cell tumors. Some of these tumors therefore resemble endometrioid adenocarcinomas with corded and nested elements. Immunohistochemistry can distinguish UTROSCT from adenocarcinoma. Uterine tumors that resemble ovarian sex cord tumors may

express cytokeratins, ER, and PR, but they lack EMA, B72.3, and Ber-EP4 expression. Uterine tumors that resemble ovarian sex cord tumors can also express inhibin and calretinin, markers that are only very seldom expressed in carcinomas (see Chapter 17).

Mesonephric adenocarcinoma

Mesonephric adenocarcinomas are known to arise in the cervix, usually in association with mesonephric remnants. However, rare mesonephric adenocarcinomas can develop within the uterus and simulate endometrial carcinoma. These tumors show the same range of features that can be encountered in cervical mesonephric adenocarcinomas: simple, round glands; small, glomeruloid papillae; and tumor cell spindling. In contrast to endometrioid adenocarcinomas, these tumors are ER negative, PR negative and frequently calretinin positive (see Chapter 9).

Metastatic colorectal adenocarcinoma

Metastatic colorectal adenocarcinomas can simulate endometrioid carcinomas to a large degree, mostly in curettage or biopsy specimens (see Chapter 16). Clues to a correct diagnosis include nuclear features that are inappropriately atypical given the overtly glandular architecture and the presence of goblet cells (Figure 7.54). Many colorectal adenocarcinomas also show dirty necrosis, but this feature is not present in all cases. This differential diagnosis can almost always be resolved with immunohistochemistry.

(A)

(B)

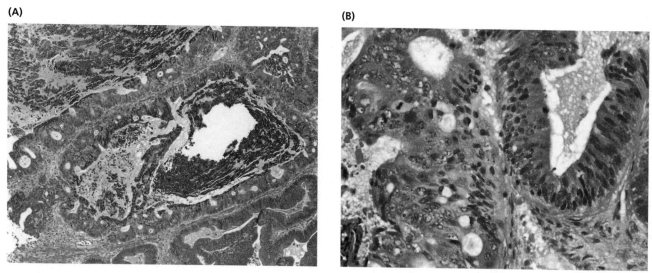

Figure 7.54 Metastatic colorectal adenocarcinoma presenting in endometrial curettage. The low-power appearance (A) may suggest endometrioid adenocarcinoma, but examination on high power (B) reveals nuclear atypia that are inappropriate for a gland-forming endometrioid adenocarcinoma.

(A)

(B)

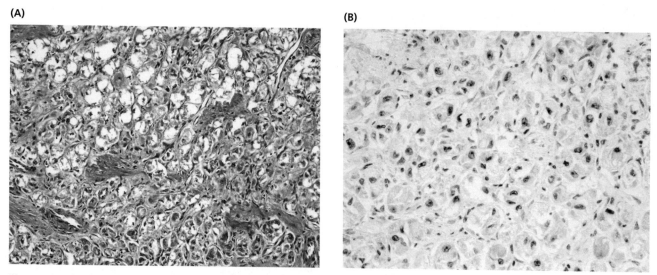

Figure 7.55 Alveolar soft part sarcoma in myometrium (A), expressing TFE3 in tumor cell nuclei (B).

Colorectal adenocarcinomas are usually CK20 positive and CK7 negative, unlike endometrioid adenocarcinomas.

Alveolar soft part sarcoma

Alveolar soft part sarcoma of the female genital tract is an uncommon and often misdiagnosed tumor (see Chapter 14). It can arise in the cervix or uterus, where it usually resides in the myometrium without continuity with the endometrial cavity. The tumor is composed of cells with abundant cytoplasm that ranges from clear to eosinophilic, growing in nests and alveoli, some of which are compressed to the point that the central empty space is obscured (Figure 7.55). The tumor cells' cytoplasm is filled with granules and crystals that are PAS positive and diastase resistant. The fibrovascular framework that supports the nests and alveoli is also a diagnostic clue. Vascular invasion may be present, but the prognosis appears to be much better than for tumors that arise in the soft tissues. The TFE3 immunohistochemical stain, with nuclear localization, can be used as a diagnostic adjunct to recognize tumors with this translocation or other abnormalities involving TFE3[38]. Alveolar soft part sarcoma shows variable, but usually weak or negative immunoreactivity for keratins, desmin, smooth muscle actin, MyoD1, S100, and HMB45.

(A)

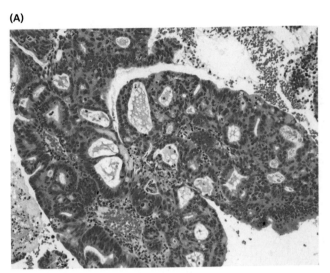

(B)

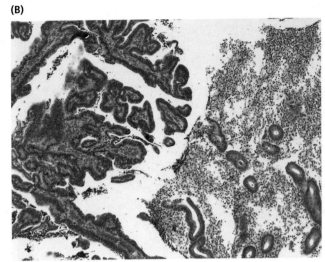

Figure 7.56 (A, B) Endocervical adenocarcinoma in endometrial curettage. Nuclear crowding and hyperchromasia, along with high mitotic rates and numerous apoptotic bodies, can suggest the correct diagnosis, especially when the background endometrium is non-neoplastic.

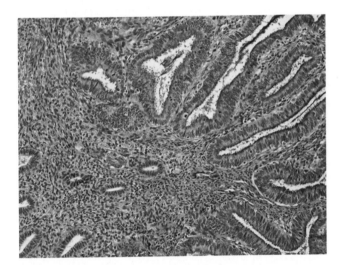

Figure 7.57 Endocervical adenocarcinoma colonizing lower uterine segment. Note nuclei resembling tubular adenoma and high mitotic rate.

Table 7.16 Characteristics of HPV-associated endocervical adenocarcinoma

Pre- or perimenopausal presentation

Evidence of previous or concomitant HPV infection or HPV-associated lesions

More lesional tissue in endocervical curettage as compared to endometrial curettage

Presence of adenocarcinoma in situ or squamous dysplasia

Tubular adenoma-like appearance
- Mucin depletion
- Pseudostratified, darkly stained, enlarged, and elongated nuclei

High mitotic index and numerous apoptotic bodies, appreciable at scanning magnification

Positive HPV in situ hybridization

Diffuse and intense expression of p16, with absent ER/PR and vimentin expression

Endocervical adenocarcinoma

Endocervical adenocarcinomas may demonstrate features that resemble those of endometrial endometrioid adenocarcinomas, but there are usually subtle histologic differences between the two (Figures 7.56 and 7.57). Striking numbers of mitotic figures and apoptotic bodies, along with monomorphous, hyperchromatic nuclei, favor endocervical adenocarcinoma. The presence of small intracytoplasmic mucin vacuoles is an additional clue that a problematic glandular lesion is endocervical in origin. Clinical presentation, precursor lesions (endocervical adenocarcinoma in situ versus endometrial hyperplasia), and

immunophenotype differ, and can be used to establish the correct diagnosis (Table 7.16). Additional details can be found in Chapter 3.

Primitive neuroectodermal tumor

Rare primitive neuroectodermal tumors (PNETs) can arise in the uterus (Figure 7.58). The presence of rosettes may mimic the appearance of glands, and nested growth patterns can suggest solid components of endometrioid adenocarcinoma. Clues to the correct diagnosis include primitive-appearing nuclei, exceedingly high mitotic indices, and

(A)

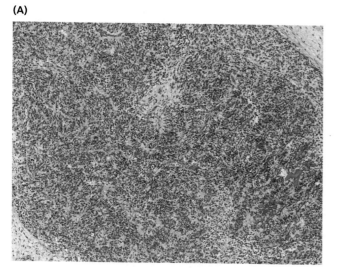

(B)

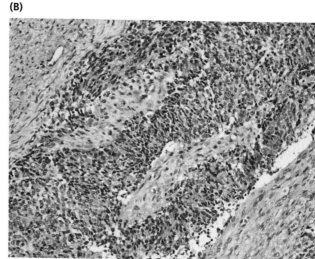

Figure 7.58 (A, B) Primitive neuroectodermal tumor of uterus (central nervous system type). Trabecular growth resembles patterns frequently seen in FIGO grade 3 endometrioid adenocarcinoma, including variants with hyalinized and corded stroma. Perivascular rosettes and primitive-appearing nuclei are clues to the correct diagnosis.

rosettes. The diagnosis can be suggested with immunohistochemical stains and confirmed with molecular testing in many cases (see Chapter 14). Primitive neuroectodermal tumors, particularly those of the peripheral variety (i.e., part of the spectrum of Ewing sarcoma), express CD99 diffusely in a membrane pattern and are usually, but not always cytokeratin negative. Given this immunophenotype, it would be reasonable to also exclude the theoretical possibility of a primitive leukemia or lymphoma with a TdT immunostain. The vast majority of peripheral primitive neuroectodermal tumors harbor t(11;22)(q24;q12), involving the *EWS* and *FLI1* genes. This can be evaluated by fluorescence in situ hybridization (FISH) assays for the translocation, or reverse-transcription polymerase chain reaction (RT-PCR) for the translocation gene product. Some uterine primitive neuroectodermal tumors are not related to the Ewing family of tumors and, instead, recall the appearance of primitive neuroectodermal tumors of the central nervous system. These tumors do not harbor the t(11;22) and frequently lack diffuse CD99 expression. Some express glial fibrillary acidic protein.

REFERENCES

1. Bokhman JV. Two pathogenetic types of endometrial carcinoma. *Gynecol Oncol* 1983;**15**(1):10–17.
2. Soslow RA, Bissonnette JP, Wilton A, *et al.* Clinicopathologic analysis of 187 high-grade endometrial carcinomas of different histologic subtypes: similar outcomes belie distinctive biologic differences. *Am J Surg Pathol* 2007;**31**(7):979–87.
3. Zaino RJ, Kurman RJ, Diana KL, Morrow CP. The utility of the revised International Federation of Gynecology and Obstetrics histologic grading of endometrial adenocarcinoma using a defined nuclear grading system: A Gynecologic Oncology Group study. *Cancer* 1995;**75**:81–6.
4. Hampel H, Frankel W, Panescu J, *et al.* Screening for Lynch syndrome (hereditary nonpolyposis colorectal cancer) among endometrial cancer patients. *Cancer Res* 2006;**66**(15):7810–17.
5. Ollikainen M, Abdel-Rahman WM, Moisio AL, *et al.* Molecular analysis of familial endometrial carcinoma: a manifestation of hereditary nonpolyposis colorectal cancer or a separate syndrome? *J Clin Oncol* 2005;**23**(21):4609–16.
6. Leitao MM, Jr., Kehoe S, Barakat RR, *et al.* Comparison of D&C and office endometrial biopsy accuracy in patients with FIGO grade 1 endometrial adenocarcinoma. *Gynecol Oncol* 2009; **113**(1):105–8.
7. Leitao MM, Jr., Kehoe S, Barakat RR, *et al.* Endometrial sampling diagnosis of FIGO grade 1 endometrial adenocarcinoma with a background of complex atypical hyperplasia and final hysterectomy pathology. *Am J Obstet Gynecol* 2010;**202**(3):278.e1–6.
8. Mariani A, Dowdy SC, Cliby WA, *et al.* Prospective assessment of lymphatic dissemination in endometrial cancer: a paradigm shift in surgical staging. *Gynecol Oncol* 2008;**109**(1):11–18.
9. Abu-Rustum NR, Khoury-Collado F, Pandit-Taskar N, *et al.* Sentinel lymph node mapping for grade 1 endometrial cancer: is it the answer to the surgical staging dilemma? *Gynecol Oncol* 2009; **113**(2):163–9.
10. Abu-Rustum NR, Zhou Q, Gomez JD, *et al.* A nomogram for predicting overall survival of women with endometrial cancer following primary therapy: toward improving individualized cancer care. *Gynecol Oncol* 2010;**116**(3):399–403.
11. Wheeler DT, Bristow RE, Kurman RJ. Histologic alterations in endometrial hyperplasia and well-differentiated carcinoma treated with progestins. *Am J Surg Pathol* 2007;**31**(7):988–98.
12. Pecorelli S. Revised FIGO staging for carcinoma of the vulva, cervix, and endometrium. *Int J Gynaecol Obstet* 2009;**105**(2):103–4.
13. Ali A, Black D, Soslow RA. Difficulties in assessing the depth of myometrial invasion in endometrial carcinoma. *Int J Gynecol Pathol* 2007;**26**(2):115–23.

14. Murray SK, Young RH, Scully RE. Unusual epithelial and stromal changes in myoinvasive endometrioid adenocarcinoma: a study of their frequency, associated diagnostic problems, and prognostic significance. *Int J Gynecol Pathol* 2003;**22**(4):324–33.

15. Longacre TA, Hendrickson MR. Diffusely infiltrative endometrial adenocarcinoma – an adenoma malignum pattern of myoinvasion. *Am J Surg Pathol* 1999;**23**(1):69–78.

16. Logani S, Herdman AV, Little JV, Moller KA. Vascular "pseudo invasion" in laparoscopic hysterectomy specimens: a diagnostic pitfall. *Am J Surg Pathol* 2008;**32**(4):560–5.

17. Kitahara S, Walsh C, Frumovitz M, Malpica A, Silva EG. Vascular pseudoinvasion in laparoscopic hysterectomy specimens for endometrial carcinoma: a grossing artifact? *Am J Surg Pathol* 2009; **33**(2):298–303.

18. Zaino RJ. FIGO staging of endometrial adenocarcinoma: a critical review and proposal. *Int J Gynecol Pathol* 2009;**28**(1):1–9.

19. Orezzoli JP, Sioletic S, Olawaiye A, Oliva E, del Carmen MG. Stage II endometrioid adenocarcinoma of the endometrium: clinical implications of cervical stromal invasion. *Gynecol Oncol* 2009; **113**(3):316–23.

20. McCluggage WG, Hirschowitz L, Wilson GE, *et al.* Significant variation in the assessment of cervical involvement in endometrial carcinoma: an interobserver variation study. *Am J Surg Pathol* 2011;**35**(2):289–94.

21. Tambouret R, Clement PB, Young RH. Endometrial endometrioid adenocarcinoma with a deceptive pattern of spread to the uterine cervix: a manifestation of stage IIb endometrial carcinoma liable to be misinterpreted as an independent carcinoma or a benign lesion. *Am J Surg Pathol* 2003;**27**(8):1080–8.

22. Walsh C, Holschneider C, Hoang Y, *et al.* Coexisting ovarian malignancy in young women with endometrial cancer. *Obstet Gynecol* 2005;**106**(4):693–9.

23. Shamshirsaz AA, Witham-Leitch M, Odunsi K, *et al.* Young patients with endometrial carcinoma selected for conservative treatment: a need for vigilance for synchronous ovarian carcinomas, case report and literature review. *Gynecol Oncol* 2007; **104**(3):757–60.

24. McKenney JK, Kong CS, Longacre TA. Endometrial adenocarcinoma associated with subtle lymph-vascular space invasion and lymph node metastasis: a histologic pattern mimicking intravascular and sinusoidal histiocytes. *Int J Gynecol Pathol* 2005;**24**(1):73–8.

25. Lax SF, Kendall B, Tashiro H, Slebos R J C, Ellenson LH. The frequency of p53, K-ras mutations, and microsatellite instability differs in uterine endometrioid and serous carcinoma – evidence of distinct molecular genetic pathways. *Cancer* 2000;**88** (4):814–24.

26. Soslow RA, Shen PU, Chung MH, Isacson C. Distinctive p53 and mdm2 immunohistochemical expression profiles suggest different pathogenetic pathways in poorly differentiated endometrial carcinoma. *Int J Gynecol Pathol* 1998;**17**:129–34.

27. Reid-Nicholson M, Iyengar P, Hummer AJ, Linkov I, Asher M, Soslow RA. Immunophenotypic diversity of endometrial adenocarcinomas: implications for differential diagnosis. *Mod Pathol* 2006;**19**(8):1091–100.

28. Kurman RJ, Norris HJ. Evaluation of criteria for distinguishing atypical endometrial hyperplasia from well-differentiated carcinoma. *Cancer* 1982;**49**:2547–59.

29. Longacre TA, Chung MH, Jensen DN, Hendrickson MR. Proposed criteria for the diagnosis of well-differentiated endometrial carcinoma: a diagnostic test for myoinvasion. *Am J Surg Pathol* 1995;**19**:371–406.

30. Young RH, Treger T, Scully RE. Atypical polypoid adenomyoma of the uterus. A report of 27 cases. *Am J Clin Pathol* 1986;**86**:139–45.

31. Longacre TA, Chung MH, Rouse RV, Hendrickson MR. Atypical polypoid adenomyofibromas (atypical polypoid adenomyomas) of the uterus – a clinicopathologic study of 55 cases. *Am J Surg Pathol* 1996;**20**:1–20.

32. Silva EG, Young RH. Endometrioid neoplasms with clear cells: a report of 21 cases in which the alteration is not of typical secretory type. *Am J Surg Pathol* 2007;**31**(8):1203–8.

33. Tafe L, Garg K, Tornos C, Soslow R. Undifferentiated carcinoma of the endometrium and ovary: a clinicopathologic correlation. *Mod Pathol* 2009;**22**(1):238A.

34. Altrabulsi B, Malpica A, Deavers MT, *et al.* Undifferentiated carcinoma of the endometrium. *Am J Surg Pathol* 2005; **29**(10):1316–21.

35. Silva EG, Deavers MT, Bodurka DC, Malpica A. Association of low-grade endometrioid carcinoma of the uterus and ovary with undifferentiated carcinoma: a new type of dedifferentiated carcinoma? *Int J Gynecol Pathol* 2006;**25**(1):52–8.

36. Ferguson SE, Tornos C, Hummer A, Barakat RR, Soslow RA. Prognostic features of surgical stage I uterine carcinosarcoma. *Am J Surg Pathol* 2007;**31**(11):1653–61.

37. Murray SK, Clement PB, Young RH. Endometrioid carcinomas of the uterine corpus with sex cord-like formations, hyalinization, and other unusual morphologic features: a report of 31 cases of a neoplasm that may be confused with carcinosarcoma and other uterine neoplasms. *Am J Surg Pathol* 2005;**29**(2):157–66.

38. Ladanyi M, Lui MY, Antonescu CR, *et al.* The der(17)t(X;17) (p11;q25) of human alveolar soft part sarcoma fuses the TFE3 transcription factor gene to ASPL, a novel gene at 17q25. *Oncogene* 2001;**20**(1):48–57.

8 SEROUS ADENOCARCINOMA

INTRODUCTION

Uterine serous carcinomas, representing approximately 15% of endometrial carcinomas, are known for being clinically aggressive tumors that disproportionately affect older women. In contrast to the more common endometrioid adenocarcinoma, serous adenocarcinoma is considered to be a type II endometrial cancer according to the Bokhman classification[1]. Type II carcinomas are estrogen independent, typically unassociated with a background of endometrial hyperplasia, and, almost by definition, high grade. Serous carcinoma is unusual in that it is frequently associated with clinically occult extrauterine metastasis, despite the absence of significant uterine enlargement and/or significant tumor volume in the uterus. Reproducible and accurate diagnosis of serous carcinoma is important, as the surgical treatment differs from that of the usual endometrioid adenocarcinoma. Fortunately, in most cases these tumors are easily recognized on an adequate endometrial sampling, but, in some cases, the distinction between serous carcinoma and endometrioid carcinoma can be problematic. Diagnostic strategies that incorporate traditional morphology, immunophenotype, genotype, and patterns of disease dissemination may be helpful, but there are some cases that defy classification; these cases should be reported as high-grade carcinomas with a note that discusses the differential diagnostic problem(s).

CLINICAL CHARACTERISTICS

Uterine serous carcinomas typically occur in the setting of endometrial atrophy, and often involve or arise from atrophic endometrial polyps. In most cases, factors known to predispose for serous carcinogenesis are not evident, but many serous carcinomas occur in patients with a history of breast cancer, including those treated with tamoxifen, and in patients who received previous pelvic radiation therapy

for rectal or cervical carcinoma. Rare serous carcinomas arise in a background of endometrial hyperplasia or low-grade endometrioid carcinoma. Despite the fact that uterine serous carcinomas morphologically resemble ovarian serous carcinoma, the risk factors are distinct. In North America, uterine serous carcinoma patients are more frequently African-American and are as much as a decade older than the typical ovarian serous carcinoma patient. Also, uterine serous carcinomas have no definitive association with nulliparity or oral contraceptive use. Uterine serous carcinomas have not been associated with *BRCA1* or *BRCA2* mutations.

Uterine serous carcinomas are well known for being highly aggressive tumors. While this is certainly true, it is perhaps even more helpful to remember that these tumors disseminate easily and widely, perhaps almost from their inception, sometimes without overt clinical signs of metastasis. In contrast to the typical endometrioid carcinoma, serous carcinomas frequently exhibit macroscopic or microscopic peritoneal dissemination and lymphovascular invasion in the absence of demonstrable myometrial invasion. This is usually explained by the observation that serous carcinomas are composed of highly dyshesive cells that are prone to detachment, disgorgement through the fallopian tubes, and implantation on tubal, ovarian, and peritoneal surfaces. They are also frequently detected in cervicovaginal Pap tests. Deep myometrial invasion in uteri that are not grossly enlarged is also common.

This predilection for presentation at high stage, combined with relative chemoresistance, means that the typical serous carcinoma patient cannot be cured at present. Survival estimates quoted for patients with serous carcinoma (all stages) are about 30–40%[1]. Patients with FIGO stage I disease are probably the only ones with a good chance of survival, in the range of 70–80%[2]. However, the threshold for qualifying for favorable prognosis stage I serous carcinoma is high. Full surgical staging, including formal lymph node dissection (not lymph node sampling), omentectomy

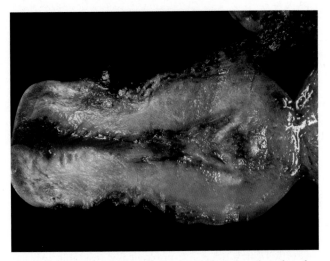

Figure 8.1 Serous carcinoma. The uterus is often not enlarged, and involvement by tumor may be subtle on gross examination.

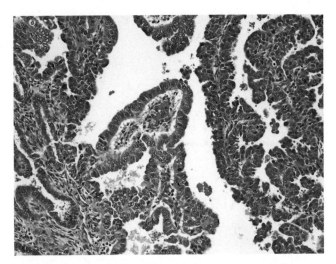

Figure 8.2 Serous carcinoma. The typical serous carcinoma forms papillae and micropapillae.

and peritoneal biopsies, is highly recommended for patients with a preoperative diagnosis of serous carcinoma. That is because as many as 50% of patients with tumor that appears confined to the uterus actually have extrauterine disease demonstrable after comprehensive staging[3]. Patients proven to have disease confined to the endometrium are at low risk of dying from disease, with survival rates estimated in the 90% range. Patients with "minimal uterine serous carcinoma" (less than 1 cm of carcinoma in the endometrium)[4], and those without residual tumor on hysterectomy and staging[5], have the best prognosis. Chemotherapy and radiotherapy are usually offered to all uterine serous carcinoma patients save for those with FIGO stage I disease limited to the endometrium. Whether all such patients benefit from chemotherapy and radiation therapy is debatable.

MORPHOLOGY

Gross pathology

Uteri harboring serous carcinomas tend to be small, contain endometrial polyps, and lack the hyperplastic endometrium that is more characteristic of endometrioid adenocarcinomas. When serous carcinoma is confined to a polyp, the tumor itself may not be grossly apparent (Figure 8.1). More advanced tumors often demonstrate obvious myometrial permeation and either extension or metastasis to regional structures included in the resection specimen. Uterine serous carcinomas have a predilection for peritoneal dissemination.

Table 8.1 Pathologic characteristics of uterine serous carcinoma

Diffuse, severe nuclear atypia, with bizarre forms being common
Nuclear atypia inappropriate for architectural grade
Serrated, irregular luminal borders
Micropapillae[a]
Dyshesion and tufting
Intraepithelial carcinoma
Background atrophy
Endometrial polyp
No hyperplasia, squamous metaplasia, or other cytoplasmic changes characteristic of endometrioid neoplasia

[a] Papillary, glandular, and solid architecture may also be present.

Microscopic pathology (Table 8.1)

The typical serous carcinoma is formed of papillae and micropapillae (Figure 8.2) lined by large, dyscohesive cells with enlarged nuclei containing macronucleoli (Figure 8.3). Compact papillae and micropapillae may give rise to the impression of slit-like spaces, another characteristic architectural feature of serous histology (Figure 8.4). Incipient micropapillae, represented by small aggregates or tufts of epithelial cells that project into lumens, are also common. Most serous carcinomas are composed of low columnar cells with eosinophilic cytoplasm, but occasional cases contain tumor cells with clear cytoplasm. Bizarre nuclear forms, multinucleated cells and nuclei with dark, smudged chromatin are typical of serous carcinoma (Figure 8.5). When serous carcinomas invade myometrium, they frequently exhibit a gaping gland appearance, sometimes with internal

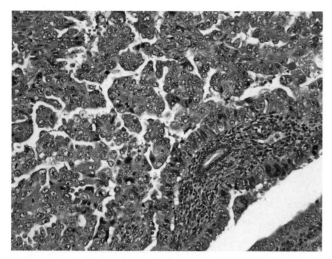

Figure 8.3 Serous carcinoma. This example exhibits innumerable micropapillae with budding and tumor cell detachment. Tumor cell nuclei are enlarged and pleomorphic relative to the entrapped, atrophic, non-neoplastic endometrial gland. Most tumor cell nuclei have vesicular chromatin with prominent nucleoli, but some are darkly stained with smudged chromatin.

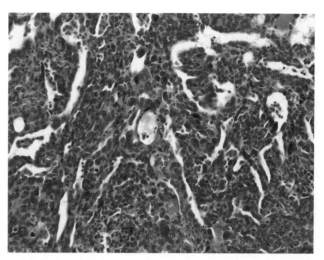

Figure 8.4 Serous carcinoma. Compression of micropapillae typically leads to the appearance of slit-like spaces.

(A)

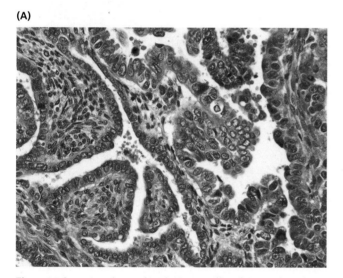

(B)

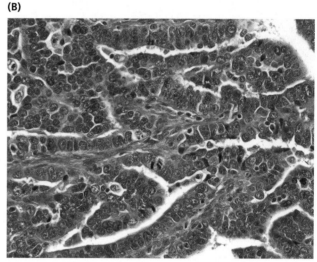

Figure 8.5 Serous carcinoma (A, B). Tumor cell nuclei are enlarged and pleomorphic relative to the stromal cell nuclei. Many tumor cell nuclei have vesicular chromatin, but some are darkly stained with smudged chromatin.

micropapillae (Figure 8.6). In most cases, there is an obvious stromal reaction to invasion, but this can be inconspicuous. Many serous carcinomas demonstrate extensive lymphovascular invasion. This can be appreciated even in cases with limited or absent myometrial invasion.

While most serous carcinomas show these features, many also grow in solid nests (Figure 8.7) or form rounded glands (Figure 8.8). Strategies that can help recognize these cases as serous carcinoma rely on identification of typical serous (and exclusion of typical endometrioid) features elsewhere, evaluation of background endometrium (should be atrophy in serous carcinoma; hyperplasia in endometrioid carcinoma), and, in some cases, the application of immunohistochemical stains.

Serous carcinomas almost always arise in a background of atrophic endometrium and atrophic endometrial polyps (Figure 8.9). Probably the only exceptions to this rule include a serous carcinoma that has entirely replaced the native endometrium with effacement of non-neoplastic structures, and the rare serous carcinoma that originates in the setting of well-differentiated or moderately differentiated endometrioid adenocarcinoma (Figure 8.10).

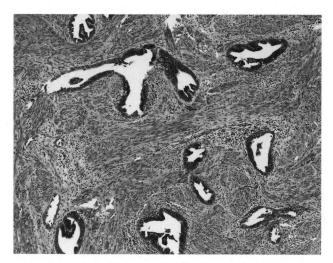

Figure 8.6 Myoinvasive serous carcinoma. These open, angulated glands, so-called "gaping glands," some with internal micropapillae, may be seen when serous carcinoma invades myometrium.

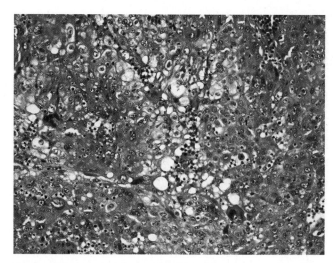

Figure 8.7 Serous carcinoma with solid architecture.

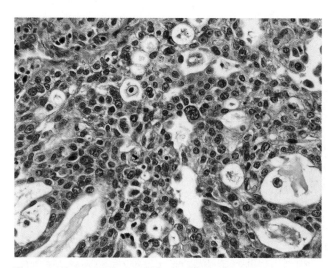

Figure 8.8 Serous carcinoma with glandular architecture.

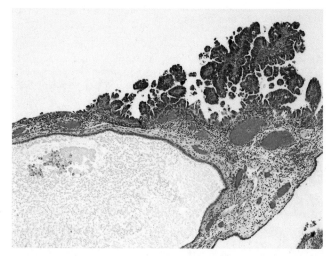

Figure 8.9 Serous carcinoma on the surface of an atrophic endometrial polyp.

To make the latter diagnosis, the serous component should be starkly different in appearance and immunophenotype from the endometrioid component. This will be discussed in more detail subsequently. Although serous carcinoma may be seen in uteri harboring foci of endometrial hyperplasia, a provisional diagnosis of serous carcinoma should be questioned if the non-neoplastic endometrium is secretory, proliferative, or hyperplastic.

Endometrioid features sufficient to exclude a diagnosis of serous carcinoma include unequivocal squamous metaplasia or squamous morules, intracytoplasmic mucin, and obvious cilia (Figure 8.11). Be aware that some serous carcinomas have cells with abundant eosinophilic cytoplasm that can mimic the appearance of squamous metaplasia (Figure 8.12). Smooth luminal borders with rounded

contours, absence of cellular dyshesion, and extensive budding are generally features of endometrioid tumors, especially when the nuclear grade is low or intermediate. With the exception of the rare mixed endometrioid and serous carcinoma, serous carcinoma should not be diagnosed when endometrioid features are evident.

Serous carcinoma in situ (intraepithelial serous carcinoma)

Many uterine serous carcinomas include an apparent non-invasive component that colonizes pre-existing, non-neoplastic, atrophic endometrium. This lesion, which has been termed endometrial intraepithelial carcinoma or "intraepithelial serous carcinoma," is a fully malignant neoplastic proliferation and may be associated with

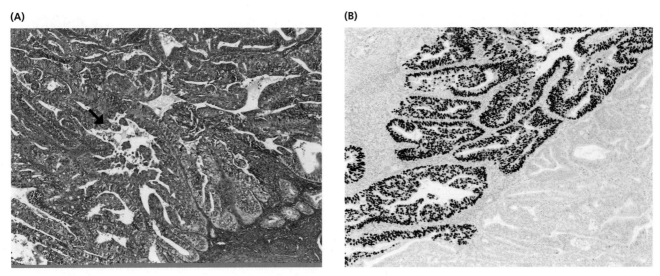

Figure 8.10 Mixed endometrioid and serous carcinoma. This endometrial carcinoma has a low-power appearance that suggests endometrioid adenocarcinoma (A). The area indicated by the arrow, however, exhibits micropapillae, budding and dyscohesion – features in keeping with serous carcinoma. The p53 immunohistochemical stain (B) shows overexpression in the serous component.

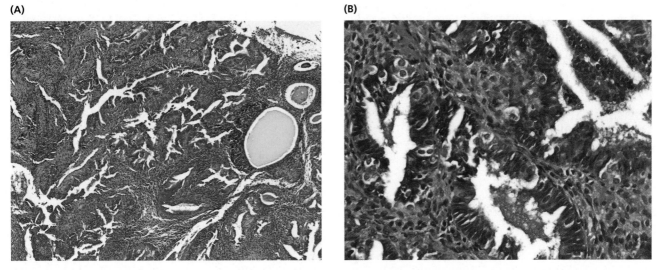

Figure 8.11 Endometrioid adenocarcinoma resembling serous carcinoma. Slit-like spaces suggest serous carcinoma (A), but high power microscopy (B) reveals that tumor cells are ciliated, with bland, small, oval nuclei. Mitotic activity is not apparent.

widespread extrauterine disease even in the absence of apparent endometrial stromal or myometrial invasion (Figure 8.13)[6]. The extrauteine disease may be manifested by other similar-appearing microscopic in situ lesions, macroscopic, histologically invasive lesions, or a combination thereof. Whether these apparent in situ foci represent true in situ carcinoma or metastases from another site, also without detectable invasion, is a currently unanswered question.

Because "intraepithelial serous carcinoma" is not mass-forming or histologically invasive, it does not exhibit the full range of architectural features that typify most serous carcinomas. Low-power clues to its presence are a dark-staining, sharply defined, linear lesion composed of tall

columnar cells, larger than those of juxtaposed atrophic endometrium, that replaces the luminal surface of flat or polypoid endometrium. Partial or complete replacement of isolated glands may also be seen. Some authors have proposed the existence of "serous dysplasia" in the uterus. This lesion, demonstrating some of the morphologic and immunohistochemical features of serous carcinoma, is thought to precede the development of "intraepithelial serous carcinoma"[7] and accompany it in some cases, but is not recommended as an independent diagnostic entity.

Since the diagnosis of "intraepithelial carcinoma" may be confused with the terminology of "intraepithelial neoplasia," this term should never be used in clinical practice

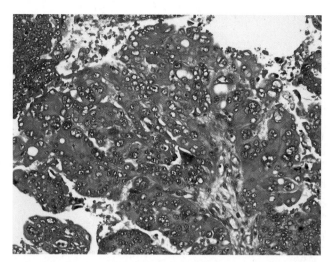

Figure 8.12 Serous carcinoma with eosinophilic cytoplasm. Abundant, eosinophilic cytoplasm may suggest the presence of squamous differentiation and a diagnosis of endometrioid adenocarcinoma. The high nuclear grade and absence of intercellular bridges are more in keeping with serous carcinoma.

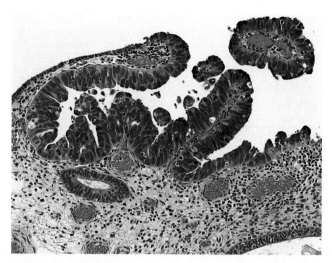

Figure 8.13 Intraepithelial serous carcinoma at the tip of an atrophic endometrial polyp.

in absence of a clear explanation of its significance; an alternative designation, and one that we endorse, is "*serous carcinoma in situ*." While we recognize that some of these lesions may represent metastases without detectable invasion, this terminology has the added advantage in that it can be used more broadly to diagnose lesions with similar appearance regardless of apparent site of origin (i.e., pelvic serous carcinoma in situ).

Table 8.2 Ancillary diagnostic tests for uterine serous carcinoma

p53 overexpression in more than 75% of tumor cell nuclei[a]
p16 overexpression in more than 90% of tumor cells
Ki-67 (MIB1) expression in more than 75% of tumor cell nuclei
Progesterone receptor (PR) expression that is weak, focal or absent

[a] About 10% of serous carcinomas show absolutely no staining with p53 antibodies. This contrasts with most endometrioid carcinomas, in which p53 antibodies stain 1–50% of tumor cell nuclei.

ANCILLARY DIAGNOSTIC TESTS (TABLE 8.2)

In many consultation practices, immunohistochemistry is used only to adjudicate cases with discrepant diagnoses or to confirm serous carcinoma when an endometrioid carcinoma is under consideration. Immunohistochemistry will support a diagnosis of serous carcinoma in approximately one-half of such problematic cases. However, since some high-grade endometrioid carcinomas may express a similar immunoprofile and not all serous carcinomas exhibit a characteristic uterine serous phenotype, immunohistochemistry is probably useful in the evaluation of fewer than 20% of such cases. Consensus diagnosis using a panel of experienced gynecologic pathologists may be as predictive of grade and cell type as immunohistochemistry[8].

Like endometrioid carcinomas, endometrial serous carcinomas commonly express pan-cytokeratins, EMA, CA125, Ber-EP4, B72.3, CK7, PAX8, and vimentin, while they are usually negative for CK20, negative or weakly positive for WT1, and lack diffuse, strong cytoplasmic expression of CEA.

Protein expression patterns in uterine serous carcinoma differ significantly from FIGO grade 1 and 2 uterine endometrioid carcinoma. However, any differences in immunohistochemical profiles become blurred when comparing FIGO grade 3 endometrioid adenocarcinoma and serous carcinoma. Therefore, the following data pertain only to differential diagnoses that involve FIGO grades 1 and 2 carcinomas and serous carcinomas.

Approximately 90% of uterine serous carcinomas shows p53 overexpression (intense nuclear expression in greater than 75% of tumor cells) as a result of *p53* mutation and the consequent accumulation of mutant protein (Figure 8.14)[9]. Most of the remaining tumors (most of which show absolutely no p53 expression) harbor *p53* mutations that result in a truncated p53 protein or a protein with conformational changes that cannot be detected using commercially available antibodies[9].

(A)

(B)

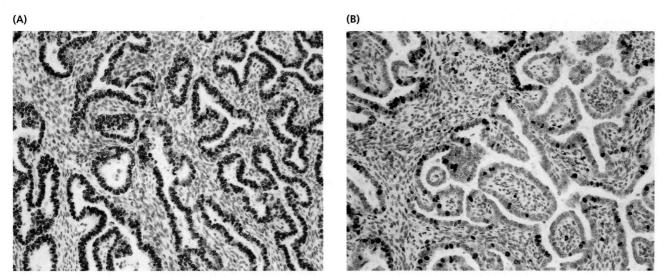

Figure 8.14 p53 expression in endometrial carcinoma. Serous carcinoma typically demonstrates p53 overexpression (A). Endometrioid adenocarcinoma usually shows p53 expression in less than 75% of tumor cells (B). This does not qualify as "p53 overexpression."

(A)

(B)

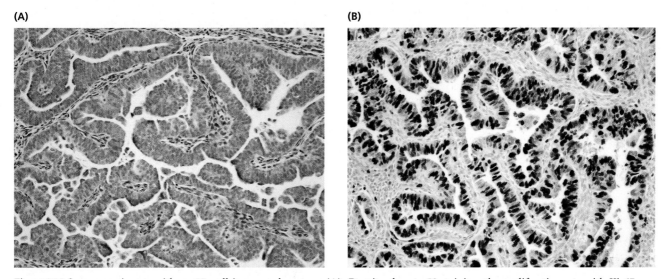

Figure 8.15 Serous carcinoma with a p53-null immunophenotype (A). Despite absent p53 staining, the proliferative rate with Ki-67 is high (B).

A serous carcinoma diagnosis can therefore be suggested, given the appropriate morphologic appearance, if the p53 shows absolutely no labeling and Ki-67 labeling is seen in greater than 75% of tumor cells (Figure 8.15). Proliferative activity, approximated with a Ki-67 labeling index, is extremely high (i.e., greater than 75% of tumor cell nuclei)[10] in uterine serous carcinoma, irrespective of the presence of p53 overexpression. Ki-67 immunohistochemistry is important given that high rates of p53 labeling have been described in certain metaplastic lesions as well as in a group of lesions that have been hypothesized to represent serous carcinoma precursors. p16 overexpression in an "every-cell pattern"

is also typical of serous carcinoma (Figure 8.16)[11]. It has been proposed that p16 is a more sensitive marker of serous differentiation as compared to p53 in the appropriate context[12]. In contrast to most endocervical carcinomas, this does not imply HPV infection; rather, it may reflect disturbances in the cell cycle that favor hyperproliferative activity. Most uterine serous carcinomas are negative for ER and PR[10,13]. Serous carcinoma in situ exhibits a similar immunoprofile.

Finally, it should be noted that, while many serous adenocarcinomas of endometrium resemble ovarian serous carcinomas, there are some important immunohistochemical differences. The most important of these is infrequent

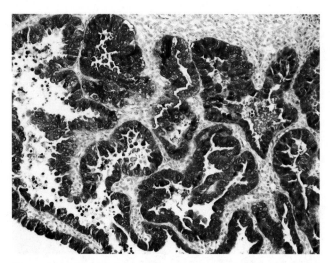

Figure 8.16 Serous carcinoma with p16 overexpression.

WT1 expression in endometrial serous carcinomas (seen in at most 20–30% of such cases) and the very common diffuse nuclear expression of WT1 in ovarian, tubal, and primary peritoneal examples (at least 70–80% of such cases)[14–16].

Table 8.3 Differential diagnosis of uterine serous carcinoma

Endometrioid adenocarcinoma

Metaplasia, reactive changes, and radiation atypia

Mixed endometrioid and serous carcinoma

Clear cell carcinoma

Ovarian, peritoneal, or fallopian tube serous carcinoma

Endocervical adenocarcinoma

Hybrid carcinomas with features of endometrioid and serous, or clear cell and serous carcinoma

Table 8.4 Pathologic characteristics of low-grade endometrioid carcinoma

Only mild or moderate nuclear atypia

Smooth luminal contours

Squamous or mucinous metaplasia or secretory change

Nuclear atypia appropriate for architectural grade

Background hyperplasia

DIFFERENTIAL DIAGNOSIS (TABLE 8.3)

Probably the most common diagnostic error involving serous carcinoma, and the one that leads to the greatest potential for clinical mismanagement and subsequent litigation, is the misdiagnosis of serous carcinoma as well-differentiated endometrioid adenocarcinoma or hyperplasia. The extent of disease may therefore be underestimated, as formal surgical staging procedures are commonly withheld for the latter two entities. This has potentially profound clinical implications because as many as 50% of serous carcinoma patients whose disease appears confined to the uterus actually have extrauterine disease demonstrable only after comprehensive surgical staging.

Endometrioid adenocarcinoma (Table 8.4)

Carcinomas should be categorized as serous when the background is atrophic, the nuclear grade is high, cellular dyshesion and tufting are present, and cytoplasmic changes associated with endometrioid differentiation are lacking (i.e., squamous, morular, or mucinous metaplasia, and the presence of cilia are absent). Although many serous carcinomas are overtly papillary, glandular[17] or, occasionally, solid patterns can be seen. Most retain, at least focally,

slit-like spaces, micropapillae or cellular tufting, dyshesion, and ragged luminal contours; all feature high-grade nuclei. Unlike most endometrioid carcinomas, serous carcinomas show dyssynchronous architectural and cytologic features. That is, although most serous carcinomas exhibit a wide range of non-solid architectural patterns, the cytologic grade remains high. In endometrioid carcinomas, the cytologic grade usually (but not always) parallels the architectural grade, with the highest grade nuclei being found in tumors with the most solid architecture. Immunohistochemistry can be used when there is diagnostic uncertainty, but this should be avoided when the tumor is otherwise high grade, because, in this situation, it is not informative. Endometrioid adenocarcinoma of FIGO grade 3 shows p53 overexpression and loss of ER and PR in as many as 30% of cases[18]. Overexpression of p53 and a high proliferative rate with Ki-67, both marking greater than 75% of tumor cell nuclei, along with absent or at most focal hormone receptor immunoreactivity, support serous carcinoma when the tumor exhibits more characteristic serous morphology. A diffusely and intensely positive p16 stain may also be useful in this distinction. Patchy p53 immunoreactivity in less than 75% of tumor cells, substantial PR expression, or p16 staining in only a subset of cells is not characteristic of uterine serous carcinoma.

(A)

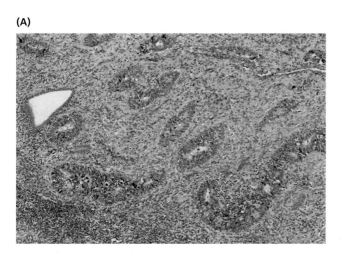

(B)

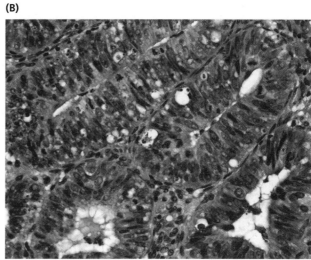

(C)

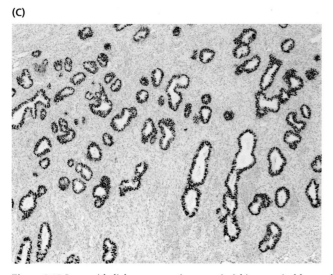

Figure 8.17 Intraepithelial serous carcinoma mimicking atypical hyperplasia or low-grade endometrioid adenocarcinoma (A, B). The lesion in panel B overexpresses p53 (C).

Serous carcinoma in situ may mimic complex atypical hyperplasia and well-differentiated endometrioid adenocarcinomas (Figure 8.17). Cellular and nuclear enlargement, the frequent presence of macronucleoli, and a high proliferative index, in addition to ragged, serrated, and uneven luminal contours with dyshesive cells and abortive micropapillae, are all features that support serous carcinoma in situ and argue against complex hyperplasia or well-differentiated adenocarcinoma.

Clear cell carcinoma

The papillae of clear cell carcinoma are often more densely hyalinized than the papillae in serous carcinoma. In contrast to clear cell carcinoma, serous carcinoma shows more substantial epithelial tufting and more extensive micropapillae (Table 8.5) (Figure 8.18). The lining epithelium is only one or two cells thick, without prominent tufting. The cells are large and cuboidal, generally contain ample clear cytoplasm filled with glycogen, and show sharply defined cytoplasmic boundaries. Hobnail cells may be seen lining a surface or a glandular lumen. The nuclei are large with prominent nucleoli.

Pelvic (non-uterine) serous carcinoma

Endometrial, ovarian, peritoneal, and tubal serous carcinomas show considerable morphologic similarity, but the background in which they occur differs[19]. There are immunophenotypic differences as well. The typical presentation of ovarian, peritoneal, or tubal serous carcinoma in an endometrial biopsy or curettage is in the

Table 8.5 Pathologic characteristics of clear cell carcinoma

Uniformly atypical nuclei with only occasional bizarre nuclear forms

Cuboidal tumor cells

Solid, tubulocystic, or papillary architecture without significant stratification (at most two or three cell layers), tufting, or extensive dyshesion

Clear cytoplasm with hobnail forms[a]

Patchy nuclear p53 expression without overexpression (exceptions occur)

Focal, weak, or absent PR expression

Serous architectural and cytoplasmic features are lacking

[a] Serous carcinomas may have clear cytoplasm and hobnail forms, and clear cell carcinoma cells may have eosinophilic cytoplasm (so-called oxyphilic variant).

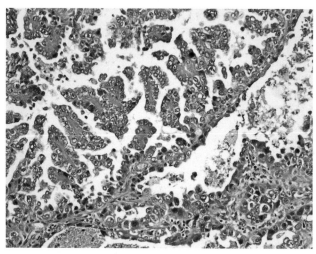

Figure 8.18 Clear cell carcinoma mimicking serous carcinoma. The papillae of clear cell carcinoma are small and round, and the stroma can be densely hyalinized. The lining epithelium is only one or two cells thick, without prominent budding.

form of small tumor cell aggregates (Figure 7.38) floating in a background of cycling or atrophic endometrium. In hysterectomy specimens, drop metastases from ovarian, peritoneal, and tubal serous carcinomas are usually superficial and unassociated with endometrial polyps; they may be multifocal. This contrasts with the typical uterine serous carcinoma, in which an atrophic background is the norm. Serous carcinomas of the ovary, peritoneum, and fallopian tube more frequently express ER and WT1 strongly and diffusely, but since as many as 30% of uterine serous carcinomas express WT1 as well, the results of this test can be misleading.

Synchronous versus metastatic serous carcinoma

It can be extremely difficult to determine whether serous carcinomas, arising in an endometrial polyp with intraepithelial serous carcinoma along with a serous carcinoma involving ovary, fallopian tube, and peritoneum, are synchronous or metastatic from one site to the other (see Table 7.8). Evidence of monoclonality[20] and immunohistochemical substantiation of endometrial serous differentiation support the idea that this scenario generally reflects a primary endometrial serous carcinoma that has metastasized to extrauterine organs[6,21]. The group from the M. D. Anderson Cancer Center, Houston[21] studied WT1 immunohistochemistry in two groups of patients, one with peritoneal carcinomatosis and no endometrial disease, and another with peritoneal carcinomatosis and serous carcinomas in endometrial polyps. Peritoneal tumors in the first group were almost always WT1 positive (supporting ovarian, tubal, or peritoneal serous carcinoma), while the endometrial and peritoneal tumors in the second group were almost always WT1 negative (supporting endometrial serous carcinoma). Given the appropriate context, then, WT1 immunostains may be useful in determining the *likelihood* that a given serous carcinoma is endometrial or extrauterine in origin. However, since as many as 20–30% of endometrial serous carcinomas have been reported to be WT1 positive, and 20–30% of ovarian, tubal, and peritoneal carcinomas may be WT1 negative, it is imprudent to claim that this test offers unqualified support for one situation over another[14–16,22]. The addition of ER immunostaining may provide some additional corroborative evidence for primary site. However, for practical purposes, serous carcinomas involving endometrium and ovary can be considered an endometrial primary if the serous carcinoma is arising in a polyp and the background endometrium is atrophic.

Endocervical adenocarcinoma

Endocervical adenocarcinomas can display papillary architecture and high nuclear grade. Small fragments of papillary endocervical adenocarcinoma in an endocervical or endometrial biopsy or curettage could therefore be confused with serous carcinoma. A general rule of thumb is to strongly consider a diagnosis of endocervical adenocarcinoma or extrauterine serous carcinoma if small fragments of a high-grade papillary tumor are admixed with cycling endometrium in a premenopausal patient.

Immunohistochemically, endocervical adenocarcinomas frequently show positive, punctate nuclear signals with high-risk HPV in situ hybridization, lack expression of WT1, ER, and PR, and fail to show overexpression of p53. Strong, diffuse CEA cytoplasmic expression, if present, also supports endocervical origin, as uterine and extra-uterine serous carcinomas do not generally exhibit strong, diffuse CEA expression. p16 immunostaining should not be used when the differential diagnosis includes endocervical and serous carcinomas, because it is typically strongly expressed in both.

Metaplasia, reactive changes, and radiation atypia

Serous carcinoma in situ can be easily confused with non-neoplastic proliferations, including atypical tubal metaplasia, eosinophilic metaplasia, benign papillary change, and reactive changes (Table 8.6) (Figures 7.8, 7.9, and 7.16). Features in favor of serous carcinoma include a mitotically active, cytologically atypical proliferation

Table 8.6 Pathologic characteristics of metaplasia, reactive change, or radiation atypia

Preserved nuclear-to-cytoplasmic ratio
Low mitotic index
No p53 overexpression
Ki-67 (MIB1) proliferative index <50%

of one cell type, with high nucleus-to-cytoplasmic ratios, and absence of cilia and stromal breakdown (Figure 8.19). Immunohistochemistry with p53 and Ki-67 (MIB1) stains together can be helpful. Overexpressed p53 with a matching Ki-67 supports serous carcinoma in situ, and low level expression of p53 with at most moderate proliferation (<50% of tumor cells) supports metaplasia or a reactive condition. Be aware that some atypical metaplastic and reactive epithelium can display a large percentage of p53 positive cells; the proliferative index in these conditions, however, typically remains below the 50% mark. In addition, p16 antibodies may be useful in this differential diagnosis, provided a diagnosis of serous carcinoma is only considered when the lesion exhibits a strong, diffuse, every-single-cell pattern, because patchy p16 expression can be seen in many examples of tubal metaplasia.

Mixed epithelial carcinomas

Rare serous carcinomas occur in a setting of well-differentiated or moderately differentiated endometrioid adenocarcinoma (Figure 8.10). In a mixed serous and endometrioid adenocarcinoma, the serous component should be starkly different in appearance and immunophenotype from the endometrioid substrate (i.e., p53 overexpression and a high proliferative index are seen in the serous carcinoma component, but not in the endometrioid component). Mixed carcinomas fitting this description are

(A) **(B)**

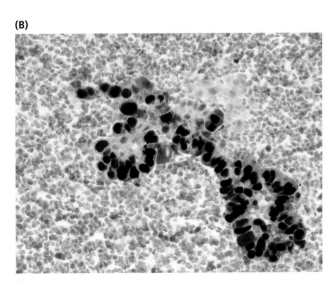

Figure 8.19 Fragments of serous carcinoma in a curettage (A); the differential diagnosis includes metaplasia and reactive changes. Significant nuclear enlargement relative to admixed atrophic endometrium, nuclear pleomorphism, and the presence of a mitotic figure support a neoplasm. p53 overexpression (B) and high proliferative rates with Ki-67 (not shown) support classification as serous carcinoma. These stains can be used when the differential diagnosis includes a metaplastic or reactive lesion.

(A)

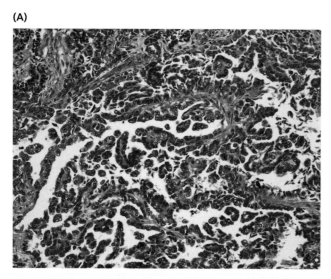

(B)

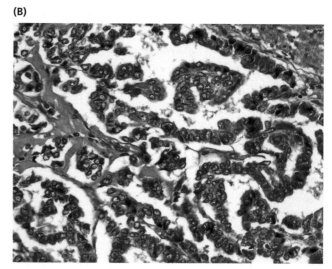

Figure 8.20 Endometrial carcinoma of uncertain histologic subtype. Papillary architecture, budding, and dyshesion suggested serous carcinoma (A), but the nuclear features (B) were uniform. Applying the Gilks' grading scheme results in classification as a low-grade carcinoma. Papillary architecture is present, but neither significant nuclear atypia nor more than 5 MF/10 HPF were noted.

very uncommon. In contrast, most carcinomas that appear to consist of two separate tumor types on examination of hematoxylin and eosin stained slides are immunophenotypically uniform.

It has been proposed that mixed tumors with a component of serous carcinoma comprising more than 25% of the tumor volume be regarded as serous carcinoma[23] from a clinical perspective, but evidence of peritoneal metastasis originating from tumors with only focal serous carcinoma are certainly on record. Therefore, although it is our practice to report the percentage of each component in a mixed carcinoma, we assign the overall grade based on the component with the highest grade.

Hybrid tumors

Histologic subtype assignment is particularly problematic when a gland-forming or papillary tumor exhibits nuclear pleomorphism and a high mitotic rate but lacks other confirmatory endometrioid or serous characteristics (Figure 8.20). Some pathologists would argue that such a tumor displays morphologic features that are not informative regarding its biology (i.e., it is a serous carcinoma masquerading as an endometrioid carcinoma), while others would say that the endometrioid component is high grade, possibly in evolution to serous carcinoma. Given those predispositions, these pathologists might base a final diagnosis on immunophenotype. However, there are pathologists who would undoubtedly counter that the immunophenotype has no diagnostic value in this setting. The

most reasonable way of approaching these hybrid proliferations is to admit that we do not know whether these tumors are endometrioid or serous or another tumor type, and that we are only now beginning to gain an insight into their prognostic assessment. Overexpression of p53, while not necessarily diagnostic of serous carcinoma given equivocal morphologic features, has been reported to be an unfavorable prognostic indicator that is independent of other variables[8].

The best diagnostic approach for these hybrid tumors depends upon whether the tumor is present in a biopsy or curettage, or in a hysterectomy specimen. In a biopsy or curettage specimen, it is probably sufficient to indicate that the tumor may be serous. This will encourage the surgeon to perform a comprehensive staging surgery that includes omentectomy, full lymph node dissection, and peritoneal biopsies. The surgeon will also expect the pathologist to assign a tumor grade. As hybrid tumors are neither obviously endometrioid nor serous, it may be misleading to assign a FIGO grade based on architecture and cytology. Using the standard FIGO grading scheme in these circumstances may result in a diagnosis of a FIGO grade 2 carcinoma, which would underestimate the aggressiveness of the tumor if in fact it is a serous carcinoma. We tend to diagnose these tumors as "high grade" and discuss the differential diagnosis of the histologic subtype in a comment. Alternatively, one could employ Gilks' binary grading scheme[24], which appears to be a prognostically informative method that can be used with any type of endometrial cancer. In this scheme, tumors that display any two of the following three features are considered "high grade:" papillary or solid architecture; high nuclear grade; more than 5 MF/10 HPF. Once the pathologist has the opportunity to fully evaluate the tumor in the hysterectomy specimen, it will be important to predict the likelihood that it will behave like a serous carcinoma. Most patients with serous carcinoma or with extrauterine disease of any histologic type are offered chemotherapy and radiation, which means that the stakes are high when the tumor is confined to the uterus and the carcinoma may be serous. We favor a diagnosis of serous carcinoma if the carcinoma is arising in an atrophic polyp and/or a background of atrophic endometrium and there are at least focal micropapillae or slit-like spaces. Diffuse ER and/or PR expression with equivocal p53 and MIB1 results, especially in the absence of atrophy, dissuade a confident diagnosis of serous carcinoma. When assignment as either serous or endometrioid is impossible, p53 immunohistochemistry along with Gilks' grading may yield valid prognostic information to assist the oncologist in devising treatment strategies.

REFERENCES

1. Soslow RA, Bissonnette JP, Wilton A, *et al.* Clinicopathologic analysis of 187 high-grade endometrial carcinomas of different histologic subtypes: similar outcomes belie distinctive biologic differences. *Am J Surg Pathol* 2007;**31**(7):979–87.

2. Fader AN, Drake RD, O'Malley DM, *et al.* Platinum/taxane-based chemotherapy with or without radiation therapy favorably impacts survival outcomes in stage I uterine papillary serous carcinoma. *Cancer* 2009;**115**(10):2119–27.

3. Carcangiu ML, Chambers JT. Uterine papillary serous carcinoma: a study on 108 cases with emphasis on the prognostic significance of associated endometrioid carcinoma, absence of invasion, and concomitant ovarian carcinoma. *Gynecol Oncol* 1992;**47**:298–305.

4. Wheeler DT, Bell KA, Kurman RJ, Sherman ME. Minimal uterine serous carcinoma: diagnosis and clinicopathologic correlation. *Am J Surg Pathol* 2000;**24**(6):797–806.

5. Hui P, Kelly M, O'Malley DM, Tavassoli F, Schwartz PE. Minimal uterine serous carcinoma: a clinicopathological study of 40 cases. *Mod Pathol* 2005;**18**(1):75–82.

6. Soslow RA, Pirog E, Isacson C. Endometrial intraepithelial carcinoma with associated peritoneal carcinomatosis. *Am J Surg Pathol* 2000;**24**(5):726–32.

7. Jarboe EA, Pizer ES, Miron A, *et al.* Evidence for a latent precursor (p53 signature) that may precede serous endometrial intraepithelial carcinoma. *Mod Pathol* 2009;**22**(3):345–50.

8. Garg K, Leitao MM, Jr., Wynveen CA, *et al.* p53 overexpression in morphologically ambiguous endometrial carcinomas correlates with adverse clinical outcomes. *Mod Pathol* 2010;**23**(1):80–92.

9. Tashiro H, Isacson C, Levine R, *et al.* p53 gene mutations are common in uterine serous carcinoma and occur early in their pathogenesis. *Am J Pathol* 1997;**150**(1):177–85.

10. Lax SF, Pizer ES, Ronnett BM, Kurman RJ. Clear cell carcinoma of the endometrium is characterized by a distinctive profile of p53, Ki-67, estrogen, and progesterone receptor expression. *Hum Pathol* 1998;**29**(6):551–8.

11. Reid-Nicholson M, Iyengar P, Hummer AJ, *et al.* Immunophenotypic diversity of endometrial adenocarcinomas: implications for differential diagnosis. *Mod Pathol* 2006;**19**(8):1091–100.

12. Chiesa-Vottero AG, Malpica A, Deavers MT, *et al.* Immunohistochemical overexpression of p16 and p53 in uterine serous carcinoma and ovarian high-grade serous carcinoma. *Int J Gynecol Pathol* 2007;**26**(3):328–33.

13. Chambers JT, Carcangiu ML, Voynick IM, Schwartz PE. Immunohistochemical evaluation of estrogen and progesterone receptor content in 183 patients with endometrial carcinoma. Part II: correlation between biochemical and immunohistochemical methods and survival. *Am J Clin Pathol* 1990;**94**(3):255–60.

14. Acs G, Pasha T, Zhang PJ. WT1 is differentially expressed in serous, endometrioid, clear cell, and mucinous carcinomas of the peritoneum, fallopian tube, ovary, and endometrium. *Int J Gynecol Pathol* 2004;**23**(2):110–18.

15. Egan JA, Ionescu MC, Eapen E, Jones JG, Marshall DS. Differential expression of WT1 and p53 in serous and endometrioid carcinomas of the endometrium. *Int J Gynecol Pathol* 2004;**23**(2):119–22.

16. Goldstein NS, Uzieblo A. WT1 immunoreactivity in uterine papillary serous carcinomas is different from ovarian serous carcinomas. *Am J Clin Pathol* 2002;**117**(4):541–5.

17. Darvishian F, Hummer AJ, Thaler HT, *et al.* Serous endometrial cancers that mimic endometrioid adenocarcinomas: a clinicopathologic and immunohistochemical study of a group of problematic cases. *Am J Surg Pathol* 2004;**28**(12):1568–78.

18. Soslow RA, Shen PU, Chung MH, Isacson C. Distinctive p53 and mdm2 immunohistochemical expression profiles suggest different pathogenetic pathways in poorly differentiated endometrial carcinoma. *Int J Gynecol Pathol* 1998;**17**:129–34.

19. Soslow RA, Slomovitz BM, Saqi A, Baergen RN, Caputo TA. Tumor suppressor gene, cell surface adhesion molecule, and multidrug resistance in mullerian serous carcinomas: clinical divergence without immunophenotypic differences. *Gynecol Oncol* 2000;**79**(3):430–7.

20. Baergen RN, Warren CD, Isacson C, Ellenson LH. Early uterine serous carcinoma: clonal origin of extrauterine disease. *Int J Gynecol Pathol* 2001;**20**(3):214–19.

21. Euscher ED, Malpica A, Deavers MT, Silva EG. Differential expression of WT-1 in serous carcinomas in the peritoneum with or without associated serous carcinoma in endometrial polyps. *Am J Surg Pathol* 2005;**29**(8):1074–8.

22. Dupont J, Wang X, Marshall DS, *et al.* Wilms Tumor Gene (WT1) and p53 expression in endometrial carcinomas: a study of 130 cases using a tissue microarray. *Gynecol Oncol* 2004;**94**(2):449–55.

23. Sherman ME, Bitterman P, Rosenshein NB, Delgado G, Kurman RJ. Uterine serous carcinoma: a morphologically diverse neoplasm with unifying clinicopathologic features. *Am J Surg Pathol* 1992;**16**:600–10.

24. Alkushi A, Abdul-Rahman ZH, Lim P, *et al.* Description of a novel system for grading of endometrial carcinoma and comparison with existing grading systems. *Am J Surg Pathol* 2005;**29**(3):295–304.

INTRODUCTION

Although endometrioid and serous adenocarcinomas comprise the majority of uterine corpus carcinomas, the less common clear cell, mucinous, and very rare squamous variants may pose considerable diagnostic problems. In addition, there are a variety of unusual carcinomas that occur in the uterus, some of which demonstrate distinctive clinical behavior as well as distinctive morphology. In contrast to the more common endometrioid and serous tumors, there are fewer data concerning these tumors.

CLEAR CELL CARCINOMA

Clear cell carcinoma currently accounts for less than 5% of all endometrial carcinomas in the United States.

Clinical characteristics

Clear cell carcinoma is considered to be a type II estrogen-independent nonendometrioid carcinoma[1]. Patients tend to be older than those with endometrioid carcinoma, but slightly younger than those with serous carcinoma, with a mean age of 62 to 67 years. As with serous carcinoma, African-American women are more frequently affected. Despite its high grade, disease is confined to the uterus at presentation in 70% of patients. Radiation and tamoxifen have been implicated in a subset of clear cell carcinomas.

Clear cell carcinoma has a worse prognosis than endometrioid carcinoma[5]. The five-year overall survival rate is 62.5% for patients with clear cell adenocarcinoma compared with 83.2% for those with endometrioid carcinoma. Stage is the most important prognostic factor; in the M. D. Anderson Center study, patients with low-stage (FIGO I and II) clear cell carcinoma had an estimated survival rate similar to that of patients with FIGO grade 3 endometrioid adenocarcinoma, and better than that of patients with serous carcinoma of similar stages[6].

In contrast to endometrioid carcinoma and uterine serous carcinoma, the molecular pathways involved in the development of clear cell carcinoma are poorly understood. The natural history and the optimal treatment of clear cell carcinoma are also not well defined, largely because most studies have combined clear cell carcinomas and serous carcinomas in their analysis. Patients with clear cell carcinoma tend to relapse in the pelvis, in para-aortic nodes, and at distant sites. In general, total abdominal hysterectomy and bilateral salpingo-oophorectomy with comprehensive surgical staging is the standard surgical treatment of patients with clear cell carcinoma of the endometrium. As with the ovarian counterpart, clear cell adenocarcinoma of the endometrium is associated with increased risk for thromboembolic events[7].

Morphology

Gross pathology

Clear cell carcinomas often form fleshy and soft masses involving most of the endometrial surface, similar to endometrioid adenocarcinoma (Figure 9.1).

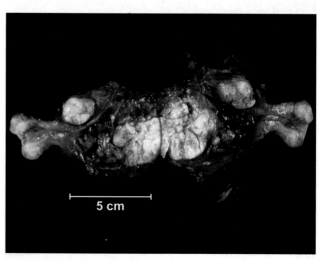

5 cm

Figure 9.1 Clear cell carcinoma.

Microscopic pathology

Microscopically, uterine clear cell carcinoma exhibits the same microscopic patterns as in the ovary; namely solid, papillary, and glandular or tubulocystic (Table 9.1; Figures

Table 9.1 Pathologic characteristics of uterine clear cell carcinoma

Histologic feature	Description
Architectural pattern(s)	Tubulocystic (glandular), papillary, solid
Cells	Polyhedral, cuboidal, flattened, hobnail
Cytoplasm	Clear or eosinophilic and granular (glycogen)
Nuclear atypia	Moderate to marked – but often focal
Mitotic index	Often low (3–4 MF/10 HPF), but may be higher
Stroma	Hyalinized or spherule-like mucoid stroma

9.2– 9.4). The papillae in clear cell carcinoma are distinctive due to the presence of prominent basement membrane material within the connective tissue core (Figure 9.3). The tumor cells are cuboidal or polygonal in contour and contain clear or eosinophilic cytoplasm with eccentric nuclei (Figure 9.5). Hobnail cells and flattened cells are also seen. The clear cytoplasm results from the presence of glycogen, but eosinophilic hyaline mucin droplets can be detected on PAS/D stain, often forming signet ring–like or targetoid structures (Figure 9.6). Nuclear atypia is usually marked (Figure 9.7); mitotic figures are often not as prominent as in serous carcinoma, but may be numerous in some cases. Foci of prominent stromal hyalinization are helpful diagnostic clues, if present. Lymphoplasmacytic or neutrophilic stromal inflammation may also be seen. Some cases of pure clear cell carcinoma may also have psammoma bodies. Clear cell

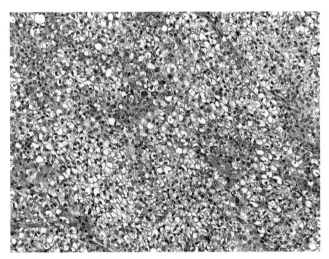

Figure 9.2 Clear cell carcinoma. Solid pattern.

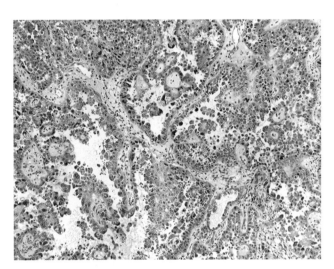

Figure 9.3 Clear cell carcinoma. Papillary pattern.

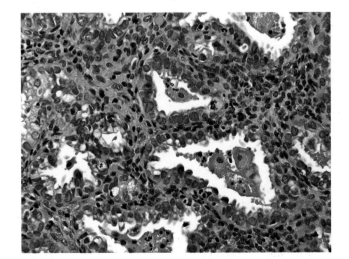

Figure 9.4 Clear cell carcinoma. Glandular pattern.

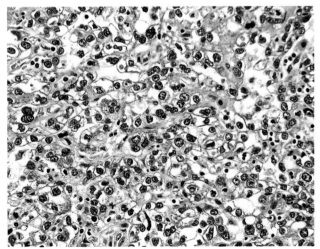

Figure 9.5 Clear cell carcinoma. The constituent cells have polyhedral or rounded contours.

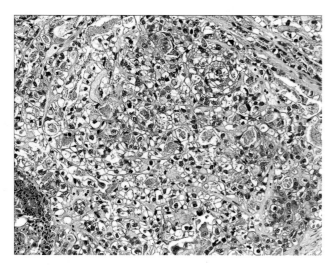

Figure 9.6 Clear cell carcinoma. Targetoid pattern.

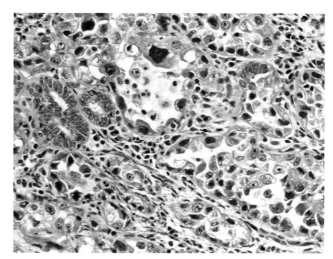

Figure 9.7 Clear cell carcinoma. Nuclear atypia is often non-uniform.

(A)

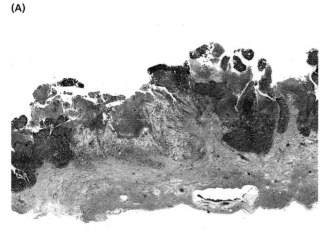

(B)

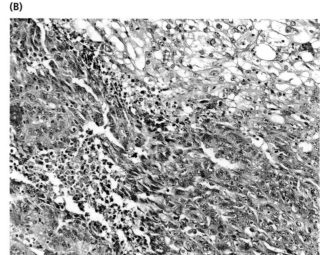

Figure 9.8 (A) Mixed clear cell carcinoma and endometrioid carcinoma. (B) The two tumors are adjacent to one another and exhibit a rather abrupt transition.

carcinoma is not assigned a FIGO grade; because of its clinical aggressiveness, it is high grade, by definition.

Pure clear cell carcinoma is rare in the uterine corpus. Some clear cell carcinomas are mixed with endometrioid carcinoma (Figure 9.8). Many uterine clear cell carcinomas have overlapping features of serous carcinoma, including hobnail forms, cell dyshesion (Figure 9.9), and eosinophilic cytoplasm (Figure 9.10), in addition to papillae, simple glands, and marked nuclear atypia. Opinion is mixed as to whether the distinction between the two has clinical impact, as both are considered high-grade tumors. However, if there is a distinct clear cell component in a tumor that otherwise appears to be uterine serous carcinoma, we diagnose the clear cell component as well, due to the

increased risk of thromboembolic events with clear cell carcinoma. The prognosis of mixed endometrioid and clear cell tumors is also not well studied, but appears to be similar for pure clear cell carcinoma. When mixed tumors occur, we diagnose both components but assign the overall grade of the higher-grade component; therefore these mixed tumors are considered high grade.

A precursor lesion for uterine clear cell carcinoma has been proposed[8]. The putative precursor cell is distributed in adjacent glands and/or surface epithelium and consists of isolated cells or patches of cells with clear or eosinophilic cytoplasm and nuclear atypia. Although of scientific interest, precursor lesions of clear cell carcinoma are of uncertain clinical significance.

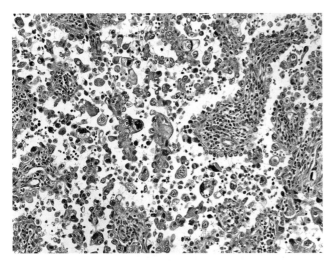

Figure 9.9 Clear cell carcinoma. Cellular dyshesion may occur in clear cell carcinomas, although it is more common in serous carcinomas.

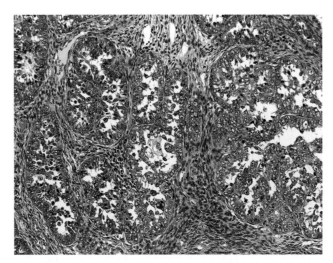

Figure 9.10 Clear cell carcinoma. Eosinophilic, granular cytoplasm is present in this variant.

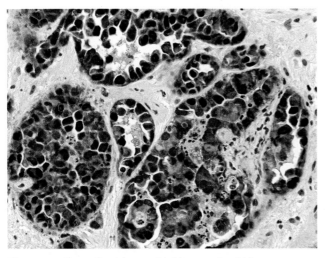

Figure 9.11 Clear cell carcinoma. In this example p16 is strong and diffuse.

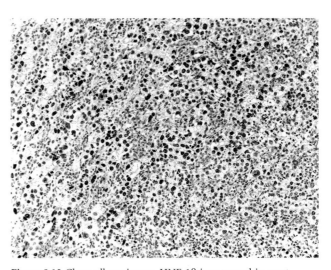

Figure 9.12 Clear cell carcinoma. HNF-1β is expressed in most clear cell carcinomas, but may be seen in yolk sac tumors, secretory and gestational endometria, and clear cell variants of renal cell carcinoma.

Ancillary diagnostic tests

The immunoprofile for uterine clear cell carcinoma is not as well defined as it is for endometrioid and serous adenocarcinoma. Most clear cell carcinomas are negative for hormone receptors ER and PR[9]. About one-half are positive for p16 (Figure 9.11). Overexpression of p53 is more common in clear cell carcinoma than in endometrioid carcinoma, but less common than in uterine serous carcinoma[9].

Transcription factor 2 gene (*TCF2*) encodes hepatocyte nuclear factor 1β (HNF-1β), which is involved in development of the urogenital system. Microarray analyses have identified up-regulation of HNF-1β in clear cell carcinoma of the ovary as well as in ovarian endometriosis, which is often associated with clear cell carcinoma. Expression of HNF-1β by immunohistochemistry is seen in clear cell carcinoma of the ovary and uterus (Figure 9.12), as well as in secretory and gestational endometrium, yolk sac tumors, and renal clear cell carcinoma (Cuff J, Salari K, Esheba GE, *et al.* Integrative bioinformatics links HNF1-β with clear cell carcinoma and tumor-associated thrombosis, personal communication, 2011)[10]. Expression of HNF-1β appears to be associated with glycogen accumulation (clear cytoplasm) and clotting factor production in ovarian and endometrioid clear cell carcinoma. In a small cohort of patients having tumors with some degree of cytoplasmic clearing, those

(A)

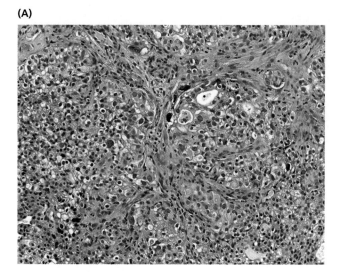

(B)

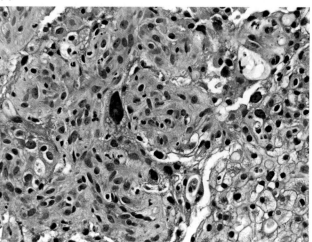

Figure 9.13 (A, B) Arias-Stella reaction.

Table 9.2 Endometrial clear cell carcinoma: differential diagnosis

Epithelial
- Arias-Stella reaction
- Serous carcinoma
- Endometrioid carcinoma
- Cervical clear cell carcinoma
- Clear cell metaplasia
- Clear cell change in pregnancy

Other
- Metastatic renal cell carcinoma

with HNF-1β expression were significantly more likely (nearly threefold) to experience a clinically significant thrombotic event (including deep venous thrombosis, pulmonary embolism, and thrombotic stroke) than those without HNF-1β expression (Cuff J, Salari K, Esheba GE, *et al.*, personal communication).

Differential diagnosis

Many tumors and tumor-like lesions in the uterus and cervix contain clear cells and may occasionally be misinterpreted as uterine corpus clear cell adenocarcinomas (Table 9.2). These conditions include clear cell carcinoma arising in the cervix, serous carcinoma, endometrioid carcinoma with secretory change, endometrioid carcinoma with other forms of cytoplasmic clear cell change, and clear cell metaplasia in the corpus. Arias-Stella change can pose diagnostic problems in both sites. Metastatic renal cell carcinoma, although uncommon, is an additional diagnostic consideration.

Arias-Stella reaction

The majority of patients with the Arias-Stella reaction are in the reproductive years; they will have experienced a recent pregnancy or be pregnant, or will have undergone hormonal therapy. In contrast, patients with clear cell carcinoma of the endometrium are almost always postmenopausal. The cells in the Arias-Stella reaction are either not mitotically active or feature only rare mitotic figures, and the nuclei show degenerative features, often with pseudoinclusions. Often, a stromal predecidual reaction is also present (Figure 9.13).

Serous carcinoma

Several of the original series of serous carcinoma contained tumors with clear cell elements[11]. Clear cell carcinoma and uterine serous carcinoma both have high-grade cytology and feature glandular and papillary architecture with hobnail cells (Figure 9.14). While uterine tumors with prototypical features of uterine serous carcinoma and clear cell carcinoma are easily distinguished, some cases have overlapping features or appear to consist of a mixture of both. There are some data to suggest mixed serous and clear cell carcinomas have a higher Ki-67 proliferation index and are more likely to harbor areas of endometrial intraepithelial carcinoma, whereas pure clear cell carcinomas are not associated with endometrial intraepithelial carcinoma[9]. Assignment to one or the other group in this circumstance is highly subjective and, from the point of view of clinical management, may be of no particular significance – both are high-grade, clinically aggressive neoplasms – and both are typically staged in a similar fashion. However, because

(A)

(B)

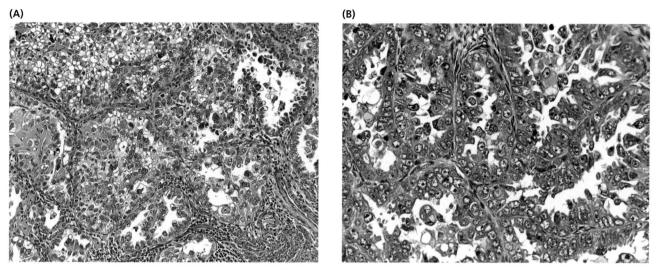

Figure 9.14 (A) Clear cell carcinoma. (B) Serous carcinoma. Both may show hobnail cells.

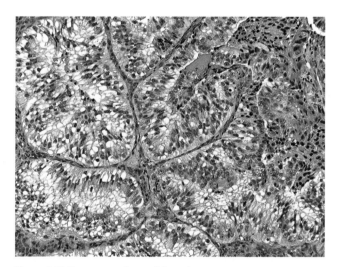

Figure 9.15 Secretory endometrial carcinoma.

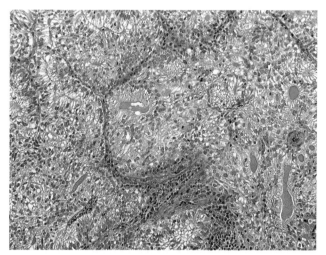

Figure 9.16 Clear cell change in endometrioid carcinoma.

of the potential increased risk for thromboembolism, tumors with any bona fide clear cell morphology should be diagnosed as clear cell carcinoma or as mixed clear cell and serous carcinoma. There are currently no discriminatory immunohistochemical markers in common usage that will reliably distinguish uterine serous carcinoma and uterine clear cell carcinoma.

Endometrioid carcinoma with secretory change

The distinction between secretory carcinoma and clear cell carcinoma is based on cytology: the tumor cell nuclei in secretory carcinoma are comparatively bland, ovoid in configuration, and do not show a hobnail or tombstone-like appearance (Figure 9.15). In contrast, uterine clear cell carcinoma has cells with nuclei with high-grade

cytologic characteristics, often protruding into glandular lumina (Figure 9.5).

Endometrioid carcinoma with other clear cell change

In addition to secretory change, endometrioid carcinomas can exhibit clear cell features due to the presence of extensively glycogenated squamous cells, lipid cells, or miscellaneous other causes not well specified[12]. Carcinomas with glycogenated squamous cells almost always have other areas with more classic features of squamous epithelium, as do most other differentiated endometrioid carcinomas with clear cells (Figure 9.16). Sometimes, a high-grade neoplasm with endometrioid features merges imperceptibly with solid cellular areas with cytoplasmic clearing;

(A)

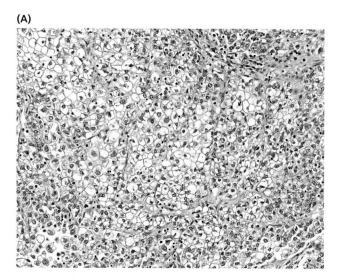

(B)

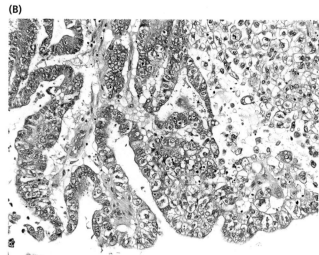

Figure 9.17 (A) Endometrial carcinoma with areas of clear cytoplasm. (B) Transition zone between endometrioid component and clear cells suggests the tumor is endometrioid with areas of cytoplasmic clearing as opposed to a true mixed tumor, although this is the type of tumor that is subject to interobserver disagreement.

in this situation, the distinction between high-grade pure endometrioid carcinoma and high-grade mixed endometrioid and clear cell carcinoma can be quite subjective (Figure 9.17). Clear cell carcinoma often has more polygonal cells with round nuclei, while endometrioid carcinoma tends to have more columnar cells with ovoid nuclei, but these distinctions are often blurred when the endometrioid component is high grade. Careful examination of the entire process in the hysterectomy specimen may yield foci of gradual transition between the endometrioid component and the component with cytoplasmic clearing (Figure 9.17). If encountered in a curettage specimen, the possibility of clear cell carcinoma should be mentioned in the report in order to guide surgical staging. If present in a hysterectomy specimen and a gradual transition is identified, the carcinoma should probably be diagnosed as high-grade endometrioid adenocarcinoma in absence of additional morphologic support for a bona fide clear cell component. Most clear cell carcinomas are negative for ER and PR hormone receptors, whereas many endometrioid carcinomas express ER and/or PR. As both tend to be negative for WT1, this is not a useful marker in this differential diagnosis.

Clear cell carcinoma of cervical origin

Clear cell carcinoma arising in the cervix has historically been linked to DES exposure in utero. However, clear cell carcinoma may develop in the cervix in absence of this teratogen (see Chapter 3). The histologic features are not dissimilar to those arising in the endometrium. As in the endometrium, these tumors are often mistaken for serous carcinoma due to their high-grade cytology, tombstone nuclear configurations, and granular, eosinophilic cytoplasm. Because of this mimicry, we suspect that at least some of the tumors that have been diagnosed in the past as rare primary cervical serous carcinoma are in fact clear cell carcinoma. Assigning primary site (e.g., cervix versus endometrium) is not possible on histology or immunohistology; localization requires correlation with ancillary clinical and imaging studies.

Clear cell metaplasia

Clear cell change in secretory and non-secretory glands (clear cell metaplasia) may be quite prominent, but the nuclei do not show significant atypia (Figure 9.18). Clear cell metaplasia may show a pseudopapillary pattern, but true papillary and solid patterns are not seen in clear cell metaplasia. However, as with endometrioid carcinoma, cytoplasmic clearing may occur in a wide variety of endometrial hyperplasias (Figure 9.19); distinction is based on the "company it keeps" – that is, adjacent areas of hyperplasia without clear cell change, foci of squamous differentiation, and so on. Most hyperplasias with clear cell change should express ER and/or PR.

Metastatic renal cell carcinoma

Metastatic renal cell carcinoma is always a consideration in the differential diagnosis of clear cell adenocarcinoma in the female genital tract, but is relatively uncommon. Active exclusion should be performed when there is (1) a prior history of renal cell carcinoma, (2) suspicion of a retroperitoneal mass, (3) family history or renal cell carcinoma or evidence of hereditary renal cell carcinoma syndrome (von Hippel–Lindau, Birt–Hogg–Dubé or possibly, hereditary leiomyomatosis), or (4) unusual distributional features (location within myometrium with minimal endometrial involvement). Imaging studies are the most useful in this distinction. Immunohistochemistry is of limited value as there is considerable overlap in expression profiles for the two tumors; PAX2 is perhaps the most useful discriminator as it is present in over 75% of renal cell carcinomas, but only in less than 10% of clear cell carcinoma of the female genital tract. Both tumors express PAX8 and HNF-1β.

MUCINOUS CARCINOMA

Focal mucinous differentiation is common in the usual endometrioid carcinoma. However, when endometrial carcinoma contains a predominant component of mucinous epithelial cells, the tumor is classified as mucinous carcinoma[13–16]. What constitutes "a predominant component of mucinous epithelial cells" has been variably defined. The WHO defines mucinous endometrial adenocarcinoma as tumors with over 90% of mucinous cells, while we and others have set a threshold of over 50%; this latter threshold is largely based on extrapolation of criteria used for diagnosing mucinous adenocarcinoma in the gastrointestinal tract. With either definition, mucinous adenocarcinoma of the endometrium is uncommon (<10% of endometrial carcinoma).

Clinical characteristics

Mucinous carcinoma is considered to be a type I estrogen-dependent tumor, and risk factors are similar to those for endometrioid adenocarcinoma. However, several lines of data suggest there may be a predilection for mucinous differentiation in tamoxifen-associated differentiated carcinomas.

Patients with mucinous carcinoma of the endometrium are essentially indistinguishable grade for grade from patients with usual endometrioid carcinoma. The importance of this variant lies instead in the challenges of (1) distinguishing mucinous carcinoma from mucinous metaplasia and complex endometrial hyperplasia with extensive

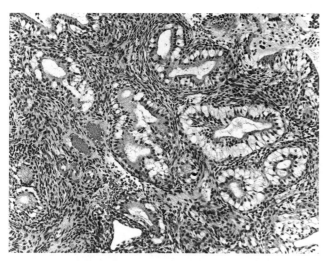

Figure 9.18 Secretory change in benign endocervical glands.

(A)
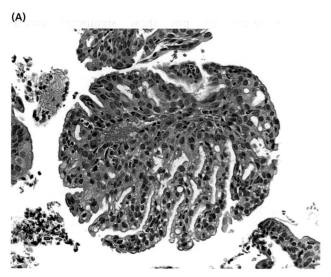

(B)
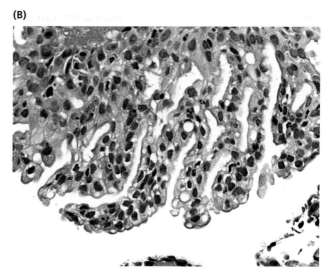

Figure 9.19 (A, B) Clear cell change in papillary metaplasia.

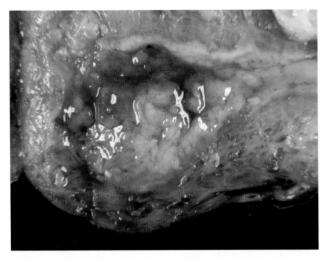

Figure 9.20 Mucinous adenocarcinoma. The gross appearance is often similar to endometrial hyperplasia; in addition, hyperplasia is often associated with this tumor type.

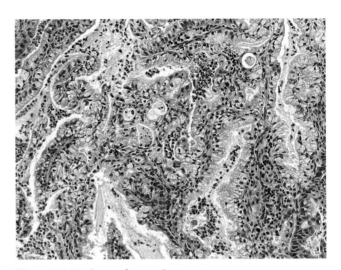

Figure 9.21 Mucinous adenocarcinoma.

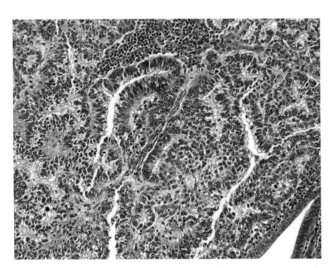

Figure 9.22 Mucinous adenocarcinoma. Glandular pattern.

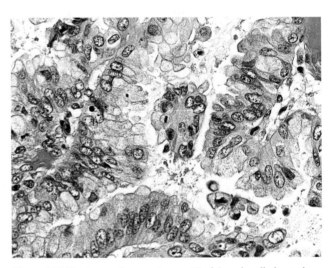

Figure 9.23 Mucinous adenocarcinoma. Nuclei are basally located, similar to endocervical-type epithelium.

mucinous metaplasia, and (2) determination of primary anatomic site when it is recovered in an endometrial sampling. Patient demographics are essentially the same as for endometrioid adenocarcinoma.

Morphology

Gross pathology

The gross pathology of mucinous adenocarcinoma is often similar to that of endometrioid adenocarcinoma (Figure 9.20). In some cases, there is copious extracellular mucin production, imparting a more gelatinous appearance to the exophytic component of the tumor. Occasional patients have mucometra.

Microscopic pathology

The neoplastic cells are morphologically similar to mucinous cells of endocervical type (Figure 9.21). Glandular, microglandular, and delicate branching papillary patterns are common; in some tumors, one pattern may predominate (Figure 9.22). The constituent cells are columnar with basal nuclei and apical cytoplasmic mucin (Figure 9.23). Mucin is also present in the gland lumens and is typically associated with a neutrophilic infiltrate (Figure 9.24). The nuclei are often banal or mildly atypical at most. Rarely, focal marked atypia may be seen. In most instances, the diagnosis is made solely on the basis of complex architecture (see Diagram 7.3). However, some mucinous carcinomas defy diagnosis on usual cytologic or architectural grounds. Some of these tumors can be recognized on the basis of voluminous extracellular mucin in the endometrial biopsy or curettage specimen (Figure 9.25)[17]. Others require hysterectomy to establish the diagnosis (Figure 9.26). We diagnose those endometrial proliferations in which the architectural complexity falls short of carcinoma (and the cytology is noninformative) as "complex mucinous endometrial proliferation, cannot exclude mucinous adenocarcinoma" with a comment that, while the sampling does not fulfill criteria for cancer, we cannot exclude the presence of a myoinvasive lesion in the uterus. Consideration should be given for hysterectomy in these cases, especially if the patient is perimenopausal or postmenopausal.

Although some authors report a low level of myoinvasion in these well-differentiated mucinous adenocarcinomas, this really depends on the threshold used for diagnosing adenocarcinoma: if the threshold is low, then fewer cases will be myoinvasive, since hyperplasias will be included in the diagnosis; if the threshold is higher, then a higher proportion of tumors diagnosed as carcinoma will be bona fide carcinomas, and the proportion of myoinvasive tumors will be higher. In our experience, the frequency of myoinvasion does not differ significantly from that of endometrioid carcinomas.

Mucinous tumors are graded on the basis of the FIGO grading scheme (see Chapter 7). Although high-grade variants of mucinous carcinoma have been described, in our experience most mucinous endometrial carcinomas are FIGO grade 1 or 2. Areas of endometrioid differentiation are commonly present. When the mucinous component is less than 50%, the tumor is classified as mixed endometrioid–mucinous adenocarcinoma, provided the mucinous epithelial cells exceed 10% of the tumor.

Ancillary diagnostic tests

The immunoprofile for uterine mucinous carcinoma is not as well defined as it is for endometrioid and serous adenocarcinoma. Most mucinous carcinomas are positive for hormone receptors ER and PR, although the degree of expression appears to be muted in comparison to equivalent-grade endometrioid carcinomas. Overexpression of p53 is not a feature of mucinous carcinoma.

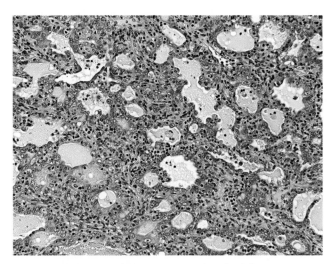

Figure 9.24 Mucinous adenocarcinoma. Microglandular pattern.

(A)

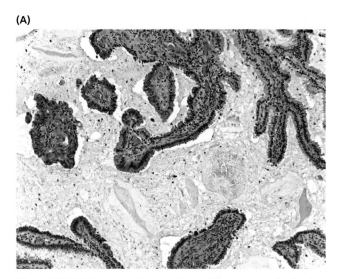

(B)

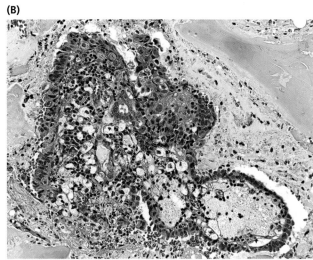

Figure 9.25 (A) Mucinous adenocarcinoma. The presence of voluminous extracellular mucin in a curettage specimen should prompt consideration for a mucinous adenocarcinoma. (B) The presence of stromal foam cells localizes this mucinous glandular proliferation to the endometrium.

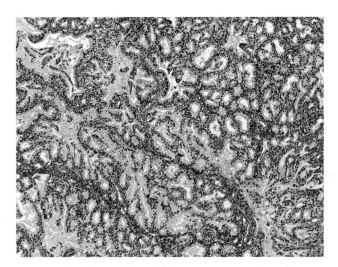

Figure 9.26 Invasive mucinous adenocarcinoma.

Differential diagnosis

This is one of the more difficult differential diagnoses in uterine sampling specimens (Table 9.3). The pathologist needs to consider site (cervix versus endometrium versus metastasis) in addition to malignant potential, and this latter consideration may involve different diagnostic criteria depending on the site of origin. For example, microglandular hyperplasia arising in the cervix is benign, while an endometrial proliferation with similar architecture may be benign, borderline, or malignant depending on the degree of complexity. Similarly, a glandular proliferation with mucinous differentiation may represent adenocarcinoma when it arises in the endocervix, but complex hyperplasia with atypia or a borderline lesion when it arises in the endometrium. To further complicate matters, the criteria used to distinguish benign from malignant are notoriously imperfect when applied to mucinous glandular lesions in the uterus.

Atypical mucinous metaplasia and hyperplasia

We are wary of interpreting predominantly mucinous processes with complex architecture as benign in curettage specimens. The distinction is usually easy to make when the architecture becomes complex or villoglandular or there is significant nuclear atypia[13,18]. However, mucinous proliferations capable of invading the myometrium may have nuclei that are not strikingly atypical and architecture that is borderline (Figure 9.27). When such tissue is recovered in perimenopausal or postmenopausal women, a hysterectomy is the best way to exclude a deceptively bland mucinous carcinoma.

Table 9.3 Differential diagnosis of mucinous epithelium in uterine sampling

Site	Clue
Cervical	
Normal endocervical elements	Basal, inconspicuous nuclei; mitotic figures rare or absent
Microglandular hyperplasia	Uniform microcystic gland pattern; small, regular nuclei; rare mitotic figures; squamous metaplasia
Other endocervical glandular hyperplasias (e.g., laminar)	Basal, inconspicuous nuclei; mitotic figures rare or absent
Endocervical adenocarcinoma (usual, intestinal, adenoma malignum)	Cytologic atypia; mitotic figures; abnormal branching architecture
Endometrium	
Metaplasia	Cytologically banal; rare or no mitotic figures; other metaplastic epithelia
Hyperplasia	Architecturally complex, but cytologically banal or only mild atypia; other hyperplastic endometria – for example, endometrioid, morular
Mucinous adenocarcinoma	Markedly complex architecture, including endometrioid areas; cytologic atypia (may be focal), abundant extracellular mucin
Microglandular proliferation – possibly overlying endometrioid adenocarcinoma[a]	Mixed macrocystic and microcystic glands; copious mucin; other metaplastic epithelia
Metastasis	
Stomach (signet ring)	Isolated signet ring cells
Colon and rectum	Dirty necrosis, segmental necrosis
Appendix	Isolated signet ring cells (goblet cell carcinoid)
Pancreas and biliary tract	Odd pattern, mixed, exuberant papillary and cribriform architecture

[a] Although this pattern is often cited as overlying endometrioid adenocarcinoma, in our experience it is simply a distinctive form of surface endometrial hyperplasia/metaplasia that may or may not be associated with underlying or adjacent adenocarcinoma.

Endocervical adenocarcinoma

Localization studies using differential curettage, hysteroscopy, or imaging studies are sometimes required to distinguish primary endometrial from primary endocervical mucinous carcinoma[19–23]. Features that favor an endometrial primary include associated endometrioid hyperplasia or metaplasia of the usual sort elsewhere in the endometrium

(A)

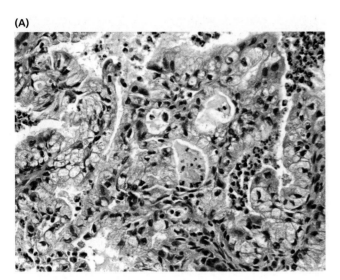

(B)

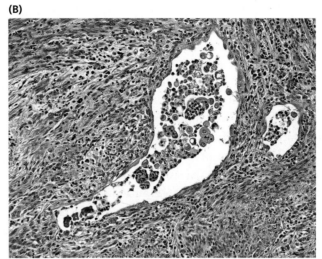

Figure 9.27 (A) Mucinous adenocarcinoma. (B) Despite the bland cytology, this tumor is associated with myometrial invasion in the subsequent hysterectomy specimen.

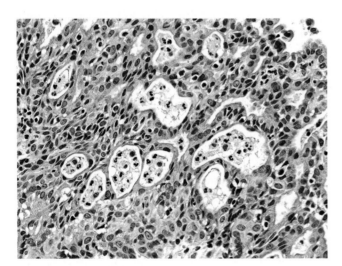

Figure 9.28 Cervical microglandular hyperplasia. It can be difficult to distinguish cervical microglandular hyperplasia from endometrial mucinous adenocarcinomas with microglandular pattern (see Figure 9.24).

(particularly hybrid mucinous endometrioid differentiation) and the presence of stromal foam cells. Most ambiguous cases can be resolved using these strategies.

In persistently ambiguous cases, immunohistochemistry can be helpful. Although a variety of markers have been proposed for this differential diagnosis over the years, we have found that a simple panel of three markers that includes vimentin, ER or PR, and an HPV marker (p16, ProEx C, or HPV in situ hybridizaton) is optimal for determining site of origin for usual endometrial and endocervical adenocarcinoma (see Chapter 3). Unfortunately, some problematic neoplasms have an intermediate or

non-specific phenotype with this panel; in most cases, incorporation of additional markers has not proven fruitful. In these cases, the uncertainty should be conveyed to the surgeon so that additional imaging studies can be pursued to help localize the tumor.

Metastatic mucinous carcinoma

Metastatic mucinous adenocarcinoma to the endometrium or cervix is rare. The gastrointestinal (colorectal or appendiceal) and pancreatobiliary tracts are the most common sources of mucinous metastases (Figures 16.5–16.7)[24,25]. Immunostains should be used judiciously in this setting. As most patients have a prior history of carcinoma and the metastasis is not the first presentation of disease, awareness of the possibility and obtaining the relevant history usually clarify matters. However, not all treating clinicians may be aware of this history at the time of evaluation. In this situation, use of a CK7/CK20 panel in conjunction with a low threshold for suspecting metastasis will prevent most misclassifications. Clues that a mucin-producing tumor may be a metastasis include isolated signet ring cells, dirty necrosis, and segmental necrosis of the malignant glands.

Cervical microglandular hyperplasia

Florid endocervical microglandular hyperplasia can be extremely difficult to distinguish from mucinous carcinoma with microglandular pattern (Figure 9.28). However, the nuclei are typically small and regular, and mitotic figures are rare; often subnuclear vacuoles are present. In contrast, microglandular mucinous proliferations in the uterus often have a mixed microcystic and distended macrocystic appearance, more copious mucin, and less pronounced squamous metaplasia, which tends to be luminal as opposed to subepithelial. The diagnosis of endometrial carcinoma with microglandular pattern is based on identification of typical endometrial adenocarcinoma merging with the microglandular pattern or the presence of significant nuclear atypia (nuclear pleomorphism and/or prominent nucleoli). Identification of specific locational attributes (e.g., stromal foam cells and vimentin expression for endometrium) is an additional useful diagnostic maneuver; these are discussed more fully below[26].

Normal endocervical mucosa

Scant strips of normal endocervix are often admixed in endometrial samplings. Basal nuclei, apical, pale-staining mucin, and the presence of basally located squamous metaplastic cells are diagnostic clues. When these fragments are numerous and there is prominent extracellular mucin, an endocervical-like endometrial carcinoma should be excluded.

SQUAMOUS CELL CARCINOMA

Pure squamous cell carcinoma of the uterine endometrium is rare[27]. Less than 0.5% of endometrial carcinomas are composed entirely of cells exhibiting squamous epithelial differentiation[28].

Clinical characteristics

Most patients with pure squamous cell endometrial carcinoma are postmenopausal (mean age: 67 years)[29]. Possible risk factors include cervical stenosis, pelvic radiation, uterine prolapse, and chronic pyometra. Many patients have extensive squamous metaplasia either preceding the development of the carcinoma or comingled with the tumor. Origin from reserve or stem cells positioned between the glandular basement membrane and the endometrial columnar epithelium has been proposed[30]. High-risk HPV has been detected in rare cases[31].

Approximately two-thirds of endometrial squamous cell carcinomas are confined to the uterus[32]. Overall survival rate is approximately 75–80% for FIGO stage I tumors, but decreases to about 25% for FIGO stage III and IV tumors. Prognosis depends on stage of disease. There is no standard treatment for endometrial squamous cell carcinoma. Treatment usually consist of total abdominal

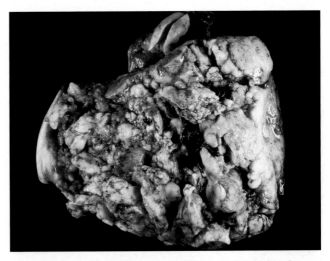

Figure 9.29 Squamous cell carcinoma. The tumor is based in the lower uterine segment, but involves the entire endometrium, with sparing of the actual endocervical mucosa.

hysterectomy with bilateral salpingo-oophorectomy followed by radiation in some patients.

Morphology

Gross pathology

The gross appearance of these tumors is often distinctive, when the uterus is replaced by the presence of well-differentiated, stratified, often keratinizing squamous epithelium (so-called ichthyosis uteri). In these cases, the uterine lining is replaced by an exophytic white-gray verrucous proliferation; necrosis and hemorrhage are absent (Figure 9.29). Other examples of uterine corpus squamous cell carcinoma may have a less distinctive appearance.

Microscopic pathology

Although varying degrees of differentiation may be present, most primary endometrial squamous cell carcinomas are well to moderately differentiated (Figure 9.30). By definition, no glandular elements can be present other than native endometrial glands[33]. Keratinization may be prominent (Figure 9.31). Foci of squamous metaplasia and dysplasia are often associated with the carcinoma (Figure 9.32), suggesting a squamous metaplasia–dysplasia–carcinoma transformation sequence. In some cases, only in situ carcinoma is present, while others show bona fide invasion into myometrium (Figure 9.33).

In order to exclude secondary involvement of the endometrium by primary cervical squamous cell carcinoma, Fluhmann proposed a series of diagnostic criteria for primary endometrial squamous cell carcinoma (Table 9.4)[33].

(A)

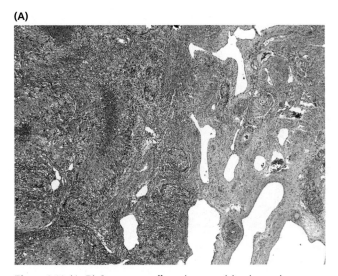

(B)

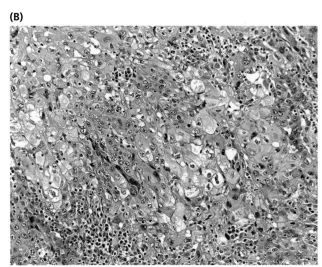

Figure 9.30 (A, B) Squamous cell carcinoma arising in uterine corpus.

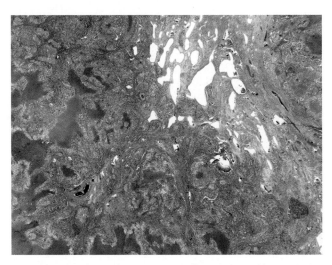

Figure 9.31 Invasive corpus squamous cell carcinoma with prominent keratinization.

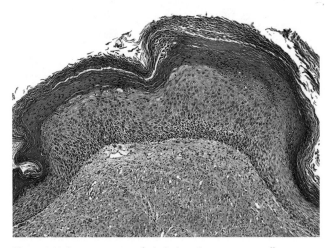

Figure 9.32 Squamous metaplasia in invasive squamous cell carcinoma of the uterine corpus.

In most respects, these criteria are valid and useful in establishing the diagnosis. However, it is well recognized that endometrial carcinoma can extend into the endocervical mucosa, occasionally even involving the squamous mucosa; whereas cervical carcinoma (both squamous and glandular types) rarely extensively replaces the endometrium. Fortunately, most of the endometrial squamous cell carcinomas that we have encountered have not demonstrated extensive replacement of cervical mucosa.

Ancillary diagnostic tests

High-risk HPV has been detected in some cases of primary endometrial squamous cell carcinoma, but not in others.

p16 has been studied in a few cases, all of which have been negative to date. Hormone receptors have not been well studied in these tumors, but occasional cases are positive for ER and PR[34]. Morular metaplasia often expresses strong nuclear CDX2[35].

Differential diagnosis

Cervical squamous cell carcinoma

Cervical squamous cell carcinoma arises in a background of high-risk HPV and is often preceded by or associated with squamous intraepithelial dysplasia or carcinoma. Also, most cervical squamous cell carcinomas occur in younger women.

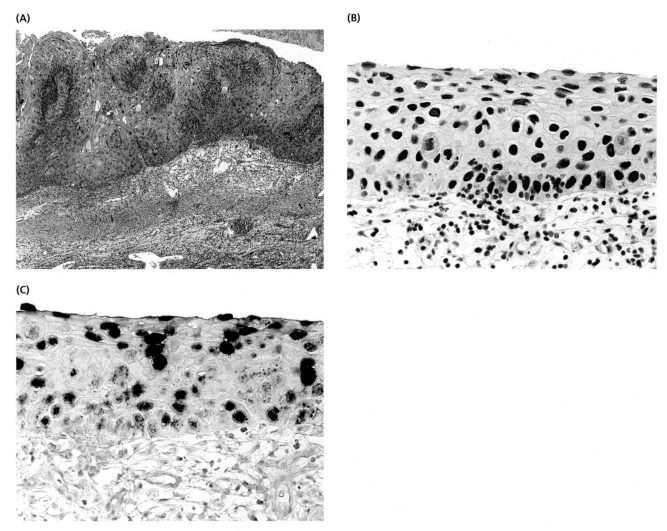

Figure 9.33 (A) Squamous cell carcinoma in situ arising in uterine corpus. (B)The tumor is ER positive. (C) Human papillomavirus in situ hybridization suggests at least some of these corpus tumors arise via the HPV pathway.

Table 9.4 Diagnostic criteria for primary uterine corpus squamous cell carcinoma[33]

(1) No coexisting endometrioid adenocarcinoma

(2) No connection between the endometrial tumor and squamous mucosa of the cervix

(3) No primary squamous cell carcinoma of the cervix

(4) If squamous cell carcinoma in situ is present in the cervix, there must be no connection between the in situ lesion and the endometrial tumor

Endometrioid adenocarcinoma with extensive squamous differentiation

Endometrioid adenocarcinoma with extensive squamous differentiation will often show morular or spindle cell areas in the differentiated tumors (formerly known as adeno-acanthoma), while the higher-grade tumors (formally

known as adenosquamous carcinomas) contain at lease some areas with glandular differentiation in addition to the malignant squamous epithelium.

Squamous metaplasia (so-called ichthyosis uteri)

The term "ichthyosis uteri" (also leukoplakia epidermidization, psoriasis uteri, epidermoid heteroplasia, cholesteometra and indirect regenerative squamous metaplasia) refers to the presence of extensive squamous metaplasia, often with abundant keratinization of the endometrium. The cytologic features are banal; mitoses may be present, but they are not particularly numerous, and atypical forms are not seen (Figure 9.34). The metaplastic epithelium often forms church spire-like exophytic fronds, resembling a verruca vulgaris, but keratohyaline granules are absent.

(A)

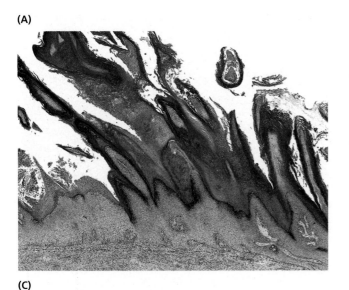

(B)

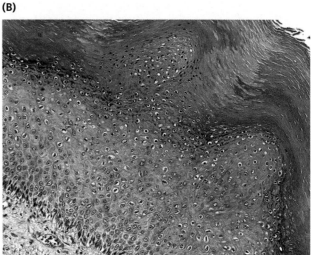

(C)

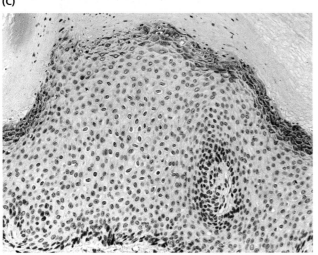

Figure 9.34 (A, B) Ichthyosis uteri. (C) p16 expression is absent.

Squamous cell carcinoma from bladder

Bladder carcinoma can secondarily involve the female genital tract, most commonly the vagina, but uterine involvement may also occur. Moreover, transitional cell carcinoma may exhibit prominent squamous differentiation, particularly in women. Therefore the presence of malignant transitional or squamous epithelium in an endometrial curetting should prompt consideration for possible extension from a bladder tumor. Clinical and imaging studies will quickly resolve this issue.

MISCELLANEOUS UTERINE CORPUS CARCINOMAS AND MALIGNANCIES

Transitional cell carcinoma

This is an extremely uncommon and poorly characterized histologic pattern in endometrial carcinomas[36–38]. The term is generally reserved for those tumors that exhibit a polypoid architecture and resemble high-grade papillary urothelial carcinoma. Areas of usual endometrioid, squamous, or serous histology are often present, and the transitional areas in these tumors likely represent an unusual cyto-architectural variation of the associated endometrial carcinoma rather than a distinct histologic variant. High-risk HPV (type 16) has been detected in some of these tumors, suggesting possible cervical origin. The immunohistochemical phenotype is usually consistent with mullerian differentiation.

Mixed carcinomas

Mixed carcinomas are common in the endometrium and are often underdiagnosed. A mixed carcinoma should be diagnosed whenever the carcinoma is composed of two or more histologic subtypes, each of which accounts for at

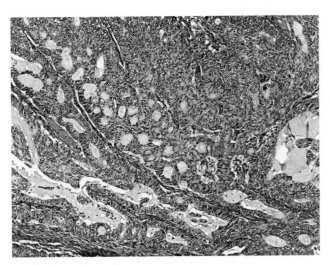

Figure 9.35 Mixed endometrioid and mucinous carcinoma.

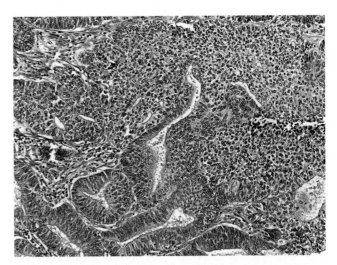

Figure 9.36 Mixed endometrioid and undifferentiated carcinoma.

least 10% of the tumor. The most common mixed tumor arising in the endometrium is endometrioid and mucinous (Figure 9.35), followed by endometrioid and undifferentiated, and endometrioid and serous or clear cell carcinoma. Many serous carcinomas in the uterus contain foci with clear cells; whether these tumors represent a variant of serous carcinoma or are in fact true mixed serous and clear cell carcinomas is currently unresolved. Since both are high-grade, aggressive neoplasms, the distinction may be moot.

Mixed endometrioid and mucinous carcinomas tend to be low grade, but not necessarily low stage. A significant proportion of endometrial cancers with microsatellite instability due to somatic methylation of the *MLH1* mismatch repair gene have mixed endometrioid and mucinous histology[39].

Mixed endometrioid and undifferentiated (also referred to as dedifferentiated endometrioid carcinoma) are diagnosed on the basis of a low-grade (typically FIGO grade 1, but occasionally grade 2) endometrioid component merging with sheets of undifferentiated cells (Figure 9.36). Some data suggest these tumors may be more aggressive than grade 2 or grade 3 endometrioid carcinoma of the same stage, but this has not yet been confirmed by other investigators[40,41]. An association with Lynch syndrome has also been observed[42].

Mixed endometrioid and serous carcinomas are rare. The diagnosis of a mixed serous and endometrioid adenocarcinoma should be made when the serous component is distinct from the endometrioid component in histologic appearance and immunophenotype. As discussed in Chapter 8, the minimum volume of true serous carcinoma that should be reported in the pathology report is poorly specified; several lines of data suggest that any component of serous carcinoma may impart a potentially adverse prognosis. Therefore, endometrioid tumors that feature foci of serous carcinoma that account for less than 10% of the total tumor should probably be diagnosed as endometrioid carcinoma with focal serous carcinoma with the percentage of the serous component in parenthesis (e.g., endometrioid adenocarcinoma with focal serous carcinoma [5%]).

Lymphoepithelioma-like carcinoma

This is also a rare tumor in the uterus[43]. It resembles lymphoepithelioma-like carcinoma elsewhere. Epstein–Barr virus has not been identified in the few tumors that have been studied. Far more common are areas of lymphoepithelioma-like carcinoma in an otherwise usual endometrioid adenocarcinoma.

Giant cell carcinoma

Endometrial carcinoma with a malignant giant cell component (endometrial giant cell carcinoma) consists of poorly cohesive sheets of bizarre multinucleated giant cells and mononuclear tumor cells (Figure 9.37)[44,45]. Minor areas of endometrioid, clear cell, serous, or carcinosarcoma histology may also be seen. A striking peritumoral and intratumoral mixed inflammatory cell infiltrate is often present. Emperipolesis has also been described. The giant cells show focal staining for epithelial markers (AE1/AE3 and CAM 5.2). Most patients are postmenopausal. The prognostic significance of the presence and extent of a giant cell component in endometrial carcinoma is uncertain.

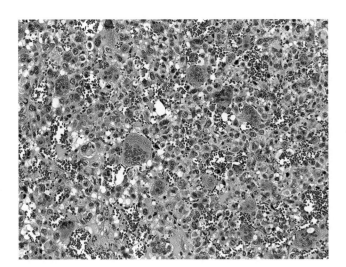

Figure 9.37 Endometrial carcinoma with osteoclast-like giant cells. Tumor giant cells are also present.

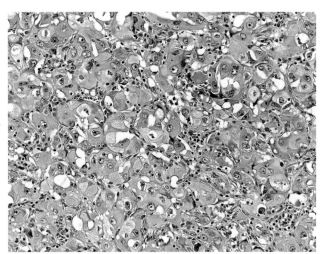

Figure 9.38 Glassy cell carcinoma.

Hepatoid carcinoma

This tumor is rare in the uterus and, when present, typically occurs in association with endometrioid carcinoma or carcinosarcoma[46–48]. The cells resemble hepatocellular carcinoma and should be positive for AFP, as well as Hepar-1 and glypican-3; in some cases, staining for pCEA may identify a canalicular pattern. The serum AFP is elevated and can be a useful tool in monitoring the disease.

Carcinoma with benign heterologous elements

Endometrial adenocarcinoma of the endometrium may rarely be associated with benign adipocytic or osteogenic elements[49]. Tumors containing these benign heterologous elements should be distinguished from the more common carcinosarcoma with heterologous elements, which have a different clinicopathologic behavior.

Carcinoma with amyloid

Most cases of uterine amyloid occur in the setting of systemic amyloidosis. Rarely, endometrioid carcinoma may be associated with amyloid in absence of systemic disease[50].

Glassy cell carcinoma

Glassy cell carcinoma is more common in the cervix, but rare examples have been described in the endometrium. As discussed in Chapter 3, the term "glassy cell carcinoma" should be reserved for those tumors containing an abundance of undifferentiated cells with ground-glass cytoplasm, distinct cell membranes, and large nuclei with prominent nucleoli (Figure 9.38). These tumors often contain a heavy inflammatory infiltrate consisting of eosinophils. Although cumulative data from case reports suggest a possibly worse prognosis for stage I disease, too few cases have been studied with sufficient detail to assign a prognosis to this histologic subtype when it arises in the endometrium. If strictly defined, glassy cell carcinoma accounts for considerably less than 1% of all endometrial carcinomas[51].

Carcinoma with yolk sac tumor

Most uterine yolk sac tumors are pure; they are more common in the cervix than the endometrium[52–56]. Occasionally, yolk sac tumor can arise in association with endometrioid adenocarcinoma or carcinosarcoma[57,58]. This is more commonly reported to occur in the ovary, but endometrial examples have also been described.

Carcinoma with immature teratoma

This is a very rare occurrence within the uterus. In one case, glial peritoneal implants were also present on the peritoneal surface of the ovaries[59].

Carcinoma with trophoblastic cells (non-gestational choriocarcinoma)

Trophoblastic cells can rarely be seen in primary uterine epithelial tumors; endometrioid, serous, and carcinosarcoma histologies have been reported[60–64]. The tumors typically occur in postmenopausal women and are associated with elevated serum hCG. The extent of trophoblastic differentiation ranges from isolated foci of syncytiotrophoblasts to fully developed non-gestational choriocarcinoma.

Undifferentiated carcinoma

Undifferentiated carcinoma, by definition, consists of sheets of cells without discernable glandular formations (Figure 9.39). One variant of this undifferentiated growth pattern has been characterized as solid sheets of monotonous medium-sized epithelial cells, with irregular myometrial permeation at the periphery[65]. Tumor cells in this latter variant are only moderately atypical and dyshesive;

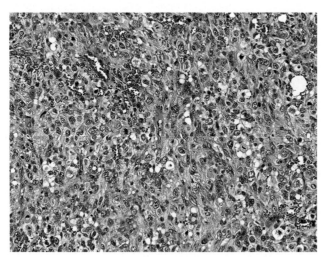

Figure 9.39 Undifferentiated large cell carcinoma.

they resemble lymphoma, plasmacytoma or rhabdoid tumor cells[40]. Immunohistochemically, rare cells express EMA or cytokeratin, but most cells lack an obviously epithelial phenotype, unlike FIGO grades 2 and 3 endometrioid carcinomas. Stains for lymphoid, rhabdomyoblastic, and rhabdoid neoplasms are negative; markers for neuroendocrine differentiation may be positive, but only focally. One-half are high stage, and the prognosis is reported to be worse than grade 3 endometrioid carcinoma[40,41].

Mesonephric carcinoma

Mesonephric (wolffian) carcinomas of the female genital tract are uncommon; they arise in sites where embryonic remnants of wolffian origin are usually detected, such as the uterine cervix, broad ligament, mesosalpinx, ovary, and, rarely, in the lateral walls of the uterus. The tumor typically exhibits retiform areas, ductal foci, and small tubules with eosinophilic secretion (Figure 9.40). The neoplastic cells are positive for cytokeratin 7, EMA, WT1, calretinin, and CD10 (Figure 9.41)[66,67].

Neuroendocrine carcinoma

This designation should be reserved for those undifferentiated tumors composed of small to intermediate cells with scant cytoplasm and hyperchromatic nuclei with a high mitotic index[68–72]. Melanoma, lymphoma, and other small cell malignancies must be excluded, and strong, diffuse immunoreactivity for one or more neuroendocrine markers,

(A)

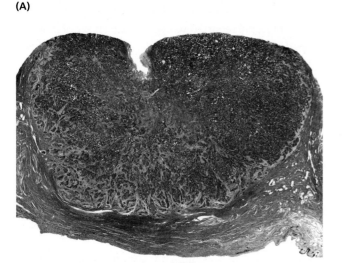

(B)

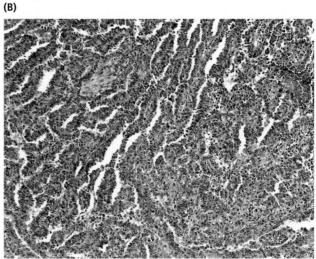

Figure 9.40 (A) Mesonephric carcinoma arising in uterine corpus. (B) The nuclei are small, cuboidal to low columnar, and monomorphic in appearance. This would be an unusual appearance for the usual endometrioid adenocarcinoma.

(A)

(B)

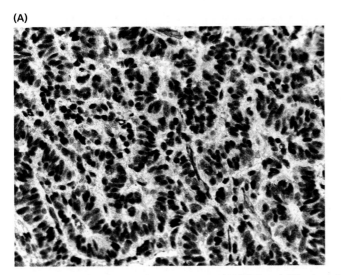

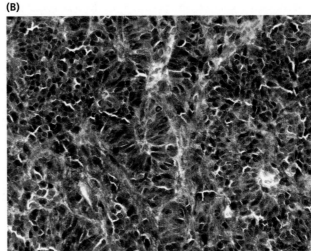

Figure 9.41 Mesonephric carcinoma expresses (A) WT1 and (B) calretinin.

particularly chromogranin and/or synaptophysin should be present. This subtype is far less common in the endometrium than in the cervix, but it is equally aggressive when it arises in the endometrium. Approximately one-half of endometrial neuroendocrine carcinomas are associated with an endometrioid component; fewer may be seen in association with carcinosarcoma. The distinction between small cell and large cell neuroendocrine carcinoma is made on the basis of the criteria used in the lung: cell size, amount of cytoplasm, and nucleoli (present in large cell; absent in small cell).

REFERENCES

1. Abeler VM, Kjorstad KE. Clear cell carcinoma of the endometrium: a histopathological and clinical study of 97 cases. *Gynecol Oncol* 1991;**40**:207–17.

2. Abeler VM, Vergote IB, Kjorstad KE, *et al.* Clear cell carcinoma of the endometrium. Prognosis and metastatic pattern. *Cancer* 1996;**78**:1740–7.

3. Kurman R, Scully R. Clear cell carcinoma of the endometrium: an analysis of 21 cases. *Cancer* 1976;**37**:872–82.

4. Lax SF. Molecular genetic changes in epithelial, stromal and mixed neoplasms of the endometrium. *Pathology* 2007;**39**:46–54.

5. Gadducci A, Cosio S, Spirito N, *et al.* Clear cell carcinoma of the endometrium: a biological and clinical enigma. *Anticancer Res* 2010;**30**:1327–34.

6. Malpica A, Tornos C, Burke TW, *et al.* Low-stage clear-cell carcinoma of the endometrium. *Am J Surg Pathol* 1995;**19**:769–74.

7. Lee L, Garrett L, Lee H, *et al.* Association of clear cell carcinoma of the endometrium with a high rate of venous thromboembolism. *J Reprod Med* 2009;**54**:133–8.

8. Fadare O, Liang SX, Ulukus EC, *et al.* Precursors of endometrial clear cell carcinoma. *Am J Surg Pathol* 2006;**30**:1519–30.

9. Lax SF, Pizer ES, Ronnett BM, *et al.* Clear cell carcinoma of the endometrium is characterized by a distinctive profile of p53, Ki-67, estrogen, and progesterone receptor expression. *Hum Pathol* 1998;**29**:551–8.

10. Yamamoto S, Tsuda H, Aida S, *et al.* Immunohistochemical detection of hepatocyte nuclear factor 1beta in ovarian and endometrial clear-cell adenocarcinomas and nonneoplastic endometrium. *Hum Pathol* 2007;**38**:1074–80.

11. Hendrickson M, Ross J, Eifel P, *et al.* Uterine papillary serous carcinoma: a highly malignant form of endometrial adenocarcinoma. *Am J Surg Pathol* 1982;**6**:93–108.

12. Silva EG, Young RH. Endometrioid neoplasms with clear cells: a report of 21 cases in which the alteration is not of typical secretory type. *Am J Surg Pathol* 2007;**31**:1203–8.

13. Nucci MR, Prasad CJ, Crum CP, *et al.* Mucinous endometrial epithelial proliferations: a morphologic spectrum of changes with diverse clinical significance. *Mod Pathol* 1999;**12**:1137–42.

14. Ross J, Eifel P, Cox R, *et al.* Primary mucinous adenocarcinoma of the endometrium. A clinicopathologic and histochemical study. *Am J Surg Pathol* 1983;**7**:715–29.

15. Vang R, Tavassoli FA. Proliferative mucinous lesions of the endometrium: analysis of existing criteria for diagnosing carcinoma in biopsies and curettings. *Int J Surg Pathol* 2003;**11**:261–70.

16. Zaloudek C, Hayashi GM, Ryan IP, *et al.* Microglandular adenocarcinoma of the endometrium: a form of mucinous adenocarcinoma that may be confused with microglandular hyperplasia of the cervix. *Int J Gynecol Pathol* 1997;**16**:52–9.

17. Fujiwara M, Longacre TA. Low grade mucinous adenocarcinoma of the uterine corpus: a rare and deceptively bland form of endometrial carcinoma. *Am J Surg Pathol* 2011;**35**:537–44.

18. Longacre TA, Chung MH, Jensen DN, *et al.* Proposed criteria for the diagnosis of well-differentiated endometrial carcinoma. A diagnostic test for myoinvasion. *Am J Surg Pathol* 1995;**19**: 371–406.

19. Cacciatore B, Lehtovirta P, Wahlstrom T, *et al.* Preoperative sonographic evaluation of endometrial cancer. *Am J Obstet Gynecol* 1989;**160**:133–7.

20. Hricak H, Lacey C, Schriock E, *et al.* Gynecologic masses: value of magnetic resonance imaging. *Am J Obstet Gynecol* 1985;**153**:31–7.

21. Posniak H, Olson M, Dudiak C, *et al.* MR imaging of uterine carcinoma: correlation with clinical and pathologic findings. *Radiographics* 1990;**10**:15–27.

22. Williams AS, Kost ER, Hermann J, *et al.* Hysteroscopy in the evaluation and treatment of mucinous adenocarcinoma. *Obstet Gynecol* 2002;**99**:509–11.

23. Zaino RJ. The fruits of our labors: distinguishing endometrial from endocervical adenocarcinoma. *Int J Gynecol Pathol* 2002;**21**:1–3.

24. Kumar A, Schneider V. Metastases to the uterus from extrapelvic primary tumors. *Int J Gynecol Pathol* 1983;**2**:134–40.

25. Kumar N, Hart W. Metastases to the uterine corpus from extragenital cancers. A clinicopathologic study of 63 cases. *Cancer* 1982;**50**:2163–9.

26. Qiu W, Mittal K. Comparison of morphologic and immunohistochemical features of cervical microglandular hyperplasia with low-grade mucinous adenocarcinoma of the endometrium. *Int J Gynecol Pathol* 2003;**22**:261–5.

27. Goodman A, Zukerberg LR, Rice LW, *et al.* Squamous cell carcinoma of the endometrium: a report of eight cases and a review of the literature. *Gynecol Oncol* 1996;**61**:54–60.

28. Abeler VM, Kjorstad KE, Berle E. Carcinoma of the endometrium in Norway: a histopathological and prognostic survey of a total population. *Int J Gynecol Cancer* 1992;**2**:9–22.

29. Bagga PK, Jaswal TS, Datta U, *et al.* Primary endometrial squamous cell carcinoma with extensive squamous metaplasia and dysplasia. *Indian J Pathol Microbiol* 2008;**51**:267–8.

30. Seltzer VL, Klein M, Beckman EM. The occurrence of squamous metaplasia as a precursor of squamous cell carcinoma of the endometrium. *Obstet Gynecol* 1977;**49**:34–7.

31. Kataoka A, Nishida T, Sugiyama T, *et al.* Squamous cell carcinoma of the endometrium with human papillomavirus type 31 and without tumor suppressor gene p53 mutation. *Gynecol Oncol* 1997;**65**:180–4.

32. Illanes D, Broman J, Meyer B, *et al.* Verrucous carcinoma of the endometrium: case history, pathologic findings, brief review of literature and discussion. *Gynecol Oncol* 2006;**102**:375–7.

33. Kay S. Squamous-cell carcinoma of the endometrium. *Am J Clin Pathol* 1974;**61**:264–9.

34. Horn LC, Richter CE, Einenkel J, *et al.* p16, p14, p53, cyclin D1, and steroid hormone receptor expression and human papillomaviruses analysis in primary squamous cell carcinoma of the endometrium. *Ann Diagn Pathol* 2006;**10**:193–6.

35. Houghton O, Connolly LE, McCluggage WG. Morules in endometrioid proliferations of the uterus and ovary consistently express the intestinal transcription factor CDX2. *Histopathology* 2008;**53**:156–65.

36. Chen KT. Extraovarian transitional cell carcinoma of female genital tract. *Am J Clin Pathol* 1990;**94**:670–1.

37. Lininger RA, Ashfaq R, Albores-Saavedra J, *et al.* Transitional cell carcinoma of the endometrium and endometrial carcinoma with transitional cell differentiation. *Cancer* 1997;**79**:1933–43.

38. Spiegel GW, Austin RM, Gelven PL. Transitional cell carcinoma of the endometrium. *Gynecol Oncol* 1996;**60**:325–30.

39. Mills A, Pai R, Liou S, *et al.* Clinicopathologic features of sporadic endometrial carcinomas with MLH1 promoter hypermethylation: a study of 54 cases. *Mod Pathol* 2011;**24**:260A.

40. Altrabulsi B, Malpica A, Deavers MT, *et al.* Undifferentiated carcinoma of the endometrium. *Am J Surg Pathol* 2005;**29**:1316–21.

41. Tafe LJ, Garg K, Chew I, *et al.* Endometrial and ovarian carcinomas with undifferentiated components: clinically aggressive and frequently underrecognized neoplasms. *Mod Pathol* 2010;**23**:781–9.

42. Garg K, Leitao MM, Jr., Kauff ND, *et al.* Selection of endometrial carcinomas for DNA mismatch repair protein immunohistochemistry using patient age and tumor morphology enhances detection of mismatch repair abnormalities. *Am J Surg Pathol* 2009;**33**:925–33.

43. Vargas MP, Merino MJ. Lymphoepitheliomalike carcinoma: an unusual variant of endometrial cancer. A report of two cases. *Int J Gynecol Pathol* 1998;**17**:272–6.

44. Jones MA, Young RH, Scully RE. Endometrial adenocarcinoma with a component of giant cell carcinoma. *Int J Gynecol Pathol* 1991;**10**:260–70.

45. Mulligan AM, Plotkin A, Rouzbahman M, *et al.* Endometrial giant cell carcinoma: a case series and review of the spectrum of endometrial neoplasms containing giant cells. *Am J Surg Pathol* 2010;**34**:1132–8.

46. Takahashi Y, Inoue T. Hepatoid carcinoma of the uterus that collided with carcinosarcoma. *Pathol Int* 2003;**53**:323–6.

47. Takeuchi K, Kitazawa S, Hamanishi S, *et al.* A case of alpha-fetoprotein-producing adenocarcinoma of the endometrium with a hepatoid component as a potential source for alpha-fetoprotein in a postmenopausal woman. *Int J Gynecol Cancer* 2006;**16**:1442–5.

48. Toyoda H, Hirai T, Ishii E. Alpha-fetoprotein producing uterine corpus carcinoma: a hepatoid adenocarcinoma of the endometrium. *Pathol Int* 2000;**50**:847–52.

49. Nogales F, Gomez-Morales M, Raymundo C, *et al.* Benign heterologous tissue components associated with endometrial carcinoma. *Int J Gynecol Pathol* 1982;**1**:286–91.

50. Kotru M, Chandra H, Singh N, *et al.* Localized amyloidosis in endometrioid carcinoma of the uterus: a rare association. *Arch Gynecol Obstet* 2007;**276**:383–4.

51. Ferrandina G, Zannoni GF, Petrillo M, *et al.* Glassy cell carcinoma of the endometrium: a case report and review of the literature. *Pathol Res Pract* 2007;**203**:217–20.

52. Clement PB, Young RH, Scully RE. Extraovarian pelvic yolk sac tumors. *Cancer* 1988;**62**:620–6.

53. Copeland LJ, Sneige N, Ordonez NG, *et al.* Endodermal sinus tumor of the vagina and cervix. *Cancer* 1985;**55**:2558–65.

54. Joseph MG, Fellows FG, Hearn SA. Primary endodermal sinus tumor of the endometrium. A clinicopathologic, immunocytochemical, and ultrastructural study. *Cancer* 1990;**65**:297–302.

55. Pileri S, Martinelli G, Serra L, *et al.* Endodermal sinus tumor arising in the endometrium. *Obstet Gynecol* 1980;**56**:391–6.

56. Spatz A, Bouron D, Pautier P, *et al.* Primary yolk sac tumor of the endometrium: a case report and review of the literature. *Gynecol Oncol* 1998;**70**:285–8.

57. Oguri H, Sumitomo R, Maeda N, *et al.* Primary yolk sac tumor concomitant with carcinosarcoma originating from the endometrium: case report. *Gynecol Oncol* 2006;**103**:368–71.

58. Patsner B. Primary endodermal sinus tumor of the endometrium presenting as "recurrent" endometrial adenocarcinoma. *Gynecol Oncol* 2001;**80**:93–5.

59. Ansah-Boateng Y, Wells M, Poole D. Coexistent immature teratoma of the uterus and endometrial adenocarcinoma complicated by gliomatosis peritonei. *Gynecol Oncol* 1985;**21**:106–10.

60. Bradley CS, Benjamin I, Wheeler JE, *et al.* Endometrial adenocarcinoma with trophoblastic differentiation. *Gynecol Oncol* 1998;**69**:74–7.

61. Horn LC, Hanel C, Bartholdt E, *et al.* Serous carcinoma of the endometrium with choriocarcinomatous differentiation: a case report and review of the literature indicate the existence of 2

prognostically relevant tumor types. *Int J Gynecol Pathol* 2006;**25**:247–51.

62. Kalir T, Seijo L, Deligdisch L, *et al.* Endometrial adenocarcinoma with choriocarcinomatous differentiation in an elderly virginal woman. *Int J Gynecol Pathol* 1995;**14**:266–9.

63. Pesce C, Merino M, Chambers J, *et al.* Endometrial carcinoma with trophoblastic differentiation. *Cancer* 1991;**68**:1799–1802.

64. Savage J, Subby W, Okagaki T. Adenocarcinoma of the endometrium with trophoblastic differentiation and metastases as choriocarcinoma: a case report. *Gynecol Oncol* 1987;**26**:257–62.

65. Abeler VM, Kjorstad KE, Nesland JM. Undifferentiated carcinoma of the endometrium. A histopathologic and clinical study of 31 cases. *Cancer* 1991;**68**:98–105.

66. Marquette A, Moerman P, Vergote I, *et al.* Second case of uterine mesonephric adenocarcinoma. *Int J Gynecol Cancer* 2006;**16**:1450–4.

67. Ordi J, Nogales FF, Palacin A, *et al.* Mesonephric adenocarcinoma of the uterine corpus: CD10 expression as evidence of mesonephric differentiation. *Am J Surg Pathol* 2001;**25**:1540–5.

68. Erhan Y, Dikmen Y, Yucebilgin MS, *et al.* Large cell neuroendocrine carcinoma of the uterine corpus metastatic to brain and lung: case report and review of the literature. *Eur J Gynaecol Oncol* 2004;**25**:109–12.

69. Huntsman DG, Clement PB, Gilks CB, *et al.* Small-cell carcinoma of the endometrium. A clinicopathological study of sixteen cases. *Am J Surg Pathol* 1994;**18**:364–75.

70. Katahira A, Akahira J, Niikura H, *et al.* Small cell carcinoma of the endometrium: report of three cases and literature review. *Int J Gynecol Cancer* 2004;**14**:1018–23.

71. Manivel C, Wick MR, Sibley RK. Neuroendocrine differentiation in mullerian neoplasms. An immunohistochemical study of a "pure" endometrial small-cell carcinoma and a mixed mullerian tumor containing small-cell carcinoma. *Am J Clin Pathol* 1986;**86**:438–43.

72. Varras M, Akrivis C, Demou A, *et al.* Primary small-cell carcinoma of the endometrium: clinicopathological study of a case and review of the literature. *Eur J Gynaecol Oncol* 2002;**23**:577–81.

10 CARCINOSARCOMA

INTRODUCTION

Carcinosarcoma, also referred to as "malignant mixed mullerian tumor" or "MMMT," is a neoplasm composed of malignant-appearing epithelial and mesenchymal elements. Although they can arise in any genital organ, carcinosarcomas are found most frequently in the uterus, where they represent less than 5% of malignant neoplasms. These tumors are increasingly thought of as carcinomas that demonstrate sarcomatoid differentiation[1,2]. Revisions to the FIGO staging system and the seventh edition of the AJCC Cancer Staging Manual now formally encourage the same staging scheme as for carcinomas[3]: tacit recognition that, in general, carcinosarcomas are closely related to carcinomas. Advances in our understanding of the interplay of tumor biology and epidemiology, along with the increasing use of comprehensive surgical staging and treatment with effective chemotherapeutic agents, have led to the conclusion that carcinosarcoma constitutes a specific clinicopathologic entity, distinct from many other biphasic uterine tumors. The typical carcinosarcoma is a biphasic, mixed epithelial and mesenchymal tumor, the clinical evolution of which is more aggressive than high-grade endometrial carcinoma.

CLINICAL CHARACTERISTICS

The mean age of patients with endometrial carcinosarcoma is in the seventh decade. Carcinosarcoma is uncommon earlier in life. Vaginal bleeding is typical, but the prototypic presentation is a polypoid mass that protrudes through the cervical os.

The five-year survival rate for carcinosarcoma is approximately 30%, and the five-year survival rate in surgical stage I disease (confined to uterus) is approximately 50%[4–6]. This very aggressive profile contrasts with that of other high-grade endometrial cancers where five-year survival rates in stage I disease are approximately 80%[7,8]. An analysis of recurrence patterns after therapy reports nearly a 60% frequency of distant recurrences, mostly involving the peritoneal cavity[9]. A study of ifosfamide with or without cisplatin for the treatment of advanced, persistent, or recurrent carcinosarcoma demonstrated that the addition of cisplatin provided a small improvement in progression-free survival but no significant survival benefit[10]. Another study favored the use of combination chemotherapy, including cisplatin, ifosfamide, and mesna, over whole abdominal radiotherapy[11]. There are no data that suggest that treating the predominant tumor component (i.e., rhabdomyosarcoma, when present) is preferable to standard therapy.

Studies that have sought to define prognostic factors are compromised by including some patients who were clinically staged and others who were surgically staged[4–6]. There is still general agreement that surgical stage is the most important prognostic indicator. In common with some of the older literature, the group at Memorial Sloan–Kettering Cancer Center, New York, has recently found that the presence of heterologous elements is a statistically significant poor prognostic factor in stage I patients[12]. In that study, 30% of patients with heterologous elements survived five years as compared to 80% of patients with homologous elements. Other prognostic factors that have been proposed include the grade of the carcinomatous and sarcomatous elements, the percentage of tumor demonstrating sarcomatous differentiation, the depth of myometrial invasion, and the presence of lymphovascular invasion, although it is not clear whether or not any of these factors have significant predictive value beyond that of surgical stage of disease[4–6].

MORPHOLOGY

Gross pathology

Many carcinosarcomas are polypoid and fill the endometrial cavity (Figure 10.1). Some are confined to polyps, whereas others invade myometrium. Polypoid tumors often protrude through the cervical os, simulating a cervical neoplasm. The tip of the polypoid mass can be necrotic, making diagnosis difficult when a biopsy samples only this part of the tumor. The tumors are variably soft to firm and tan with areas of necrosis and hemorrhage.

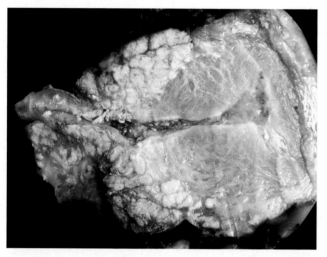

Figure 10.1 Carcinosarcoma is typically large and polypoid with areas of necrosis.

Microscopic pathology

The cardinal rule of carcinosarcoma is that it is a biphasic tumor, composed of distinct, malignant-appearing epithelial and mesenchymal elements (Table 10.1; Figure 10.2). This definition essentially excludes from consideration all monophasic tumors, such as undifferentiated carcinomas and undifferentiated sarcomas, and tumors that display *either* malignant-appearing epithelial elements (such as endometrioid adenocarcinoma with spindle cell features) *or* malignant-appearing mesenchymal elements (such as mullerian adenosarcoma).

Both malignant epithelial and mesenchymal components are conspicuous in most tumors, but occasional cases show sarcoma or carcinoma almost exclusively (Figure 10.3). That being said, both epithelial and mesenchymal components are required for diagnosis. About one-third of carcinosarcomas harbor a carcinoma with endometrioid differentiation (Figure 10.4), and two-thirds contain a carcinoma that is serous (Figure 10.5) or too poorly

Table 10.1 Pathologic characteristics of carcinosarcoma

Biphasic tumor
Epithelial component is histologically high grade
Mesenchymal component is histologically high grade
Mimics are excluded[a]

[a] Mimics include endometrioid carcinoma with spindle cell elements, adenosarcoma, dedifferentiated endometrial carcinoma, poorly differentiated carcinoma, and combined adenocarcinoma and neuroendocrine carcinoma.

(A)

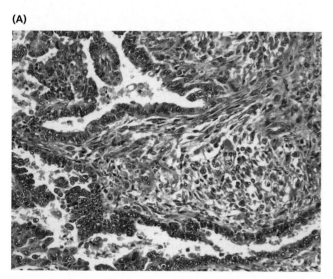

(B)

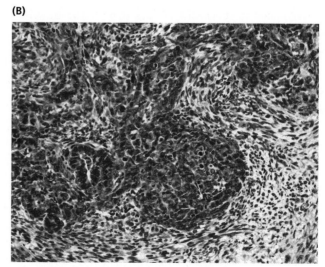

Figure 10.2 Carcinosarcomas demonstrate a biphasic appearance with distinct, malignant-appearing, and histologically high-grade epithelial and mesenchymal elements (A and B).

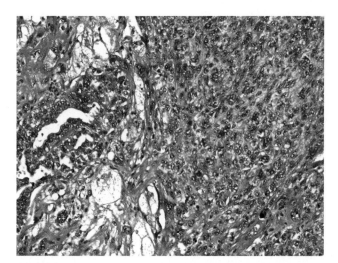

Figure 10.3 Carcinosarcoma with only focal evidence of epithelial differentiation.

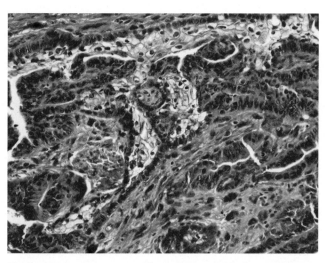

Figure 10.4 Carcinosarcoma with an endometrioid adenocarcinoma component. Reproduced with permission from Soslow RA. Mixed mullerian tumors. In Oliva E, ed. *Current Concepts in Gynecologic Pathology: Mesenchymal Tumors of the Female Genital Tract* in the series Surgical Pathology Clinics, Goldblum JR, ed. Philadelphia, PA: Saunders; 2009:**2**(4):707–30, Figure 4.

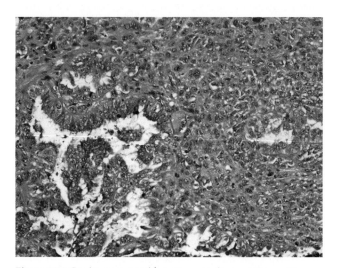

Figure 10.5 Carcinosarcoma with a serous carcinoma component.

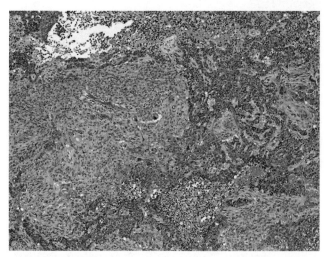

Figure 10.6 Carcinosarcoma in which the carcinoma is too poorly differentiated to subclassify.

differentiated to subclassify (Figure 10.6)[12]. The endometrioid tumors may be associated with complex atypical hyperplasia, and the two latter tumors may contain foci of intraepithelial serous carcinoma. Many carcinosarcomas contain epithelial tumor cells with clear cytoplasm, but the architectural and cytologic features of these tumors often have more in common with serous or endometrioid carcinoma than with pure clear cell carcinoma. Mucinous and squamous carcinomas have also been described, but these are rare. In the Memorial Sloan–Kettering series[12], more than 80% were grade 3 endometrioid, serous, or undifferentiated. The sarcomatous components vary in appearance. The homologous sarcomatous regions of carcinosarcoma are usually spindle cell tumors without obvious differentiation, often resembling fibrosarcoma or pleomorphic undifferentiated sarcoma (Figure 10.7). Very

few carcinosarcomas contain a mesenchymal proliferation that looks like leiomyosarcoma or endometrial stromal sarcoma. Essentially all are histologically high grade (Figure 10.8). Guidelines, admittedly subjective and empirical, that are used to separate "high grade" from "low grade" mesenchymal elements in the context of a biphasic uterine tumor include: nuclear pleomorphism recognizable at scanning magnification (nuclear enlargement three-times that of non-neoplastic myometrial smooth muscle or non-neoplastic endometrial stromal cells) and easily found mitotic figures. A diagnosis of carcinosarcoma should be reconsidered if the malignant mesenchymal component

(A)

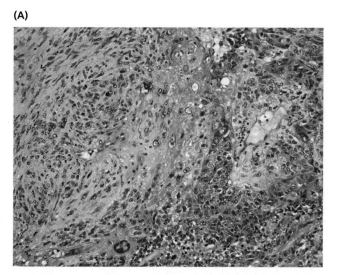

(B)

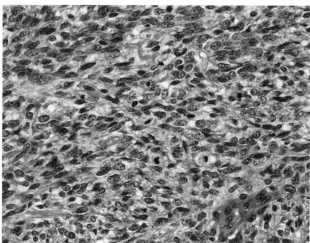

Figure 10.7 Carcinosarcomas with homologous sarcoma (A and B).

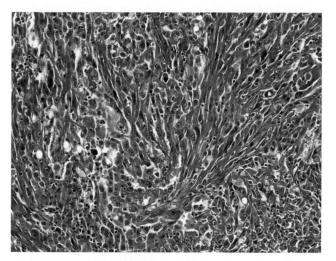

Figure 10.8 Histologically high-grade sarcoma in carcinosarcoma.

cannot be circled with a pen and measured; it would prefer-ably measure more than 1 or 2 mm. These practices are valid only when the lesion is well sampled, and reasonable only when the pathologist and clinician understand one another's thresholds for diagnosis and therapeutic decisions.

The most common heterologous elements are cartilagin-ous or rhabdomyoblastic (i.e., resembling pleomorphic rhabdomyosarcoma or embryonal rhabdomyosarcoma) (Figure 10.9). Occasional cases with fatty, osteoid, neural/neuroectodermal, and vasoformative elements have been described.

Most carcinosarcoma metastases are epithelial only or, less commonly, epithelial predominant. It is extraordinary to find sarcoma-only metastases from carcinosarcoma, but this can occur when heterologous sarcomatous compon-ents predominate.

ANCILLARY DIAGNOSTIC TESTS

Immunohistochemistry does not play a major role in the diagnosis of carcinosarcoma since diagnostic criteria are based on review of hematoxylin and eosin slides. Further-more, the mesenchymal components frequently demonstrate coexpression of epithelial-associated and mesenchymal-associated markers, which can be diagnostically confusing. Pleomorphic, monophasic neoplasms with patchy keratin expression that fail to meet diagnostic criteria for carcino-sarcoma cannot be diagnosed as carcinosarcoma. That being said, the immunophenotype of carcinosarcoma gen-erally follows that of the individual elements present in the tumor. For example, serous regions express keratins and generally overexpress p53, while the rhabdomyoblastic constituents express desmin and myogenin. Useful appli-cations of immunohistochemistry in this setting include verification of the presence of a specific heterologous element, particularly rhabdomyosarcoma (Figures 10.9C and 10.10), or a malignant epithelial component (i.e., p53 overexpression) when the epithelium looks neoplastic and probably malignant (Figure 10.11).

DIFFERENTIAL DIAGNOSIS

As mentioned earlier, most monophasic tumors should not be considered candidates for a carcinosarcoma diagnosis; although it is possible that some uterine pleomorphic rhabdomyosarcomas represent carcinosarcomas in which

(A)

(B)

(C)

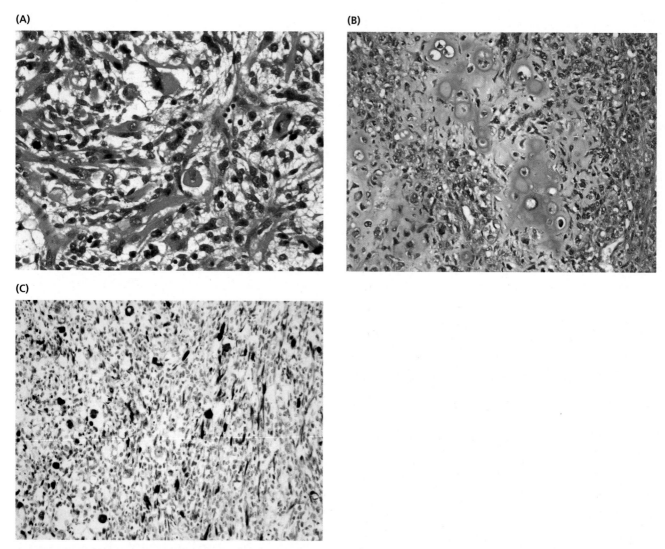

Figure 10.9 Carcinosarcoma with heterologous sarcoma (A and B). Myogenin immunostain marking rhabdomyoblasts is illustrated in C.

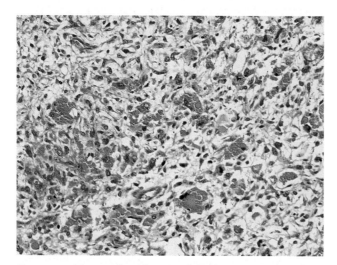

Figure 10.10 Tumor cells with eosinophilic globules – a mimic of rhabdomyoblastic differentiation.

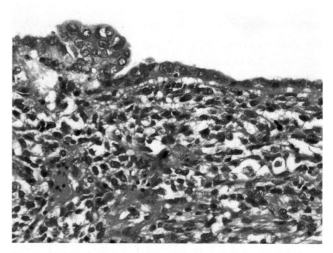

Figure 10.11 Biphasic tumor with malignant stroma and atypical epithelium. Lack of p53 overexpression in the epithelial compartment and the focal presence of cilia (at right) supported classification as adenosarcoma rather than carcinosarcoma.

Table 10.2 Differential diagnosis of carcinosarcoma

Adenosarcoma

Endometrioid carcinoma with spindle cell elements

Dedifferentiated endometrial carcinoma

Poorly differentiated carcinoma

Combined adenocarcinoma and neuroendocrine carcinoma

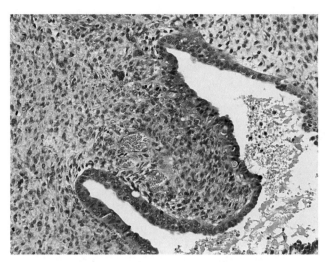

Figure 10.12 Adenosarcomatous area within carcinosarcoma. The presence of histologically high-grade malignant epithelium supports classification as carcinosarcoma instead of adenosarcoma.

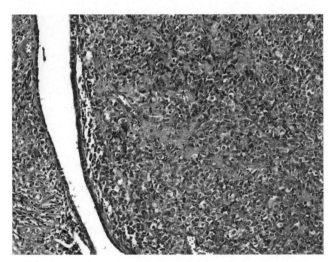

Figure 10.13 Adenosarcoma with high-grade stromal overgrowth.

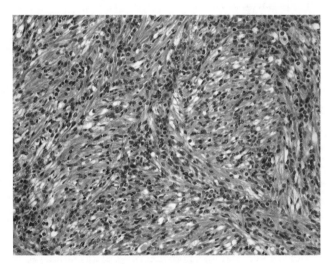

Figure 10.14 Rhabdomyosarcoma in heterologous adenosarcoma (typical biphasic pattern was evident elsewhere).

the epithelial component has not been sampled or has been overgrown by sarcoma. This leaves the biphasic tumors. The four most important biphasic tumors to consider in the differential diagnosis are adenosarcoma, endometrioid adenocarcinoma with spindle cell elements[13,14], so-called dedifferentiated endometrial carcinoma[15], and combined adeno- and neuroendocrine carcinoma (Table 10.2).

Mullerian adenosarcoma

Mullerian adenosarcomas are polypoid tumors featuring club-like fronds and papillary projections onto the tumor's surface and into entrapped cysts. The epithelial component is benign appearing and frequently metaplastic; whereas the mesenchymal component is malignant, although it is usually low grade in appearance. The typical adenosarcoma, therefore, does not resemble carcinosarcoma, although occasional carcinosarcomas can contain areas that are histologically indistinguishable from adenosarcoma (Figure 10.12)[16]. Diagnostic problems are sometimes encountered when adenosarcomas display sarcomatous stromal overgrowth. Adenosarcomas with sarcomatous stromal overgrowth are usually histologically high grade and may exhibit effacement of epithelial components; unlike carcinosarcoma, these tumors do not feature malignant epithelial components. Very rare adenosarcomas can manifest complex atypical hyperplasia or even well-differentiated endometrioid adenocarcinoma in the epithelial compartment[17], but these tumors should not be diagnosed as carcinosarcoma. Phyllodes-like growth patterns with epithelium showing low histologic grade are all against a carcinosarcoma diagnosis. Last, be aware that adenosarcomas, particularly those containing histologically high-grade sarcoma (Figure 10.13), can include heterologous elements (Figure 10.14).

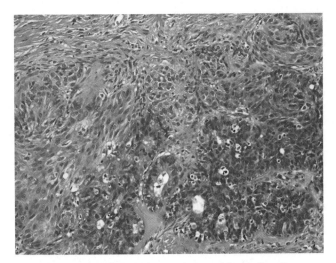

Figure 10.15 Endometrioid adenocarcinoma with spindle cell elements. Glandular and spindle cell components are histologically low grade and are fused.

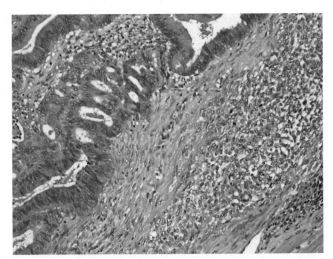

Figure 10.16 Dedifferentiated endometrial carcinoma, showing a combination of well-differentiated adenocarcinoma (left) and undifferentiated carcinoma (right). Carcinosarcomas only very rarely contain well-differentiated endometrioid adenocarcinoma.

Endometrioid adenocarcinoma with spindle cell elements

Endometrioid adenocarcinomas with spindle cell elements have been reported in the uterus and ovary[13,14]. The endometrioid elements, frequently showing squamous metaplasia, fuse seamlessly with spindle cell elements that are not histologically high grade, by definition (Figure 10.15). The endometrioid component is FIGO grade 1 or 2, and the spindle cell component is cellular, but not markedly atypical. It is usually difficult to find appreciable mitotic activity in the spindle cell component at scanning magnification. Mature-appearing osteoid and chondroid elements can also be encountered, but rhabdomyoblasts have not been reported. The distinction between this entity and carcinosarcoma is based on the tumor's grade and the presence of element fusion. It is thought that FIGO grade 1 and 2 endometrioid carcinomas with spindle cell elements are clinically similar to low-grade endometrioid carcinomas that lack spindle cell elements. In small endometrial samplings, the distinction between a low-grade endometrioid carcinoma with spindle elements and a carcinosarcoma may be difficult; such cases may require a guarded comment in the pathology report with a deferral to the hysterectomy specimen for final classification.

"Dedifferentiated" endometrial carcinoma

"Dedifferentiated" endometrial carcinoma is a recently described entity with a moderately or well-differentiated endometrioid adenocarcinoma juxtaposed against an undifferentiated carcinoma (Figure 10.16)[15,18,19]. These biphasic tumors feature an undifferentiated component that is distinct from the differentiated component, theoretically leading to confusion with carcinosarcoma. In contrast to FIGO grade 3 endometrioid carcinoma, the undifferentiated component is composed of expansive sheets of monomorphic, dyshesive, round tumor cells without any gland formation, obviously nested architecture, or squamous differentiation. A rhabdoid appearance is frequently encountered, as is myxoid stroma. In contrast to the mesenchymal component of carcinosarcoma, the cells are not overtly pleomorphic, nor are they spindle shaped. The undifferentiated component characteristically shows only focal or weak keratin expression, potentially compounding difficulties with the differential diagnosis. Although expression of EMA and CK18 has been documented in most examples, this does not provide explicit support for this entity when carcinosarcoma is in the differential diagnosis. The presence of a well-differentiated endometrioid component and the appearance of the undifferentiated areas permit distinction from carcinosarcoma. Although the reported clinical follow-up is limited, it appears that dedifferentiated carcinoma is even more clinically aggressive than carcinosarcoma, with nearly every affected patient suffering rapid recurrence or death. Another difference with carcinosarcoma concerns the apparent more frequent loss of expression of DNA mismatch repair (MMR) proteins in dedifferentiated carcinomas[20]; suggesting that some of these tumors are part of the Lynch syndrome/hereditary non-polyposis colorectal carcinoma spectrum[21].

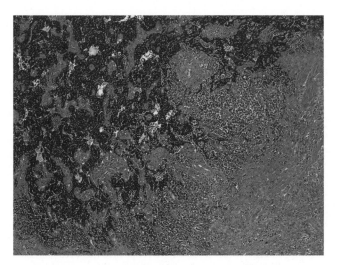

Figure 10.17 Small cell carcinoma: the characteristic histologic features of small cell carcinoma differ from the pleomorphic and spindle cell features typical of the sarcomatous component of carcinosarcoma.

Poorly differentiated carcinoma

Monophasic tumors should not be diagnosed as carcinosarcoma, although there are certain scenarios when it is reasonable to suggest the possibility of carcinosarcoma. Carcinomas with anaplastic features are sometimes found in biopsy specimens that precede a hysterectomy containing carcinosarcoma. Poorly differentiated carcinomas may also demonstrate incomplete mesenchymal differentiation or "epithelial–mesenchymal transition" (subtle tumor cell spindling or myxoid stroma, for example) at the periphery of infiltrating nests and glands. It is best to withhold a diagnosis of carcinosarcoma until one is sure that two distinctive components are present.

Combined adenocarcinoma and neuroendocrine carcinoma

Combined adenocarcinoma and neuroendocrine carcinoma can mimic carcinosarcoma. The gland-forming elements have a similar appearance in both tumors, but the diffuse areas display some differences. Specifically, diffuse areas in tumors with neuroendocrine differentiation should resemble histologically similar tumors in lung (Figure 10.17). The criteria for diagnosing pulmonary small cell and large cell neuroendocrine carcinomas can be used in the gynecologic tract. While the diagnosis of small cell carcinoma is generally reproducible, the diagnosis of large cell neuroendocrine carcinoma can be subject to difference in opinion. To establish the latter diagnosis, the

diffuse zones should display obviously organoid, palisading, trabecular, or rosette-like growth patterns; large tumor cells with a polygonal shape; frequent nucleoli; a high mitotic rate; and neuroendocrine features by immunohistochemistry. The extent of neuroendocrine marker expression sufficient to support an impression of a large cell neuroendocrine carcinoma should be diffuse and strong if the morphologic features are not entirely characteristic. It should be noted that dedifferentiated endometrial carcinomas can show focal and weak neuroendocrine marker expression[19] (as can the epithelial components of carcinosarcomas), but the morphologic features of the undifferentiated component of dedifferentiated carcinomas do not include organoid, palisading, trabecular, or rosette-like growth patterns.

REFERENCES

1. McCluggage WG. Uterine carcinosarcomas (malignant mullerian tumors) are metaplastic carcinomas. *Int J Gynecol Cancer* 2002;**12**(6):687–90.
2. Sreenan JJ, Hart WR. Carcinosarcomas of the female genital tract: a pathologic study of 29 metastatic tumors: further evidence for the dominant role of the epithelial component and the conversion theory of histogenesis. *Am J Surg Pathol* 1995;**19**:666–74.
3. Pecorelli S. Revised FIGO staging for carcinoma of the vulva, cervix, and endometrium. *Int J Gynaecol Obstet* 2009;**105**(2):103–4.
4. Silverberg SG, Major FJ, Blessing JA, et al. Carcinosarcoma (malignant mixed mesodermal tumor) of the uterus. A Gynecologic Oncology Group pathologic study of 203 cases. *Int J Gynecol Pathol* 1990;**9**:1–19.
5. Yamada SD, Burger RA, Brewster WR, et al. Pathologic variables and adjuvant therapy as predictors of recurrence and survival for patients with surgically evaluated carcinosarcoma of the uterus. *Cancer* 2000;**88**(12):2782–6.
6. Major FJ, Blessing JA, Silverberg SG, et al. Prognostic factors in early-stage uterine sarcoma: a Gynecologic Oncology Group study. *Cancer* 1993;**71** Suppl:1702–9.
7. Soslow RA, Bissonnette JP, Wilton A, et al. Clinicopathologic analysis of 187 high-grade endometrial carcinomas of different histologic subtypes: similar outcomes belie distinctive biologic differences. *Am J Surg Pathol* 2007;**31**(7):979–87.
8. Alektiar KM, McKee A, Lin O, et al. Is there a difference in outcome between stage I–II endometrial cancer of papillary serous/clear cell and endometrioid FIGO grade 3 cancer? *Int J Radiat Oncol Biol Phys* 2002;**54**(1):79–85.
9. Callister M, Ramondetta LM, Jhingran A, Burke TW, Eifel PJ. Malignant mixed mullerian tumors of the uterus: analysis of patterns of failure, prognostic factors, and treatment outcome. *Int J Radiat Oncol Biol Phys* 2004;**58**(3):786–96.
10. Sutton G, Brunetto VL, Kilgore L, et al. A phase III trial of ifosfamide with or without cisplatin in carcinosarcoma of the uterus: a Gynecologic Oncology Group study. *Gynecol Oncol* 2000;**79**(2):147–53.

11. Wolfson AH, Brady MF, Rocereto T, *et al.* A Gynecologic Oncology Group randomized phase III trial of whole abdominal irradiation (WAI) vs. cisplatin-ifosfamide and mesna (CIM) as post-surgical therapy in stage I–IV carcinosarcoma (CS) of the uterus. *Gynecol Oncol* 2007;**107**(2):177–85.

12. Ferguson SE, Tornos C, Hummer A, Barakat RR, Soslow RA. Prognostic features of surgical stage I uterine carcinosarcoma. *Am J Surg Pathol* 2007;**31**(11):1653–61.

13. Murray SK, Clement PB, Young RH. Endometrioid carcinomas of the uterine corpus with sex cord-like formations, hyalinization, and other unusual morphologic features: a report of 31 cases of a neoplasm that may be confused with carcinosarcoma and other uterine neoplasms. *Am J Surg Pathol* 2005;**29**(2):157–66.

14. Tornos C, Silva EG, Ordonez NG, *et al.* Endometrioid carcinoma of the ovary with a prominent spindle-cell component, a source of diagnostic confusion – a report of 14 cases. *Am J Surg Pathol* 1995;**19**:1343–53.

15. Silva EG, Deavers MT, Bodurka DC, Malpica A. Association of low-grade endometrioid carcinoma of the uterus and ovary with undifferentiated carcinoma: a new type of dedifferentiated carcinoma? *Int J Gynecol Pathol* 2006;**25**(1):52–8.

16. Seidman JD, Chauhan S. Evaluation of the relationship between adenosarcoma and carcinosarcoma and a hypothesis of the histogenesis of uterine sarcomas. *Int J Gynecol Pathol* 2003;**22**(1):75–82.

17. Clement PB, Scully RE. Mullerian adenosarcoma of the uterus: a clinicopathologic analysis of 100 cases with a review of the literature. *Hum Pathol* 1990;**21**:363–81.

18. Tafe L, Garg K, Tornos C, Soslow R. Undifferentiated carcinoma of the endometrium and ovary: a clinicopathologic correlation. *Mod Pathol* 2009;**22**(1):238A.

19. Altrabulsi B, Malpica A, Deavers MT, *et al.* Undifferentiated carcinoma of the endometrium. *Am J Surg Pathol* 2005;**29**(10):1316–21.

20. Broaddus RR, Lynch HT, Chen LM, *et al.* Pathologic features of endometrial carcinoma associated with HNPCC: a comparison with sporadic endometrial carcinoma. *Cancer* 2006;**106**(1):87–94.

21. Garg K, Leitao MM, Jr., Kauff ND, *et al.* Selection of endometrial carcinomas for DNA mismatch repair protein immunohistochemistry using patient age and tumor morphology enhances detection of mismatch repair abnormalities. *Am J Surg Pathol* 2009;**33**(6):925–33.

11   ADENOFIBROMA AND ADENOSARCOMA

INTRODUCTION

The adenofibroma–adenosarcoma spectrum of biphasic mullerian tumors in the female gynecologic tract resembles the fibroadenoma–phyllodes spectrum in the breast. As in the breast, zones of histologic overlap exist and, on occasion, areas of adenofibromatous and adenosarcomatous differentiation may be seen in the same neoplasm. Classification of these tumors is ultimately based on the most histologically malignant area, but it should not be surprising that, just as there are gradations of histologic malignancy amongst these tumors, gradations of clinical behavior may also occur. However, unlike the situation in the breast, most (some authorities have maintained all) of these biphasic tumors in the uterus fall well within the low-grade sarcoma spectrum. In contrast, adenofibromas, if they exist, are clinically benign with little risk for recurrence once they are completely excised.

ADENOSARCOMA

Adenosarcoma is uncommon; it is a predominantly low-grade malignant tumor that is composed of sarcomatous stroma and benign epithelial elements. This tumor often represents a challenge for the pathologist due to significant overlap with benign polyps on the one hand and with carcinosarcoma and sarcoma entrapping benign glands on the other. Indeed, the low-grade forms of adenosarcoma account for a significant proportion of malignant lesions within the female genital tract and peritoneum that are underdiagnosed by pathologists[1].

Most adenosarcomas occur in the uterine corpus, but they may arise in cervical, vaginal, tubal, ovarian, and peritoneal sites. Involvement of additional extragenital sites in women has been linked to endometriosis. An association with unopposed estrogen and tamoxifen therapy has been reported in uterine adenosarcoma[2]. As with carcinosarcoma, a prior history of pelvic radiation has also been implicated in a few cases[3].

CLINICAL CHARACTERISTICS

Most patients with uterine corpus adenosarcoma are post-menopausal, although approximately 30% of affected women are premenopausal. Adenosarcomas most often present as polyps or polypoid lesions arising in the uterine body, which may protrude through the cervical os or appear to arise from the cervix or lower uterine segment. Abnormal vaginal bleeding, pelvic pain, and uterine enlargement are not unusual. Often there is a history of recurrent polyps, which on retrospect may morphologically represent adenofibroma or early or subtle forms of adenosarcoma. A history of tamoxifen therapy or prior pelvic radiation may be present.

Most patients with uterine adenosarcoma are FIGO stage I and are cured by hysterectomy. Approximately one-fourth of uterine corpus adenosarcomas are myoinvasive. Deep myoinvasion, lymphovascular invasion, high-grade heterologous stroma, stromal overgrowth, and extrauterine spread are associated with disease recurrence. Almost 30% of adenosarcomas with stromal overgrowth have spread beyond the uterus at presentation. The overall recurrence rate is 15–25% for tumors without stromal overgrowth and 45–70% for those with stromal overgrowth. Recurrent disease typically appears in the pelvis, although distant recurrences may develop many years after pelvic recurrence(s). Approximately 10–25% of patients with uterine adenosarcoma die of their disease. This figure rises to as high as 75% for those whose tumors contain stromal overgrowth.

Cervical adenosarcomas tend to occur at a younger age than their uterine counterparts. Patients with primary cervical adenosarcomas range in age from 13 to 67 years (mean: 37 years). Most present during the reproductive years with abnormal bleeding, which is initially attributed to benign endocervical polyps. The polyps may be exocervical or endocervical and range in size from 2 to 8 cm or more. A sarcoma botyroides appearance has been reported.

Data are limited, but most cases appear to be cured by hysterectomy, possibly due to the early detection of low-stage disease in the majority of patients. To date, less than 50 patients have been reported with endocervical adenosarcoma. As in uterine corpus tumors, depth of invasion and sarcomatous overgrowth are adverse prognostic indicators.

Surgery, including complete staging, is the mainstay of therapy for uterine adenosarcoma with or without sarcomatous overgrowth. It has been suggested that complete resection of the polyp alone may be adequate initial therapy for cervical adenosarcoma when it occurs in younger women, provided there is a stalk that is clearly uninvolved and there is no histologic evidence of invasion. Although this is still controversial and there is little supporting data, conservation of reproduction and/or hormonal function should always be considered in these cases. Additional therapy in the form of radiation, chemotherapy, or both has been reported for more advanced disease; however, the superiority of any one modality has not been determined. Hormonal therapy has also been tried in the adjuvant setting in low-stage disease, but there appears to be no justification for oophorectomy in younger patients at this time.

Adenosarcomas are typically slowly growing, indolent tumors, but recurrences at five or more years following diagnosis are not unusual. In some instances, recurrence may not occur until 13 or more years following definitive therapy. Recurrences tend to be local, with distant metastases following initial local recurrence(s). It has been suggested that these hematogenous metastases almost always contain only sarcomatous elements[4]. A subset of tumors may exhibit a more aggressive clinical course; these tumors often have stromal overgrowth or other features of a high-grade sarcoma, and may resemble carcinosarcoma in their clinical behavior. Foci of adenosarcoma may be seen in some carcinosarcomas, which suggests possible evolution to carcinosarcoma in some cases[5].

MORPHOLOGY

Gross pathology

Adenosarcoma is a mucosal-based polypoid mass arising in the corpus (90%) or cervix (10%). The polyps vary in size from 1 to 17 cm (mean: 5 cm), may be multiple, and typically exhibit microcystic architecture on cut section.

Microscopic pathology

Most adenosarcomas feature uniformly distributed, often cystic, and irregularly contoured glandular elements, often with internal papillations scattered throughout a variably cellular stroma (Figure 11.1). The stroma forms a characteristic hypercellular collar or cuff (so called "cambium layer") around the glands (Figure 11.2), which often exhibit mixed differentiation, including endometrioid, endocervical, ciliated, eosinophilic, and squamous (Figure 11.3). The epithelium typically appears benign or, less often, atypical,

(A)

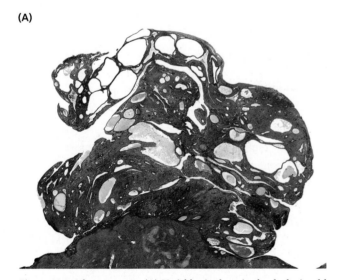

(B)

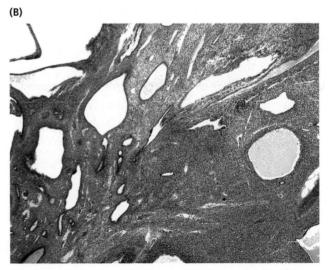

Figure 11.1 Adenosarcoma. (A) Variably sized cystic glands depicted here account for the cystic gross appearance of some low-grade adenosarcomas. (B) Adenosarcoma merges with adenofibroma (left). Inadvertent sampling of the adenofibroma component may lead to delayed therapy if the polyp is not completely removed and fully evaluated.

simulating complex hyperplasia or adenocarcinoma in situ (Figures 11.4–11.6). Asymmetric growth of stroma may compress the epithelial component to produce irregular stellate glandular configurations; sometimes, when this asymmetry is extreme, polypoid invaginations are produced (Figure 11.7). Stromal foam cells may be present. The classic adenosarcoma exhibits a frond-like growth pattern, resembling phyllodes tumor of the breast (Figure 11.8). The stroma may exhibit a variety of specific and non-specific differentiated types, including endometrial stromal, smooth muscle (Figure 11.9), fibrous, and myxoid (Figure 11.10). Approximately 20% have heterologous stroma, consisting of islands of fat, cartilage, or

skeletal muscle (rhabdomyoblasts), which then may be mistaken for carcinosarcoma or pure sarcoma in a limited sampling. Foci of sex cord–like elements may also be present (Figure 11.11). Adenosarcomas fall into three general groups, depending on the atypicality of the stroma and the presence of stromal overgrowth:

Group 1: the first and most common type of adenosarcoma resembles adenofibroma, but possesses more cellular and more mitotically active stroma (= low-grade adenosarcoma). In most cases, the stromal component is nondescript, but in some instances the stromal cells are arranged in cordlike patterns reminiscent of sex cord elements in uterine tumors resembling sex cord stromal tumors. The recommended mitotic index thresholds for classifying a tumor as adenosarcoma vary between 2 MF/10 HPF and 4 MF/10 HPF[3,6]. The latter criterion is recommended, unless a particular tumor exhibits prominent stromal cellularity or cytologic atypia; in which case the tumor should be classified as of uncertain malignant potential. An alternative approach is to classify these tumors as low-grade adenosarcoma (or low malignant potential [LMP]), with the understanding that such tumors will probably either not recur at all or may only recur many years after diagnosis. The distinction is most important in women of reproductive age, for whom a hysterectomy may not be the treatment of choice.

Group 2: the second group features histologically malignant stroma (= high-grade adenosarcoma), most often

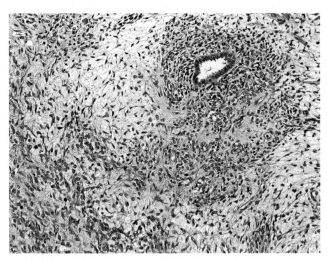

Figure 11.2 Adenosarcoma. Stromal cuffing due to increased stromal proliferation in the immediate vicinity of the constituent glands is a diagnostic feature of adenosarcoma.

(A)

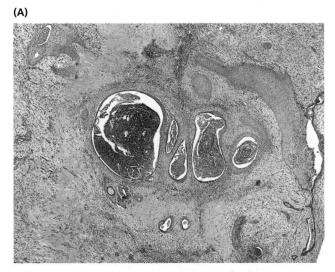

(B)

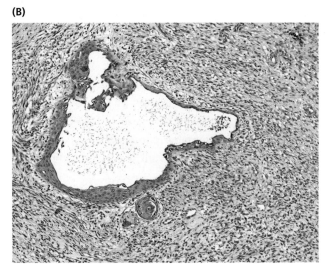

Figure 11.3 Adenosarcoma. (A, B) The constituent glands in low-grade adenosarcoma often exhibit a varied pattern of mucinous and squamous, as well as endometrioid, differentiation. These various forms of metaplasia may be mistaken for metaplasia in a benign endometrial polyp in lesions with lesser degrees of stromal proliferation.

(A)

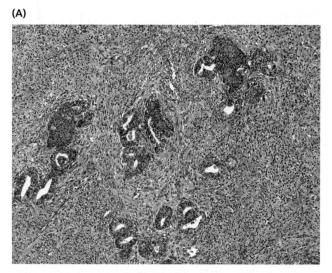

(B)

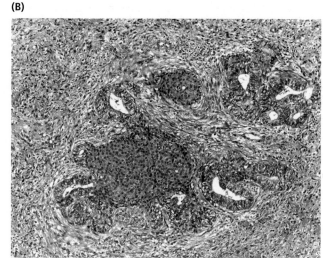

Figure 11.4 (A, B) Atypical polypoid adenomyoma–like area in adenosarcoma.

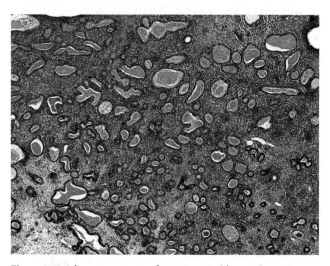

Figure 11.5 Adenosarcoma may feature areas with prominent glands, which may be misinterpreted as endometrial hyperplasia in a limited sampling.

manifested by rhabdomyosarcomatous differentiation, but chondroid, smooth muscle, and undifferentiated sarcoma may also be seen (Figure 11.12). This group of tumors often contains numerous mitotic figures, including atypical mitoses. Stromal overgrowth is not present.

Group 3: the third group features stromal overgrowth (= adenosarcoma with stromal overgrowth). By definition, tumors with stromal overgrowth should contain pure stroma comprising more than 25% of the tumor volume (Figure 11.13). Most, but not all, of this group also contain high-grade sarcomatous stroma, often with heterologous differentiation

(typically rhabdomyosarcoma). These latter tumors are associated with a uniformly poor prognosis. In some tumors, the stroma in the areas of stromal overgrowth is low grade or bland as in the first type of adenosarcoma, and these tumors, despite the presence of stromal overgrowth, may be associated with a more indolent disease course, with long disease-free intervals punctuated by intermittent localized recurrences. The mitotic count almost always exceeds 4 MF/10 HPF in tumors with stromal overgrowth, although exceptions do rarely occur, typically in the group with low-grade sarcomatous overgrowth. Since stromal overgrowth is such a poor prognostic indicator, foci of stromal overgrowth that do not meet the 25% volume criterion should still be reported as a volume percentage to signify that the adenosarcoma may represent a somewhat more aggressive tumor than the usual adenosarcoma.

Recurrent adenosarcomas may continue to exhibit a biphasic phenotype or may be composed of stroma only (Figure 11.14). In some instances, recurrences may transform to higher-grade sarcoma or develop heterologous elements that were not apparent in the primary tumor[7]. The transformation to higher-grade sarcoma or sarcomatous overgrowth is usually associated with increased tempo of disease with increased frequency of recurrence and involvement of multiple sites. Hematogenous metastases, typically to the lung, may occur and are often comprised only of stromal elements.

(A)

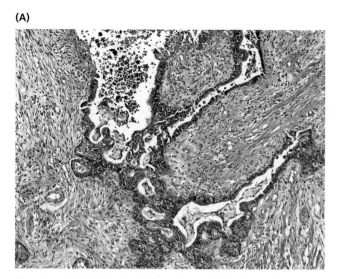

(B)

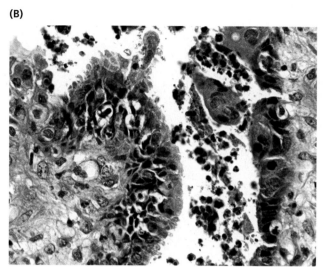

Figure 11.6 (A, B) Focal area of carcinoma in situ in adenosarcoma.

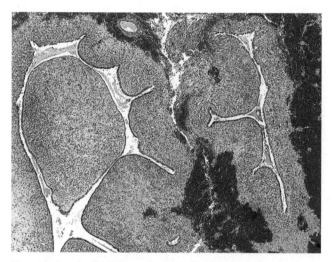

Figure 11.7 A distinctive feature of low-grade adenosarcoma is the presence of compressed glands due to stromal condensation.

ANCILLARY DIAGNOSTIC TESTS

The immunophenotype of most adenosarcomas resembles that of endometrial stromal tumors (positive for ER, PR, WT1, and CD10, with variable expression of muscle markers, androgen receptors, and cytokeratin). Expression of ER, PR, and CD10 is commonly lost in cases showing stromal overgrowth[8]. The stroma of adenosarcomas, particularly the low-grade tumors, is often CD10 positive, and so this marker cannot be used to differentiate endometrial stromal sarcoma with benign glands from a low-grade adenosarcoma.

A complex karyotype involving multiple chromosomes was identified by cytogenetic and molecular cytogenetic analysis of an adenosarcoma from a 15-year-old girl[9]. Neither p53 nor HER2 appear to play a significant role in this disease[8].

DIFFERENTIAL DIAGNOSIS

The differential diagnosis of adenosarcoma includes adenofibroma and other clinically benign processes with little or no recurrent potential at the benign end of the spectrum, and carcinosarcoma and other clinically malignant processes with significant recurrent and metastatic potential at the malignant end of the spectrum (Tables 11.1 and 11.2).

Adenofibroma

The diagnosis of adenofibroma has been historically reserved for mixed glandular and stromal polyps composed of benign glands set in a paucicellular, fibromatous or fibrotic, and mitotically inactive stroma (Figure 11.15). As mentioned earlier, an unqualified diagnosis of adenofibroma is currently discouraged, particularly in uterine sampling specimens; this is in part due to the inherent inability to predict clinical behavior with these lesions, and in part due to the issues associated with incomplete sampling. A variety of diagnostic approaches have been proposed, each of which is imperfect. A default diagnosis of "adenosarcoma" for all such lesions generally entails hysterectomy, which is often curative; however the risk–benefit ratio for this approach is obviously lower in an

(A)

(B)

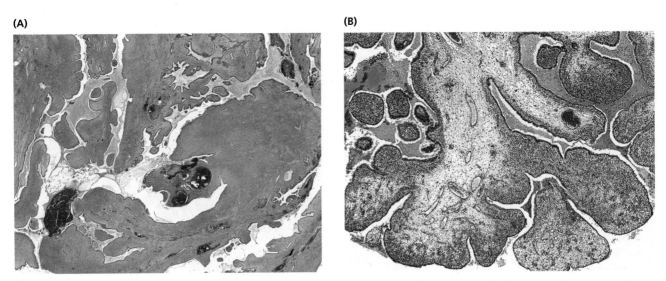

Figure 11.8 (A, B) Frond-like papillary configurations, similar to those encountered in phyllodes tumors of the breast, are characteristic of adenosarcoma.

(A)

(B)

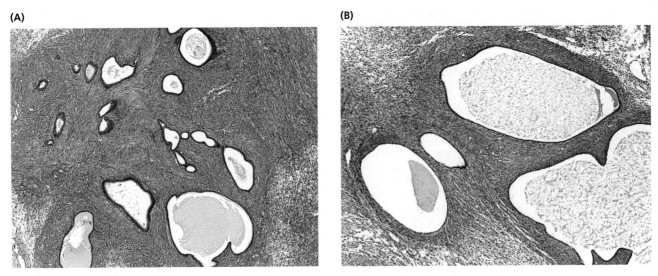

Figure 11.9 (A) Smooth muscle differentiation in low-grade adenosarcoma. (B) Intraperitoneal recurrence at eight years.

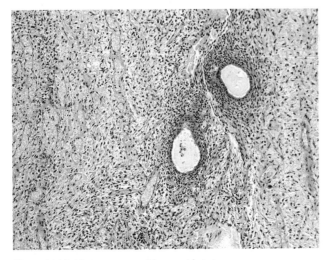

Figure 11.10 Adenosarcoma with myxoid stroma.

otherwise healthy postmenopausal woman than in a younger woman who wishes to preserve fertility. Alternative diagnoses, such as "at least adenofibroma, cannot exclude low-grade adenosarcoma" offer a more accurate assessment of the situation; especially if the pathologist provides a comment that discusses the difficulties in establishing a definitive diagnosis. In these latter cases, imaging studies and repeat hysteroscopic directed sampling should be considered. Although adenofibroma may have the typical gross and low-power microscopic appearance of adenosarcoma, the presence of any periglandular stromal condensation, increased stromal cellularity, and/or increased mitotic index warrants consideration for the diagnosis of adenosarcoma. Also, the presence of heterologous stromal elements is

(A)

(B)

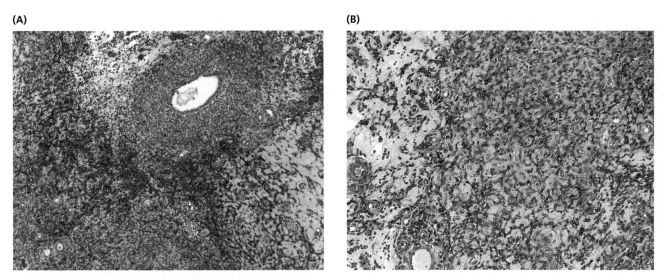

Figure 11.11 (A, B) Areas of sex cord differentiation are not uncommon in low-grade adenosarcoma.

(A)

(B)

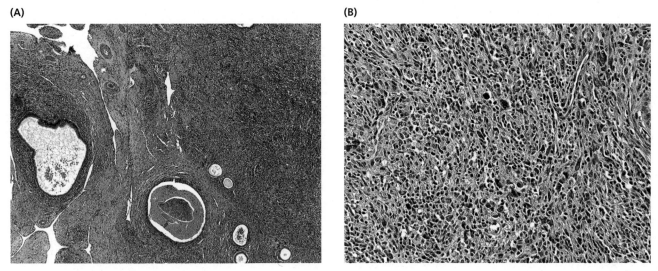

Figure 11.12 (A, B) High-grade sarcoma in adenosarcoma. Adenosarcomas with high-grade sarcoma tend to exhibit a more aggressive clinical course than usual low-grade adenosarcoma.

highly unusual in adenofibroma; to date, only one case with mature fat has been described. When issuing a diagnosis of adenosarcoma, it is important to remember that tumors falling within the low-grade end of the spectrum (i.e., no high-grade sarcoma, no stromal overgrowth) are considered clinically low grade, and it is advisable to append the "low grade" descriptor to the diagnosis (low-grade adenosarcoma).

The distinction between adenofibroma and adenosarcoma can usually be made when the entire uterus is available for examination, although there is some controversy concerning the level of mitotic activity that predicts potential for recurrence in the absence of high-grade sarcomatous elements. Clement and Scully proposed

a threshold of 2 MF/10 HPF; whereas Zaloudek and Norris presented evidence to support a threshold of 4 MF/10 HPF[3,6]. This controversy largely reflects the observation that these predictors are far from perfect and occasional adenofibromatous lesions, even with minimal or no mitotic activity, are associated with myoinvasion and/or local recurrence on clinical follow-up[10,11]. Since authorities differ on the appropriate mitotic index for distinguishing adenofibroma from adenosarcoma, uterine tumors with particularly cellular stroma, more than minimal stromal cell atypia, and/or borderline mitotic counts should be considered as being of at least uncertain malignant potential, particularly if subepithelial condensation is present.

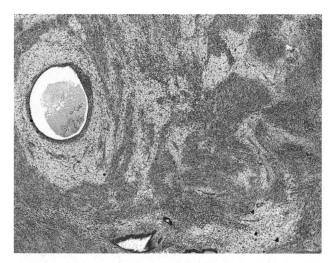

Figure 11.13 Sarcomatous overgrowth in adenosarcoma is associated with a worse prognosis than the usual low-grade adenosarcoma.

Distinction between adenofibroma and adenosarcoma in the ovary and other extragenital sites can be more difficult, due to the exuberant stromal component that may accompany some of the epithelial neoplasms in these sites. Problems most often arise when the adenosarcoma exhibits predominantly fibromatous stromal overgrowth, inconspicuous periglandular cuffs, or few, abortive intraglandular projections. To circumvent these problems, all cases with any ambiguous histologic features falling within the adenofibroma–adenosarcoma spectrum should be thoroughly sampled, especially when encountered in an extragenital site. If the problematic lesion still defies classification after thorough sectioning, consideration should be given for imaging studies and/or repeat sampling, particularly if the patient is of reproductive age.

(A)

(B)

(C)

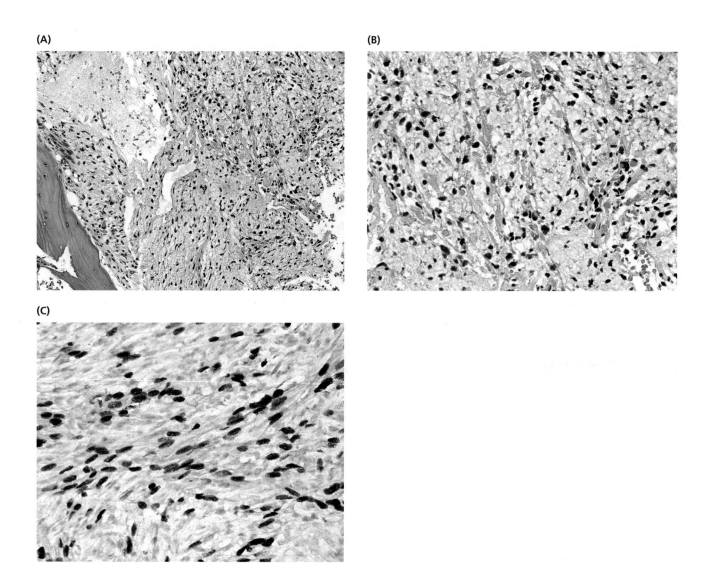

Figure 11.14 (A) Metastatic adenosarcoma; only the sarcomatous component is present (bone metastasis). (B) Stellate cells set in myxoid matrix are rhabdomyoblasts. (C) Myogenin demonstrates rhabdomyosarcomatous differentiation.

Table 11.1 Histopathologic features of adenosarcoma

Biphasic tumor

Epithelial component is histologically benign – may be atypical or rarely low-grade carcinoma in situ

Mesenchymal component is histologically malignant – may be low grade (most common) or high grade, with or without stromal overgrowth[a]

Mimics are excluded (see Table 11.2)

[a] Stromal overgrowth is defined as over 25% of the tumor volume – this may be an inaccurate assessment when made on a uterine sampling specimen. Therefore, foci of stromal overgrowth that do not meet the 25% volume criterion should still be reported as a volume percentage to signify that the adenosarcoma may represent a somewhat more aggressive tumor than the usual adenosarcoma.

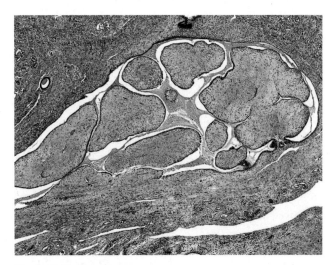

Figure 11.15 Adenofibroma.

Table 11.2 Differential diagnosis of adenosarcoma

	Benign glands	*Malignant glands*
Benign stroma	Endometrial (or cervical) polyp	(Carcinofibroma)[a]
	Adenofibroma	Adenocarcinoma with spindled and corded stroma
	Adenomyoma	
	Atypical polypoid adenomyoma	
	Polypoid endometriosis	
Malignant stroma	Adenosarcoma	Carcinosarcoma
	With sarcomatous stroma	Homologous stroma
	With stromal overgrowth	Heterologous stroma
	Endometrial stromal sarcoma with glandular elements	
	Sarcoma entrapping benign glands	
	Embryonal rhabdomyosarcoma	

[a] Carcinofibroma, a term reported in the older literature to describe the presence of adenocarcinoma in an adenofibromatous process, is not a standard diagnostic entity. It is used to refer to the rare uterine tumor that consists of obviously malignant epithelial elements set in abundant fibroblastic stroma or admixed with benign smooth muscle, adipose tissue, or cartilage (so called "carcinomesenchymoma").

Endometrial polyp

Endometrial polyps may contain atypical stromal cells with cytologic features similar to the atypical stromal cells observed in the vulva, vagina, and cervix (Figure 5.37)[12].

However, the characteristic intraglandular polypoid projections and periglandular stromal cuffs of adenosarcoma are not present in benign polyps. Large endometrial polyps may harbor increased stromal mitotic figures (up to 5 MF/10 HPF), but these polyps do not have significant stromal atypia nor do they have a marked increase in stromal cellularity. Such polyps are distinguished from adenofibromas on the basis of inactive glands in the endometrial polyp and the characteristic papillary or intraglandular polypoid projections in the adenofibroma.

Endocervical polyp

Endocervical polyps occur over a wide age range, but the majority occur in women 40 years of age or more. Most are small (<1 cm) and single. Patients are often asymptomatic, but may present with vaginal bleeding. A variety of secondary patterns can be seen in endocervical polyps, including cysts, stromal edema, stromal fibrosis, stromal myofibrosis, stromal calcification, and increased stromal vascularity (Figure 4.2). Heterologous elements (fat, cartilage, bone, glia) can be present. In addition, the epithelium may show squamous metaplasia, squamous dysplasia (squamous intraepithelial lesion, carcinoma in situ), or even invasive carcinoma. Microglandular hyperplasia, endocervical glandular hyperplasia, and Arias-Stella reaction are also quite common. However, the characteristic intraglandular polypoid projections and periglandular stromal cuffs of adenosarcoma are not present in benign endocervical polyps.

Polypoid adenomyoma/atypical polypoid adenomyoma

Polypoid adenomyoma or adenomyo*fibro*ma (PA) is a circumscribed aggregate of fibromuscular tissue containing small, architecturally simple glands without branching or budding; while atypical polypoid adenomyoma (APA) contains architecturally complex glands with prominent squamous (or morular) metaplasia[13]. The constituent stromal cells in both lesions are cytologically bland. They present as an exophytic or endophytic polypoid growth in the lower uterine segment or, less commonly, cervix, and are thought to represent endometrial polyps or submucosal leiomyomas until they are examined histologically (Figures 5.40 and 5.41). Trichrome stain often confirms the impression of a mixture of spindled smooth muscle cells and collagen. Polypoid adenomyoma lesions are benign, while atypical polypoid adenomyoma may, rarely, demonstrate superficial myometrial invasion by foci that morphologically meet criteria for well-differentiated adenocarcinoma (Figure 5.42). These lesions do not typically pose a significant diagnostic problem unless they feature an especially prominent fibromyomatous stroma or foci of alternate stromal differentiation.

However, occasionally, focal increased stromal mitotic figures (3–5 MF/10 HPF) may be present in polypoid adenomyoma and atypical polypoid adenomyoma, raising the differential diagnosis of adenosarcoma. The problem may be compounded by foci of squamous epithelial differentiation, which are present in most cases of atypical polypoid adenomyoma. Unlike uterine adenosarcoma, polypoid adenomyoma and atypical polypoid adenomyoma occur predominantly in premenopausal or perimenopausal women. Many of the patients are nulliparous, and a clinical history of infertility is not uncommon. Although tumors in the adenofibroma–adenosarcoma spectrum may feature stromal smooth muscle, the stroma elsewhere is usually also either highly cellular and resembles endometrial stroma, or paucicellular and populated by spindled fibroblastic cells with abundant collagen. Rarely, we have encountered adenosarcomas with a predominant low-grade smooth muscle stroma, but, even in these tumors, areas of classic periglandular stromal condensation and intraluminal polypoid projections are seen.

Adenomyomas of endocervical type may also occur[17]. The patient demographics tend to be similar to those for the usual endometrioid atypical polypoid adenomyoma. Most are cervical, polypoid, less than 8 cm, and, when

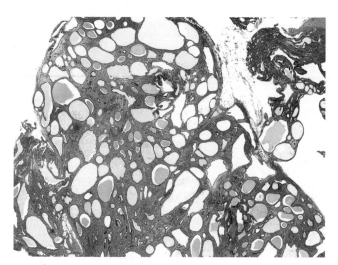

Figure 11.16 Polypoid endometriosis.

macroscopic, resemble a myoma with mucin-filled cysts. Rarely, the lesion may be situated entirely within the cervical wall, forming a mural mass. Microscopically, the glands are arranged in a loose, lobular pattern, which may also feature endometrioid or tubal-type glands (Figure 4.3). The surrounding stroma is myomatous or, more accurately, fibromyomatous. No stromal condensation is present. These polyps are benign; no recurrences or extrauterine extension have been reported.

Polypoid endometriosis

Polypoid endometriosis (Figure 11.16) is a rare manifestation of endometriosis that may simulate a neoplasm on clinical, intraoperative, or pathologic assessment[18]. Some cases may be attributable to exogenous hormones or hyperestrinism, and, like conventional endometriosis, some may represent a premalignant or neoplastic process. Unlike conventional endometriosis, polypoid endometriosis affects a slightly older age group, with 60% of cases occurring in women over 50 years of age. Clinical follow-up in the largest series of cases reported to date indicates a benign course, although follow-up is limited in that only seven of the reported patients had more than five years follow-up, and only four had seven or more years[18].

Like adenosarcoma, polypoid endometriosis often features various types of epithelial metaplasia (tubal, mucinous, squamous, papillary syncytial metaplasia), but, unlike adenosarcoma, it usually does not exhibit the characteristic stromal cellularity or stromal atypia of adenosarcoma. Some cases may feature intraglandular stromal papillae and focal periglandular stromal hypercellularity,

(A)

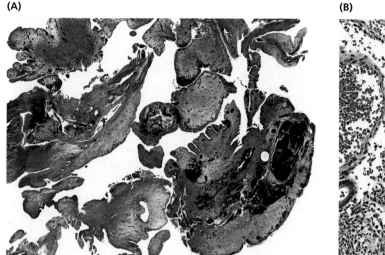

(B)

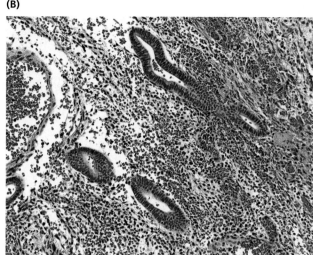

Figure 11.17 (A, B) Extragenital adenosarcoma arising in pre-existing polypoid endometriosis.

and the point at which these lesions cease to be polypoid endometriosis and warrant classification as adenosarcoma is not always easy to define. Because of this potential for histologic overlap, the distinction between these two processes can be very difficult on frozen section as well as on permanent sections in some cases. Given the diagnostic difficulties and the limited data concerning the clinical behavior of polypoid endometriosis, the possibility of adenosarcoma should be mentioned during intraoperative consultation for any endometriotic lesion presenting as an unusual mass-like process. Whenever possible, complete conservative excision is probably warranted. In problematic cases, examination of multiple sections should be performed.

Conventional endometriosis can give rise to a number of malignant processes. Ovarian clear cell carcinoma and endometrioid adenocarcinoma are the most notable examples of tumors arising in association with endometriosis in the ovary. In extragenital sites, adenosarcoma and endometrial stromal sarcoma are also prominent (Figure 11.17). A significant proportion of extragenital adenosarcomas that have been reported in the literature are diagnosed only after repeated biopsies and/or multiple clinical recurrences of endometriosis. While it is likely that some of these cases are histologically non-informative and possibly responsible for the historic designation of "aggressive endometriosis," it is also possible that at least some cases may contain more diagnostic foci that can only be identified when extensively sampled. Adenosarcoma should be given strong consideration in the differential diagnosis of any new pelvic or abdominal

mass in a patient with a history of endometriosis, and such masses should be subjected to extensive sectioning and histologic evaluation.

Adenocarcinoma with spindled and corded stroma

Low-grade endometrial carcinomas may contain a prominent spindled epithelial cell component, hyalinized osteoid-like stroma, or a cellular corded and hyalinized stromal pattern. In most such cases, the malignant glandular component is readily apparent and the tumor resembles a "low-grade carcinosarcoma" (Figure 11.18). However, in some cases (particularly in endometrial curettage specimens), the malignant gland pattern may not be as apparent and the cellular stroma may suggest an adenosarcoma. Both tumors may present as polyps and occur in a comparatively similar age range. Adenocarcinoma with spindled stroma tends to show more prominent squamous differentiation (up to 70% of cases), but in other respects these two tumors may resemble one another in absence of bona fide malignant glands and/or definitive periglandular cellular stromal condensation. Since a diagnosis of either lesion should result in similar management (e.g., additonal sampling and/or imaging studies in a reproductive-age woman, or total hysterectomy with possible staging), it should be sufficient to mention the differential diagnosis in a comment section of the report and defer final classification to the anticipated additional material in difficult cases.

(A)

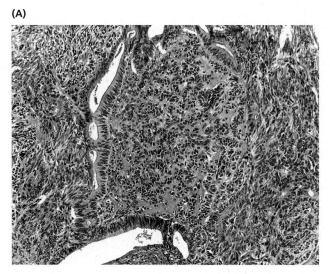

(B)

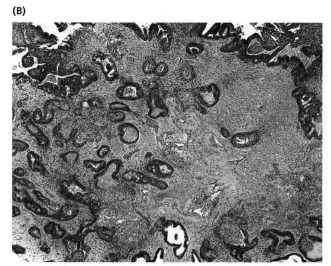

Figure 11.18 (A, B) Low-grade endometrial carcinoma with spindled stroma.

Carcinosarcoma

This distinction is based on the epithelial component. The malignant epithelial component in carcinosarcoma is typically high grade and is usually not confused with the atypical glands that may occur in adenosarcoma (Figure 10.2). Uncertainty in a curettage or biopsy specimen may occur due to inadequate sampling, and many of these ambiguous cases can be resolved on hysterectomy. However, foci of atypical glands (Figure 11.6) and even well-differentiated adenocarcinoma may rarely occur in tumors that are otherwise indistinguishable from adenosarcomas. Tumors with these features should be diagnosed as adenosarcomas with focal low-grade adenocarcinoma, provided the foci are relatively small. Since such tumors are uncommon, there are no outcome data (other than anecdotal) that support this classification, but one would expect that these tumors would behave more like typical adenosarcoma unless there is associated high-grade carcinoma, high-grade sarcoma, or stromal overgrowth. Recent data suggest that the distinction between uterine carcinosarcoma and adenosarcoma with high-grade sarcomatous overgrowth may be moot, given the observed equivalent poor prognosis[19].

Sarcoma entrapping benign glands

In adenosarcoma, the glands are typically scattered throughout the tumor and they are large, irregular, and cystic in contour with stromal cuffing. Often, they feature papillations and various types of metaplastic epithelium. In contrast, glands that are entrapped by a sarcomatous

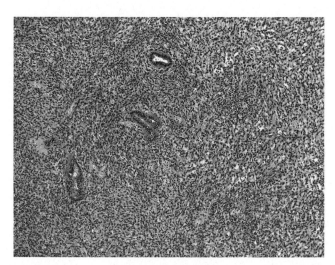

Figure 11.19 Sarcoma entrapping benign glands.

proliferation are typically small and inconspicuous or form focal aggregates of residual glands surrounded by sarcoma (Figure 11.19). This pattern can be observed with endometrial stromal sarcoma, undifferentiated endometrial sarcoma, and high-grade endocervical sarcoma, as well as in a variety of other pure sarcomas (see discussion in Chapter 14). Obviously, adenosarcomas with stromal overgrowth may also entrap benign glands in the areas of stromal overgrowth. The key to the diagnosis is the presence elsewhere of typical adenosarcoma.

Endometrial stromal sarcoma with glandular elements

Adenosarcoma may exhibit overlapping histologic features with that of endometrial stromal sarcoma with prominent

(A)

(B)

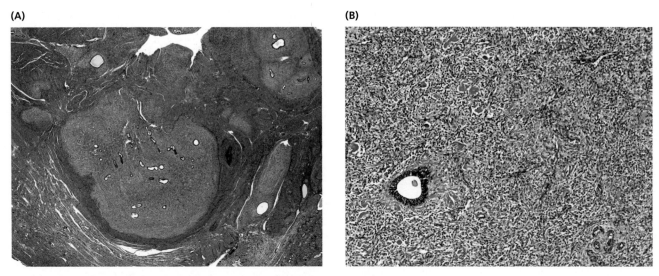

Figure 11.20 (A, B) Low-grade endometrial stromal sarcoma with benign glands.

(A)

(B)

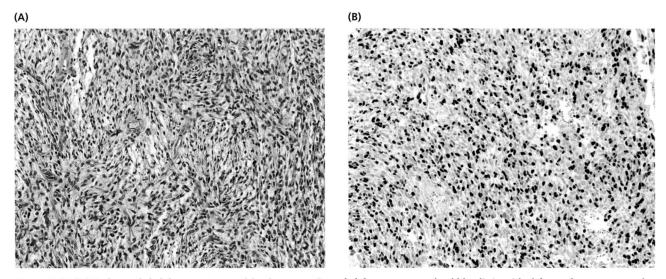

Figure 11.21 (A) Embryonal rhabdomyosarcoma arising in corpus. Pure rhabdomyosarcoma should be distinguished from adenosarcoma and carcinosarcoma, both of which are more common in the uterus. (B) Myogenin confirms the diagnosis.

glandular elements (Figure 11.20). Over a certain range of appearances there is no sharp distinction between the two, but features favoring adenosarcoma include dilated, irregularly shaped glands with intraluminal polypoid protrusions, a variety of mullerian epithelial types, and the characteristic periglandular stromal condensation.

If epithelium is present in endometrial stromal sarcoma, it usually takes the form of poorly circumscribed, but regularly contoured small tubular glands or cords of epithelial-like cells. The epithelial type in stromal sarcoma is almost always endometrioid, while a variety of epithelial types with mucinous, squamous, and syncytial metaplasia are often present in adenosarcoma. The stroma in endometrial stromal sarcoma is also more monomorphous and

does not exhibit the periglandular condensation around glands that is so characteristic of adenosarcoma. Sex cord elements may be seen in both.

Embryonal rhabdomyosarcoma

Although most uterine adenosarcomas arise in the uterine corpus, occasional tumors arise in the cervix. When they occur in the cervix of postmenarchal teenagers they often pose a clinical differential diagnosis of embryonal rhabdomyosarcoma (sarcoma botryoides) (Figure 11.21). This differential diagnosis may continue at the macroscopic level, since a botryoides appearance has been reported in some cases of cervical adenosarcoma. Furthermore, when these cervical adenosarcomas feature microscopic rhabdomyosarcomatous differentiation, they can be especially difficult to distinguish from embryonal rhabdomyosarcoma. Since the treatment and prognosis of cervical embryonal rhabdomyosarcomas may differ substantially from that of an adenosarcoma, the diagnosis of adenosarcoma in this setting should be made with caution and only after complete histologic evaluation. Embryonal rhabdomyosarcoma usually occurs in a younger premenarchal age group as opposed to the postmenarchal age group.

REFERENCES

1. Young RH, Clement PB. Malignant lesions of the female genital tract and peritoneum that may be underdiagnosed. *Semin Diagn Pathol* 1995;**12**:14–29.

2. Clement PB, Oliva E, Young RH. Mullerian adenosarcoma of the uterine corpus associated with tamoxifen therapy: a report of six cases and a review of tamoxifen-associated endometrial lesions. *Int J Gynecol Pathol* 1996;**15**:222–9.

3. Clement P, Scully R. Mullerian adenosarcoma of the uterus: a clinicopathologic analysis of 100 cases with a review of the literature. *Hum Pathol* 1990;**21**:363–81.

4. Murugasu A, Miller J, Proietto A, *et al.* Extragenital mullerian adenosarcoma with sarcomatous overgrowth arising in an endometriotic cyst in the pouch of Douglas. *Int J Gynecol Cancer* 2003;**13**:371–5.

5. Seidman JD, Chauhan S. Evaluation of the relationship between adenosarcoma and carcinosarcoma and a hypothesis of the histogenesis of uterine sarcomas. *Int J Gynecol Pathol* 2003;**22**:75–82.

6. Zaloudek CJ, Norris HJ. Adenofibroma and adenosarcoma of the uterus: a clinicopathologic study of 35 cases. *Cancer* 1981;**48**:354–66.

7. Tackin S, Bozaci EA, Sonmezer M, *et al.* Late recurrence of uterine mullerian adenosarcoma as heterologous sarcoma: three recurrences in 8 months increasing in number and grade of sarcomatous components. *Gynecol Oncol* 2006;**101**:179–82.

8. Soslow RA, Ali A, Oliva E. Mullerian adenosarcomas: an immunophenotypic analysis of 35 cases. *Am J Surg Pathol* 2008;**32**:1013–21.

9. Chen Z, Hong B, Drozd-Borysiuk E, *et al.* Molecular cytogenetic characterization of a case of mullerian adenosarcoma. *Cancer Genet Cytogenet* 2004;**148**:129–32.

10. Clement P, Scully R. Mullerian adenofibroma of the uterus with invasion of myometrium and pelvic veins. *Int J Gynecol Pathol* 1990;**9**:363–71.

11. Czernobilsky B, Hohlweg-Majert P, Dallenbach-Hellweg G. Uterine adenosarcoma: a clinicopathologic study of 11 cases with a re-evaluation of histologic criteria. *Arch Gynecol* 1983;**233**:281–94.

12. Tai LH, Tavassoli FA. Endometrial polyps with atypical (bizarre) stromal cells. *Am J Surg Pathol* 2002;**26**:505–9.

13. Gilks CB, Clement PB, Hart WR, *et al.* Uterine adenomyomas excluding atypical polypoid adenomyomas and adenomyomas of endocervical type: a clinicopathologic study of 30 cases of an underemphasized lesion that may cause diagnostic problems with brief consideration of adenomyomas of other female genital tract sites. *Int J Gynecol Pathol* 2000;**19**:195–205.

14. Longacre TA, Chung MH, Rouse RV, *et al.* Atypical polypoid adenomyofibromas (atypical polypoid adenomyomas) of the uterus. A clinicopathologic study of 55 cases. *Am J Surg Pathol* 1996;**20**:1–20.

15. Mazur M. Atypical polypoid adenomyomas of the endometrium. *Am J Surg Pathol* 1981;**5**:473–82.

16. Young R, Treger T, Scully R. Atypical polypoid adenomyoma of the uterus. A report of 27 cases. *Am J Clin Pathol* 1986;**86**:139–45.

17. Gilks CB, Young RH, Clement PB, *et al.* Adenomyomas of the uterine cervix of endocervical type: a report of ten cases of a benign cervical tumor that may be confused with adenoma malignum [corrected]. *Mod Pathol* 1996;**9**:220–4.

18. Parker RL, Dadmanesh F, Young RH, *et al.* Polypoid endometriosis: a clinicopathologic analysis of 24 cases and a review of the literature. *Am J Surg Pathol* 2004;**28**:285–97.

19. Krivak TC, Seidman JD, McBroom JW, *et al.* Uterine adenosarcoma with sarcomatous overgrowth versus uterine carcinosarcoma: comparison of treatment and survival. *Gynecol Oncol* 2001;**83**:89–94.

12 UTERINE SMOOTH MUSCLE TUMORS

INTRODUCTION

Uterine leiomyomas are the most common mesenchymal tumor in the female genital tract; the vast majority are easily diagnosed. Most uterine leiomyosarcomas, although much less common, are also readily diagnosed. Diagnostic problems arise when uterine mesenchymal tumors exhibit (1) altered or non-standard forms of smooth muscle differentiation (myxoid, epithelioid, etc.), (2) variant or ambiguous histologic features (e.g., increased cellularity, cytologic atypia, increased mitotic figures, or necrosis), (3) a mixture of smooth muscle and stromal differentiation, or (4) unusual anatomic distribution.

The diagnosis of uterine smooth muscle tumors depends on: the degree of experience with that entity (i.e., uterine leiomyomas are very common and, therefore, histologic criteria are well defined and well recognized for the vast majority of these tumors); the extent to which the specimen under evaluation is representative of the entire tumor (a particular issue with uterine samplings and myomectomy specimens); and the extent to which the tumor exhibits non-ambiguous morphologic or anatomical distributional features. Uterine smooth muscle tumors that are rarely encountered and therefore have less reported clinical follow-up data are often more correctly referred to as "with limited experience," while those that defy classification using standard criteria are more appropriately labeled as "uncertain malignant potential." Most uterine tumors of "uncertain malignant potential" may prove, over time and accumulated experience, to have low recurring potential (recurrences to local pelvic or intra-abdominal sites) or low malignant potential (delayed metastases to lung, bone, etc., with prolonged clinical course following excision of the metastases – i.e., low-grade leiomyosarcoma), in which case one or the other of these terms would be the more appropriate designation.

LEIOMYOMA

The conventional (usual) leiomyoma is the most common tumor to occur in the uterus, involving up to 75% of hysterectomy specimens. Often, more than one leiomyoma is present in any given patient. There are no well-defined predisposing factors (other than hereditary leiomyomatosis), but an increased incidence is observed in African-American women.

Clinical characteristics

Leiomyomas tend to occur in the fourth and fifth decade. Clinical manifestations depend on size, secondary changes such as infarction, and location. The most common symptoms are pain, abnormal vaginal bleeding, and a pelvic mass. Rarely, patients present with erythrocytosis, clinical features similar to Meig's syndrome, or fever and leukocytosis due to secondary infection of the leiomyoma. Most patients with leiomyomas are asymptomatic.

Leiomyomas are benign. Rare instances of leiomyosarcomas apparently arising in or adjacent to a leiomyoma have been reported (see below), but this is exceedingly uncommon.

Morphology

Gross pathology

The typical leiomyoma is a well-circumscribed, firm, pale tan or white intramyometrial, submucosal, or subserosal nodule that bulges from the surrounding myometrium on cut section (Figure 12.1). A polypoid configuration is also seen, particularly in the submucosal tumors. Leiomyomas exhibit a broad spectrum of sizes ranging from <1.0 cm to >10.0 cm, with the majority falling between 5 and 10 cm. Multiple leiomyomas are common.

The usual leiomyoma has a tan–white whorled appearance, whereas more cellular and/or mitotically active

(A)

(B)

(C)

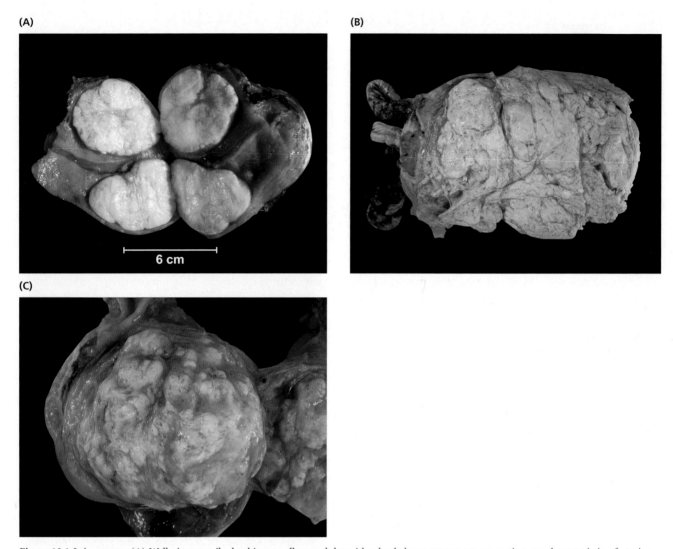

Figure 12.1 Leiomyoma. (A) Well-circumscribed, white or yellow nodules with whorled appearance on cut section are characteristic of uterine leiomyomas. (B) Degenerative change in leiomyoma. (C) Necrosis in infarcted leiomyoma.

variants may be tan or pale yellow, with a more fleshy consistency. Foci of central hemorrhage, cystic degeneration, yellow softening, calcification, or, rarely, ossification may be seen; these changes are attributed to ischemia, degeneration, and senescence (Figure 12.1). Leiomyomas with hydropic change exude a pale, watery or slightly mucoid fluid on cut section. In pregnant and postmenopausal women, leiomyomas may become secondarily infected with resultant abscess formation (so called pyomyoma).

The *cotyledonoid* variant of smooth muscle tumor has a very distinctive sinuous growth pattern that imparts an exophytic placenta-like appearance ("Sternberg tumor"). Cotyledonoid dissecting leiomomyas often bulge from the serosal surface (Figure 12.2), but may be confined to the uterus and "pop out" on cut section (see below).

Microscopic pathology

The usual leiomyoma exhibits the histologic features of conventional smooth muscle cells. Elongated spindle cells with eosinophilic cytoplasm are arranged in fascicles, often with variable amounts of intercellular collagen (Figure 12.3). Epithelioid cells may be present, but do not usually comprise more than 50% of the tumor in the usual leiomyoma. Cytologic atypia is minimal or absent, and mitotic figures are few or, when increased, are often confined to regions of infarction or ulceration. Most are well circumscribed, but an irregular interface with the surrounding myometrium may occur and is not a sign of malignancy. Foci of infarction with hyaline necrosis, dystrophic calcification, or acellular fibrosis can be seen in many leiomyomas (Figure 12.4). Necrosis secondary to infarction (so-called hyaline necrosis) exhibits

(A)   **(B)**

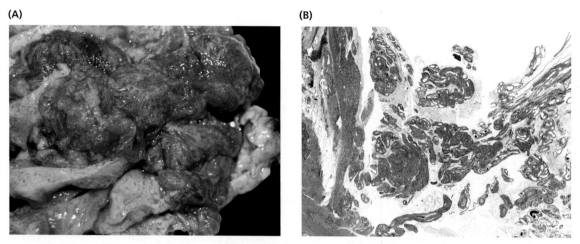

Figure 12.2 (A) Cotyledonoid leiomyoma ("Sternberg tumor") resembles placenta extruding from the myometrium.
(B) Cotyledonoid leiomyoma forms nodular aggregates of smooth muscle that extrude into cystic cavity.

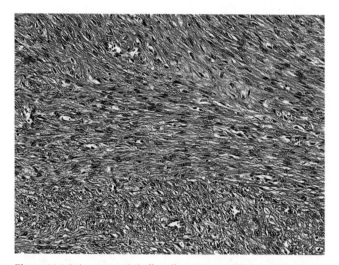

Figure 12.3 Leiomyoma. Spindle cells are arranged in elongate
fascicles. The cytoplasm is eosinophilic and the nuclei are blunt ended.
Mitotic figures are absent in this example, but may be present,
particularly in areas near infarction.

a characteristic zonation effect due to the presence of a
layer of organizing fibrosis and/or granulation tissue separating the necrotic lesional cells from the surrounding
viable cells (Figure 12.4). Often, only ghost outlines of the
necrotic lesional cells, blood vessels, and supporting
stroma are visualized in the necrotic zone. Residual
islands of preserved, viable tumor cells are typically
absent[1]. Necrosis secondary to ulceration of a mucosal
leiomyoma may additionally contain numerous inflammatory cells within the fibrotic zone, but true abscess
formation is not seen unless the leiomyoma is secondarily
infected.

A variety of changes have been attributed to treatment
with gonadotropin-releasing hormone, including fibrinoid
degeneration of vessel walls, decreased vessel number,

(A)

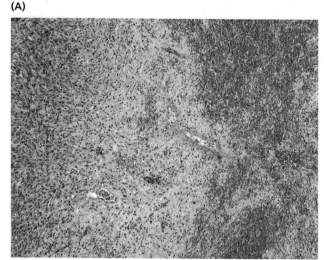

(B)

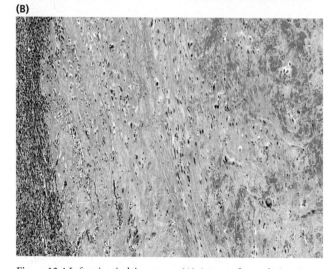

Figure 12.4 Infarction in leiomyoma. (A) A zone of granulation tissue
separates the central necrotic and hemorrhagic tissue from the
surrounding viable smooth muscle. (B) In this example, a zone of
hyalinized fibrous tissue separates the central necrotic and
hemorrhagic tissue from the surrounding viable smooth muscle.

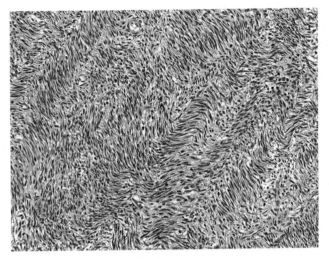

Figure 12.5 Neurilemmoma-like leiomyoma.

decreased vessel size, focal hypercellularity, hyalinization, lymphocytic infiltrate, and decreased cellular proliferation, but the specificity of these changes is untested[2].

Patients treated by prior embolectomy may harbor intravascular or extravascular material in the surrounding myometrial vessels. Hyaline necrosis, suppurative necrosis, and early ischemic necrosis may be seen in the embolized leiomyomas[2].

A variety of other interesting and unusual patterns and/or secondary changes may be seen in uterine leiomyomas with conventional histology (Figures 12.5–12.8), most of which have no bearing on prognosis (Table 12.1). The more commonly encountered and/or clinically relevant variant patterns are discussed further below.

(A)   **(B)**

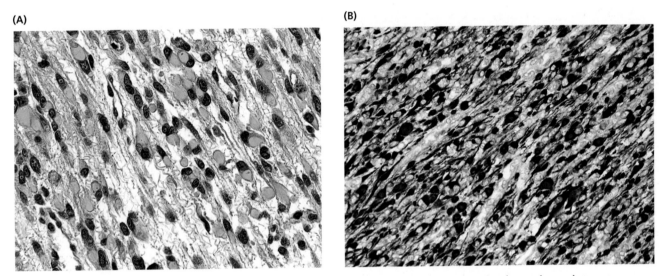

Figure 12.6 (A) Rhabdoid-like cells with globular eosinophilic cytoplasmic inclusions in otherwise conventional smooth muscle tumor. (B) Desmin highlights the rhabdoid-like cells. These cells may occur in benign and malignant uterine smooth muscle tumors.

(A)   **(B)**

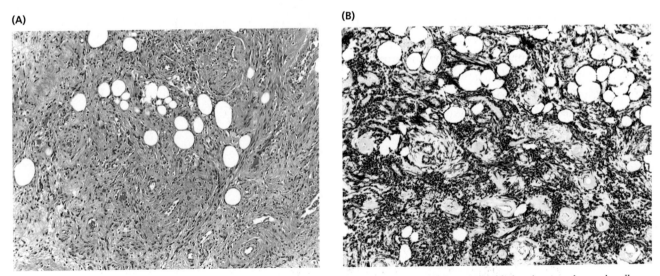

Figure 12.7 Lipoleiomyoma. (A) Mature fat is present in otherwise conventional leiomyoma. (B) Desmin highlights the smooth muscle cells.

Figure 12.8 Leiomyoma with osteoid-like matrix.

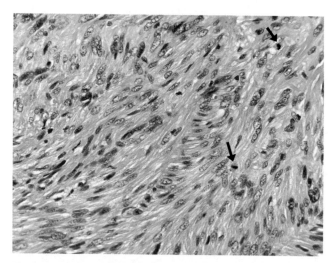

Figure 12.9 Mitotically active (see arrows) leiomyoma.

Table 12.1 Unusual patterns in uterine smooth muscle tumors[2]

Histologic feature	Descriptive term
Mature fat[3]	Lipoleiomyoma
Brown fat[4]	Leiomyohibernoma
Nuclear palisading	Neurilemmoma-like leiomyoma
Acellular fibrosis	Hyalinized leiomyoma
Edema	Hydropic leiomyoma
Highly vascularized[5]	Angioleiomyoma
Extensive hemorrhage[6]	Apoplectic leiomyoma
Plexiform pattern	Plexiform leiomyoma
Skeletal muscle-like and rhabdoid-like cells[7]	Leiomyoma or leiomyosarcoma (may be epithelioid) with rhabdoid-like cells
Clear cells	Leiomyoma or leiomyosarcoma (may be epithelioid) with clear cells
Inclusion bodies[8]	Leiomyoma, epithelioid or myxoid, rarely leiomyosarcoma with inclusion bodies
Calcification	Leiomyoma with dystrophic calcification
Mature bone or cartilage	Leiomyoma with osseous or cartilaginous metaplasia
Massive inflammatory infiltrate	Leiomyoma with inflammatory cell infiltrate
Massive lymphoid infiltrate[9]	Leiomyoma with massive lymphoid infiltrate
Massive histiocytic (xanthomatous) infiltrate	Leiomyoma or leiomyosarcoma with histiocytic (xanthomatous) infiltrate
Massive eosinophilic infiltrate	Leiomyoma with eosinophilic infiltrate
Massive mast cell infiltrate	Leiomyoma with mast cell infiltrate
Abscess	Pyomyoma (suppurative leiomyoma)
Osteoclast-like giant cells	Leiomyoma or leiomyosarcoma with osteoclast-like giant cells

Cotyledonoid dissecting leiomyoma ("Sternberg tumor")

The *cotyledonoid dissecting* leiomyoma is quite uncommon, but often mistaken for intravenous leiomyomatosis or diffuse leiomyomatosis because of its unusual growth pattern; it is composed of multiple nodules of vascularized benign smooth muscle with a swirling growth pattern (as opposed to a fascicular pattern), set in a hydropic or edematous paucicellular matrix (Figure 12.2)[10]. The cotylenoid leiomyoma is benign.

Mitotically active leiomyoma

It has become apparent that mitotic indices as high as 20 MF/10 HPF may be encountered in clinically benign smooth muscle neoplasms, provided there is no significant nuclear atypia and/or tumor cell necrosis[1,2]. Most of these mitotically active leiomyomas exhibit conventional smooth muscle morphology with variable degrees of hypercellularity (Figure 12.9). By definition, mitotic figures are increased to at least 5 MF/10 HPF, but higher counts are not uncommon in these tumors, and in occasional tumors the mitotic count exceeds 20 MF/10 HPF[1]. Atypical mitotic figures are absent. The distribution of the mitotic figures varies; in most cases, they are scattered throughout the tumor, but in some cases, they are concentrated to several distinct foci and appear to form proliferation centers.

Cellularity varies in mitotically active tumors; marked hypercellularity may be present. Uterine smooth muscle tumors exhibiting such features are designated mitotically active leiomyoma or cellular mitotically active leiomyoma, depending on the degree of cellularity.

Mitotically active leiomyoma is benign. When encountered in a myomectomy specimen, it can be treated in a conservative fashion if it has been adequately sampled and is thought to be representative of the uterine mass on clinical or imaging studies. What counts as "adequate sampling" of a myomectomy specimen is seldom addressed in the literature; in absence of evidence to the contrary, we recommend the one section per centimeter rule be applied unless the tumor exhibits any unusual clinical, macroscopic, or microscopic findings. In the presence of unusual features (particularly necrosis, increased numbers of mitotic figures, cellular atypia, and possible infiltrative margins), additional sections should be sufficient to establish a definitive diagnosis of leiomyoma or leiomyosarcoma; if there is any uncertainty, the entire lesion should be evaluated before rendering a diagnosis of smooth muscle tumor of uncertain malignant potential (STUMP; see below). Histologically similar tumors with mitotic indices that exceed 20 MF/10 HPF are also considered clinically benign, but since collective experience is more limited with this type of tumor, a comment should accompany the diagnosis indicating that there is less experience with this type of tumor and the patient should receive continued clinical follow-up[1].

Atypical leiomyoma (symplastic leiomyoma, leiomyoma with bizarre nuclei)

Atypical leiomyomas are morphologically striking tumors due to the presence of numerous bizarre and atypical, often multinucleated cells. These tumors have alternatively been referred to by the terms "bizarre" and "symplastic" leiomyomas, owing to their conspicuous nuclear atypia. Although there is considerable evidence that supports their innocuous behavior, atypical leiomyomas continue to pose diagnostic concern because of their histologic similarity to leiomyosarcoma.

Atypical leiomyoma is defined by the presence of moderate to severe cytologic atypia in the absence of significant mitotic activity or tumor cell necrosis (Figure 12.10). The atypia in atypical leiomyoma consists of nuclear hyperchromasia with marked nuclear pleomorphism, irregular nuclear membranes, and abnormal nucleoli. Multinucleate cells reminiscent of osteoclasts may be encountered. Rarely, extremely bizarre chromatin abnormalities can resemble atypical mitotic figures in atypical leiomyomas (Figure 12.11); in the absence of an increased background mitotic activity, this finding should not raise concern for a more aggressive neoplasm. The degree of atypia present

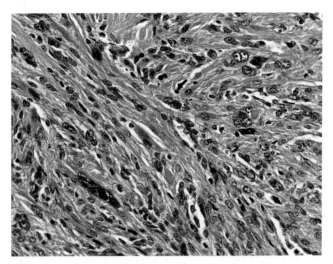

Figure 12.10 Atypical leiomyoma is characterized by markedly atypical cells, often with monstrous nuclei. Tumor cell necrosis is absent and mitotic figures are either absent or only focally increased in most cases.

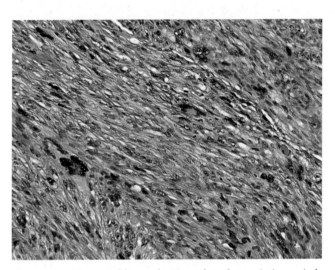

Figure 12.11 Bizarre and karyorrhectic nuclear chromatin in atypical leiomyoma may simulate atypical mitotic figures.

in these tumors is reminiscent of that seen in atypical fibroxanthoma. In most cases, the mitotic count is less than 4 MF/10 HPF; focal increased mitotic counts may be seen in some tumors, but they should not exceed 10 MF/10 HPF[1]. Atypical leiomyomas have been subdivided based on the distribution of atypia throughout the neoplasm. Tumors with "focal atypia" are defined as those with only patches of atypical cells set in a background of otherwise bland smooth muscle cells; while those with "diffuse atypia" demonstrate widespread pleomorphism[1]. In the Bell et al. study[1], leiomyomas with focal atypia and a mitotic index of ≤10 MF/10 HPF were classified as "leiomyoma with atypia, but limited experience." We currently classify both groups of tumors (with focal or

(A)

(B)

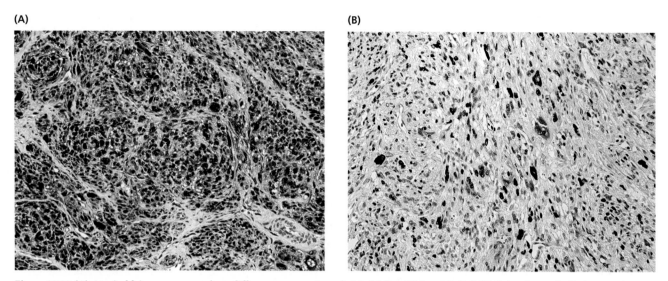

Figure 12.12 (A) Atypical leiomyoma may show diffuse overexpression of p16. (B) In addition, Ki-67 (MIB1) may be markedly increased.

(A)

(B)

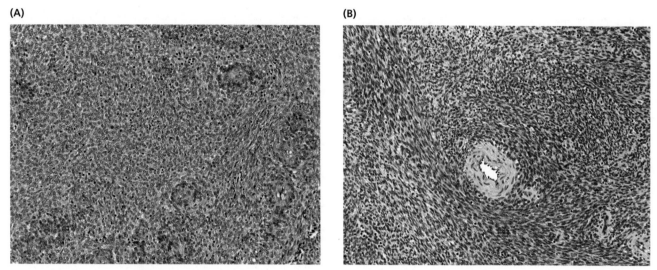

Figure 12.13 Cellular leiomyoma. (A) This highly cellular tumor is composed of a dense proliferation of spindle cells in a vague fascicular pattern. (B) A thick-walled blood vessel is present.

diffuse cytologic atypia) as "atypical leiomyoma," based on recent additional follow-up data[11].

Despite the disturbing cytology, current evidence supports a benign course for the vast majority of these neoplasms; rare patients have had intrauterine recurrence following myomectomy and several have had local recurrence following hysterectomy. Given this data, at present the most practical treatment approach to classic atypical leiomyomas remains complete removal to facilitate full evaluation of the lesion and limit the chance of recurrence. Hysterectomy is appropriate treatment for women for whom parity is not an issue, but myomectomy with close clinical follow-up is an acceptable alternative, especially for patients who prefer to maintain fertility. Several patients so treated have had successful pregnancies with no evidence of local recurrence.

A variety of cell markers have been employed to help differentiate atypical leiomyoma from leiomyosarcoma, but these should always be interpreted with caution as atypical leiomyomas may strongly express p16, and there may be a high Ki-67 labeling index in these tumors (Figure 12.12).

Cellular (hypercellular) leiomyoma

Microscopically, cellular leiomyomas are almost entirely composed of closely spaced cells that have lost much of their characteristic eosinophilic, fibrillary cytoplasm (Figure 12.13); because of their marked cellularity they may be mistaken for endometrial stromal tumors

(A)

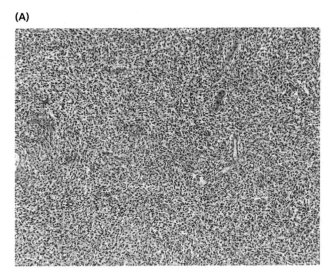

(B)

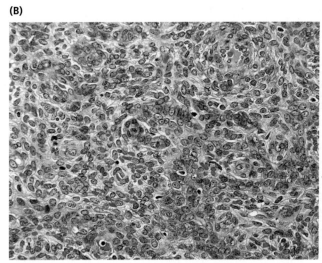

Figure 12.14 Low-grade endometrial stromal neoplasm. (A) The cells form whorls around small arterioles, which may be inconspicuous or hyalinized. (B) Endometrial stromal cells are stubbier than smooth muscle cells and have oval to fusiform nuclei (compare with Figure 12.13).

(Figure 12.14). In some instances, the mitotic index is increased (= mitotically active cellular leiomyoma), but there should be no atypical mitotic figures, and cytologic atypia is minimal or absent. Tumor cell necrosis is absent. Cellular leiomyomas are benign and can be adequately treated by myomectomy, provided they have been adequately sampled.

Diffuse leiomyomatosis

Diffuse, symmetrical enlargement of the uterus by numerous, often cellular, confluent leiomyomatous mural nodules is classified as diffuse leiomyomatosis. This is a rare condition. Since intravenous leiomyomatosis may impart a similar morphologic appearance, any uterus suspected of harboring a diffuse leiomyomatous proliferation should be carefully examined grossly and microscopically for the presence of intravascular involvement.

Hydropic leiomyoma

In some leiomyomas, hydropic, edematous, or myxoid change can be so extensive that it is difficult to discern the underlying smooth muscle elements. The extensive hydropic change results in replacement of most of the smooth muscle elements by pale-staining, very paucicellular fibrous tissue. Unlike myxoid leiomyoma, the intercellular matrix in hydropic leiomyoma is edema fluid and does not stain positively on colloidal iron or alcian blue stains. The classic microscopic appearance of perinodular hydropic degeneration is that of large-caliber vessels suspended in hydropic or myxomatous areas (Figure 12.15)[12]. Often, foci of collagenization are also present. These relatively common hydropic

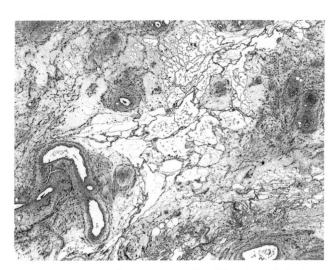

Figure 12.15 Hydropic leiomyoma. Small nodules of vascularized smooth muscle are suspended in an edematous, pale-staining matrix.

leiomyomas are important only in so far as they may simulate the much rarer myxoid leiomyosarcoma.

Myxoid leiomyoma

True myxoid leiomyomas are uncommon. They are characterized by spindled and, often, stellate cells separated by abundant, weakly basophilic material that is positive on colloidal iron or alcian blue stains (Figure 12.16). However, the true margins of a myxoid leiomyoma are circumscribed, and cytologic atypia and necrosis are absent. Myxoid leiomyoma may be more frequently encountered during pregnancy.

Small foci of myxoid change can be seen in leiomyomas that otherwise exhibit usual spindle cell morphology. When myxoid degeneration is focal it may interdigitate with the

(A)

(B)

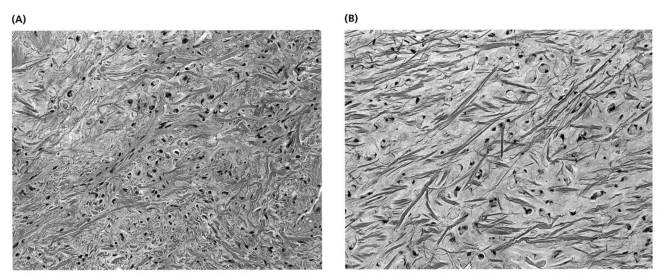

Figure 12.16 (A) Myxoid leiomyoma. (B) Myxoid degeneration in leiomyoma. Spindle cells in this leiomyoma are pushed aside by basophilic mucoid material containing stellate cells with minimal cytoplasm. Note the absence of cytologic atypia.

(A)

(B)

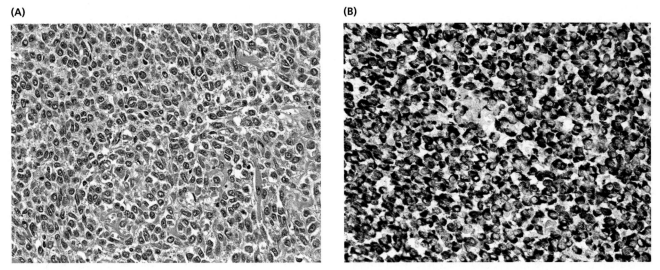

Figure 12.17 Epithelioid smooth muscle tumor. (A) The cells have rounded contours with eosinophilic, slightly granular cytoplasm. (B) Desmin expression is strong in this example, but not all epithelioid smooth muscle tumors will express desmin to this extent.

constituent usual smooth muscle cells of an otherwise conventional leiomyoma, simulating invasion. In these situations, contextual clues (adjacent ischemic infarction, banal features, etc.) and, if necessary, additional sampling almost always resolve diagnostic problems. We generally and somewhat arbitrarily reserve the diagnosis of myxoid leiomyoma only for those tumors that are predominantly or extensively myxoid.

Epithelioid leiomyoma

These tumors are predominantly or entirely composed of ovoid or rounded polygonal cells with eosinophilic, granular, or clear cytoplasm (Figure 12.17)[13]. The cells are distributed in sheets, nests, or cords, and may form a plexiform pattern. In most cases, the nuclei are centrally placed, small,

and regular (Figure 12.17); rarely, osteoclast-like cells or large, bizarre cells similar to those in atypical leiomyoma may be present. Mitotic figures are rare, and tumor cell necrosis is absent. Epithelioid foci are not uncommon in leiomyomas that otherwise exhibit usual spindle cell morphology. As with myxoid leiomyomas, we reserve the diagnosis of epithelioid leiomyoma only for those tumors that are predominantly or extensively epithelioid.

Ancillary diagnostic tests

Uterine smooth muscle cells express desmin, h-caldesmon, smooth muscle actin, and occasionally, CD10. When CD10 expression is present in a uterine smooth muscle tumor exhibiting usual morphology, it is usually weaker and less extensive than the smooth muscle markers, but on occasion the CD10 expression may be as strong and diffuse as desmin expression; in these cases, the classification of the smooth muscle tumor should not be altered unless the tumor exhibits an unusual pattern of differentiation (increased cellularity, possible stromal elements, etc.). Cytokeratin and EMA expression is often seen in uterine smooth muscle tumors. Almost all benign and low-grade smooth muscle neoplasms in the uterine corpus and elsewhere in the female genital tract express hormone receptors (estrogen receptor and progesterone receptor). Uterine smooth muscle tumors with usual and epithelioid morphology may also express HMB45; a subset of these latter tumors has been classified as uterine perivascular epithelioid cell tumors (PEComas) – although this is a subject of ongoing controversy (see *Perivascular epithelioid cell tumor*, below).

Differential diagnosis

The diagnosis of usual leiomyoma is straightforward and generally poses no difficulty. Leiomyomas with secondary changes, increased mitotic activity, hypercellularity, or variant histology (epithelioid or myxoid) can pose significant differential diagnostic problems, especially in limited samplings or myomectomy specimens[14,15]. When these latter changes occur, the key differential diagnoses are leiomyosarcoma, endometrial stromal tumor (nodule or sarcoma), primary or metastatic carcinoma, perivascular epithelioid cell tumor, uterine tumor resembling ovarian sex cord tumor (UTROSCT), and placental site trophoblastic tumor (PSTT). Each of these entities is discussed in the relevant sections below.

Leiomyosarcoma, usual type

In addition to severe cytologic atypia, leiomyosarcoma has an increased mitotic index (frequently >20 MF/10 HPF) and tumor cell necrosis (see *Leiomyosarcoma*, page 230). The presence of severe atypia, and/or any tumor cell necrosis, and/or mitotic index >10 MF/10 HPF are diagnostic of leiomyosarcoma. However, due to the pyknotic and karyorrhectic debris that is present, the mitotic index can be difficult to assess in some cases.

To resolve this problem there has been interest in the use of cell cycle markers to predict those tumors that are likely to recur or behave in a clinically aggressive fashion[16,17]. However, recent work on the expression of cell cycle markers in atypical leiomyoma has failed to show a clear relationship between recurrence and increased cell cycle marker expression by immunohistochemistry[2]. Clinically benign atypical leiomyoma (classic "symplastic leiomyoma") may exhibit a high Ki-67 index or express strong p16; neither marker is useful in distinguishing atypical leiomyoma from leiomyosarcoma (Figure 12.12). We recommend caution in interpreting these stains.

Endometrial stromal neoplasm, either nodule or sarcoma

Endometrial stromal tumors may resemble cellular and epithelioid leiomyomas and vice versa. Prolapsed leiomyomas may be particularly prone to demonstrate small foci of hypercellular stroma mimicking endometrial stromal differentiation. If the mesenchymal tumor is well circumscribed, the differential diagnosis is stromal nodule versus cellular leiomyoma; since both are benign, there is little at stake. If the tumor is not well circumscribed, the possibility of a low-grade endometrial stromal sarcoma must be excluded, since the latter entity is associated with extension beyond the uterus and disease recurrence. Endometrial stromal sarcomas have thin-walled arching vessels, a diffuse growth pattern, and shorter, stubbier cells (Figure 12.14). In contrast, smooth muscle tumors have thick-walled blood vessels within the tumor, a fascicular growth pattern, cleft-like spaces, and more elongate, spindle-shaped cells. Endometrial stromal tumors express CD10, but not h-caldesmon, while smooth muscle tumors express desmin and/or h-caldesmon[18,19]. However, since smooth muscle tumors may also express CD10, a panel of markers consisting of CD10, desmin, and h-caldesmon is most useful in confirming smooth muscle differentiation. Strong desmin or h-caldesmon staining with weak or absent CD10 favors a smooth muscle tumor; whereas strong CD10 staining and weak or absent desmin and h-caldesmon staining provides support for endometrial stromal differentiation[18,19]. Caution should be exercised when relying on expression of smooth muscle markers in epithelioid smooth muscle tumors, since this group of tumors may show keratin expression with weak or absent expression for desmin and h-caldesmon.

Hypercellular myometrium

Hypercellular myometrium may mimic a cellular leiomyoma, but there is no discrete mass, and the region of hypercellularity often merges imperceptibly with surrounding myometrium. Hypercellular foci may occur in the superficial myometrium and simulate a cellular leiomyoma in uterine sampling specimens. It has been suggested that uterine leiomyomas may arise from these hypercellular zones[20]. Should this pose a clinical or diagnostic problem, correlation with imaging studies can be useful.

Intravenous leiomyomatosis

The prominent nodular architecture in nodular hydropic degeneration may simulate intravenous leiomyomatosis on gross examination; absence of an intravascular growth pattern on microscopic examination excludes the latter diagnosis.

Non–smooth muscle, myxoid-appearing mesenchymal lesions

A variety of other myxoid-appearing mesenchymal lesions may mimic leiomyoma with myxoid change; they are all uncommon but include neurilemmoma and neurofibroma, as well as inflammatory myofibroblastic tumor. The first two neoplasms are positive for S100 protein. Inflammatory myofibroblastic tumor contains a characteristic plasma cell infiltrate and a more fascicular or hyalinized pattern. Intrauterine myxoma may rarely occur in association with Carney's complex; expression of smooth muscle markers is absent (see Chapter 14). Additional sectioning will disclose characteristic features of smooth muscle in almost all hydropic and myxoid uterine leiomyomas.

Myxoid leiomyosarcoma

Myxoid leiomyomas are uncommon and should be carefully evaluated for the presence of infiltration, cytologic atypia, or the presence of mitotic figures (see **Myxoid leiomyosarcoma**, page 233).

Superficial cervicovaginal myofibroblastoma

This is an uncommon benign mesenchymal proliferation composed of spindle and stellate-shaped cells separated by a collagenous or myxoid stroma[21]. This lesion is typically small (mean: 2.3 cm), well circumscribed, and spares the surface epithelium by a rim of intervening normal stroma. Because it is immunoreactive for desmin and hormone receptors, it may be mistaken for a smooth muscle tumor on limited sampling. However, unlike conventional leiomyoma, superficial cervicovaginal myofibroblastoma has a patternless arrangement; a fascicular pattern, if present, is minor. Positive staining for CD34 is often present.

Epithelioid plexiform tumorlet

When nests of epithelioid smooth muscle cells are entirely plexiform and small (<1 cm), these tumors are referred to as plexiform tumorlets ($\leq$1 MF/10 HPF)[22]. They may be single or multiple; when multiple they may be mistaken for a stromal tumor or, possibly, a uterine tumor resembling ovarian sex cord tumor (UTROSCT). Some tumorlets may exhibit biphenotypic smooth muscle – stromal differentiation. Tumorlets are benign and almost always incidental findings in a patient who is undergoing evaluation for another unrelated reason (Chapter 14). Therefore, if a uterine sampling is obtained for a suspected uterine mass and the sole finding is a plexiform tumorlet, further evaluation would be indicated.

Undifferentiated carcinoma

Cellular smooth muscle tumors, both benign and malignant, may mimic an undifferentiated carcinoma in an endometrial sampling, especially if the specimen is partially crushed or limited in volume. Since both tumors can express cytokeratin and some undifferentiated endometrial carcinomas may lose keratin (and gain vimentin), the distinction relies on histology and demonstration of the presence of smooth muscle markers – desmin and h-caldesmon.

Metastases

Metastatic lobular carcinoma and melanoma can often be distinguished on the basis of an infiltrative pattern that appears to preserve pre-existing endometrial glands. Diagnosis can be confirmed by demonstration of cytokeratin and EMA in carcinoma and S100 protein and other melanocytic markers in melanoma.

Uterine tumor resembling ovarian sex cord tumor

Uterine tumor resembling ovarian sex cord tumor (UTROSCT) may superficially resemble an epithelioid leiomyoma, but the sex cord elements – cords, trabeculae, hollow tubules, retiform structures, and prominent foam cells – are much more pronounced in UTROSCT, and the smooth muscle cells are often inconspicuous (see Chapter 14)[23]. Diffuse expression for smooth muscle markers desmin and h-caldesmon favors a smooth muscle neoplasm; while coexpression of muscle markers with inhibin and calretinin favors UTROSCT[24,25].

PEComa

Epithelioid uterine smooth muscle tumors that express HMB45 and other melanocytic markers have been designated as perivascular epithelioid cell tumors (PEComas); the relationship between epithelioid leiomyoma, epithelioid leiomyosarcoma, and perivascular epithelioid cell tumor is controversial and is discussed separately (see ***Perivascular epithelioid cell tumor***, below).

LEIOMYOSARCOMA

Uterine leiomyosarcoma is rare, but accounts for the majority of uterine sarcomas. The term leiomyosarcoma is used here to refer to those smooth muscle tumors that exhibit morphologic features that have been shown to correlate with aggressive clinical behavior: that is, systemic metastases (typically lung, liver, brain, etc.), typically within the first five years of diagnosis. Other, less common uterine smooth muscle tumor variants that do not exhibit these morphologic features may on occasion exhibit high stage or recurrent disease, but the clinical course is typically more protracted. The term *low-grade leiomyosarcoma* has been proposed for some of these variants, but data are limited for these types of tumors and this term is currently not considered a standard diagnosis in gynecologic pathology. The recommended approach to these variants is addressed in the following discussion.

An insufficient number of cervical leiomyosarcomas have been studied to develop site-specific criteria similar to those that are in routine use for uterine smooth muscle tumors. Our current approach extrapolates diagnostic criteria from the corpus tumors to predict malignant potential. Since cervical leiomyosarcoma is rare, secondary involvement by uterine corpus leiomyosarcoma arising in the isthmus or lower uterine segment should be excluded. Primary tumors exhibit the same histologic features as those in the uterine corpus.

Clinical characteristics

Most uterine leiomyosarcomas occur after age 40, although they may be seen in younger women. A prior history of pelvic radiation may be present. Presenting symptoms do not differ significantly from leiomyoma. Often, there is a history of rapid growth, although this may be seen with leiomyoma. Rapid growth during treatment with gonadotropin-releasing hormone agonists should be viewed with concern. Approximately one-third of patients present with disease beyond the confines of the uterus.

Uterine leiomyosarcoma is an aggressive tumor and most patients die of disease despite aggressive therapy. Prognosis depends chiefly on stage (Table 12.2). Stage I tumors have the best prognosis. *Am J Surg Pathol.* 2011;**35**(11):1626–37. Tumor

Table 12.2 International Federation of Gynecology and Obstetrics (FIGO) staging for uterine leiomyosarcoma[27]

Stage	Definition
I	Tumor limited to uterus
IA	Tumor ≤ 5 cm
IB	Tumor > 5 cm
II	Tumor extends to the pelvis
IIA	Adnexal involvement
IIB	Tumor extends to extrauterine pelvic tissue
III	Tumor invades abdominal tissues (not just protruding into the abdomen)
IIIA	One site
IIIB	More than one site
IVA	Tumor invades bladder and/or rectum
IVB	Distant metastasis

size, and stage, in addition to other factors, have been found to be prognostically significant in a recent single-institution series of cases. The data indicate that uterine leiomyosarcomas that meet Stanford criteria are high grade sarcomas. Data from the same group also indicate that ER/PR expression in Stage I leiomyosarcoma is prognostically favorable[26]. However, small leiomyosarcomas are very rare, and there are limited outcome data using current diagnostic criteria for these tumors. Recurrences are primarily hematogenous, but local pelvic recurrences are not uncommon. Sites of recurrence include lung, pelvis, and abdomen, liver, brain, bone, and kidney. Most patients develop recurrence within two years of initial diagnosis.

Morphology

Gross pathology

USUAL LEIOMYOSARCOMA
In contrast to the usual leiomyoma, the usual leiomyosarcoma is often single, large, and grossly soft and fleshy, with areas of necrosis and hemorrhage. Most are greater than 5 cm. When present in association with other smooth muscle tumors, it is often the dominant mass.

MYXOID LEIOMYOSARCOMA
Myxoid leiomyosarcoma is a large, gelatinous neoplasm that may appear circumscribed or uncircumscribed on gross examination. Foci of necrosis or hemorrhage may be present.

EPITHELIOID LEIOMYOSARCOMA
These tumors often form large, fleshy intrauterine masses. Hemorrhage is common.

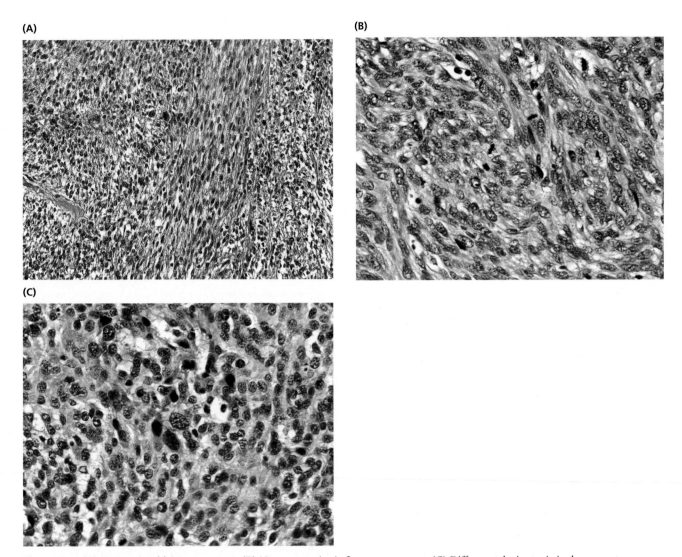

Figure 12.18 (A) Conventional leiomyosarcoma. (B) Numerous mitotic figures are present. (C) Diffuse cytologic atypia is also present.

Microscopic pathology

USUAL LEIOMYOSARCOMA

The usual uterine leiomyosarcoma is composed of hypercellular fascicles of spindle cells possessing abundant eosinophilic cytoplasm with longitudinal cytoplasmic fibrils (Figure 12.18). The nuclei are fusiform, usually have rounded ends, and are hyperchromatic, with coarse chromatin and prominent nucleoli. Cellular pleomorphism is marked in poorly differentiated neoplasms (Figure 12.19). Multinucleated tumor cells are found in 50% of leiomyosarcomas. Osteoclast-like giant cells, xanthomatous change, rhabdoid, or skeletal muscle-like cells with inclusion bodies may also be present[2]. Leiomyosarcomas invade the surrounding myometrium, but a leiomyosarcoma with a circumscribed margin can give rise to metastases. Vascular invasion is identified in 10–20%.

Any two of the following three diagnostic criteria warrant diagnosis of usual leiomyosarcoma: diffuse moderate to marked cytologic atypia; mitotic index $\geq$ 10 MF/10 HPF, and/or tumor cell necrosis[1].

Tumor cell necrosis, as well as infarction necrosis, is often present. Tumor cell necrosis is characterized by abrupt transition of viable tumor cells to necrotic tumor cells, often with ghost outlines and perivascular islands of residual, viable tumor cells (Figure 12.20)[1]. It is important to bear in mind that infarct (hyaline) necrosis may occur in leiomyosarcomas (Figure 12.21), and, on occasion, early infarct (hyaline) necrosis may also show abrupt transition from necrotic tumor cells and viable tumor cells without a characteristic zonation. Therefore, in clinical practice, a diagnosis of leiomyosarcoma should not rest solely on the presence of necrosis. Single apoptotic cells may occur in infarct (hyaline) necrosis and tumor cell necrosis, and are non-specific.

The mitotic index is often in excess of 20 MF/10 HPF. It is important to provide an accurate assessment of the mitotic

(A)

(B)

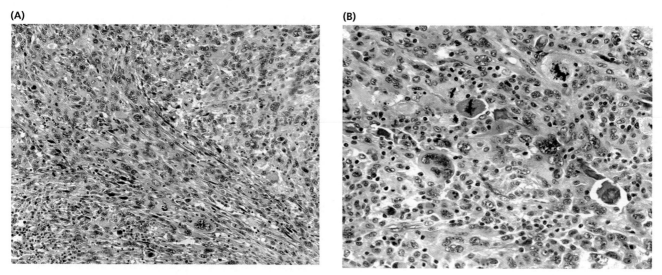

Figure 12.19 Leiomyosarcoma. (A) There is severe cytologic atypia with nuclear pleomorphism that is easily detectable on low magnification. (B) The degree of atypia resembles that seen in atypical leiomyoma (Figure 12.10).

(A)

(B)

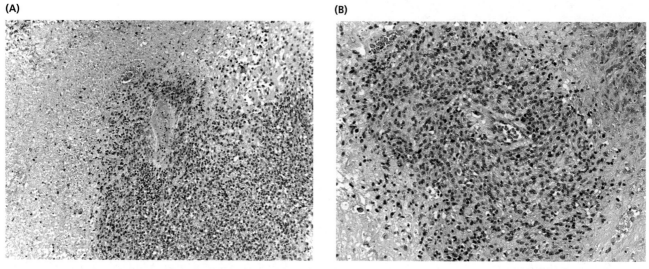

Figure 12.20 Tumor cell necrosis in leiomyosarcoma. (A) Islands of viable tumor surround blood vessels within the zone of necrosis. (B) Abrupt transition from necrotic tumor to viable tumor is present. A similar abrupt transition may also be seen in early ischemic infarcts.

index. Increased mitoses can be seen in smooth muscle tumors immediately adjacent to foci of infarction; this can artificially yield a higher mitotic index. Other areas away from the infarction site should be counted. Poor fixation and thick sections may prevent adequate assessment of mitotic count in smooth muscle tumors. Pyknotic nuclei, infiltrating lymphocytes, and precipitated hematoxylin may mimic mitotic figures. Only those nuclei exhibiting a clearly defined spindle apparatus should be scored. Moreover, bizarre and karyorrhectic nuclei may mimic atypical mitotic figures. This is especially common in atypical leiomyoma (symplastic leiomyoma, leiomyoma with bizarre nuclei) and does not portend a worse prognosis. If a uterine smooth muscle tumor exhibits features that are concerning for leiomyosarcoma on other grounds (e.g.,

moderate to severe atypia or tumor cell necrosis) and the mitotic index is in question, the diagnosis of smooth muscle tumor of uncertain malignant potential should be considered. Ki-67 index is not a substitute for mitotic index in uterine smooth muscle tumors. The use of phospho-histone H3 (pHH3), a specific marker of cells undergoing mitosis, provides a more accurate reflection of mitotic index[2]. Leiomyosarcoma may express p16 in a strong, diffuse pattern, but this is neither sensitive nor specific (Figure 12.22).

In most cases, moderate to severe atypia is recognized by nuclear hyperchromatism and pleomorphism that is visible at low power. However, there are occasional leiomyosarcomas in which the atypia is diffuse and rather uniform from cell to cell; such cases may be overlooked if

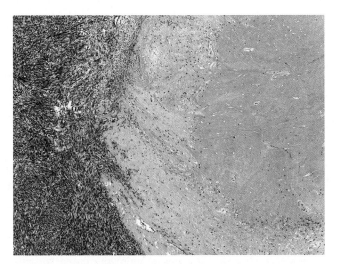

Figure 12.21 Infarction necrosis in leiomyosarcoma. Note zonation phenomenon similar to that depicted in Figure 12.4. The transition is not abrupt as in tumor cell necrosis.

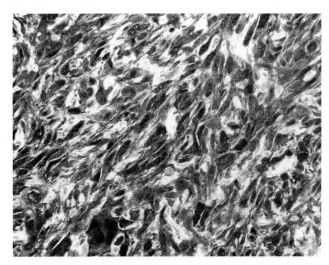

Figure 12.22 Leiomyosarcoma often has diffuse overexpression of p16, but this is neither sensitive nor specific (see Figure 12.12).

(A) **(B)**

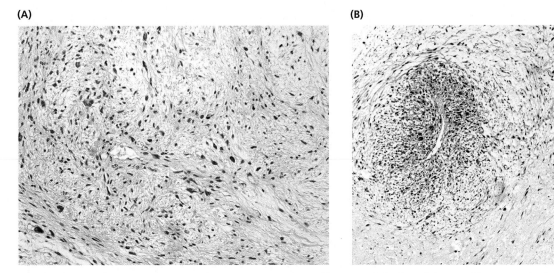

Figure 12.23 Myxoid leiomyosarcoma. (A) Spindle cells are separated by paucicellular, basophilic myxoid stroma. Mitotic figures are often sparse. (B) Stellate cells form cuffs around vessels.

one relies solely on a low-power assessment of variation in nuclear size and shape.

MYXOID LEIOMYOSARCOMA

Myxoid leiomyosarcoma is very rare. The classic microscopic appearance of myxoid leiomyosarcoma consists of small, oval or stellate cells with scant cytoplasm set in abundant, amorphous pale-staining, basophilic extracellular mucoid matrix; tumor cell necrosis is often also present (Figure 12.23). An extensive, well-developed, cellular fascicular pattern is usually absent. This characteristic low cellularity partly accounts for the low mitotic index in most myxoid leiomyosarcomas, although, in some cases, the mitotic index is high. Often, there is a substantial degree of cytologic atypia, at least focally.

The most useful features in diagnosing myxoid leiomyosarcoma, based on data from the Stanford series, are coagulative tumor cell necrosis and mitotic index >2 MF/10 HPF[28]. Since the threshold for mitotic index differs significantly from that of usual leiomyosarcoma, these criteria should only be applied to tumors that exhibit a predominant (50% or more) or exclusive myxoid pattern; uterine smooth muscle tumors with small foci of myxoid change should be evaluated using standard criteria. In the absence of significant cytologic atypia in the myxoid areas, infiltrative margins, vascular invasion, or more pronounced cytologic atypia in non-myxoid areas are additional helpful microscopic features in identifying a predominantly myxoid uterine tumor as a leiomyosarcoma[29]. Myxoid tumors with moderate to severe atypia, a mitotic index of less than

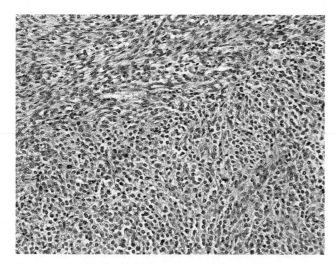

Figure 12.24 Epithelioid leiomyosarcoma. Diffuse atypia is present and there are scattered mitotic figures.

2 MF/10 HPF, and no tumor cell necrosis should be classified as being of uncertain malignant potential, because experience is too limited to be certain about their aggressive potential.

Most myxoid leiomyosarcomas do not resemble smooth muscle tumors or do so only focally; in fact, recent data from our laboratory as well as others indicate that many of these tumors fail to express desmin or other smooth muscle markers except in areas of more usual smooth muscle differentiation; this raises the obvious question of histogenesis and whether or not these tumors are true leiomyosarcoma or some other type of sarcoma. Currently this issue is unresolved, but operationally we continue to employ the diagnosis of leiomyosarcoma for these tumors given the historical use of the term and the circumstantial data that at least a subset of these tumors exhibits foci of unequivocal, smooth muscle differentiation.

EPITHELIOID LEIOMYOSARCOMA

Epithelioid leiomyosarcoma exhibits the pattern of epithelioid differentiation (e.g., round cells with eosinophilic and granular or clear cytoplasm forming nests, cords, or gland-like spaces) in addition to the usual features of malignancy seen in the more conventional leiomyosarcoma[13]. However, epithelioid leiomyosarcomas are often not as mitotically active as usual leiomyosarcoma (Figure 12.24). The nuclei in epithelioid tumors are round or slightly angular, and often occupy the center of the cell. Eccentric nuclei may impart a signet ring appearance.

In the Stanford series, tumor cell necrosis, moderate to severe atypia, and mitotic index >5 MF/10 HPF were most predictive of adverse outcome[30]. Epithelioid tumors with moderate to severe atypia, but without tumor cell necrosis and a mitotic index of less than 5 MF/10 HPF should be classified as being of uncertain malignant potential.

Epithelioid leiomyosarcoma is diagnosed by the combination of diffuse moderate to severe cytologic atypia, 5 MF/10 HPF or more, or tumor cell necrosis. These criteria are applicable only to tumors that exhibit at least 50% epithelioid morphology, as defined above.

Grading leiomyosarcoma

There is no universally accepted grading scheme for uterine leiomyosarcoma. Historically, mitotic index was used as a surrogate for aggressive behavior. However, using current criteria, all uterine leiomyosarcomas are histologically and clinically high-grade sarcomas[26]. Low-grade leiomyosarcomas of the uterus are currently not well defined. Some pathologists diagnose low-grade leiomyosarcoma for any smooth muscle tumor that histologically falls short of leiomyosarcoma but that appears to have recurred or to have spread beyond the uterus. In this scheme, benign metastasizing leiomyoma as well as recurrent smooth muscle tumor of uncertain malignant potential (STUMP) and recurrent atypical leiomyoma (bizarre leiomyoma) are all considered low-grade leiomyosarcoma[26]. However, other pathologists prefer to maintain the smooth muscle tumor of uncertain malignant potential or atypical leiomyoma designation unless on review it is felt the diagnosis is in error. Hovering in the background of these considerations are the additional issues of multicentricity and implantation (see discussion on morcellation below). In our experience, many tumors that pathologists think might be "low-grade leiomyosarcoma" are much more likely to be something else – that is, smooth muscle tumor of uncertain malignant potential, stromal tumor, etc[26]. Therefore, until more data are available, pathologists should refrain from assigning a definitive grade for bona fide uterine leiomyosarcomas, with the understanding that *all* are clinically high grade, based on current criteria. The remaining tumors that exhibit lesser degrees of clinically aggressive, but otherwise uncertain or unpredictable behavior should continue to be designated as separate entities with a comment that addresses an estimate of the likelihood (and expected tempo) for recurrence and/or metastasis; if there is uncertainty, this should also be so stated, preferably with an explicit reason for the uncertainty (see *Smooth muscle tumors of uncertain malignant potential*, below).

Differential diagnosis

The key differential diagnoses for the conventional uterine corpus leiomyosarcoma are atypical leiomyoma and other leiomyoma variants, other high-grade sarcomas (see Chapter 14), including undifferentiated endometrial sarcoma, and epithelial-poor carcinosarcoma or epithelial-poor adenosarcoma. Distinction between atypical leiomyoma, mitotically active leiomyoma, cellular leiomyoma, and other problematic leiomyoma variants is discussed under the appropriate headings.

An observed overexpression of p16, p53, and Ki-67 (MIB1) in leiomyosarcoma compared to leiomyoma and leiomyoma variants has led to the suggestion that these markers may be of utility in diagnosing problematic uterine smooth muscle tumors[16,31]. Although we too have observed significantly higher levels of expression in uterine leiomyosarcoma of the conventional type (Figure 12.22), not all leiomyosarcomas demonstrate this feature and some clinically benign leiomyoma variants exhibit similar levels of overexpression, particularly for p16 (Figure 12.12).

Myxoid leiomyoma

Leiomyoma with myxoid and/or hydropic change is vastly more prevalent than myxoid leiomyosarcoma. In the former, the constituent cells are small and uniform with minimal atypia and the mitotic index is low. A well-circumscribed uterine leiomyoma with myxoid change and no cytologic atypia may contain up to 5 MF/10 HPF, provided none of the division figures are atypical. Sometimes, the distinction cannot be made on a curettage specimen; in these cases, imaging studies to determine extent of involvement and a myomectomy procedure may provide sufficient data for a more informed evaluation. Those cases that continue to defy classification should be designated as myxoid smooth muscle tumors of uncertain malignant potential (myxoid STUMP).

Pleomorphic rhabdomyosarcoma

Rhabdomyosarcoma is uncommon in the uterus in pure form. The pleomorphic subtype is most common, but, occasionally, a spindle cell component is prominent[32,33]. The presence of brightly eosinophilic cytoplasm and cross-striations favor rhabdomyosarcoma, but because these features may be somewhat subjective, this diagnosis should be confirmed by myogenin or MyoD1.

Undifferentiated endometrial sarcoma

A fascicular growth pattern and desmin and/or h-caldesmon expression distinguish leiomyosarcoma from an undifferentiated endometrial sarcoma (high-grade undifferentiated uterine sarcoma) (Figure 12.25). On occasion, a high-grade tumor may exhibit vague or focal fascicular architecture and/or focal, weak, or minimal staining

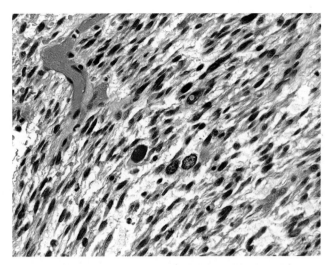

Figure 12.25 Undifferentiated sarcoma. No specific evidence of smooth muscle differentiation is present. Tumors with this histology should be evaluated for foci of high-grade carcinoma to exclude a carcinosarcoma.

for smooth muscle markers; in absence of more convincing evidence of smooth muscle differentiation, we classify these as high-grade sarcoma. Whether such tumors demonstrate any substantive difference in clinical behavior and/or response to adjuvant therapy is currently unknown.

Carcinosarcoma or adenosarcoma

The sarcomatous component of carcinosarcoma or, rarely, adenosarcoma may resemble leiomyosarcoma; judicious sampling to identify the epithelial component often resolves most diagnostic problems. In biopsy or curettage specimens containing limited tissue, the distinction between sarcoma and carcinosarcoma or adenosarcoma may not be possible; in these instances it is appropriate to mention the possibility of a biphasic tumor in which the epithelial element is not represented in the uterine sampling.

Inflammatory myofibroblastic tumor

Inflammatory myofibroblastic tumor has been reported to occur in the uterus and may be mistaken for a myxoid leiomyosarcoma; however, the former tumor is clinically less aggressive and may be treated more conservatively if recognized on a uterine sampling or myomectomy specimen[34]. The presence of a lymphoplasmacytic infiltrate in a low-grade, often myxoid-appearing mesenchymal lesion that exhibits a hypocellular, fascicular, or hyalinized pattern may suggest the diagnosis (Figure 12.26). Expression of ALK1 protein may confirm the diagnosis, but only about 50% of inflammatory myofibroblastic tumors express ALK1, and these ALK1-positive tumors typically occur in younger individuals (see Chapter 14)[34].

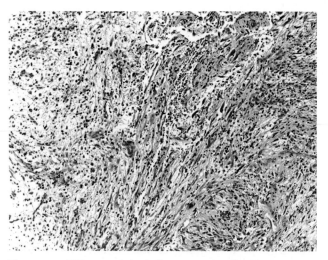

Figure 12.26 This non-uterine inflammatory myofibroblastic tumor consists of myofibroblastic spindle cells with intermingled plasma cells and small lymphocytes.

Melanoma

Primary or metastatic melanoma may mimic an epithelioid leiomyosarcoma, especially on a limited sampling. Immunostains for S100 protein and other melanoma markers are helpful. Also, pigment may be present.

Gastrointestinal stromal tumor

Primary gastrointestinal stromal tumor (GIST) is rare in the uterine corpus[35]. More frequently, gastrointestinal stromal tumor extends from the bowel wall or an adjacent location and simulates a uterine smooth muscle tumor. Distinction from the usual leiomyosarcoma is based on the presence of stubbier, more fusiform cells without a well-developed fascicular pattern (Figure 12.27). In addition, the mitotic index is often low in gastrointestinal stromal tumor. An immunohistochemistry panel that

(A)

(B)

(C)

(D)

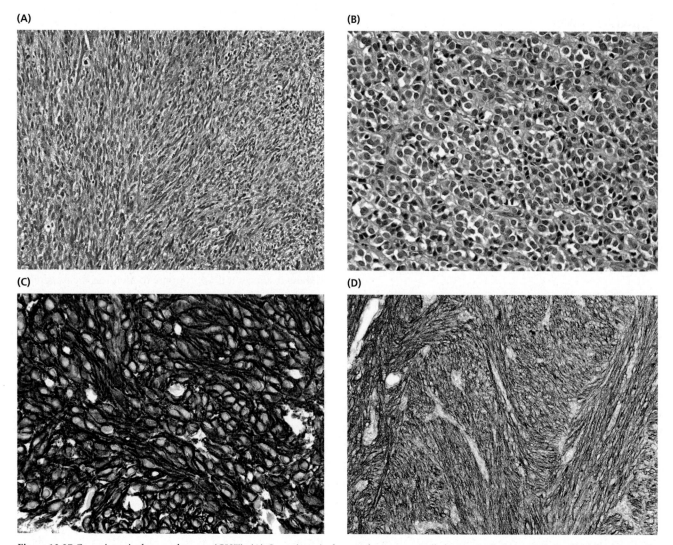

Figure 12.27 Gastrointestinal stromal tumor (GIST). (A) Gastrointestinal stromal tumor typically has a spindled morphology, which in this case is arranged in fascicles, simulating a conventional smooth muscle tumor. (B) Epithelioid gastrointestinal stromal tumor may mimic epithelioid leiomyoma. (C) DOG1 expression is not typically seen in smooth muscle tumors. (D) Typical pattern of CD117 in gastrointestinal stromal tumor.

(A)

(B)

(C)

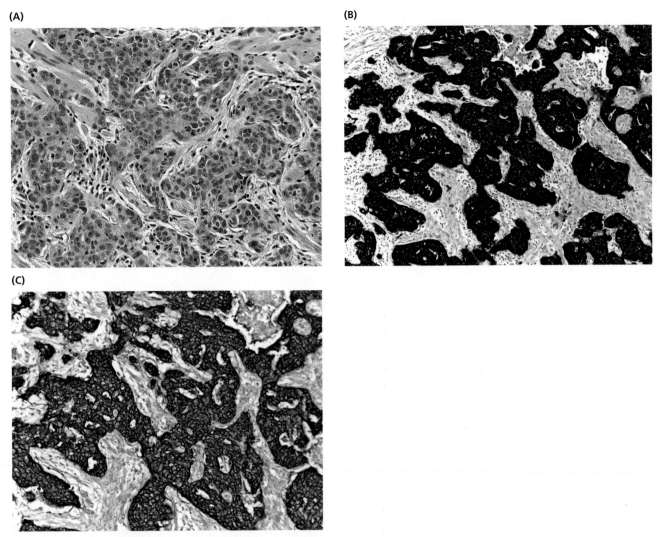

Figure 12.28 (A) Placental site trophoblastic tumor (PSTT) infiltrates between uterine smooth muscle cells, unlike epithelioid smooth muscle tumors. (B) Cytokeratin expression is diffuse and strong. (C) Expression of hPL is often prominent.

includes desmin, CD117 (c-kit) and DOG1 should be helpful, but care must be taken in the evaluation of such tumors, as strong CD117 expression in absence of a detectable c-kit mutation can occasionally be seen in uterine leiomyosarcoma, as well as other primary uterine mesenchymal neoplasms[36].

Undifferentiated carcinoma

Epithelioid leiomyosarcoma should be distinguished from poorly differentiated or undifferentiated carcinoma. A diagnosis of carcinoma is favored when there is an endometrial-based lesion, associated endometrial hyperplasia, or gland-forming areas of usual adenocarcinoma. Squamous elements are additional supportive histologic features. Although some experts recommend immunohistochemistry in difficult cases, this maneuver may not resolve the problem. Undifferentiated uterine carcinomas may lose cytokeratin expression, and leiomyosarcomas may exhibit considerable expression of cytokeratin

and EMA. Demonstration of desmin or h-caldesmon in leiomyosarcoma is useful, but many epithelioid leiomyosarcomas exhibit negligible expression for smooth muscle markers.

Placental site trophoblastic tumor

Placental site trophoblastic tumor (PSTT) and epithelioid trophoblastic tumor (ETT) occur during the reproductive years and are typically diagnosed in curettage specimens obtained for abnormal vaginal bleeding[37–39]. A prior history of pregnancy may not be apparent. Serum β-hCG is usually only moderately elevated. Even though epithelioid cells are prominent in placental site trophoblastic tumor and epithelioid trophoblastic tumor, the epithelioid cells infiltrate between myometrial muscle fibers (Figure 12.28) instead of forming a mass that replaces myometrium as in epithelioid smooth muscle tumors. Placental site trophoblastic tumor is also strongly cytokeratin positive, but negative for muscle markers. Additional markers, such as human placental lactogen (hPL), Mel-CAM, and inhibin help confirm the diagnosis of placental site trophoblastic tumor (Figure 12.28). Epithelioid trophoblastic tumor additionally expresses p63[39].

Benign myxoid change of the myometrium and cervical stroma

This pseudoneoplastic change, which has been recently reported in late-reproductive aged women, consists of conspicuous replacement of the myometrium or cervical stroma by an accumulation of hypocellular myxoid stromal material containing bland, spindle-shaped cells and small blood vessels[40]. Some cases may show multifocal or infiltrative patterns, simulating an invasive myxoid smooth muscle tumor. However, cytologic atypia, tumor cell necrosis, and mitotic activity are absent. An association with NF-1 has been observed in some patients.

PEComa

The distinction between perivascular epithelioid tumor and epithelioid leiomyosarcoma is discussed separately (see *Perivascular epithelioid cell tumor*).

SMOOTH MUSCLE TUMORS OF UNCERTAIN MALIGNANT POTENTIAL

In rare uterine smooth muscle tumors, the histologic features are not sufficiently developed to allow classification into benign or malignant categories[1]. Type of differentiation, type of necrosis, mitotic index, degree of atypia, or the degree of representation of the entire tumor mass in a limited biopsy or myomectomy specimen may be ambiguous or otherwise in doubt. For this group of tumors, the designation of uncertain malignant potential is an appropriate diagnosis (Figure 12.29). The most common situations in which this designation (STUMP) is used include the following.

(1) Smooth muscle tumors in which tumor cell necrosis cannot be distinguished from early infarction necrosis.
(2) Smooth muscle tumors in which the type of differentiation (conventional vs. epithelioid) is unclear and the mitotic index is in the range where, depending on the pattern assignment, the tumor would be leiomyoma or leiomyosarcoma.
(3) Smooth muscle tumors with usual histology but a mitotic index that, depending on the stringency of the mitotic determination, straddles the border between leiomyoma and leiomyosarcoma.

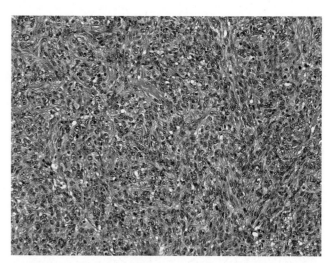

Figure 12.29 Smooth muscle tumor of uncertain malignant potential (STUMP).

(4) Purely epithelioid tumors with moderate to severe atypia, but no tumor necrosis and a mitotic index <5 MF/10 HPF.
(5) Purely myxoid tumors with moderate to severe atypia, a mitotic index of less than 2 MF/10 HPF, and no tumor cell necrosis.

Recent studies suggest that at least some of these smooth muscle tumor of uncertain malignant potentials recur, often following a prolonged disease-free interval. Most of the tumors that have recurred have had focal or multifocal moderate to severe atypia with no tumor cell necrosis and mitotic index ≤10 MF/10 HPF[17]; these tumors have elsewhere been referred to as atypical leiomyomas with limited experience[1].

LEIOMYOSARCOMA ARISING IN LEIOMYOMA

Rare cases of leiomyosarcoma apparently arising in a pre-existing leiomyoma have been reported[41]. While it is certainly possible for this to occur, it appears to be exceedingly uncommon; those cases that do appear to have a bona fide associated leiomyoma have been small, and demonstrated a favorable prognosis.

MIXED SMOOTH MUSCLE AND STROMAL NEOPLASMS

Some uterine mesenchymal tumors exhibit a mixed smooth muscle and endometrial stromal histology[42,43]. These tumors may be mixed in a patchwork quilt pattern or gradually merge with one another. A distinctive starburst pattern of smooth muscle differentiation merging with short or long fascicles of smooth muscle or endometrial stromal cells may also be seen (Figure 12.30)[43]. Since at least some of these mixed tumors have behaved in an aggressive fashion, all mixed stromal and smooth muscle tumors should be regarded as variants of endometrial stromal neoplasms and diagnosed as endometrial stromal nodule or endometrial stromal sarcoma, depending on circumscribed or infiltrative margins and absence or presence of vascular invasion, respectively[43].

SMOOTH MUSCLE TUMORS OF THE FEMALE GENITAL TRACT WITH UNUSUAL ANATOMIC DISTRIBUTION

Most uterine leiomyosarcomas are clinically confined to the uterus on presentation; when extrauterine disease is present it is likely to involve the lung, liver, or bone[14,15]. However, advanced-stage leiomyosarcomas may also exhibit intraperitoneal and regional lymph node involvement. In either situation, the pathologist may be faced with a diagnostic dilemma if the tumor in question does not exhibit classical features of a sarcoma, as there are a variety of smooth muscle proliferations that can simulate leiomyosarcoma by virtue of their distribution of disease. These include disseminated peritoneal leiomyomatosis (DPL), benign metastasizing leiomyoma (BML), intravenous leiomyomatosis (IVL), and lymphangioleiomyomatosis (LAM), as well as retroperitoneal leiomyomas and leiomyosarcomas. With the exception of the latter, most of these entities do not exhibit morphologic features of leiomyosarcoma, but are of concern due to their distributional attributes.

Disseminated peritoneal leiomyomatosis

Disseminated peritoneal leiomyomatosis (DPL) is a rare condition (Table 12.3) characterized by widespread nodules of histologically benign smooth muscle in the omentum and peritoneum, often numbering in the tens to hundreds. The intraoperative appearance of disseminated peritoneal leiomyomatosis is often so alarming that an intraoperative pathologic examination with frozen section is requested to exclude abdominal carcinomatosis.

Table 12.3 Disseminated peritoneal leiomyomatosis (DPL)

Multiple, small (most <2 cm) nodules of benign smooth muscle on peritoneal surface
Reproductive-age patient
History of recent pregnancy or other source of estrogen stimulation (endogenous or exogenous)
Concomitant uterine leiomyomas
Decidual reaction and/or endometriosis may be present in smooth muscle nodules
Spontaneous regression following removal of estrogen stimulus

(A)

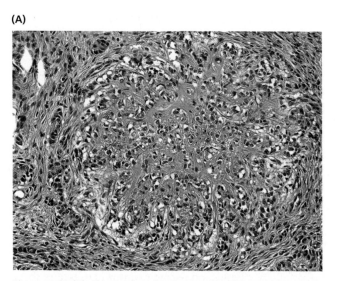

(B)

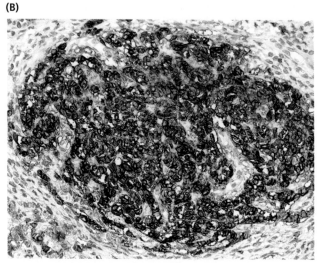

Figure 12.30 (A) Characteristic "starburst pattern" in mixed stromal and smooth muscle tumor. (B) Desmin highlights the smooth muscle component. Mixed tumors should be evaluated as if they were pure endometrial stromal neoplasms: presence of myometrial invasion or vascular invasion is diagnostic of low-grade endometrial stromal sarcoma.

(A)

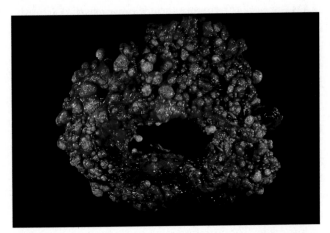

(B)

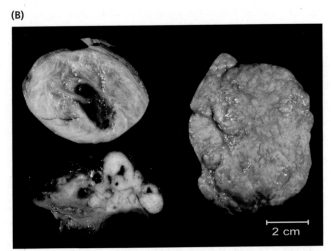

2 cm

Figure 12.31 Disseminated peritoneal leiomyomatosis (DPL). (A) The omentum is covered by multiple, small nodules of smooth muscle tumors. (B) Endometriois is present in this smooth muscle nodule in disseminated peritoneal leiomyomatosis.

Despite the alarming appearance, disseminated peritoneal leiomyomatosis is usually associated with an indolent clinical course and can be treated conservatively with long-term follow-up. The condition is rare; less than 150 cases have been reported in the literature[2].

Clinical characteristics

Disseminated peritoneal leiomyomatosis is most common in women of reproductive age (mean: 37 years), who are pregnant or have a long-term history of oral contraceptive use or endogenous increased estrogen production. Most cases are discovered incidentally at laparotomy. Ascites may be present.

Disseminated peritoneal leiomyomatosis appears to either regress or show no growth once hormonal stimulus is removed (cessation of pregnancy, removal of estrogen-secreting ovarian tumors, etc.). Therefore, extensive surgery is not usually recommended, except for symptomatic relief for patients who have completed child-bearing. Because of the strong association with increased hormonal production in some cases, treatment with gonadotropin-releasing hormone agonists (GnRH) has been advocated[44].

Almost all reported cases of "malignant disseminated peritoneal leiomyomatosis" have had atypical clinical or histologic features. Women who present with multiple peritoneal smooth muscle tumors in *absence* of any of the following features should be regarded as harboring potentially malignant tumors and followed closely: (1) concomitant uterine leiomyomas, (2) exogenous or increased endogenous estrogen exposure, or (3) hormone receptor expression on immunohistochemistry studies. Similarly, presentation in the postmenopausal years is

unusual and other, possibly more aggressive neoplasms should be considered.

Morphology

GROSS PATHOLOGY

The nodules are usually small, firm, gray to white, and cover the peritoneal surfaces and omentum, clinically simulating a disseminated malignancy (Figure 12.31). In most cases, the nodules in disseminated peritoneal leiomyomatosis measure 2 to 3 mm in size, but nodules measuring 3 to 4 cm may occur, and nodules as large as 10 cm have been reported, but, in each case, the nodules are situated immediately beneath the peritonealized surfaces and unattached to blood vessels. Lymph node involvement may also be present[2]. Many patients have uterine leiomyomas at the time of diagnosis.

MICROSCOPIC PATHOLOGY

Disseminated peritoneal leiomyomatosis is composed of histologically benign-appearing smooth muscle (Figure 12.32); occasionally, foci of endometriosis or sex cord–like elements are present. Estrogen and progesterone receptors are present.

Differential diagnosis

LEIOMYOSARCOMA

Because of the extensive disease within the peritoneum, the unwary pathologist may confuse disseminated peritoneal leiomyomatosis with metastatic leiomyosarcoma. However, the typical gross appearance of metastatic leiomyosarcoma is that of large, fleshy and necrotic tumor masses, and there is significant cytologic atypia and mitotic activity on microscopic examination. In addition, in most cases of

(A)

(B)

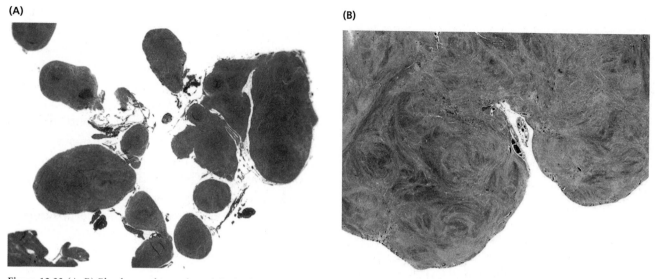

Figure 12.32 (A, B) Bland smooth muscle nodules in disseminated peritoneal leiomyomatosis arise in the subperitoneal tissue.

metastatic leiomyosarcoma there will be a history of a previously resected leiomyosarcoma or a concomitant, large uterine mass. Metastatic leiomyosarcoma is often concentrated in the pelvis with distribution in the vicinity of the round ligament and iliac veins.

BENIGN METASTASIZING LEIOMYOMA

Benign metastasizing leiomyoma usually presents as one or more pulmonary nodules; when it occurs within the pelvis and abdomen, there are usually only one or two nodules, the nodules are larger, and they tend to be distributed near the region of the round ligament or iliac veins. Extension into the smaller pelvic veins by intravenous leiomyomatosis may simulate the peritoneal distribution of disseminated peritoneal leiomyomatosis on initial inspection, but disseminated peritoneal leiomyomatosis only involves subperitoneal surfaces, and invasion or involvement of the lumens of blood vessels does not occur. Although intravenous leiomyomatosis has been reported to occur in association with benign metastasizing leiomyoma, there is no clear association with disseminated peritoneal leiomyomatosis[45].

"PARASITIC" LEIOMYOMA

Pedunculated leiomyomas have been reported to detach from their subserosal point of uterine attachment due to torsion and necrosis of the pedicle. Reattachment to other sites in the pelvis or omentum then generates a secondary parasitic vascular supply. This phenomenon, if it occurs at all, is uncommon and is not associated with the presence of multiple smooth muscle nodules scattered throughout the

abdomen. Typically, there is one or only a few such tumor nodules in parasitic leiomyoma, and the nodules are often larger than those usually seen in disseminated peritoneal leiomyomatosis.

GASTROINTESTINAL STROMAL TUMOR

Gastrointestinal stromal tumor (GIST) may be multiple, but is usually not as extensive as disseminated peritoneal leiomyomatosis. Whereas disseminated peritoneal leiomyomatosis is centered on the peritoneal surface, gastrointestinal stromal tumor is centered on the bowel. Although approximately 10% of gastrointestinal stromal tumors arise in the mesentery, omentum, pelvis, or retroperitoneum, most gastrointestinal stromal tumors are large and 85–90% are positive for CD117.

MESENTERIC FIBROMATOSIS

Mesenteric fibromatosis may present as multiple confluent mesenteric nodules, but the individual nodules are usually large and infiltrative and exhibit nuclear accumulation of β-catenin.

NODULAR AND DIFFUSE PERITONEAL DECIDUAL REACTION

Nodular and diffuse peritoneal decidual reaction may be visible at cesarean section as multiple small peritoneal nodules. Microscopic presence of subperitoneal decidual cells, often with admixed lymphocytes and admixed smooth muscle cells, may simulate disseminated peritoneal leiomyomatosis. The nodules are smaller in decidual reaction and lack the characteristic fascicular arrangement of

Table 12.4 Benign metastasizing leiomyoma

Histologically benign smooth muscle tumor in lung, pelvis, or abdomen

Histologically benign smooth muscle tumor in the uterus, either concurrently or, more commonly, in uterus removed during prior hysterectomy procedure[a]

No retroperitoneal, gastrointestinal, or other smooth muscle tumors

[a] Confirmation of a benign uterine smooth muscle tumor may not always be possible, since the uterus has often been removed many years prior to development of the benign metastases, and material is no longer available for review.

the smooth muscle cells in disseminated peritoneal leiomyomatosis. The two disorders likely represent opposite ends of a spectrum of hormonal mediated changes in the subperitoneal tissue.

Benign metastasizing leiomyoma

Benign metastasizing leiomyoma (BML) is a condition consisting of histologically benign smooth muscle tumors in the lungs, lymph nodes, or abdomen that appear to originate from a benign uterine leiomyoma, which typically is removed many years prior to the development of extrauterine disease (Table 12.4)[46].

The diagnosis of benign metastasizing leiomyoma should only be made when the metastasis and the putative primary uterine tumor (if available for review) are histologically banal – that is, they meet criteria for leiomyoma (not smooth muscle tumor of uncertain malignant potential or sarcoma). Rare tumors with a clinical history suggesting benign metastasizing leiomyoma represent histologic and clinical progression from atypical leiomyoma, in which case "benign metastasizing leiomyoma" should not be diagnosed. If the recurrence is atypical leiomyoma/smooth muscle tumor of uncertain malignant potential, it should be diagnosed as recurrent atypical leiomyoma/smooth muscle tumor of uncertain malignant potential, but when the recurrence is sarcoma morphologically, it should be diagnosed as leiomyosarcoma.

A variety of hypotheses have been proposed to explain the pathogenesis of benign metastasizing leiomyoma, including: (1) lymphovascular dissemination of a benign uterine leiomyoma; (2) metastasis from a low-grade uterine leiomyosarcoma, which is undersampled or, if adequately sampled, morphologically uninformative; (3) hormonally induced smooth muscle metaplasia and hyperplasia; and (4) multifocality of primary smooth muscle neoplasia. Rare

hybrids of benign metastasizing leiomyoma and intravenous leiomyomatosis have been observed, suggesting that in these instances pulmonary spread has occurred via the intravenous leiomyomatosis[45]. Some experts maintain that benign metastasizing leiomyoma is a form of low-grade leiomyosarcoma and should be so designated. However, the parameters of the term "low-grade leiomyosarcoma" have not been well defined with respect to uterine smooth muscle tumors, and the term benign metastasizing leiomyoma is well entrenched in the clinical literature; we employ the benign metastasizing leiomyoma diagnostic terminology, particularly since complete excision of the smooth muscle nodules, often in association with hormonal therapy, is associated with prolonged survival.

Clinical characteristics

Benign metastasizing leiomyoma most commonly presents in women during their late reproductive years. There is usually a history of prior hysterectomy, often many years prior to presentation. Lung nodules, which may be single or multiple (usually no more than three to four) are the most common presentation, but some women present with pelvic nodules or, in some cases, lymph node involvement.

Morphology

GROSS PATHOLOGY

The tumors in benign metastasizing leiomyoma are well circumscribed, firm, and exhibit the characteristic whorled pattern on cut section. Secondary hemorrhage may be present.

MICROSCOPIC PATHOLOGY

The tumors in benign metastasizing leiomyoma are composed of a proliferation of bland smooth muscle cells, without nuclear pleomorphism, necrosis, or significant mitotic activity. In the lung, the tumor nodules usually contain entrapped benign lung epithelial elements, consistent with an indolent growth process (Figure 12.33).

Ancillary diagnostic tests

Two consistent chromosomal aberrations have been observed in lung tumors from patients with benign metastasizing leiomyoma (19q and 22q terminal deletion in all cases studied). This cytogenetic profile is also found in approximately 3% of uterine leiomyoma, but has not been described in other types of benign or malignant neoplasia[47].

(A)

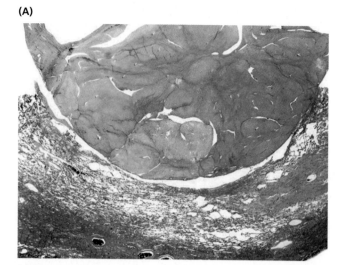

(B)

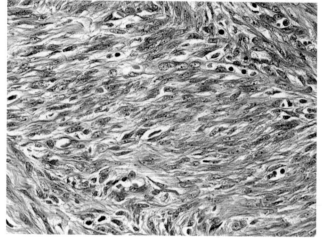

Figure 12.33 (A) Benign metastasizing leiomyoma in lung. (B) There is no cytologic atypia.

Differential diagnosis

LEIOMYOSARCOMA

The usual leiomyosarcoma is bulky, necrotic, and hemorrhagic. Cellular atypia, numerous mitotic figures, and tumor cell necrosis are almost always present.

LYMPHANGIOLEIOMYOMATOSIS

Nodules of smooth muscle in lymphangioleiomyomatosis are intimately associated with lymphatics and often form discrete packets or nests of cells with clear or slightly granular cytoplasm. The lungs may show prominent cysts on imaging studies. The muscle cells in lymphangioleiomyomatosis express HMB45.

GASTROINTESTINAL STROMAL TUMOR

Gastrointestinal stromal tumor typically metastasizes to intra-abdominal sites and liver before metastasizing to

Table 12.5 Intravenous leiomyomatosis (IVL)

Venous distention by smooth muscle imparts wormy appearance to the uterus. Extension into extrauterine veins may be seen at the time of hysterectomy
Uterine mass typically also present
Veins distended by smooth muscle, which can show conventional, epithelioid, or myxoid histology
Complete resection is curative in vast majority of cases (rare cases associated with benign metastasizing leiomyoma)

the lung. Staining for CD117 and DOG1 identifies most gastrointestinal stromal tumors.

Intravenous leiomyomatosis

Intravenous leiomyomatosis (IVL) occurs in women over 50 ears of age, but may present during the reproductive years (Table 12.5). Patients may be asymptomatic, but more commonly present with a pelvic mass clinically indistinguishable from a typical uterine leiomyoma. Intravenous leiomyomatosis is notorious for its ability to grow into the right heart, causing cardiopulmonary insufficiency. Intravenous leiomyomatosis is treated by complete removal of the intravenous tumor, which often includes excision of involved veins. Prognosis depends on the extent of venous involvement. If completely excised, patients have a very favorable prognosis; recurrence is uncommon.

Morphology

GROSS PATHOLOGY

When confined to the pelvis, the condition is recognized as worm-like protrusions of smooth muscle from veins at the parametrial margin of hysterectomy specimens.

MICROSCOPIC PATHOLOGY

Intravenous leiomyomatosis is characterized by intravenous intrusion of histologically benign smooth muscle (Figure 12.34). The smooth muscle in intravenous leiomyomatosis resembles smooth muscle tumors in the uterus in every respect, and may feature epithelioid, myxoid, or sex cord features[48]. The presence of vessels within vessels in the normal uterus may provide an anatomic basis for the pathogenesis of intravenous leiomyomatosis.

Ancillary diagnostic tests

Rearrangements of the *HMGA2* gene have been reported in intravenous leiomyomatosis[49]. It has also been suggested

(A)

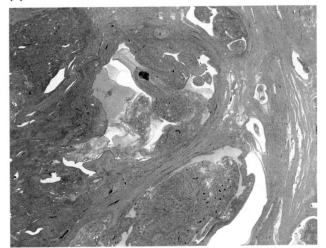

(B)

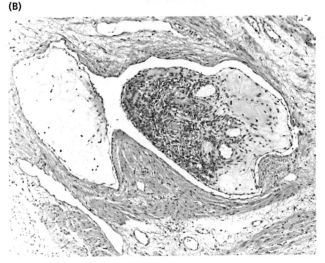

Figure 12.34 (A) Intravenous leiomyomatosis. (B) The intravascular tumor has numerous thick-walled blood vessels and a clefted contour.

that intravenous leiomyomatosis may arise from a uterine leiomyoma with a t(12;14)(q15;q24)[50].

Differential diagnosis

ENDOMETRIAL STROMAL SARCOMA

Endometrial stromal sarcoma (ESS) is more cellular than the smooth muscle in the usual intravenous leiomyomatosis. The individual cells are small and stubby, and there is a fine plexiform vascular pattern in stromal neoplasms that is not typically seen in intravenous leiomyomatosis. The endometrium is primarily involved in endometrial stromal sarcoma, whereas the dominant site of involvement is the myometrium in intravenous leiomyomatosis. Also, most stromal sarcomas are associated with an intrauterine mass, whereas intravenous leiomyomatosis may not have a distinct mass lesion.

Table 12.6 Lymphangioleiomyomatosis (LAM)

Small nodular, often widespread proliferations of HMB45-positive myoid cells along lymphatic channels and lymph nodes
Sites of affected lymph nodes include pelvis, retroperitoneum, and mediastinum, where enlarged masses forming lymphangiomyomas may be seen
Uterine tumors may be present, and there is overlap between this condition and perivascular epithelioid cell tumor (see *Perivascular epithelioid cell tumor*)
The most serious form of this disease involves pulmonary lymphatic channels
Association with tuberous sclerosis complex
Most cases are incidental findings, with no associated pulmonary disease, but imaging studies are recommended

HYDROPIC LEIOMYOMA

Hydropic leiomyoma may simulate intravenous leiomyomatosis on macroscopic examination, but characteristic hydropic change without intravascular intrusion is seen.

DIFFUSE LEIOMYOMATOSIS

Diffuse leiomyomatosis does not involve lymphatic or venous channels.

Lymphangioleiomyomatosis

Lymphangioleiomyomatosis (LAM) is a rare condition occurring in women of reproductive age, characterized by nodular, often widespread proliferations of myoid cells along lymphatic channels and lymph nodes (Table 12.6). Sites of affected lymph nodes include pelvis, retroperitoneum, and mediastinum, where enlarged masses forming lymphangiomyomas may be seen. Rare uterine tumors are also seen, and there is overlap between this condition and perivascular epithelioid cell tumor (see *Perivascular epithelioid cell tumor*). The most serious form of this disease involves pulmonary lymphatic channels.

Clinical characteristics

Lymphangioleiomyomatosis is usually sporadic, but patients with tuberous sclerosis complex are often affected[51,52]. Most cases of lymphangioleiomyomatosis are incidental findings in patients undergoing surgery for other, often unrelated causes; they may be focal and apparently unicentric or multifocal, involving multiple lymph nodes. Pulmonary involvement is often absent, even in cases of apparent multifocal and/or diffuse pelvic lymphangioleiomyomatosis. Prognosis depends on extent of involvement. Pulmonary disease is often associated with a progressive clinical course;

(A)

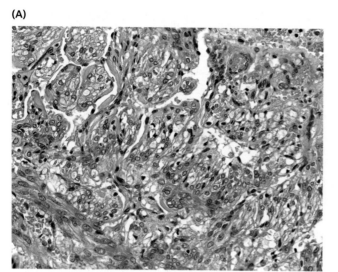

(B)

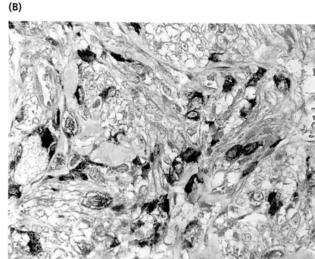

Figure 12.35 (A) Lymphangioleiomyomatosis has spindled and epithelioid cells with clear to slightly granular eosinophilic cytoplasm arranged in distinctive packets. (B) HMB45 expression is typically patchy in distribution.

lung transplantation is often effective. Stigmata of tuberous sclerosis may be present in affected patients.

Morphology

GROSS PATHOLOGY

Macroscopic lesions appear tan, solid or solid and cystic. Often, no distinct gross abnormality is present.

MICROSCOPIC PATHOLOGY

Ill-defined nodules of spindle and clear cells with epithelioid features abut lymphatics and the hilar regions of lymph nodes, often replacing large portions of the node (Figure 12.35). Immunoreactivity for HMB45 and desmin is present (Figure 12.35)[51].

Differential diagnosis

DISSEMINATED PERITONEAL LEIOMYOMATOSIS

The predominant involvement of lymph nodes and association with lymphatic channels distinguishes lymphangioleiomyomatosis from disseminated peritoneal leiomyomatosis, where the nodules are scattered throughout the peritoneum and associated with the subperitoneum. Involvement of pulmonary parenchyma is not a feature of disseminated peritoneal leiomyomatosis.

PELVIC (EXTRAUTERINE) AND RETROPERITONEAL
SMOOTH MUSCLE TUMORS

Pelvic (extrauterine) and retroperitoneal smooth muscle tumors in women always raise the differential diagnosis of possible spread from a uterine primary. In most instances, this can be resolved by examining the uterus and confirming either

(1) the absence of concomitant uterine smooth muscle tumor, or (2) the presence of a smooth muscle tumor with histologic features of leiomyoma. In those cases in which the uterus has been previously removed, an effort should be made to review the slides from the hysterectomy specimen. If the prior procedure involved morcellation of a uterus containing leiomyomas, consideration should be given for "iatrogenic" implantation of the uterine smooth muscle tumor (see below). Since most benign or low-grade pelvic and retroperitoneal smooth muscle tumors express hormone receptors and most uterine leiomyosarcomas cease to express hormone receptors, the use of immunohistochemistry is very limited in this setting, other than to confirm smooth muscle differentiation.

Once a tumor is determined to be highly likely of retroperitoneal origin, the pathologist should use the criteria recommended for distinguishing retroperitoneal leiomyoma from leiomyosarcoma, as these criteria differ from those in the uterus (Table 12.7). A general rule of thumb in the evaluation of extrauterine smooth muscle tumors is that gynecologic smooth muscle tumors, unless high-grade, express the hormone receptors ER and/or PR; whereas smooth muscle tumors of soft tissue or cutaneous origin do not.

"IATROGENIC" PELVIC LEIOMYOMAS

In recent years, we and others have encountered a number of so-called "recurrent uterine smooth muscle tumors" in women who have undergone vaginal hysterectomy or, more commonly, laparoscopic hysterectomy with morcellation of the uterus[54,55]. In most cases, the "recurrent" tumor is

Table 12.7 Diagnostic approach to retroperitoneal smooth muscle tumors[2,53]

	Leiomyoma[a]	*Leiomyosarcoma*
Age	Perimenopausal	Peak in seventh decade
Site	Pelvic sites	Retroperitoneum, pelvis, abdomen
Size	Often small, but may be large and multiple (usually two to five at most)	Large: 5 to >10 cm
Mitotic index	<3–4 MF/10 HPF	>3–4 MF/10 HPF
Cellular atypia	No atypia	Atypia, often severe
Necrosis	Hyaline necrosis, but no tumor cell necrosis	Tumor cell necrosis[b]
Hormone receptor status	ER+/PR+	ER−/PR−

[a] Pelvic retroperitoneal leiomyoma may occur in women with uterine leiomyomas and mimic benign metastasizing leiomyoma. Pelvic retroperitoneal leiomyoma exhibits the same histologic and immunochemical features as benign metastasizing leiomyoma, except that pelvic retroperitoneal leiomyoma is not associated with lung or lymph node involvement. Pelvic retroperitoneal leiomyoma may present as a single or multiple (usually two or three) nodules, but the nodules are often regionally confined.

[b] Hyaline necrosis may also be seen.

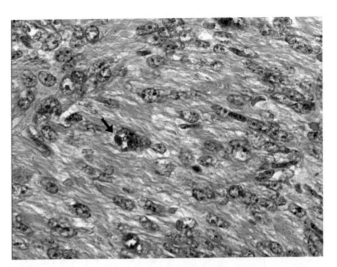

Figure 12.36 Uterine leiomyoma in hereditary leiomyomatosis. The prominent, eosinophilic nucleolus is characteristic of germline mutation in the fumarate hydratase gene. These patients often also have multiple cutaneous leiomyomas. There is a high risk for developing type II papillary renal cell carcinoma in hereditary leiomyomatosis. (Courtesy of Dr. Karuna Garg.)

histologically benign and probably resulted from growth of missed fragments of uterine tissue after the prior morcellation procedure, culminating in development of symptomatic iatrogenic parasitic myomas. Although follow-up is limited and case numbers are few, it appears that these tumors are not clinically aggressive and are adequately treated by surgical excision. Therefore, until there is data that indicate otherwise, iatrogenic parasitic leiomyoma should be considered in the differential diagnosis of all new pelvic smooth muscle tumors in patients with a history of morcellation. On rare occasions, we have encountered smooth muscle tumors in this setting that exhibited one or more concerning histologic features – that is, increased mitotic figures, cellular atypia, marked cellularity, necrosis, and so on – in this situation, it is appropriate to consider a diagnosis of smooth muscle tumor of uncertain malignant potential and recommend continued follow-up.

HEREDITARY LEIOMYOMATOSIS

Mutations in the fumarase hydratase gene, an enzyme that is involved in the mitochondrial tri-carboxylic acid cycle,

are associated with a dominantly inherited susceptibility to uterine leiomyomas and multiple cutaneous smooth muscle neoplasms. Recognition of this autosomal-dominant disorder is important since these patients are at risk for the development of type II papillary renal cell carcinoma[56]. The leiomyomas in this condition are histologically similar to usual uterine leiomyomas, but often exhibit unusually prominent eosinophilic nucleoli (Figure 12.36). The cutaneous tumors may be diffuse or segmental, and may develop before or after the uterine leiomyomas.

PERIVASCULAR EPITHELIOID CELL TUMOR

Perivascular epithelioid cell tumor (PEComa) is a rare epithelioid mesenchymal tumor in the female genital tract composed of histologically and immunohistochemically distinctive epithelioid cells. Perivascular epithelioid cell tumor of the gynecologic tract accounts for almost 40% of all cases. Most occur in the uterus, with smaller numbers reported to arise in the uterine cervix, vagina, and pelvic soft tissues.

Clinical characteristics

Most perivascular epithelioid cell tumors occur in perimenopausal women (mean: 51 years), but the age range of reported cases is 19 to 79 years[57]. Folpe *et al.* have classified perivascular epithelioid cell tumor into benign, uncertain malignant potential, and malignant categories based on tumor size (>5 cm); infiltrative margins; high-grade nuclear atypia and cellularity; mitotic index (>1 MF/50 HPF); necrosis; and vascular invasion[57]. Perivascular epithelioid cell tumors with nuclear pleomorphism and/or multinucleated giant cells *only* or size over 5 cm are of uncertain malignant potential; while perivascular epithelioid cell tumor with two or more worrisome features are considered to be malignant or at high risk for aggressive behavior. In general, any perivascular epithelioid cell tumor with significant pleomorphism, easily found mitotic figures, and necrosis is likely to be clinically malignant. Clinically aggressive tumors typically spread to the lungs, although local recurrences, bone metastases, and, rarely, lymph node metastases have also been reported.

Morphology

Gross pathology

The uterine tumors are 0.5 to 13 cm in size (mean: 3.5 cm) and usually single, although several additional, smaller tumors are occasionally identified at the time of hysterectomy. In some patients with uterine perivascular epithelioid cell tumor, additional perivascular aggregates of HMB45-positive epithelioid cells are seen in the adjacent ovary, pelvic tissue, and lymph nodes ("PEComatosis")[58]. A subset of perivascular epithelioid cell tumor, angiomyolipoma, and lymphangioleiomyomatosis is associated with tuberous sclerosis complex, although this appears to be less common for the tumors that arise in the gynecologic tract[57,59].

Microscopic pathology

Perivascular epithelioid cell tumor exhibits a variable spindled and epithelioid morphology; the spindled cells are arranged in characteristic short fascicles and cell nests, while the epithelioid cells are arranged in a nested or sheet-like pattern (Figure 12.37)[57,59]. The cells are clear to slightly eosinophilic with granular cytoplasm, and can be seen radiating from blood vessels. Nuclear atypia may be present, but the nuclei in most cases are ovoid and normochromic with small nucleoli. Some tumors contain scattered multinucleated cells or cells with so-called "spider cell" morphology – giant cells with a central eosinophilic zone surrounded by a peripheral clear zone (Figure 12.38)[57]. A sclerosing variant has also been reported[60]. Mitotic

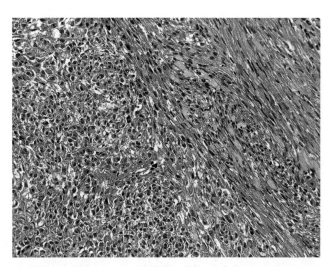

Figure 12.37 Perivascular epithelioid cell tumor with epithelioid and spindle morphology in uterus. The epithelioid features and granular cytoplasm overlap with epithelioid smooth muscle tumor.

activity varies, ranging from 0 MF/50 HPF to 50 MF/50 HPF, with most cases exhibiting few mitoses.

Ancillary diagnostic tests

Perivascular epithelioid cell tumor expresses at least one melanocytic marker (Figure 12.38), with HMB45 most frequently expressed (92%), followed by Melan-A (72%), and MiTF (50%)[57]. Up to 80% of perivascular epithelioid cell tumors will stain positive for smooth muscle actin; desmin and h-caldesmon expression is less common. The tumors frequently express hormone receptors.

Differential diagnosis

Perivascular epithelioid cell tumor is a controversial entity, particularly when it occurs in the uterus. Since conventional benign and malignant smooth muscle neoplasms may rarely express HMB45, and perivascular epithelioid cell tumor may rarely express desmin and h-caldesmon, it is possible that these tumors represent a morphologic continuum of uterine mesenchymal differentiation, rather than a distinct entity[61,62]. However, because of the potential association with tumors in the tuberous sclerosis complex and the more uncertain clinical behavior of perivascular epithelioid cell tumor, the distinction between the two tumors should probably be made until more information is available. In general, any epithelioid mesenchymal neoplasm in the uterus with prominent clear or eosinophilic pale granular cytoplasm should be evaluated by a panel of markers that includes HMB45, desmin, and h-caldesmon. CD10 should also be included in those problematic cases in which stromal differentiation is also a consideration.

(A)

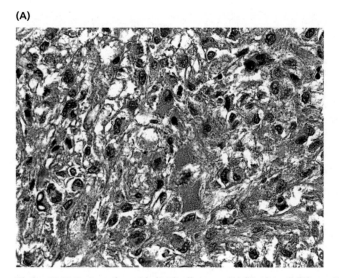

(B)

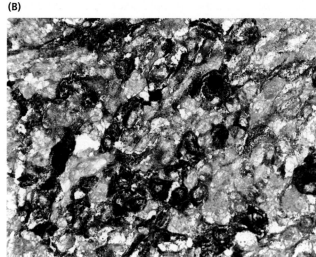

Figure 12.38 Perivascular epithelioid cell tumor (A) "Spider cells" formed by dense aggregates of eosinophilic material surrounded by a peripheral clear zone in perivascular epithelioid cell tumor. (B) Spindle and "spider cells" cells are positive for HMB45 in perivascular epithelioid cell tumor, often in a patchy distribution.

Epithelioid leiomyosarcoma

Perivascular epithelioid cell tumor and epithelioid leiomyosarcoma have overlapping histologic features. The presence of HMB45 or other melanocytic marker is required for perivascular epithelioid cell tumor. However, HMB45 is variably present in epithelioid leiomyosarcoma, as well as in the conventional and myxoid types. In addition, variable expression of other smooth muscle markers may be present in perivascular epithelioid cell tumors. We reserve the diagnosis of perivascular epithelioid cell tumor for those tumors that exhibit characteristic histologic features: epithelioid and/or epithelioid and spindled cells, clear cytoplasm, arranged in a short fascicular and nested or sheet-like pattern. However, the presence of HMB45 in any epithelioid mesenchymal tumor of the uterus should raise the possibility of lymphangioleiomyomatosis or tuberous sclerosis.

Melanoma

Melanoma and clear cell sarcoma can be distinguished from perivascular epithelioid cell tumor by the presence of strong and diffuse S100 expression. On occasion, clear cell sarcoma may express only HMB45 and, in these instances, identification of the t(12;22)(q13;q13)(*EWS; ATF1*) gene fusion will confirm the diagnosis.

Undifferentiated carcinoma

Perivascular epithelioid cell tumor can be confused with a variety of epithelial neoplasms such as undifferentiated carcinoma, clear cell carcinoma, and metastatic lobular carcinoma of the breast, particularly when present in a small biopsy specimen. Although a rare perivascular epithelioid cell tumor may express cytokeratin, diffuse keratin expression has not been observed in perivascular epithelioid cell tumor, and EMA expression is typically absent.

REFERENCES

1. Bell SW, Kempson RL, Hendrickson MR. Problematic uterine smooth muscle neoplasms. A clinicopathologic study of 213 cases. *Am J Surg Pathol* 1994;**18**:535–58.
2. Mills AM, Longacre TA. Smooth muscle tumors of the female genital tract. *Surg Pathol Clin* 2009;**2**(4):625–77.
3. Wang X, Kumar D, Seidman JD. Uterine lipoleiomyomas: a clinicopathologic study of 50 cases. *Int J Gynecol Pathol* 2006;**25**: 239–42.
4. Chen KT. Uterine leiomyohibernoma. *Int J Gynecol Pathol* 1999; **18**:96–7.
5. McCluggage WG, Boyde A. Uterine angioleiomyomas: a report of 3 cases of a distinctive benign leiomyoma variant. *Int J Surg Pathol* 2007;**15**:262–5.
6. Myles J, Hart W. Apoplectic leiomyomas of the uterus. A clinicopathologic study of five distinctive hemorrhagic leiomyomas associated with oral contraceptive usage. *Am J Surg Pathol* 1985;**9**:798–805.
7. Parker RL, Young RH, Clement PB. Skeletal muscle-like and rhabdoid cells in uterine leiomyomas. *Int J Gynecol Pathol* 2005; **24**:319–25.
8. Dundr P, Povysil C, Tvrdik D, *et al.* Uterine leiomyomas with inclusion bodies: an immunohistochemical and ultrastructural analysis of 12 cases. *Pathol Res Pract* 2007;**203**:145–51.
9. Ferry JA, Young RH. Malignant lymphoma, pseudolymphoma, and hematopoietic disorders of the female genital tract. *Pathol Annu* 1991;**26**:227–63.

13 ENDOMETRIAL STROMAL TUMORS

INTRODUCTION

Endometrial stromal neoplasms consist of endometrial stromal nodule and low-grade endometrial stromal sarcoma. Low-grade endometrial stromal sarcomas (ESSs) are uncommon uterine malignancies that constitute less than 20% of uterine sarcomas. Although a relatively rare disease, endometrial stromal sarcoma can pose many diagnostic problems, including the necessity to distinguish it from endometrial stromal nodule on the one hand and high-grade sarcoma on the other. These issues have an important impact on surgical management and selection of adjuvant therapy. That they are indolent tumors makes studying the natural history of these tumors complex; many patients become lost to follow-up or die of unrelated causes, which complicates surveillance for recurrence. Low-grade endometrial stromal sarcoma is distinguished from undifferentiated endometrial sarcoma on the basis of morphology and substantial differences in clinical presentation and survival.

CLINICAL CHARACTERISTICS

The mean age of patients with low-grade endometrial stromal sarcoma is in the fifth decade. At least half of affected patients are premenopausal. The disease tends to present like other endometrial tumors, with vaginal bleeding being common. Another typical presentation is a polypoid mass. There are occasional reports of endometrial stromal sarcoma developing after tamoxifen therapy.

Most low-grade endometrial stromal sarcomas are diagnosed in hysterectomy specimens. The diagnosis can also sometimes be suggested in myomectomy and curettage specimens and on imaging studies, but a firm diagnosis of endometrial stromal sarcoma can only be substantiated when the tumor/myometrial interface is available for examination. If a curettage shows a low-grade endometrial stromal neoplasm and the tumor/myometrial interface cannot be examined histologically, it can be impossible to make a diagnosis of sarcoma. Many patients are therefore subjected to hysterectomy in an attempt to provide both diagnostic tissue and therapeutic excision. There are case reports describing alternative approaches for motivated and informed patients who desire uterine preservation.

The 5-year, disease-specific survival rate for low-grade endometrial stromal sarcoma is approximately 80–90%, and the 10-year disease-specific survival rate is about 70%[1]. Patients who present with FIGO stage I (organ-confined) disease have superior outcomes, with 5-year survival rates approaching 100% and 10-year survival rates in the 90% range. In contrast, patients who present with high-stage disease have only a 40% probability of survival that remains constant at 10 years. Therefore, patients who present with low-stage tumors probably continue to experience recurrence decades after diagnosis, whereas patients diagnosed with high-stage tumors experience recurrence and frequently die of disease within five years of diagnosis. Stage is therefore the most powerful prognostic indicator in endometrial stromal sarcoma. Undifferentiated endometrial sarcomas, some of which may represent an endometrial stromal sarcoma that has undergone progression, have significantly worse survival rates as compared to low-grade endometrial stromal sarcomas[2].

Surgery is the mainstay of therapy for patients with endometrial stromal sarcoma, and numerous anecdotal reports of the beneficial effects of progestational therapy are on record. Radiation therapy can be used in selected cases where surgery is difficult or impossible and local control of disease is sought.

MORPHOLOGY

Gross pathology

Endometrial stromal sarcomas are soft, glistening, and yellow (Figure 13.1). They almost always demonstrate an

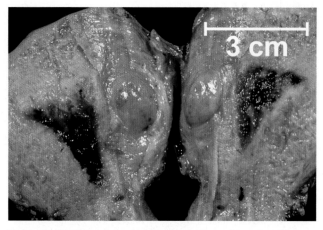

Figure 13.1 Endometrial stromal neoplasms are often soft, pale tan or yellow, and are either grossly well circumscribed (endometrial stromal nodule), or irregularly infiltrate the surrounding myometrium (low-grade endometrial stromal sarcoma).

Table 13.1 Pathologic characteristics of endometrial stromal neoplasms

Tumor cells resemble those of non-neoplastic proliferative-phase endometrium

No nuclear pleomorphism; scant cytoplasm

Presence of spiral arteriole-like blood vessels and delicate, branching capillaries, some with staghorn shapes

Many examples contain prominent stromal hyaline and/or foam cells

Mitotic index generally under 10 MF/10 HPF

Histologic variants may contain benign-appearing smooth muscle, fibroblasts and myofibroblasts, sex cord–like arrangements, and endometrioid-like glands

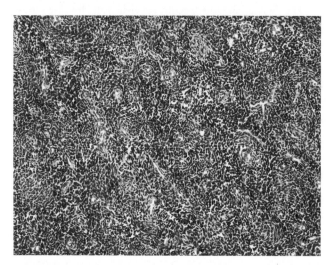

Figure 13.2 Endometrial stromal neoplasm. Tumor cells are small with scant cytoplasm. Note the characteristic vasculature.

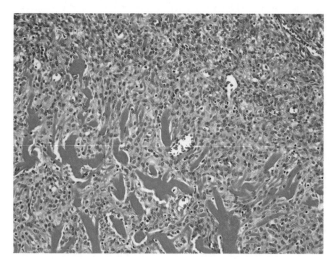

Figure 13.3 Endometrial stromal neoplasm with thick collagen deposition.

infiltrative growth pattern that contrasts with circumscribed growth that is more typical of leiomyomas and endometrial stromal nodules. Gross evidence of vascular invasion may also be appreciated. Endometrial stromal nodules and the polypoid portions of endometrial stromal sarcomas may show hemorrhage and necrosis. Rare endometrial stromal neoplasms exhibit smooth muscle differentiation. The gross appearance of such tumors is typically a combination of the glistening, yellow appearance of stromal neoplasms and the tan, whorled appearance of smooth muscle tumors.

Microscopic pathology

The typical low-grade endometrial stromal sarcoma is a microscopically infiltrative neoplasm composed of cells resembling non-neoplastic proliferative endometrial stroma, invested in a capillary and arteriolar-rich vascular network (Table 13.1). The tumor cells are small, with inapparent cytoplasm and oval nuclei without striking irregularities or nucleoli (Figure 13.2). Many cases exhibit dense stromal collagen (Figure 13.3). Progestational therapy may result in a pseudodecidualized appearance. Low-grade endometrial stromal sarcomas almost never contain pleomorphic cells, although rare cases have exhibited bizarre nuclei, similar to those occasionally encountered in endometrial polyps. Mitotic figures may be numerous (see discussion of undifferentiated endometrial sarcoma below). Two types of vessels are found: spiral arteriole-like vessels and delicate, arborizing capillaries that sometimes take on a pericytomatous or staghorn appearance (Figure 13.4). The pattern of infiltration is

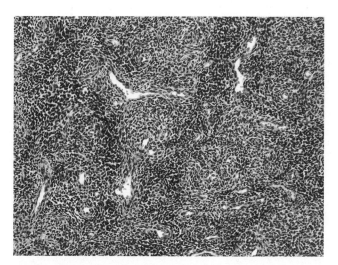

Figure 13.4 Endometrial stromal neoplasm showing spiral arteriole-like vessels and delicate, branching capillaries.

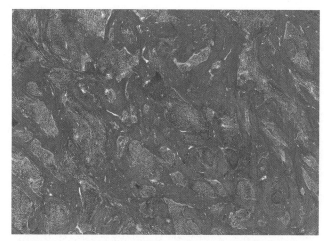

Figure 13.5 Low-grade endometrial stromal sarcoma with a permeative growth pattern.

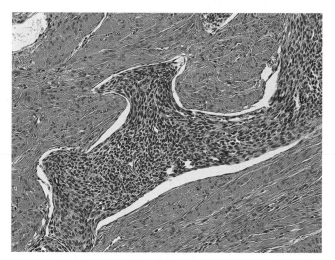

Figure 13.6 Lymphatic invasion in endometrial stromal sarcoma.

usually described as "tongue-like" on microscopic examination (Figure 13.5). Prominent lymphatic invasion is also very typical of this tumor (Figure 13.6).

There are several histologic variants of low-grade endometrial stromal sarcoma. They include otherwise typical endometrial stromal sarcomas that incorporate smooth muscle cells (Figure 13.7), myofibroblasts, fibroblasts (with or without myxoid stroma)(Figure 13.8), sex cord–like elements (Figure 13.9), endometrioid glands (Figure 13.10), epithelioid cells (Figure 13.11), and, very rarely, skeletal muscle, fat, bone, rhabdoid cells, and osteoclastic-type giant cells. Other very uncommon variants have been reported. These include low-grade endometrial stromal sarcomas that coexist or recur as histologically high-grade sarcoma (so-called dedifferentiated stromal sarcoma[3]) and mixed endometrial stromal

and smooth muscle tumors in which the smooth muscle component resembles leiomyosarcoma[4]. The clinical correlates of these histologic variants have not been studied in detail. Emerging cytogenetic data suggest that tumors containing both stromal and smooth muscle elements should be considered in essence endometrial stromal tumors, not mixed endometrial stromal and smooth muscle tumors[5].

Diagnosing metastatic endometrial stromal sarcoma can sometimes be difficult, particularly when metastasis is unsuspected (the history and attendant diagnosis of a hysterectomy performed decades prior to the metastasis may not be forthcoming), or when the histologic appearance of the metastasis differs from that of the primary[7]. Otherwise conventional low-grade endometrial stromal sarcomas may recur with predominantly fibroblastic or smooth muscle histology (Figure 13.12). An occasional endometrial stromal sarcoma with smooth muscle differentiation has been misdiagnosed as "low-grade leiomyosarcoma." Metastatic endometrial stromal sarcoma in the lung is frequently paucicellular and can resemble solitary fibrous tumors, benign metastasizing leiomyomas, or hamartomas (Figure 13.13).

ANCILLARY DIAGNOSTIC TESTS

Endometrial stromal neoplasms, both nodules and sarcomas, express CD10, ER, PR, and WT1[8] in most cases (Table 13.2). Many also express β-catenin[12]. Smooth muscle actin[9,11,13] and cytokeratin expression[11] is common, as is patchy expression of androgen receptors[14]. Endometrial stromal sarcomas and stromal nodules with conventional features

(A)

(B)

(C)

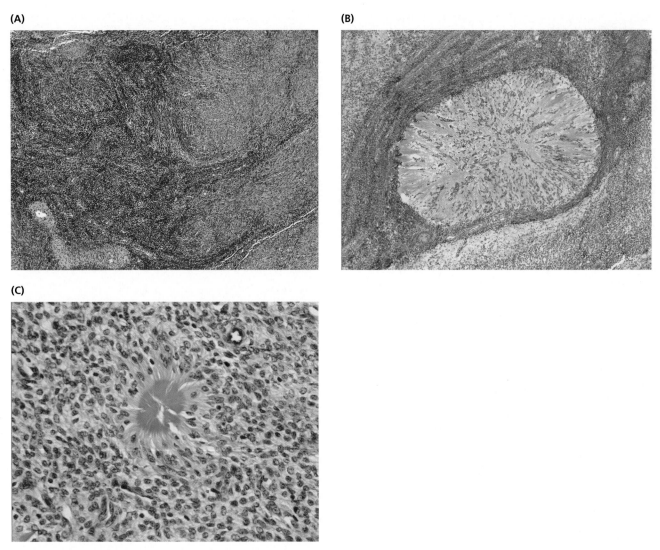

Figure 13.7 Endometrial stromal neoplasm showing smooth muscle differentiation (at right; A). Round aggregates of epithelioid cells (B) with a starburst of fibrocollagenous material at center (C) are seen in some examples of endometrial stromal tumors with smooth muscle differentiation. Illustrations B and C are courtesy of Karuna Garg, MD.

(A)

(B)

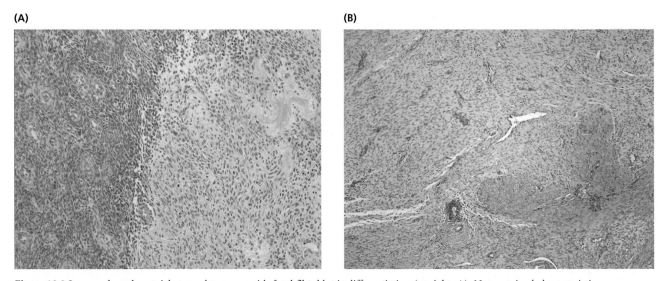

Figure 13.8 Low-grade endometrial stromal sarcoma with focal fibroblastic differentiation (at right; A). Note retained characteristic vasculature in fibroblastic tumor infiltrating myometrium (B). Illustration A is courtesy of Karuna Garg, MD.

(A)

(B)

(C)

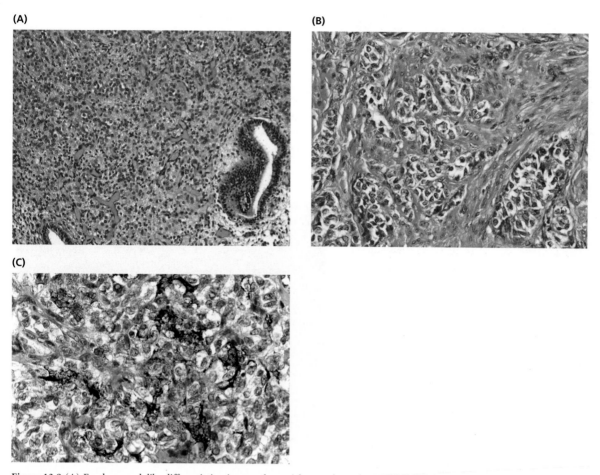

Figure 13.9 (A) Focal sex cord–like differentiation in an endometrial stromal neoplasm. This subtle pattern may occasionally prompt consideration for metastatic breast carcinoma (see Figure 13.22). More obvious examples of sex cord–like differentiation (B) usually prompt consideration for uterine tumor resembling ovarian sex cord tumor (UTROSCT; Figure 13.26), a lesion that, by definition should lack typical examples of endometrial stromal neoplasia. (C) The sex cord elements may express CD10, desmin, keratin, or inhibin (depicted here).

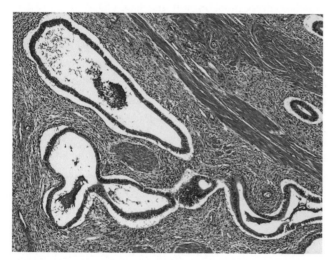

Figure 13.10 Low-grade endometrial stromal sarcoma containing endometrioid glands. Reproduced with permission from Soslow RA. Mixed mullerian tumors. In Oliva E, ed. *Current Concepts in Gynecologic Pathology: Mesenchymal Tumors of the Female Genital Tract* in the series Surgical Pathology Clinics, Goldblum JR, ed. Philadelphia, PA: Saunders 2009;**2**(4):707–30, Figure 24.

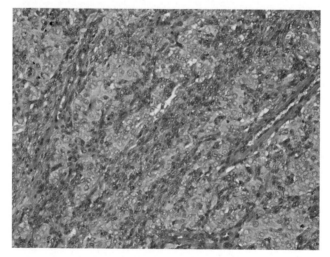

Figure 13.11 Endometrial stromal neoplasm with plump, epithelioid cells in a background of spindle cells. This finding has been described in tumors with t(10;17).

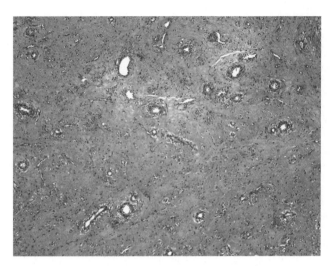

Figure 13.12 Metastatic low-grade endometrial stromal sarcoma showing myofibroblastic differentiation.

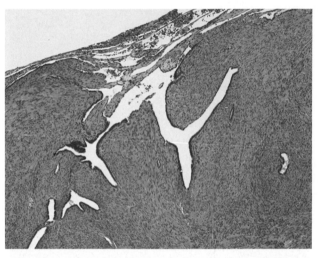

Figure 13.13 Metastatic low-grade endometrial stromal sarcoma with smooth muscle differentiation in lung. Note alveoli at the periphery and entrapment of non-neoplastic pulmonary glandular epithelium, which is typical of many metastatic mesenchymal tumors in lung. The uterine primary showed convincing evidence of endometrial stromal differentiation.

(i.e., those resembling proliferative phase endometrial stroma) and lacking smooth muscle differentiation only very rarely express desmin[7,15] and CD34. Diffuse desmin and h-caldesmon[15] expression supports smooth muscle differentiation. The Ki-67 labeling index usually falls below 10–15%.

The variant tumors usually demonstrate an immunophenotype that is concordant with the type of differentiation seen in the constituent non-stromal elements. For example, in an endometrial stromal sarcoma with smooth muscle differentiation, components resembling conventional endometrial stromal sarcoma express CD10 but not h-caldesmon; while components resembling smooth

Table 13.2 Ancillary diagnostic tests for endometrial stromal neoplasms

Diffuse expression of CD10 in most examples, but not all
Diffuse ER and PR nuclear expression
CD34 expression generally lacking
Desmin and h-caldesmon expression lacking in tumors without smooth muscle differentiation
Assays for t(7;17) or *JAZF1-JJAZ1* translocation

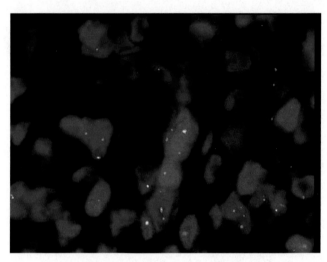

Figure 13.14 Fluorescence in situ hybridization. Reproduced with permission from Oliva E, de Leval L, Soslow RA, Herens C. High frequency of JAZF1-JJAZ1 gene fusion in endometrial stromal tumors with smooth muscle differentiation by interphase fluorescence in situ hybridization detection. *Am J Surg Pathol* 2007;**31**(8):1277–84, Fig. 2B.

muscle express h-caldesmon and lack CD10 or express it weakly. Variants showing sex cord differentiation often exhibit a variety of phenotypes; the areas resembling ovarian sex cord tumors typically coexpress keratins and smooth muscle actin, and sometimes show inhibin, calretinin, CD99, and desmin expression as well.

Approximately 50% of low-grade endometrial stromal sarcomas and stromal nodules possess a typical translocation, t(7p;17q), involving JAZF1and *JJAZ1* (the latter now referred to as *SUZ12*)[5]. The prevalence of this translocation is much lower in the fibroblastic variants[17] and in so-called high-grade endometrial stromal sarcoma[5]. Assays detecting this translocation include classical cytogenetics and fluorescence in situ hybridization (Figure 13.14). Reverse-transcription polymerase chain reaction has also been used to detect the translocation gene product. Alternate translocations that can be encountered include t(6p;7p) involving *PHF1* and *JAZF1*, t(6p;10q;10p) involving *PHF1* and *EPC1*[18], and t(10;17), involving *YWHAE* and *FAM22*[19].

DIFFERENTIAL DIAGNOSIS

The differential diagnosis of endometrial stromal neoplasms is featured in Table 13.3.

Endometrial stromal nodule

Low-grade endometrial stromal sarcomas and stromal nodules have identical histologic features. Like endometrial stromal sarcomas, stromal nodules may also display smooth muscle, fibroblastic, myofibroblastic, and sex cord–like differentiation. Endometrial stromal nodules are well-circumscribed tumors without significant myometrial invasion or any lymphovascular invasion (Figure 13.15); whereas stromal sarcomas are almost always diffusely infiltrative.

There are occasional examples of predominantly well-circumscribed nodules with minimal involvement of myometrium (Figure 13.16). Sections from the periphery of these tumors show up to three minor interdigitations at the tumor/myometrial junction and/or isolated tongues of tumor that protrude no more than 3 mm into myometrium[20]. Clinical follow-up for these kinds of cases is very limited, but the available evidence suggests that these tumors have more in common with stromal nodules than with stromal sarcomas. The term "endometrial stromal nodule with limited myometrial infiltration" is acceptable as long as the significance of the finding is described in the pathology report. Tumors with irregularities at the tumor/myometrial interface exceeding this are classified as endometrial stromal sarcoma.

Endometrial stromal nodules with smooth muscle differentiation can be confused with endometrial stromal sarcoma, especially when sections are taken through the center of the tumor instead of at the periphery. In these cases, the smooth muscle component of the nodule is mistaken for myometrium, leading to the erroneous conclusion that the stromal neoplasm has invaded myometrium (Figure 13.17). In general, the smooth muscle components of these stromal nodules are characterized by fibrillary, wispy, and disorganized smooth muscle fibers and myofibroblasts, or rounded, almost hyalizined, whorls. Myometrium, in contrast, is generally composed of thick, organized muscle bundles. Examination of tumor in a hysterectomy specimen allows mapping of the location of sections taken, and correlation between gross and

Table 13.3 Differential diagnosis of endometrial stromal sarcoma

Endometrial stromal nodule
Adenomyosis
Endometrial stromal breakdown
Undifferentiated endometrial sarcoma
Highly cellular leiomyoma
Intravenous leiomyomatosis
Spindle cell leiomyosarcoma
Epithelioid leiomyoma/sarcoma
Adenosarcoma
Uterine tumor resembling ovarian sex cord tumor (UTROSCT)
Solitary fibrous tumor/hemangiopericytoma

(A)

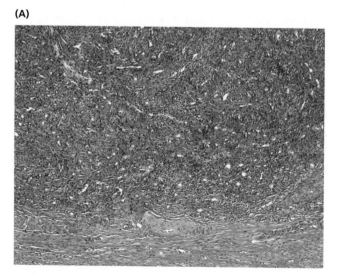

(B)

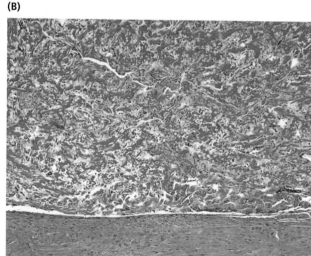

Figure 13.15 Endometrial stromal nodules. (A, B) Well-circumscribed proliferations of neoplastic endometrial stroma, can demonstrate the same range of variant morphologies as low-grade endometrial stromal sarcoma.

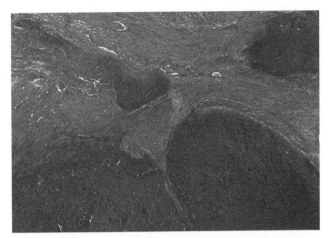

Figure 13.16 Endometrial stromal nodule with limited myometrial infiltration. This lesion, almost entirely well circumscribed, showed two foci of myometrial infiltration measuring no more than 3mm. No lymphovascular invasion was identified.

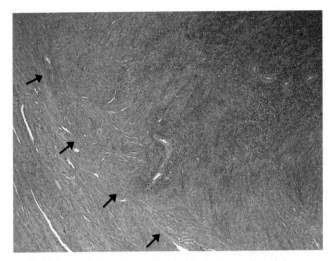

Figure 13.17 Endometrial stromal nodule with smooth muscle differentiation mimicking endometrial stromal sarcoma. Irregularly shaped zones of smooth muscle differentiation (to the right of the arrows) give the impression of myometrial invasion. This lesion, however, is well circumscribed and does not invade myometrium (left of arrows).

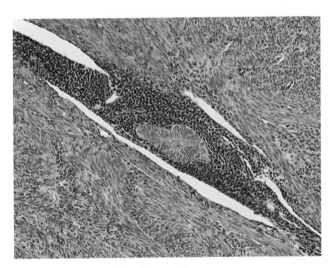

Figure 13.18 Intravascular adenomyosis.

microscopic characteristics. Sections of the tumor's periphery that include myometrium can be assessed for invasion, whether or not metaplastic smooth muscle is present. Distinguishing a stromal nodule with extensive smooth muscle differentiation and a myoinvasive endometrial stromal sarcoma can sometimes be impossible in curettage material and in myomectomy specimens that have been enucleated without a rim of uninvolved myometrium.

Non-neoplastic endometrial stroma

Adenomyosis in a hysterectomy specimen may lead to concern about the presence of an endometrial stromal neoplasm, especially if glands are sparse or absent; this pattern of adenomyosis typically occurs in postmenopausal

patients and is recognized by the absence of a definite mass. The stromal cells in gland-poor adenomyosis are typically atrophic. In addition, adenomyosis is generally surrounded by hypertrophic smooth muscle, which is typically not present in endometrial stromal sarcomas demonstrating myometrial permeation. Low-grade endometrial stromal sarcoma with endometrioid-like glandular differentiation may be more difficult to distinguish from prominent adenomyosis; however, the former is generally not associated with adjacent smooth muscle hypertrophy, and features more prominent stroma with the characteristic plexiform vascular network. The presence of prominent vascular invasion is an additional diagnostic clue. Intravascular adenomyosis (Figure 13.18) may be encountered occasionally, but this should not prompt a diagnosis of endometrial stromal sarcoma if the background myometrium shows typical adenomyosis. In almost all cases of benign endometrial stromal sarcoma mimics, the mimics are identified incidentally and the uterus has not been removed for a suspected mass lesion.

Endometrial stromal breakdown (Figure 13.19) or fragments of benign endometrial polyps may also suggest an endometrial stromal neoplasm in a curettage specimen. In contrast to endometrial stromal sarcoma, endometrial stromal breakdown is seldom found when the clinical scenario indicates the presence of a mass lesion. Histologically, fragments of compact stroma with associated fibrin are more consistent with endometrial stromal breakdown. The presence of compact, inactive stroma with thick-walled vessels

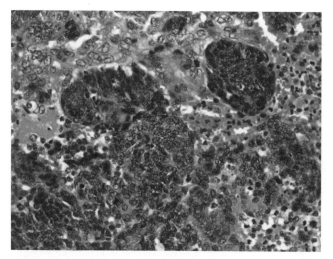

Figure 13.19 Endometrial stromal breakdown.

helps to distinguish a benign cellular endometrial polyp from a stromal neoplasm.

Undifferentiated endometrial sarcoma

It was previously reported that mitotic indices exceeding 10 MF/10 HPF separated low and high-grade endometrial stromal sarcomas, but when typical cytologic features of endometrial stroma are present and the tumor is confined to the uterus, mitotic index does *not* separate indolent from aggressive tumors (Tables 13.4 and 13.5). Sarcomas with or without an endometrial stromal sarcoma growth pattern that are highly cytologically atypical and mitotically active, and fail to show features commonly seen in differentiated uterine sarcomas such as leiomyosarcoma or adenosarcoma, are currently considered "undifferentiated endometrial sarcomas"[1,21]. Most undifferentiated endometrial sarcomas contain obviously pleomorphic tumor cells and are often referred to as "undifferentiated endometrial sarcomas with nuclear pleomorphism"[1]. These tumors are unrelated to low-grade endometrial stromal sarcoma, frequently harbor p53 mutations, and lack expression of CD10, ER, and PR[1].

Monomorphic variants of undifferentiated sarcoma have also been reported (Table 13.5)[2]. Some investigators have suggested that these "undifferentiated endometrial sarcomas with nuclear monomorphism" represent high-grade endometrial stromal sarcoma, but criteria for distinguishing these tumors from low-grade endometrial stromal sarcoma have not yet been confirmed in large studies. Emerging data suggest that these high-grade, monomorphic tumors have t(10;17), involving *YWHAE* and *FAM22,* may express CD10

Table 13.4 Pathologic characteristics of undifferentiated endometrial sarcoma with pleomorphism

Nuclear pleomorphism recognizable at scanning magnification

Mitotic index greater than 10 MF/10 HPF[a]

Focal, very weak or absent CD10, ER, and PR staining

p53 overexpression

Absence of benign or malignant glandular components (e.g., adenosarcoma or carcinosarcoma)

[a] Mitotic index greater than 10 MF/10 HPF is not an absolute criterion, as the occasional low-grade endometrial stromal sarcoma may exhibit mitotic activity in this range. Rather, a high mitotic index along with nuclear pleomorphism, large nuclear size, and focal, weak, or absent CD10, ER, and PR staining, with p53 overexpression, is characteristic of undifferentiated endometrial sarcoma.

Table 13.5 Pathologic characteristics of undifferentiated endometrial sarcoma with monomorphism

Uniform cells at scanning magnification

Mitotic index greater than 10 MF/10 HPF[a]

Large nuclei with irregular contours

Only patchy CD10, ER, and PR expression, particularly in more spindle cells

Absence of benign or malignant glandular components (e.g., adenosarcoma or carcinosarcoma)

YWHAE rearrangement

[a] Mitotic index greater than 10 MF/10 HPF is not an absolute criterion, as the occasional low-grade endometrial stromal sarcoma may exhibit mitotic activity in this range. Rather, a high mitotic index along with large nuclear size, and focal, weak, or absent CD10, and PR staining, with p53 overexpression, is characteristic of undifferentiated endometrial sarcoma.

and ER/PR, but levels of expression are relatively deficient compared to usual low-grade endometrial stromal sarcoma[19]. Despite the nuclear uniformity in undifferentiated endometrial sarcoma with nuclear monomorphism, the mitotic index is significantly in excess of 10 MF/10 HPF, the absolute nuclear size is increased relative to proliferative phase endometrium and low-grade endometrial stromal sarcoma, and tumor cell necrosis is almost always present (Figure 13.20). Anecdotal data suggest that Ki-67 indices significantly exceed 15% in undifferentiated sarcomas. Rare examples of undifferentiated sarcomas arising in a background of low-grade endometrial stromal sarcoma have been reported (so-called dedifferentiated stromal sarcoma)[3]. The clinical outcomes for both pleomorphic and monomorphic undifferentiated endometrial sarcomas are substantially worse than for low-grade endometrial stromal

(A)

(B)

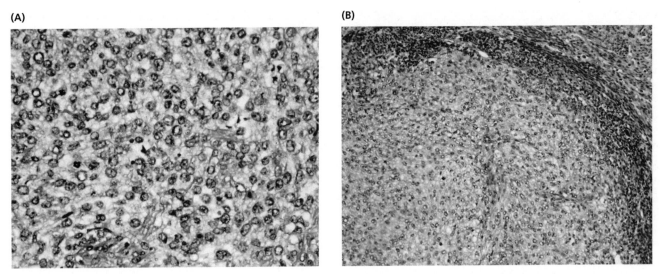

Figure 13.20 Undifferentiated endometrial sarcoma with monomorphic features (A), associated with low-grade endometrial stromal sarcoma at its periphery (B).

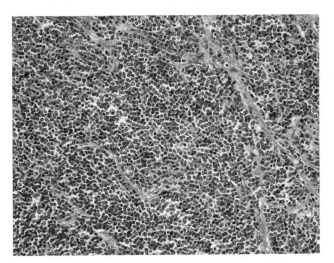

Figure 13.21 Undifferentiated carcinoma lacking characteristic endometrial stromal sarcoma vasculature. Immunohistochemical stains (not shown) demonstrated evidence of epithelial differentiation.

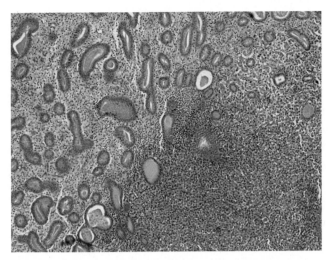

Figure 13.22 Metastatic lobular carcinoma in endometrial stroma.

sarcoma, with presentation at high stage, early recurrence, and frequent mortality being common[1].

Undifferentiated carcinoma

Undifferentiated carcinoma often grows in solid sheets, with dyshesive tumor cells that may resemble lymphoma, plasmacytoma, or rhabdoid tumor cells (Figure 13.21)[22–23]. The appearance of a diffuse, malignant, small-to-intermediate cell neoplasm may also prompt consideration for endometrial stromal sarcoma or undifferentiated endometrial sarcoma. The strikingly high mitotic rate, without the characteristic endometrial stromal sarcoma vasculature, permits

distinction from endometrial stromal sarcoma. Immunohistochemical evidence of epithelial differentiation, when present, permits differentiation from undifferentiated endometrial sarcoma. Immunohistochemically, rare cells express EMA or CK18 strongly, but most cells lack an obviously epithelial phenotype. Metastatic lobular breast carcinoma (Figure 13.22) typically also features a monomorphic appearance, but strong expression of cytokeratin, ER, and PR is typical.

Highly cellular leiomyoma and leiomyosarcoma

Highly cellular leiomyomas characteristically display at least focal fascicular architecture with more abundant eosinophilic

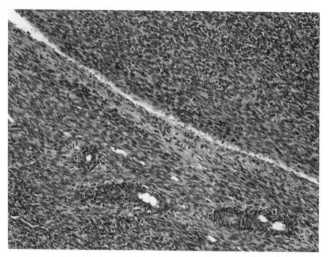

Figure 13.23 Highly cellular leiomyomas may superficially resemble an endometrial stromal tumor, but frequently feature thick-walled vessels, clefted spaces, and fascicular growth patterns; all of which are less commonly encountered in endometrial stromal tumors.

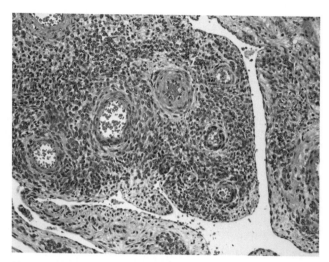

Figure 13.24 Intravenous leiomyomatosis may simulate endometrial stromal sarcoma on gross examination, but microscopically will show more prominent cleft-like spaces and thick-walled vessels.

cytoplasm, have a cleft-like zone at their periphery, and contain thick-walled blood vessels (Figure 13.23)[13]. Smooth muscle tumors may also contain numerous mast cells, which are uncommon in endometrial stromal neoplasms. Uterine leiomyosarcoma is almost never a cytologically low-grade neoplasm, in contrast to endometrial stromal neoplasms. Immunohistochemically, CD10 expression without desmin or h-caldesmon expression supports endometrial stromal differentiation, but staining with SMA can be encountered in both tumor types. Any convincing desmin or h-caldesmon staining, with or without CD10, supports smooth muscle differentiation. The presence of t(7;17) would also support an endometrial stromal neoplasm.

Intravenous leiomyomatosis and leiomyosarcoma

Vessel invasion is characteristic of intravenous leiomyomatosis (Figure 13.24) and is frequently found in endometrial stromal sarcoma and leiomyosarcoma. Intravenous leiomyomatosis resembles leiomyoma or highly cellular leiomyoma; while leiomyosarcoma is almost always a histologically high-grade tumor. Immunohistochemical studies, as detailed previously, will help distinguish cellular variants from endometrial stromal sarcoma.

Epithelioid smooth muscle tumor

Epithelioid smooth muscle tumors can resemble endometrial stromal neoplasms when tumor cells are rounded

instead of spindled. As compared to endometrial stromal sarcoma, epithelioid smooth muscle neoplasms are composed of larger cells with more abundant pink cytoplasm, and they lack the characteristic vasculature of endometrial stromal tumors. Thick-walled vessels are almost always present. The nuclei are typically more rounded and centrally positioned in epithelioid smooth muscle tumors. However, endometrial stromal tumors with epithelioid cells may be particularly difficult to distinguish from an epithelioid smooth muscle tumor in a limited uterine sampling. Immunohistochemistry can be helpful for this differential diagnosis, although epithelioid smooth muscle tumors may lack desmin and/or h-caldesmon expression. The differential diagnosis of epithelioid mesenchymal tumors also includes PEComa (perivascular epithelioid cell tumor); this entity is discussed elsewhere (Chapter 12).

Mullerian adenosarcoma

The stromal component of adenosarcoma can be morphologically and immunohistochemically identical to endometrial stromal sarcoma, leading to difficulties distinguishing these entities, especially in a limited uterine sampling specimen. When sufficient tumor tissue is present for evaluation, adenosarcoma can be recognized by the presence of a more variable appearance of the epithelial component, often with cystically dilated glands, while the glands in stromal sarcomas are generally few and haphazardly placed. Most importantly, adenosarcomas

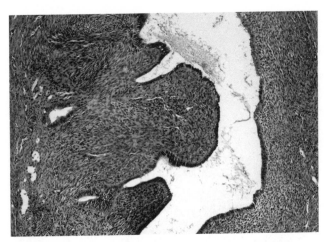

Figure 13.25 Low-grade mullerian adenosarcoma. The stromal component of these tumors resembles endometrial stromal sarcoma. Adenosarcoma can be diagnosed in the presence of phyllodes-like architecture and subepithelial stromal condensation.

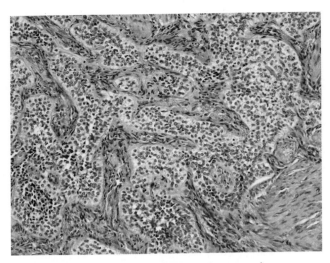

Figure 13.26 Uterine tumor resembling ovarian sex cord tumor. Conventional endometrial stromal differentiation is absent.

have, at least focally, a phyllodes-like appearance, with stroma condensing around epithelium with a leaf-like growth pattern (Figure 13.25). This pattern is absent in endometrial stromal sarcoma.

Uterine tumor resembling ovarian sex cord tumor

Endometrial stromal tumors can display prominent, even extensive, sex cord–like differentiation. These tumors essentially always retain an appreciable component of endometrial stromal tumor cells. In contrast, UTROSCT is, by definition, devoid of endometrial stromal differentiation (Figure 13.26)[24]. When so defined, UTROSCTs are mostly, but not exclusively, well-circumscribed tumors (like endometrial stromal nodule), with very limited recurring potential. Sex cord–like areas in endometrial stromal tumors and UTROSCT would both be expected to show varying combinations of CD10, inhibin, cytokeratin, desmin, and SMA expression. The translocation t(7;17) has not been detected in UTROSCT[24].

Solitary fibrous tumor/hemangiopericytoma

From a theoretical standpoint, most tumors previously thought to represent uterine hemangiopericytomas are, in fact, endometrial stromal tumors. However, rare solitary fibrous tumors probably do arise in the uterus on occasion. In extrauterine sites, particularly lung and

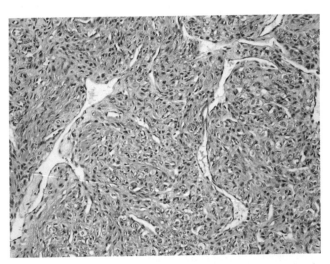

Figure 13.27 Solitary fibrous tumor. This lesion may be confused with metastatic endometrial stromal sarcoma because of its cellularity and pericytomatous vessels. However, there are morphologic and also immunohistochemical differences between these two entities. Alternating cellular and sclerotic zones may be seen in both tumors, but they are more common in solitary fibrous tumor. CD34 marks most solitary fibrous tumors and it is almost always absent in endometrial stromal sarcoma.

retroperitoneum, this differential diagnosis has practical importance; endometrial stromal sarcoma, solitary fibrous tumor, and hemangiopericytoma may all demonstrate fibroblast-like cells, with collagen deposition and staghorn vessels (Figure 13.27). Further adding to confusion is the expression of CD10 and PR in solitary fibrous tumor/ hemangiopericytoma. Unlike stromal sarcoma, however, the vast majority of solitary fibrous tumors/hemangiopericytomas expresses CD34 and are ER negative[11].

REFERENCES

1. Chang KL, Crabtree GS, Lim-Tan SK, Kempson RL, Hendrickson MR. Primary uterine endometrial stromal neoplasms. A clinicopathologic study of 117 cases. *Am J Surg Pathol* 1990;**14**:415–38.

2. Kurihara S, Oda Y, Ohishi Y, *et al.* Endometrial stromal sarcomas and related high-grade sarcomas: immunohistochemical and molecular genetic study of 31 cases. *Am J Surg Pathol* 2008; **32**(8):1228–38.

3. Malpica A, Deavers MT, Silva EG. High-grade sarcoma in endometrial stromal sarcoma: dedifferentiated endometrial stromal sarcoma. *Mod Pathol* 2006;**19**(Suppl 1):188A.

4. Oliva E, Clement PB, Young RH, Scully RE. Mixed endometrial stromal and smooth muscle tumors of the uterus – a clinicopathologic study of 15 cases. *Am J Surg Pathol* 1998;**22**:997–1005.

5. Koontz JI, Soreng AL, Nucci M, *et al.* Frequent fusion of the JAZF1 and JJAZ1 genes in endometrial stromal tumors. *Proc Natl Acad Sci USA* 2001;**98**(11):6348–53.

6. Oliva E, de Leval L, Soslow RA, Herens C. High frequency of JAZF1-JJAZ1 gene fusion in endometrial stromal tumors with smooth muscle differentiation by interphase FISH detection. *Am J Surg Pathol* 2007;**31**(8):1277–84.

7. Yilmaz A, Rush DS, Soslow RA. Endometrial stromal sarcomas with unusual histologic features: a report of 24 primary and metastatic tumors emphasizing fibroblastic and smooth muscle differentiation. *Am J Surg Pathol* 2002;**26**(9):1142–50.

8. Chu PG, Arber DA, Weiss LM, Chang KL. Utility of CD10 in distinguishing between endometrial stromal sarcoma and uterine smooth muscle tumors: an immunohistochemical comparison of 34 cases. *Mod Pathol* 2001;**14**(5):465–71.

9. Oliva E, Young RH, Amin MB, Clement PB. An immunohistochemical analysis of endometrial stromal and smooth muscle tumors of the uterus – a study of 54 cases emphasizing the importance of using a panel because of overlap in immunoreactivity for individual antibodies. *Am J Surg Pathol* 2002;**26**(4):403–12.

10. McCluggage WG, Sumathi VP, Maxwell P. CD10 is a sensitive and diagnostically useful immunohistochemical marker of normal endometrial stroma and of endometrial stromal neoplasms. *Histopathology* 2001;**39**(3):273–8.

11. Bhargava R, Shia J, Hummer AJ, *et al.* Distinction of endometrial stromal sarcomas from 'hemangiopericytomatous' tumors using a panel of immunohistochemical stains. *Mod Pathol* 2005; **18**(1):40–7.

12. Jung CK, Jung JH, Lee A, *et al.* Diagnostic use of nuclear beta-catenin expression for the assessment of endometrial stromal tumors. *Mod Pathol* 2008;**21**(6):756–63.

13. Oliva E, Young RH, Clement PB, Bhan AK, Scully RE. Cellular benign mesenchymal tumors of the uterus: a comparative morphologic and immunohistochemical analysis of 33 highly cellular leiomyomas and six endometrial stromal nodules, two frequently confused tumors. *Am J Surg Pathol* 1995;**19**:757–68.

14. Moinfar F, Regitnig P, Tabrizi AD, Denk H, Tavassoli FA. Expression of androgen receptors in benign and malignant endometrial stromal neoplasms. *Virchows Arch* 2004;**444**(5):410–14.

15. Rush DS, Tan JY, Baergen RN, Soslow RA. h-Caldesmon, a novel smooth muscle-specific antibody, distinguishes between cellular leiomyoma and endometrial stromal sarcoma. *Am J Surg Pathol* 2001;**25**(2):253–8.

16. Nucci MR, O'Connell JT, Huettner PC, *et al.* h-Caldesmon expression effectively distinguishes endometrial stromal tumors from uterine smooth muscle tumors. *Am J Surg Pathol* 2001;**25**(4): 455–63.

17. Huang HY, Ladanyi M, Soslow RA. Molecular detection of JAZF1-JJAZ1 gene fusion in endometrial stromal neoplasms with classic and variant histology: evidence for genetic heterogeneity. *Am J Surg Pathol* 2004;**28**(2):224–32.

18. Micci F, Panagopoulos I, Bjerkehagen B, Heim S. Consistent rearrangement of chromosomal band 6p21 with generation of fusion genes *JAZF1/PHF1* and *EPC1/PHF1* in endometrial stromal sarcoma. *Cancer Res* 2006;**66**(1):107–12.

19. Lee CH, Marino-Enriquez A, van de Rijn M, *et al.* The histologic features of endometrial stromal sarcomas characterized by *YWHAE* rearrangement – distinction from usual low-grade endometrial stromal sarcoma with *JAZF1* rearrangement. *Mod Pathol* 2011;**24**: 255A (abstract 1081).

20. Dionigi A, Oliva E, Clement PB, Young RH. Endometrial stromal nodules and endometrial stromal tumors with limited infiltration – a clinicopathologic study of 50 cases. *Am J Surg Pathol* 2002; **26**(5):567–81.

21. Evans HL. Endometrial stromal sarcoma and poorly differentiated endometrial sarcoma. *Cancer* 1982;**50**:2170–82.

22. Tafe LJ, Garg K, Chew I, Tornos C, Soslow RA. Endometrial and ovarian carcinomas with undifferentiated components: clinically aggressive and frequently underrecognized neoplasms. *Mod Pathol* 2010;**23**(6):781–9.

23. Altrabulsi B, Malpica A, Deavers MT, *et al.* Undifferentiated carcinoma of the endometrium. *Am J Surg Pathol* 2005;**29**(10): 1316–21.

24. Staats PN, Garcia JJ, Dias-Santagata DC, *et al.* Uterine tumors resembling ovarian sex cord tumors (UTROSCT) lack the JAZF1-JJAZ1 translocation frequently seen in endometrial stromal tumors. *Am J Surg Pathol* 2009;**33**(8):1206–12.

14 OTHER UTERINE MESENCHYMAL TUMORS

INTRODUCTION

Endometrial stromal and smooth muscle proliferations are the most common mesenchymal proliferations in the uterus and, when combined, account for the vast majority of mesenchymal uterine processes in the cervix and corpus. However, there are a number of other mesenchymal lesions that the pathologist may encounter, either in the curettage or, more commonly, in the hysterectomy specimen. Most of these are benign, but occasionally lesions with intermediate or frankly malignant clinical behavior may also occur.

UTERINE TUMOR RESEMBLING OVARIAN SEX CORD TUMOR

Uterine tumors resembling ovarian sex cord tumor (UTROSCTs) are rare tumors that continue to pose diagnostic challenges for pathologists. Since Clement and Scully first drew attention to this group of unusual neoplasms, they have been variously grouped with the endometrial stromal, smooth muscle, or "other" categories of uterine mesenchymal tumors[1]. Because they do not clearly exhibit smooth muscle or stromal features, we place them in the "other" category unless they exhibit significant endometrial stromal elements. Tumors with any significant endometrial stromal component are grouped with endometrial stromal tumors and classified as benign or malignant depending on the presence of infiltrative margins and/or vascular invasion (see Chapter 13).

Clinical characteristics

Uterine tumors resembling ovarian sex cord tumor occur in the reproductive and postmenopausal age groups. The clinical presentation is similar to that of uterine smooth muscle tumors. Patients often present with a uterine mass, abnormal vaginal bleeding, and/or pelvic pain. Some patients are asymptomatic.

Most UTROSCTs are confined to the uterus at presentation and are clinically benign. Rare recurrences have been reported at intervals of 2–12 years. Most of these clinically more aggressive tumors have been associated with serosal rupture, a predominance of endometrial stroma (and thus, likely represent endometrial stromal sarcoma), prominent vascular invasion, and cytologic atypia. Few UTROSCTs have been sufficiently studied to know whether they have additional morphologic features that would reliably predict aggressive behavior. Given the absence of data, we use the same criteria for distinguishing stromal nodule from endometrial stroma sarcoma for these tumors: that is, only tumors with circumscribed borders, a low mitotic index, and uniform, cytologically bland cells should be diagnosed as UTROSCT. All others should either be grouped with endometrial stromal sarcoma or, if high grade, with undifferentiated endometrial sarcoma.

Morphology

Gross pathology

Most tumors are myometrial-based, solid, and well-circumscribed masses arising within the uterine corpus. Occasional tumors form submucosal or subserosal polypoid masses, similar to smooth muscle tumors. Rare tumors are predominantly cystic. Depending on the lipid content, the sectioned surface may be tan and firm, or yellow and soft. Necrosis and hemorrhage are uncommon.

Microscopic pathology

The constituent cells are arranged in cords, hollow tubules, trabeculae, and/or sheets resembling sex cord elements (adult granulosa cell or Sertoli cell tumors) (Figures 14.1 and 14.2) or, in some cases, glandular epithelial elements (endometrioid tumor) (Figure 14.3). The cells typically have scanty cytoplasm, indistinct cell margins, and round

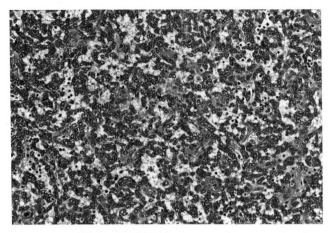

Figure 14.1 UTROSCT. Sex cord elements are reminiscent of cords seen in some granulosa cell tumors.

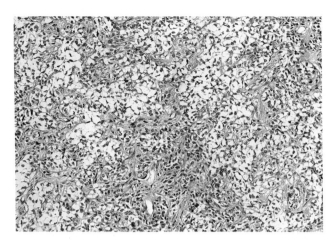

Figure 14.2 UTROSCT. Sertoliform pattern.

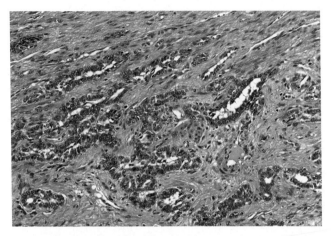

Figure 14.3 UTROSCT. Glandular pattern.

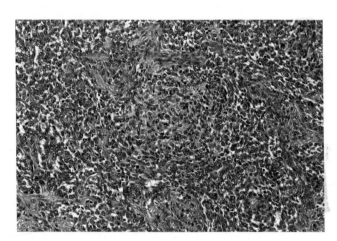

Figure 14.4 UTROSCT. Cells are small and uniform and show no significant mitotic activity.

(A)

(B)

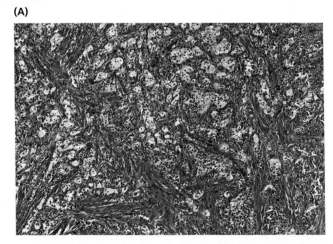

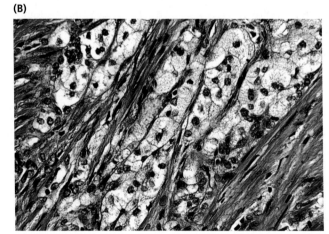

Figure 14.5 UTROSCT (A) Prominent foam cell pattern. (B) The cells resemble foamy histiocytes.

nuclei (Figure 14.4). In some tumors, however, the constituent cells may have abundant eosinophilic, clear, or foamy cytoplasm (Figure 14.5). Despite the resemblance to granulosa cell elements, nuclear grooves may not be conspicuous. Mitotic figures are rare or absent. The stroma between the epithelioid structures varies from paucicellular and fibroblastic to an appearance similar to normal myometrium (Figure 14.6). A significant endometrial stromal

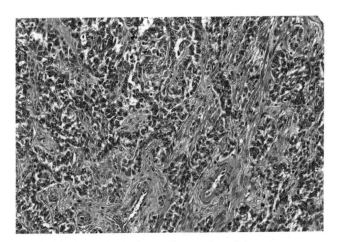

Figure 14.6 UTROSCT. Background mesenchymal tissue demonstrates smooth muscle differentiation.

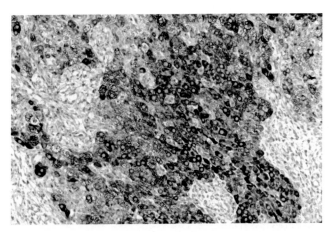

Figure 14.7 Inhibin expression in UTROSCT.

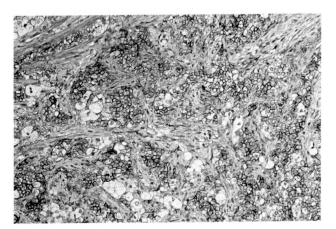

Figure 14.8 Cytokeratin expression in UTROSCT.

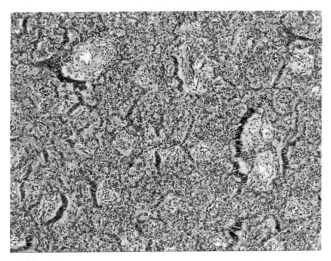

Figure 14.9 Low-grade endometrial stromal sarcoma with sex cord elements.

component should be absent, unless entrapped by the tumor. Hyaline matrix may be prominent. Although most tumors have pushing margins, vascular intrusion has been observed in rare cases. This latter feature, if focal and confined to the vicinity of the main tumor, does not appear to confer an adverse prognosis.

Ancillary diagnostic tests

The cells composing the sex cord–like areas are often calretinin and/or inhibin positive (Figure 14.7), and may express keratin (Figure 14.8), smooth muscle actin, or desmin, or a combination thereof [1,56]. Other markers reported to be positive in these tumors include CD99, Melan-A, WT1, CD10, h-caldesmon, and smooth muscle myosin heavy chain. Most tumors express ER and PR. Uterine tumors resembling ovarian sex cord tumor do not exhibit the t(7;17) translocation resulting in a *JAZF1-JJAZ1* gene fusion that occurs in endometrial stromal neoplasms[7].

Differential diagnosis

The chief differential diagnosis is endometrial stromal sarcoma and, on occasion, endometrial carcinoma with spindled, corded, and nested elements.

Endometrial stromal tumor (endometrial stromal nodule, endometrial stromal sarcoma)

Endometrial stromal tumors may contain glands and sex cord–like elements, but these are generally a small component of the neoplasm, whereas UTROSCTs are composed almost entirely of sex cord–like structures. In fact, in the majority of UTROSCTs, the resemblance to an ovarian sex cord stromal tumor is so striking that the pathologist may initially question whether the tumor is of uterine origin. Problems arise when occasional endometrial stromal tumors exhibit a more pronounced complement of sex cord–like structures (Figure 14.9),

(A)

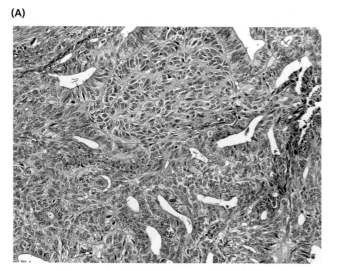

(B)

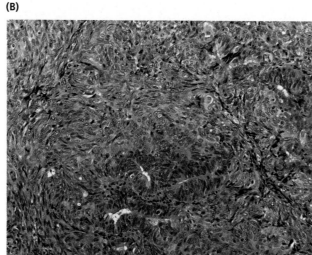

Figure 14.10 (A, B) Low-grade endometrioid adenocarcinoma with corded elements

or when occasional suspected UTROSCTs contain cellular areas resembling endometrial stromal cells. If the problematic tumor is well circumscribed, cytologically banal, and shows no evidence of vascular invasion, the distinction between an endometrial stromal tumor (which in this situation would be a benign stromal nodule) and UTROSCT is probably inconsequential in terms of patient prognosis and treatment. However, to prevent misdiagnosis of a potentially malignant, albeit low-grade endometrial stromal sarcoma, we limit the diagnosis of UTROSCT to tumors that do not exhibit any of the features typically associated with stromal sarcoma; tumors that exhibit the presence of a significant component of endometrial stroma are diagnosed as either endometrial stromal sarcoma or, if well circumscribed after assiduous sampling, as stromal nodule.

Since the diagnosis of UTROSCT requires no clear-cut areas of endometrial stromal neoplasia, extensive sampling is mandatory to identify any area with the pattern of typical endometrial stromal neoplasia. The distinction is important, as patients with a UTROSCT as defined here appear to have an excellent prognosis if completely excised[1,2].

Endometrioid adenocarcinoma with spindled, corded, and nested elements

Endometrioid adenocarcinomas with corded and nested elements may resemble UTROSCTs (Figure 14.10). Most of such tumors also harbor large areas of squamous or morular differentiation, which is not a feature of UTROSCT. Immunohistochemistry can help distinguish UTROSCT from adenocarcinoma. Like endometrioid

adenocarcinomas, UTROSCTs may express cytokeratins and hormone receptors, but they also express inhibin and calretinin – markers that are only very seldom expressed in carcinomas.

Adenofibroma/adenosarcoma

Adenofibroma and adenosarcoma contain benign and, most often, cystically dilated glands uniformly distributed throughout the tumor, rather than the cords, trabeculae, or tubules characteristic of sex cord–like tumors. In addition, a papillary architecture is often seen in adenofibroma/adenosarcoma, but is absent in UTROSCT. Moreover, the stroma in UTROSCT is paucicellular and cytologically banal; while, in adenosarcoma, the stroma is cellular and mitotically active, and the spindled stromal cells form a concentric, entrapping layer around the dilated glands.

Epithelioid smooth muscle tumor

Epithelioid leiomyoma with a prominent plexiform pattern (Figure 14.11) may superficially resemble UTROSCT, but the sex cord elements – cords, trabeculae, hollow tubules, retiform structures, and prominent foam cells – are much more pronounced in UTROSCT, and the smooth muscle cells are often inconspicuous. In addition, epithelioid smooth muscle tumors are generally more cellular and impart a more uniform, monomorphous appearance than UTROSCT. Diffuse expression for smooth muscle markers desmin and h-caldesmon favors a smooth muscle neoplasm; while coexpression of muscle markers with inhibin and calretinin favors UTROSCT[5,6,8]. Both can coexpress cytokeratin, hormone receptors, and CD10.

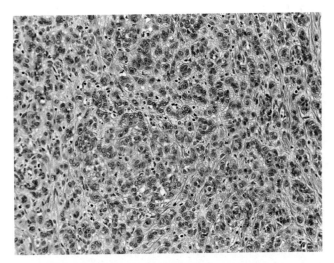

Figure 14.11 Plexiform smooth muscle tumor.

PLEXIFORM TUMORLET

Plexiform tumorlets are small aggregates of epithelioid mesenchymal cells that appear to represent smooth muscle, although occasional examples are positive for CD10 as well as desmin (Figure 14.12). They often occur along the endo-myometrial junction and are often incidental findings in curettage specimens. Occasionally, tumorlets arise deeper in the myometrium (Figure 14.13). They may be single or multiple. When multiple nodules are present in an endometrial sampling, they may pose concern for a more extensive smooth muscle or endometrial stromal proliferation, but the small size and circumscription are typically apparent even in limited samplings. Plexiform tumorlets are benign.

(A)   (B)

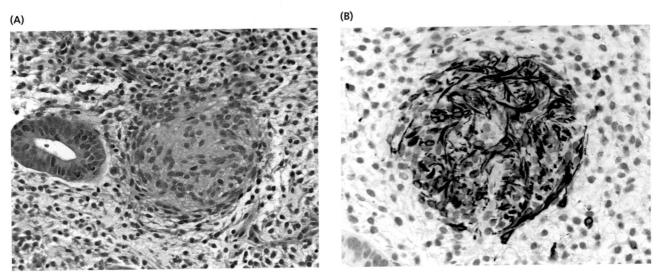

Figure 14.12 (A) Tumorlet in endometrial curettage (B) Desmin highlights spindle cells.

(A)   (B)

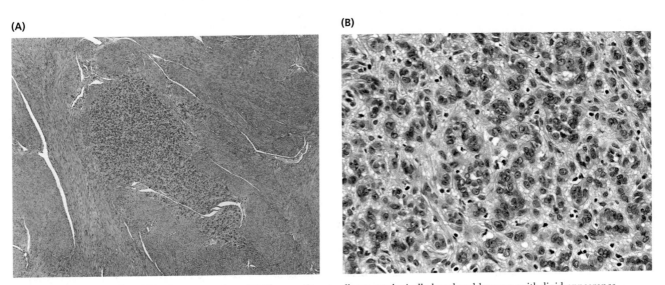

Figure 14.13 (A) Tumorlet within the myometrium. (B) The constituent cells are cytologically banal and have an epithelioid appearance.

MISCELLANEOUS UTERINE MESENCHYMAL TUMORS

A variety of other benign and malignant mesenchymal tumors other than smooth muscle and endometrial stromal have been reported in the uterus. Most of the benign tumors are rarely encountered and of little clinical consequence, but they may pose difficulty for the pathologist due to unusual presentation and/or mimicry of more common uterine mesenchymal tumors. The cervix is the more commonly affected site. For convenience, both cervix and corpus sites are discussed together.

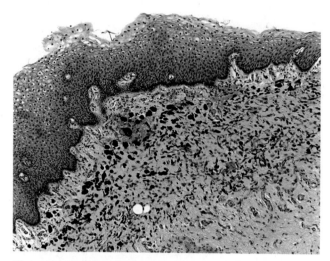

Figure 14.14 Spindle cell blue nevus in cervix.

MISCELLANEOUS BENIGN MESENCHYMAL TUMORS

Blue nevus

Common spindle and, rarely, cellular blue nevi occur in the cervix and corpus of the uterus. The common spindle cell nevus is usually seen in the cervix, ranges from 0.1 to 2.0 cm in size, is blue to gray in coloration, and is usually solitary, although multiple lesions have been reported[9]. Many are incidental findings in biopsy, curettage, or hysterectomy specimens performed for another unrelated condition; incidental involvement of endometrial stroma in an endometrial curettage specimen has been reported. Microscopically, blue nevi consist of fascicles of spindle, dendritic melanocytes associated with pigmented macrophages (Figure 14.14). The less common cellular variant has been reported in the cervix and corpus, and is also small, being discovered in uteri removed for leiomyomas. The cellular variant contains some spindle cells, but, in addition, there are prominent epithelioid cells with clear cytoplasm; both cell types contain intracytoplasmic melanin[10]. As in the cutaneous cellular blue nevus, the nuclei of the tumor cells are either rounded or elongate with minimal atypia; intranuclear inclusions may be seen, but nucleoli are inconspicuous and mitotic figures are rare or absent. Both types are positive for S100 protein (Figure 14.15); the cellular variant will often also express HMB45 and other melanocytic markers[10]. Mucosal melanosis is more often detected clinically; it is not a true neoplasm, but consists of pigmentation of the basal epithelial cells, with or without basal melanocytes[11]. A pigmented myomatous neurocristoma of the uterus composed of pigmented and non-pigmented melanocytes

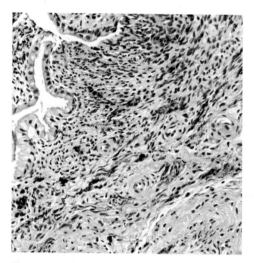

Figure 14.15 S100 protein in blue nevus.

in a matrix of altered smooth-muscle cells has also been reported[12]. All are clinically benign.

Glomus tumor

Glomus tumor has been observed in the cervix and uterus[13]. The cervical tumors, when described, are small, situated deep in the cervical wall, and asymptomatic; only one was recognized on macroscopic exam. The histologic features are the same as elsewhere in the body; the typical nesting pattern and uniform, cytologically bland small cells can be confused with a well-differentiated neuroendocrine tumor, but positive immunohistochemical studies with smooth muscle actin on the one hand and chromogranin and synaptophysin on the other will resolve this problem.

On occasion, uterine leiomyomas may assume a particularly prominent vascular pattern resembling

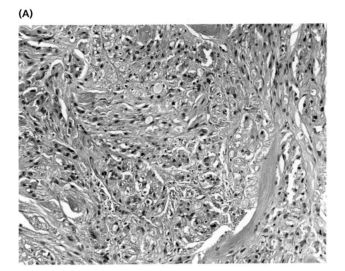

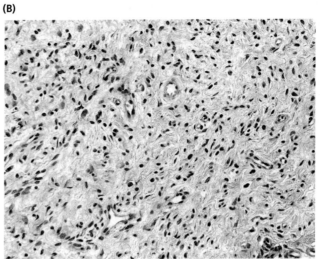

Figure 14.16 (A) Schwannoma in cervix. (B) Neurofibroma.

glomangiomyoma and angiomyoma, respectively. We consider these tumors to be variants of uterine smooth muscle tumors and do not separately classify them.

Lipoma

More than two-dozen pure lipomas have been reported in the uterus, most of which occurred in postmenopausal women. The uterine corpus is the most commonly affected site, and the clinical symptoms and physical signs are similar to those associated with leiomyomas. Most of the reported cases are postoperative diagnoses in hysterectomy specimens removed for suspected leiomyomas. In recent years, computed tomography and magnetic resonance imaging studies have assisted in the preoperative diagnosis[14]. Rarely, spindle cell lipoma may arise in the cervix[15].

Myxoma

Intrauterine myxoma may rarely occur in association with Carney's complex. An unusual "myxoid uterine leiomyoma" and an "unusual mesenchymal cervical neoplasm" have been reported in patients with Carney's syndrome[16]. Benign myxoid change may also be seen in the myometrium and cervical stroma unassociated with Carney's syndrome[17].

Nerve sheath tumors (benign)

Schwannomas, neurofibromas, and plexiform neurofibromas can arise in the uterus, but the frequency is at the case report level. The cervix is preferentially involved

(Figure 14.16). The histologic features are similar to those of their soft tissue counterparts. Some of the schwannomas have been pigmented[18]. The plexiform neurofibromas have been associated with NF1.

Rhabdomyoma

Rhabdomyoma rarely occurs in the cervix and corpus. The lesion is similar to fetal rhabdomyoma encountered elsewhere. Lesional tissue contains spindle cells with abundant eosinophilic cytoplasm, and regular vesicular nuclei with conspicuous nucleoli. The cytoplasm of the cells is rich in longitudinal myofibrils, and cross-striations are readily seen (Figure 14.17). Mitotic figures are absent.

Solitary fibrous tumor

Rare examples of solitary fibrous tumor have been reported in the uterine cervix and corpus[19,20]. All of the reported cases had classic features: bland spindle cells arranged in a patternless pattern, interspersed ropy collagen, branching "stag horn" vessels, CD34 positivity, etc. Solitary fibrous tumor in the uterus has been associated with production of high-molecular-weight insulin-like growth factor II. All followed a benign clinical course.

Vascular tumors

Hemangiomas can arise at all levels of the uterus and cervix, including endometrium, myometrium, and serosa[21]. Most corpus hemangiomas diffusely involve the myometrium.

(A)

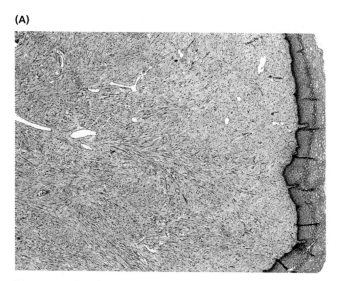

(B)

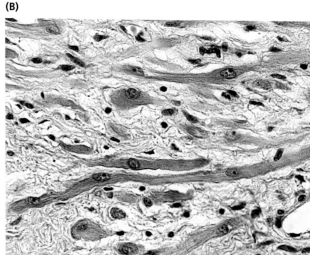

Figure 14.17 (A, B) Cervicovaginal rhabdomyoma.

(A)

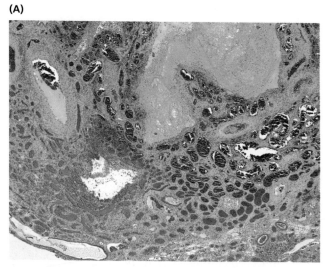

(B)

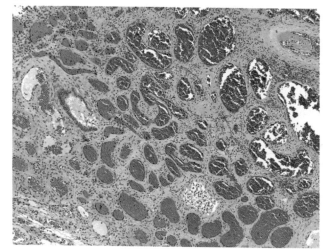

Figure 14.18 (A, B) Hemangioma arising in endometrial polyp.

Both cavernous and, less commonly, capillary or spindle cell subtypes are seen (Figure 14.18). Patients may present with vaginal bleeding and obstetric complications, ranging from infertility to maternal and fetal demise from pronounced bleeding of the gravid uterus. Most patients are asymptomatic and the hemangiomas are found incidentally. Despite the reported complications, many patients have had successful vaginal or cesarean deliveries even in the presence of extensive myometrial involvement. Because of the variable clinical manifestations, the appropriate treatment for uterine hemangiomas is unclear. Although hysterectomy is the primary mode of therapy in most symptomatic cases, conservative treatment has been advocated for all others. Estrogen receptors have been identified in the endothelial cells of the hemangiomas.

Arteriovenous malformations (AVMs) are exceedingly rare in the uterus[22]. Congenital arteriovenous malformations are the result of abnormal development of primitive blood vessels, resulting in connections between pelvic arteries and veins in the uterus without an intervening capillary bed. The most common clinical presentation is abnormal uterine bleeding, which may be aggravated by therapeutic curettage. Three-dimensional CT angiography can be helpful in identifying the underlying lesions. Embolization followed by surgical excision has been performed for rare cases of refractory and diffuse cervicovaginal and uterine lesions.

True congenital arteriovenous malformation should be distinguished from acquired arteriovenous fistula or arteriovenous shunt, which consists of communications between the uterine arteries and myometrial veins, secondary to another pathologic condition or an iatrogenic event.

Uterine lymphangioma is extremely rare; theoretically, capillary or cavernous types could occur, but reported cases have exhibited a cavernous pattern[23]. These tumors are recognized on the basis of expression of lymphatic endothelial markers, such as D2-40/podoplanin. An unusual lymphangiomatous-like growth pattern of vascular and lymphatic channels has been reported in the uterus in blue rubber bleb nevus syndrome[24].

MISCELLANEOUS MESENCHYMAL LESIONS WITH INTERMEDIATE CLINICAL BEHAVIOR

Gastrointestinal stromal tumor

Primary gastrointestinal stromal tumor is rare in the uterine corpus. Several cases have been reported, at least two of which have been confirmed by mutational analysis[25,26]. Patients have been older – the two patients with *KIT* mutations were 74 and 77 years of age – and had no evidence of gastrointestinal tract involvement. The tumors appeared to be attached to the posterior uterine fundus in both cases, analogous to subserosal leiomyoma. One tumor ruptured. Both had spindle cell morphology with minimal atypia and low mitotic index (3–4 MF/50 HPF). As in the gastrointestinal tract, the tumor cells in uterine gastrointestinal stromal tumors are positive for CD117 (c-kit), CD34, and likely DOG1, but negative for desmin (although rare gastrointestinal stromal tumors may show focal desmin expression). Derivation from primitive mesenchymal cells or, perhaps, rare CD117-positive interstitial Cajal-like mesenchymal cells within the myometrium has been proposed.

Inflammatory myofibroblastic tumor

This lesion has been reported to occur in the uterus[27]. The classic lesion is characterized by the presence of a lymphoplasmacytic infiltrate in a low-grade, often myxoid-appearing mesenchymal lesion exhibiting a variably cellular, fascicular, or, occasionally, hypocellular fibrous pattern (Figure 14.19). The constituent cells are spindled with uniform vesicular nuclei. The spindle cell pattern in conjunction with coexpression of smooth muscle markers (desmin, but not h-caldesmon) and

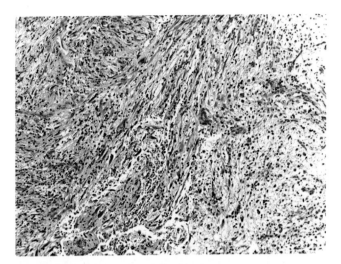

Figure 14.19 Inflammatory myofibroblastic tumor.

keratin may lead to misdiagnosis of myxoid smooth muscle tumor. Expression of ALK1 protein can provide confirmatory evidence of the diagnosis, but only 50% of inflammatory myofibroblastic tumors express ALK1, and most are in younger patients. Approximately 25% of intra-abdominal inflammatory myofibroblastic tumors recur, but less than 5% metastasize; outcome data is too limited to predict behavior for those that arise in the uterus.

Paraganglioma

Uterine paraganglioma (three cases, two of which were clinically malignant) and melanotic paraganglioma (two cases) have been reported in the literature[28]. All have arisen in the corpus. The histologic features are identical to those that occur elsewhere. The melanotic tumors were small, incidental findings; both were associated with psammomatous calcifications[29].

MISCELLANEOUS SARCOMAS

With the exception of leiomyosarcoma, pure sarcomas are quite rare in the uterus.

These include homologous (angiosarcoma, neurogenic sarcoma) and heterologous (embryonal rhabdomyosarcoma, alveolar rhabdomyosarcoma, pleomorphic rhabdomyosarcoma, osteosarcoma, chondrosarcoma, liposarcoma, Ewing/primitive neuroectodermal tumor, and myxofibrosarcoma) tumors, as well as several neoplasms of uncertain lineage (alveolar soft part sarcoma, epithelioid sarcoma). Most uterine corpus sarcomas present in postmenopausal women, while most cervical sarcomas – for example, embryonal rhabdomyosarcoma – occur in younger patients. Until recently, pelvic radiation therapy has been considered an etiologic factor in some cases, but, over the past decade, a variety of uterine corpus sarcomas have been reported following tamoxifen therapy. In the discussion that follows, it is important to keep in mind that the diagnosis of pure sarcoma, particularly the heterologous variant, requires exclusion of carcinomatous elements, since carcinosarcoma is far more common. The extent of sampling is not always clearly stated in the literature, which always raises the possibility that some of the reported cases may have been sarcomatous overgrowth in a carcinosarcoma or adenosarcoma.

Homologous sarcomas

Angiosarcoma

This is a rare, but highly aggressive tumor in the uterus. Less than 25 cases have been described in the literature[32]. Affected patients have ranged in age from 17 to 81 years, but most are in perimenopausal or postmenopausal women. An association with ovarian and tubal angiomatosis has been reported in a single patient. Prior exposure to radiation for cervical squamous cell carcinoma has been reported in another. No clear predisposing factors have been identified in the remaining patients. Most patients present with vaginal bleeding, pelvic mass, and/or weight loss. Extrauterine spread to ovarian and other pelvic sites is common; many patients also have evidence of distant metastases at the time of diagnosis. Uterine angiosarcoma does not appear to involve pelvic or para-aortic lymph nodes, even in cases with extrauterine disease. Survival is poor.

Grossly, uterine angiosarcomas are fleshy, hemorrhagic, and necrotic (Figure 14.20). The tumors range from <5 cm to 30 cm when size has been documented. They form polypoid or intramural masses. They are often mistaken for leiomyosarcoma in the intraoperative setting. Microscopically, they are composed of varying amounts of poorly differentiated, epithelioid, or spindle cells (Figure 14.21). Multiple sectioning may be required in order to identify a vascular pattern (Figure 14.21). The diagnosis is confirmed by immunostaining for CD31, CD34, and FRG. In most cases that have been studied, the tumor cells have been negative for desmin, actin, and h-caldesmon. As in other sites, uterine angiosarcoma may express cytokeratins.

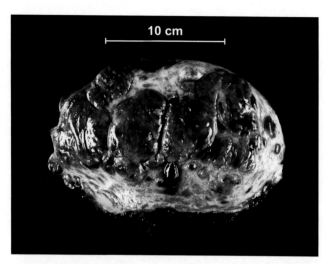

Figure 14.20 Angiosarcoma in uterus. (Courtesy of Jenifer Zisken, MD, PhD, Stanford University Medical Center.)

Melanoma

Primary melanoma can occur in the cervix, although primary vaginal and vulvar melanoma is far more common (Figure 14.22)[36]. Most patients are 50 to 70 years of age, but women as young as 26 years have been reported. Presenting symptoms are abnormal Pap smear, abnormal bleeding or discharge, or symptoms related to distant metastases. When an exophytic mass is present and can be biopsied, the diagnosis is relatively straightforward. Almost one-half of cases have had grossly apparent pigment. However, occasional cases are more deeply infiltrative, and biopsy material may be scant and/or poorly representative. In situ melanoma is often absent, and up to 25% are amelanotic[37]. In these situations, a high index of suspicion is required, with use of a broad panel of antibodies that includes melanoma markers as well as S100 protein. The prognosis is poor[38]. The differential diagnosis is spindle cell squamous cell carcinoma, undifferentiated carcinoma, malignant neuroectodermal tumor, leiomyosarcoma, nerve sheath sarcomas, perivascular epithelioid cell tumor, and benign melanotic lesions (mucosal melanosis, blue nevus).

Nerve sheath sarcomas (neurofibrosarcoma)

Uterine malignant peripheral nerve sheath tumors present at a wide age range (21 to 73 years; mean 44 years), but more than 50% of reported cases have been in women less than 50 years of age[39]. In contrast to leiomyosarcomas, almost all occur in the uterine cervix. The spindled cells in these lesions are arranged in vague

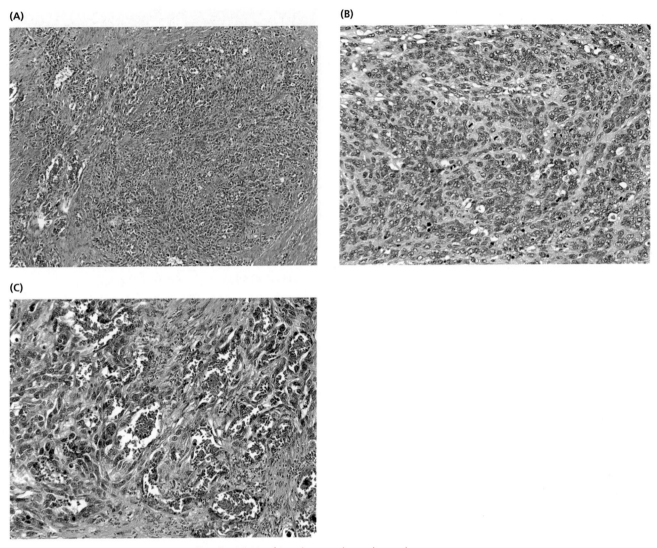

Figure 14.21 (A) Angiosarcoma. (B) Spindle cells. (C) Vasoformative areas in uterine angiosarcoma.

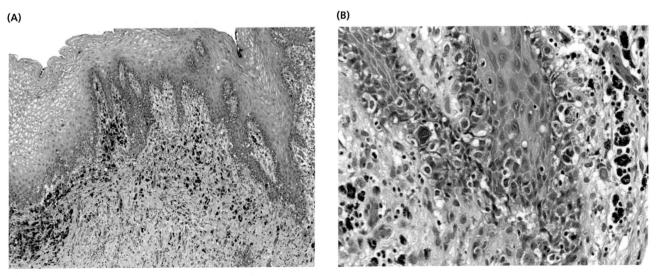

Figure 14.22 (A) Cervical melanoma. (B) Pagetoid component.

herringbone, nodular, or storiform patterns (Figure 14.23) and tend to infiltrate but not destroy the native endocervical glands. Alternating hypocellular areas that may be myxoid, fibrous, or edematous may focally simulate myxoid leiomyosarcoma, but the tumor cells are negative for smooth muscle markers, and all tumors show markedly cellular areas in addition to the paucicellular foci. In most cases, S100 protein expression is focal or weak; CD34 expression in those cases that have been studied (Figure 14.24) suggests that neurofibrosarcoma may be a more appropriate diagnosis[41]. A possible relationship to the endocervical CD34-positive stromal fibrocyte has been proposed[41]. None of the cervical malignant peripheral nerve sheath sarcomas have been associated with neurofibromatosis.

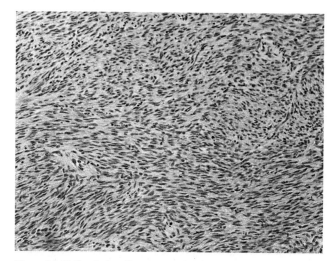

Figure 14.23 Cervical malignant peripheral nerve sheath sarcoma (neurofibrosarcoma).

(A)

(B)

(C)

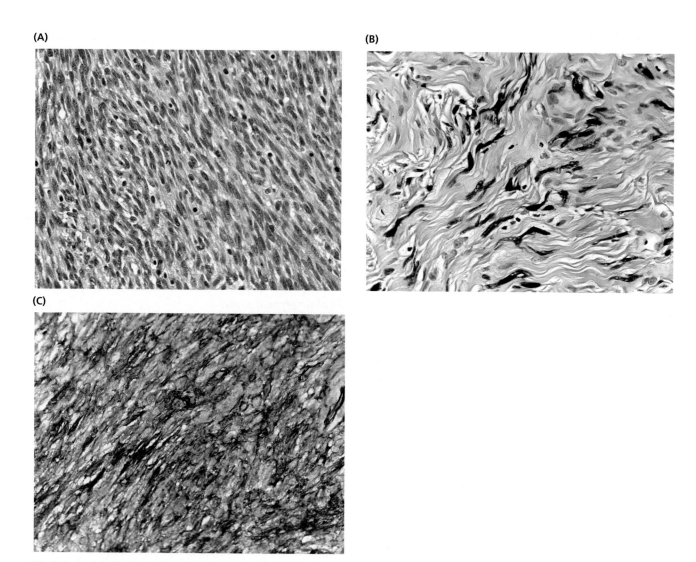

Figure 14.24 (A) Cervical malignant peripheral nerve sheath sarcoma (neurofibrosarcoma). (B) S100 expression is focal. (C) CD34 expression is more extensive.

Heterologous sarcomas

Chondrosarcoma

Pure primary chondrosarcoma of the uterus is an extremely rare uterine tumor (<4% of all uterine sarcomas)[42–44]. Less than 20 cases have been reported in the literature. Chondrosarcomas of the uterus most commonly take the form of a heterologous component of carcinosarcoma. Patients are usually postmenopausal women, with a range of 41 to 66 years (mean: 53 years). The most common presenting symptom of these tumors is vaginal bleeding, followed by abdominal distention, abdominal pain, and postcoital bleeding. One patient in the literature was asymptomatic. The uterus is typically enlarged by an intramural and polypoid mass, that often protrudes through the external os into the vagina. The treatment of choice is total abdominal hysterectomy with bilateral salpingo-oophorectomy. Chondrosarcoma of the uterus is an aggressive malignant tumor with high risk of early recurrence and/or metastases. Extrauterine spread to lungs, the abdominal and pelvic cavities, and urinary bladder is common.

Liposarcoma

As with other types of pure sarcoma, adequate sampling is important to exclude the presence of an epithelial component in any suspected case of pure liposarcoma in the uterus. Pure liposarcoma develops in perimenopausal and postmenopausal women (age range 23–78 years). Patients present with uterine bleeding or pelvic pain. The tumors are generally large (9 cm or larger), with only one of eight cases with a reported size measuring 4 cm in a recent literature review[45]. Approximately 50% arise in the cervix. The tumor varies from fleshy to friable in consistency, and may have myxoid, hemorrhagic, or necrotic areas. Well differentiated, myxoid, and round cell or pleomorphic types have been reported (Figure 14.25). Typical lipoblasts may not be readily identifiable. The recommended treatment is complete surgical excision with clear margins; the efficacy of adjuvant radiation or chemotherapy has not been established.

Osteosarcoma

Patients with primary pure uterine osteosarcoma present with vaginal bleeding, abdominal pain, and uterine enlargement. The mean age is 64 years (range 41–82 years). Two-thirds of patients have metastatic disease at presentation (50% are distant metastases)[46,47]. Uterine osteosarcomas

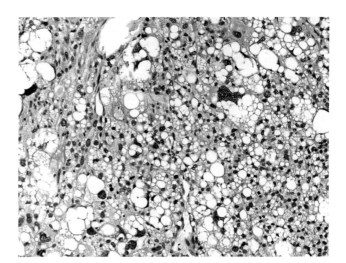

Figure 14.25 Pleomorphic liposarcoma in uterus.

demonstrate similar features to their soft tissue counterpart, although a cartilagenous component appears to be less common in the uterine tumors. Multinucleated osteoclast-like giant cells are frequently observed.

Although pure primary uterine osteosarcoma exhibits a microscopic appearance indistinguishable from that of osteosarcomas of soft tissue and bone, the mean survival time (8.5 months) of uterine osteosarcoma is approximately half that of cases of osteosarcoma of soft tissue (16 months). Extensive sampling for the search for epithelial elements is important, since osteosarcomas are also more aggressive and have a significantly worse outcome than carcinosarcoma. Treatment includes hysterectomy with or without bilateral salpingo-oophorectomy, followed by radiation therapy and/or chemotherapy.

Rhabdomyosarcoma

Although the vagina is the more common site in the female genital tract, embryonal rhabdomyosarcoma (so-called sarcoma botryroides) may arise in the cervix and, rarely, in the corpus. In contrast to vaginal rhabdomyosarcoma, which is more common in children, cervical rhabdomyosarcoma tends to occur in young adults (mean age: 18 years). The tumors form polypoid masses, usually 3 to 4 cm in size, and exhibit a similar gross and microscopic appearance to their vaginal counterpart. Most are embryonal (Figure 14.26), but spindle and alveolar variants may also be seen[48]. Almost one-half of cases have had islands of cartilage, which may make the distinction between adenosarcoma with heterologous elements, and rhabdomyosarcoma difficult in small biopsies. The prognosis is favorable unless the tumor has alveolar histology.

(A)

(B)

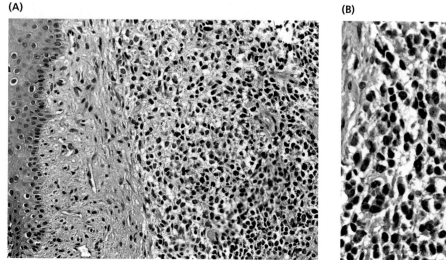

Figure 14.26 (A, B) Embryonal rhabdomyosarcoma arising in cervix.

(A)

(B)

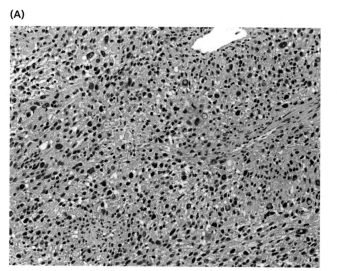

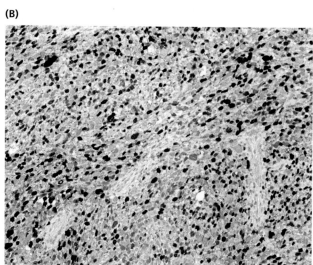

Figure 14.27 (A) Pleomorphic rhabdomyosarcoma arising in corpus. (B) Myogenin highlights neoplastic cells.

When rhabdomyosarcoma develops in the corpus, it usually occurs in an older age group and exhibits a pleomorphic or alveolar appearance (Figure 14.27)[49,50]. Most patients present with uterine bleeding. The tumors are often large (>5 cm) and solid, with areas of hemorrhage and necrosis. The tumors are highly cellular and composed of pleomorphic cells admixed with multinucleated tumor giant cells[49]. Since rhabdomyosarcoma is a common constituent of carcinosarcoma, all suspected pure rhabdomyosarcomas occurring in older women should be adequately sampled to exclude high-grade malignant glandular elements. If pure, the presence of rhabdomyoblasts and positivity for myogenin excludes the diagnosis of leiomyosarcoma. Pleomorphic rhabdomyosarcomas are aggressive neoplasms with poorer

prognosis than carcinosarcoma; surgery, radiation, and chemotherapy may improve survival.

Undifferentiated pleomorphic sarcoma

The older literature contains approximately a dozen case reports of malignant fibrous histiocytoma in the uterus[51,52]. It is likely that most of these would currently be classified as either undifferentiated pleomorphic sarcoma or undifferentiated endometrial sarcoma (high-grade uterine sarcoma; see Chapter 12). Affected patients range in age from 43 to 75 years and present with vaginal bleeding and a pelvic mass. Distant metastases may be present. The tumors are large, fleshy, and necrotic polypoid masses that involve endometrium and myometrium. The constituent cells are pleomorphic spindled and epithelioid cells, often with interspersed tumor giant cells and osteoclast-like giant cells. The prognosis is poor.

Differential diagnosis

The chief differential diagnostic considerations for all of these tumors are carcinosarcoma and adenosarcoma with stromal overgrowth and an inconspicuous epithelial component. Since all of these sarcomas are high grade and treated similarly, the distinction between pure high-grade sarcoma and adenosarcoma with high-grade sarcoma may not be of great importance. However, since adjuvant therapy may differ for carcinosarcoma, the pathologist should make a good faith effort to adequately section these tumors to identify malignant epithelial elements should they be present.

OTHER MESENCHYMAL NEOPLASMS

Alveolar soft part sarcoma

Alveolar soft part sarcoma of the female genital tract is an uncommon and often misdiagnosed tumor. It can arise in the cervix or uterus, where it usually resides in the myometrium (often in the lower uterine segment) without continuity with the endometrial cavity[53–55]. Most are small (≤5 cm) when diagnosed. Unlike their soft tissue counterpart, the prognosis appears to be much better for these tumors when they arise in the uterus, even in the presence of vascular invasion.

Because of the predominant intramural uterine involvement, alveolar soft part sarcoma can simulate an epithelioid leiomyosarcoma. The former tumor is composed of cells with abundant cytoplasm that ranges from clear, to eosinophilic and granular, growing in nests and alveoli, some of which may be compressed to the point that the central empty space is obscured (Figure 14.28). The typical alveolar growth pattern and PAS-positive diastase resistant crystals seen in alveolar soft part sarcoma distinguish it from epithelioid leiomyosarcoma. The fibrovascular framework that supports the nests and alveoli is also a diagnostic clue.

Alveolar soft part sarcoma is characterized by fusion of the TFE3 transcription factor gene on Xp11 to a novel gene on 17q25 and will demonstrate nuclear staining with TFE3. Alveolar soft part sarcomas may show weak

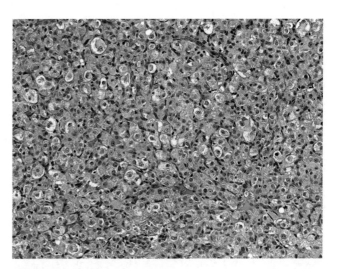

Figure 14.28 Alveolar soft part sarcoma.

immunoreactivity for keratins, desmin, smooth muscle actin, myogenin, S100, and HMB45.

Epithelioid sarcoma

Classic (distal type) epithelioid sarcoma may rarely present in the female genital tract (Figure 14.29). However, the proximal type of epithelioid sarcoma, which is a highly aggressive neoplasm, is more commonly encountered in this region (Figure 14.30). The latter variant has been reported to arise in the cervix[56]. Prior reports of malignant rhabdoid tumor involving the uterine corpus likely represent additional examples of proximal epithelioid sarcoma[57]. The histology of these proximal types of epithelioid sarcoma is often more epithelioid and carcinomatous than in epithelioid sarcoma of the distal extremities. The constituent cells are also often larger and may have a rhabdoid appearance[60]. Although the reported age range for these tumors is 39 to 71 years, most of the proximal type occurs in younger women. These tumors are highly aggressive and often misdiagnosed as poorly differentiated or undifferentiated carcinoma. The single cervical case that has been reported was initially diagnosed as glassy cell carcinoma.

As in the classic distal type of epithelioid sarcoma, the proximal type is positive for cytokeratin and EMA, and approximately 50% are positive for CD34. Almost 95% of both types of epithelioid sarcoma also exhibit loss of INI1 expression, which is a useful confirmatory stain when used in the appropriate clinical context (Figure 14.30)[61]. Other tumors, such as malignant rhabdoid tumor, epithelioid

(A)

(B)

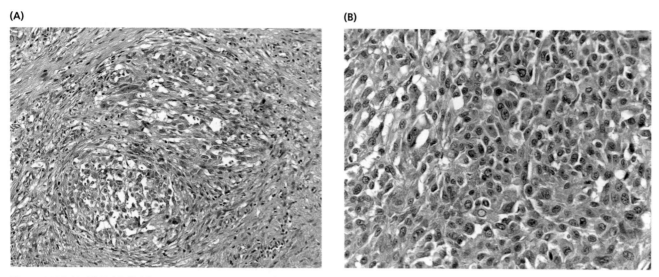

Figure 14.29 (A, B) Epithelioid sarcoma arising in cervix (distal type).

(A)

(B)

(C)

(D)

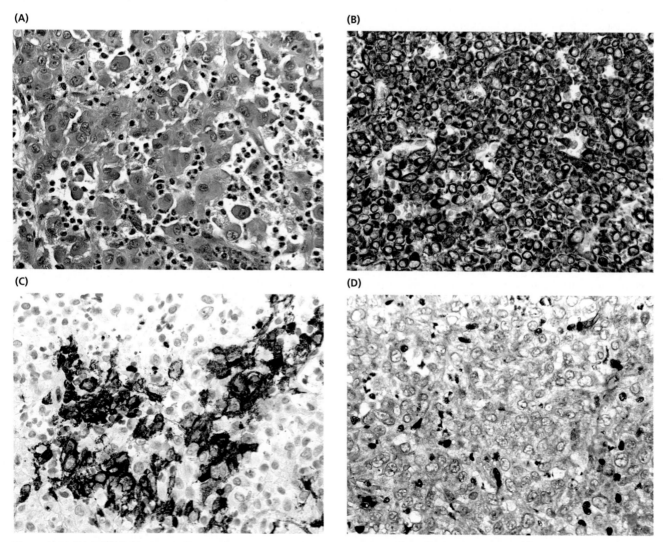

Figure 14.30 (A) Epithelioid sarcoma (proximal type). (B) Cytokeratin is strong and diffuse in these tumors. (C) CD34 expression is seen in approximately 40% of tumors. (D) INI1 is absent (normal internal control lymphocytes and stroma show nuclear positivity).

malignant peripheral nerve sheath tumor, renal medullary carcinoma, and a subset of myoepithelial carcinomas may also lose INI1 expression, but most of these tumors do not pose a significant differential diagnostic problem in the uterus.

Primitive neuroectodermal tumor/Ewing sarcoma

Rarely, primitive neuroectodermal tumor (PNET)/Ewing sarcoma can arise in the uterus[62]. Most arise in the corpus, but about one-third develop in the cervix. Admixed well-differentiated endometrioid carcinoma (endometrium), squamous carcinoma (cervix), or undifferentiated carcinoma (cervix) is seen in some cases[65]. The presence of rosettes may mimic the appearance of glands, and nested growth patterns can suggest solid components of endometrioid adenocarcinoma. Clues to the correct diagnosis include primitive-appearing nuclei and high mitotic index. The diagnosis can be suggested by immunohistochemical stains and confirmed by molecular testing in many cases. Primitive neuroectodermal tumor/Ewing sarcoma expresses CD99 diffusely in a membrane pattern, and they are usually, but not always cytokeratin negative. Given this immunophenotype, it would be reasonable to also exclude the theoretical possibility of a primitive leukemia or lymphoma with a TdT immunostain. The vast majority of peripheral primitive neuroectodermal tumors harbor t(11;22)(q24;q12), involving the *EWS* and *FLI1* genes. This can be evaluated by fluorescence in situ hybridization assays for the translocation or reverse-transcription polymerase chain reaction for the translocation gene product.

Some uterine neuroectodermal tumors more closely resemble primitive neuroectodermal tumors of the central nervous system. These tumors are not related to the PNET/Ewing sarcoma family and do not harbor t(11;22). CD99 expression is weak or absent; many express synaptophysin and glial fibrillary acidic protein.

REFERENCES

1. Baker RJ, Hildebrandt RH, Rouse RV, et al. Inhibin and CD99 (MIC2) expression in uterine stromal neoplasms with sex-cord-like elements. *Hum Pathol* 1999;**30**:671–9.
2. Clement P, Scully R. Uterine tumors resembling ovarian sex-cord tumors. A clinicopathologic analysis of fourteen cases. *Am J Clin Pathol* 1976;**66**:512–25.
3. Fekete PS, Vellios F, Patterson BD. Uterine tumor resembling an ovarian sex-cord tumor: report of a case of an endometrial stromal tumor with foam cells and ultrastructural evidence of epithelial differentiation. *Int J Gynecol Pathol* 1985;**4**:378–87.
4. Kantelip B, Cloup N, Dechelotte P. Uterine tumor resembling ovarian sex cord tumors: report of a case with ultrastructural study. *Hum Pathol* 1986;**17**:91–4.
5. Irving JA, Carinelli S, Prat J. Uterine tumors resembling ovarian sex cord tumors are polyphenotypic neoplasms with true sex cord differentiation. *Mod Pathol* 2006;**19**:17–24.
6. Krishnamurthy S, Jungbluth AA, Busam KJ, et al. Uterine tumors resembling ovarian sex-cord tumors have an immunophenotype consistent with true sex-cord differentiation. *Am J Surg Pathol* 1998;**22**:1078–82.
7. Staats PN, Garcia JJ, Dias-Santagata DC, et al. Uterine tumors resembling ovarian sex cord tumors (UTROSCT) lack the JAZF1-JJAZ1 translocation frequently seen in endometrial stromal tumors. *Am J Surg Pathol* 2009;**33**:1206–12.
8. Hildebrandt RH, Rouse RV, Longacre TA. Value of inhibin in the identification of granulosa cell tumors of the ovary. *Hum Pathol* 1997;**28**:1387–95.
9. Patel DS, Bhagavan BS. Blue nevus of the uterine cervix. *Hum Pathol* 1985;**16**:79–86.
10. Eskue K, Prieto VG, Malpica A. Cellular blue nevus of the uterus: a case report and review of the literature. *Int J Gynecol Pathol* 2010;**29**:583–6.
11. Yilmaz AG, Chandler P, Hahm GK, et al. Melanosis of the uterine cervix: a report of two cases and discussion of pigmented cervical lesions. *Int J Gynecol Pathol* 1999;**18**:73–6.
12. Martin PC, Pulitzer DR, Reed RJ. Pigmented myomatous neurocristoma of the uterus. *Arch Pathol Lab Med* 1989;**113**:1291–5.
13. Albores-Saavedra J, Gilcrease M. Glomus tumor of the uterine cervix. *Int J Gynecol Pathol* 1999;**18**:69–72.
14. Fujimoto Y, Kasai K, Furuya M, et al. Pure uterine lipoma. *J Obstet Gynaecol Res* 2006;**32**:520–3.
15. Zahn CM, Kendall BS, Liang CY. Spindle cell lipoma of the female genital tract. A report of two cases. *J Reprod Med* 2001;**46**:769–72.
16. Clement PB, Young RH, Scully RE. Clinical syndromes associated with tumors of the female genital tract. *Semin Diagn Pathol* 1991;**8**:204–33.
17. McCluggage WG, Young RH. Myxoid change of the myometrium and cervical stroma: description of a hitherto unreported non-neoplastic phenomenon with discussion of myxoid uterine lesions. *Int J Gynecol Pathol*;**29**:351–7.
18. Terzakis JA, Opher E, Melamed J, et al. Pigmented melanocytic schwannoma of the uterine cervix. *Ultrastruct Pathol* 1990;**14**:357–66.
19. Rahimi K, Shaw PA, Chetty R. Solitary fibrous tumor of the uterine cervix. *Int J Gynecol Pathol* 2010;**29**:189–92.
20. Wakami K, Tateyama H, Kawashima H, et al. Solitary fibrous tumor of the uterus producing high-molecular-weight insulin-like growth factor II and associated with hypoglycemia. *Int J Gynecol Pathol* 2005;**24**:79–84.
21. Virk RK, Zhong J, Lu D. Diffuse cavernous hemangioma of the uterus in a pregnant woman: report of a rare case and review of literature. *Arch Gynecol Obstet* 2009;**279**:603–5.
22. Wang S, Lang JH, Zhou HM. Venous malformations of the female lower genital tract. *Eur J Obstet Gynecol Reprod Biol* 2009;**145**:205–8.
23. Furui T, Imai A, Yokoyama Y, et al. Cavernous lymphangioma arising from uterine corpus. *Gynecol Oncol* 2003;**90**:195–9.
24. Patel RC, Zynger DL, Laskin WB. Blue rubber bleb nevus syndrome: novel lymphangiomatosis-like growth pattern within

the uterus and immunohistochemical analysis. *Hum Pathol* 2009;**40**:413–17.

25. Terada T. Gastrointestinal stromal tumor of the uterus: a case report with genetic analyses of c-kit and PDGFRA genes. *Int J Gynecol Pathol* 2009;**28**:29–34.

26. Wingen CB, Pauwels PA, Debiec-Rychter M, *et al.* Uterine gastrointestinal stromal tumour (GIST). *Gynecol Oncol* 2005;**97**:970–2.

27. Rabban JT, Zaloudek CJ, Shekitka KM, *et al.* Inflammatory myofibroblastic tumor of the uterus: a clinicopathologic study of 6 cases emphasizing distinction from aggressive mesenchymal tumors. *Am J Surg Pathol* 2005;**29**:1348–55.

28. Beham A, Schmid C, Fletcher CD, *et al.* Malignant paraganglioma of the uterus. *Virchows Arch A Pathol Anat Histopathol* 1992;**420**:453–7.

29. Tavassoli F. Melanotic paraganglioma of the uterus. *Cancer* 1986;**58**:942–8.

30. van Leeuwen J, van der Putten HW, Demeyere TB, *et al.* Paraganglioma of the uterus. A case report and review of literature. *Gynecol Oncol* 2011;**121**:418–19.

31. Young T, Thrasher T. Nonchromaffin paraganglioma of the uterus. A case report. *Arch Pathol Lab Med* 1982;**106**:608–9.

32. Ongkasuwan C, Taylor J, Tang C, *et al.* Angiosarcomas of the uterus and ovary: clinicopathologic report. *Cancer* 1982;**49**:1469–75.

33. Schammel DP, Tavassoli FA. Uterine angiosarcomas: a morphologic and immunohistochemical study of four cases. *Am J Surg Pathol* 1998;**22**:246–50.

34. Tallini G, Price FV, Carcangiu ML. Epithelioid angiosarcoma arising in uterine leiomyomas. *Am J Clin Pathol* 1993;**100**:514–18.

35. Witkin G, Askin F, Geratz J, *et al.* Angiosarcoma of the uterus: a light microscopic, immunohistochemical, and ultrastructural study. *Int J Gynecol Pathol* 1987;**6**:176–84.

36. Clark KC, Butz WR, Hapke MR. Primary malignant melanoma of the uterine cervix: case report with world literature review. *Int J Gynecol Pathol* 1999;**18**:265–73.

37. Duggal R, Srinivasan R. Primary amelanotic melanoma of the cervix: case report with review of literature. *J Gynecol Oncol*; **21**:199–202.

38. Pusceddu S, Bajetta E, Carcangiu ML, *et al.* A literature overview of primary cervical malignant melanoma: an exceedingly rare cancer. *Crit Rev Oncol Hematol* 2011; in press. doi: 10.1016/j.critrevonc.2011.03.008

39. Bernstein HB, Broman JH, Apicelli A, *et al.* Primary malignant schwannoma of the uterine cervix: a case report and literature review. *Gynecol Oncol* 1999;**74**:288–92.

40. Keel SB, Clement PB, Prat J, *et al.* Malignant schwannoma of the uterine cervix: a study of three cases. *Int J Gynecol Pathol* 1998;**17**:223–30.

41. Mills AM, Karamchandani JR, Vogel H, *et al.* Endocervical fibroblastic malignant peripheral nerve sheath tumor (neurofibrosarcoma): report of a novel entity possibly related to endocervical CD34 fibrocytes. *Am J Surg Pathol* 2011;**35**:404–12.

42. Clement P. Chondrosarcoma of the uterus: report of a case and review of the literature. *Hum Pathol* 1978;**9**:726–32.

43. Kofinas A, Suarez J, Calame R, *et al.* Chondrosarcoma of the uterus. *Gynecol Oncol* 1984;**19**:231–7.

44. Namizato CS, Muriel-Cueto P, Baez-Perez JM, *et al.* Chondrosarcoma of the uterus: case report and literature review. *Arch Gynecol Obstet* 2008;**278**:369–72.

45. Moinfar F, Azodi M, Tavassoli FA. Uterine sarcomas. *Pathology* 2007;**39**:55–71.

46. Kempson RL, Bari W. Uterine sarcomas. Classification, diagnosis, and prognosis. *Hum Pathol* 1970;**1**:331–49.

47. Su M, Tokairin T, Nishikawa Y, *et al.* Primary osteosarcoma of the uterine corpus: case report and review of the literature. *Pathol Int* 2002;**52**:158–63.

48. Baiocchi G, Cestari LA, Macedo MP, *et al.* Surgical implications of mesenteric lymph node metastasis from advanced ovarian cancer after bowel resection. *J Surg Oncol* 2011;**104**(3):250–4.

49. Fadare O, Bonvicino A, Martel M, *et al.* Pleomorphic rhabdomyosarcoma of the uterine corpus: a clinicopathologic study of 4 cases and a review of the literature. *Int J Gynecol Pathol*;**29**:122–34.

50. Ferguson SE, Gerald W, Barakat RR, *et al.* Clinicopathologic features of rhabdomyosarcoma of gynecologic origin in adults. *Am J Surg Pathol* 2007;**31**:382–9.

51. Chou ST, Fortune D, Beischer NA, *et al.* Primary malignant fibrous histiocytoma of the uterus – ultrastructural and immunocytochemical studies of two cases. *Pathology* 1985;**17**:36–40.

52. Fujii S, Kanzaki H, Konishi I, *et al.* Malignant fibrous histiocytoma of the uterus. *Gynecol Oncol* 1987;**26**:319–30.

53. Burch DJ, Hitchcock A, Masson GM. Alveolar soft part sarcoma of the uterus: case report and review of the literature. *Gynecol Oncol* 1994;**54**:91–4.

54. Gray GF, Jr., Glick AD, Kurtin PJ, *et al.* Alveolar soft part sarcoma of the uterus. *Hum Pathol* 1986;**17**:297–300.

55. Roma AA, Yang B, Senior ME, *et al.* TFE3 immunoreactivity in alveolar soft part sarcoma of the uterine cervix: case report. *Int J Gynecol Pathol* 2005;**24**:131–5.

56. Jeney H, Heller DS, Hameed M, *et al.* Epithelioid sarcoma of the uterine cervix. *Gynecol Oncol* 2003;**89**:536–9.

57. Cattani MG, Viale G, Santini D, *et al.* Malignant rhabdoid tumour of the uterus: an immunohistochemical and ultrastructural study. *Virchows Arch A Pathol Anat Histopathol* 1992;**420**:459–62.

58. Cho KR, Rosenshein NB, Epstein JI. Malignant rhabdoid tumor of the uterus. *Int J Gynecol Pathol* 1989;**8**:381–7.

59. Niemann TH, Goetz SP, Benda JA, *et al.* Malignant rhabdoid tumor of the uterus: report of a case with findings in a cervical smear. *Diagn Cytopathol* 1994;**10**:54–9.

60. Tholpady A, Lonergan CL, Wick MR. Proximal-type epithelioid sarcoma of the vulva: relationship to malignant extrarenal rhabdoid tumor. *Int J Gynecol Pathol*;**29**:600–4.

61. Hornick JL, Dal Cin P, Fletcher CD. Loss of INI1 expression is characteristic of both conventional and proximal-type epithelioid sarcoma. *Am J Surg Pathol* 2009;**33**:542–50.

62. Daya D, Lukka H, Clement PB. Primitive neuroectodermal tumors of the uterus: a report of four cases. *Hum Pathol* 1992;**23**:1120–9.

63. Malpica A, Moran CA. Primitive neuroectodermal tumor of the cervix: a clinicopathologic and immunohistochemical study of two cases. *Ann Diagn Pathol* 2002;**6**:281–7.

64. Varghese L, Arnesen M, Boente M. Primitive neuroectodermal tumor of the uterus: a case report and review of literature. *Int J Gynecol Pathol* 2006;**25**:373–7.

65. Sinkre P, Albores-Saavedra J, Miller DS, *et al.* Endometrial endometrioid carcinomas associated with Ewing sarcoma/peripheral primitive neuroectodermal tumor. *Int J Gynecol Pathol* 2000;**19**:127–32.

15 MISCELLANEOUS PRIMARY UTERINE TUMORS

INTRODUCTION

With the exception of adenomatoid tumor and lymphoma, the most commonly encountered primary uterine tumors other than those presented in the prior chapters are gestational neoplasms or metastases. The latter two disease processes are discussed elsewhere.

ADENOMATOID TUMOR

Adenomatoid tumor is a benign tumor of mesothelial origin that can be mistaken clinically and histologically for a leiomyoma[1–3]. Patients are usually of reproductive age and are undergoing evaluation for another, unrelated disorder. The tumors often form a distinct, solid pale yellow gross mass that may appear less well circumscribed than a leiomyoma. An intramural cystic component or exophytic serosal component may rarely be seen. Most adenomatoid tumors are incidental findings in hysterectomy specimens, but presentation in uterine curettings

has been reported[4]. Histology is variable and includes adenoid, angiomatoid, cystic, glandular, solid, tubular, and, rarely, oncocytic patterns (Figures 15.1–15.5). An infiltrative pattern of growth is common, but direct extrauterine extension, marked cytologic atypia, tumor cell necrosis, and mitotic figures are typically absent. Signet ring cell morphology is common, but it is typically focal. Vacuolated, lipoblast-like cells are also a frequent finding, as are distinctive thread-like bridging strands crossing tubular spaces[5,6]. Lymphoid aggregates may also be present. Adenomatoid tumors express WT1, CK5/6, and caldesmon, although calretinin and D2-40 demonstrate the highest sensitivity (Figure 15.6)[6,7]. The differential diagnosis is leiomyoma, hemangioma, and metastatic adenocarcinoma, especially signet ring cell type.

YOLK SAC TUMOR

Uterine yolk sac tumor is rare, and when it occurs it is typically seen in the cervix and/or vagina of infants[8].

(A) **(B)**

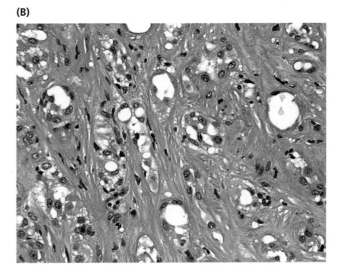

Figure 15.1 (A, B) Adenomatoid tumor. Tubular and glandular pattern. Aggregates of lymphoid cells are often associated with uterine adenomatoid tumors.

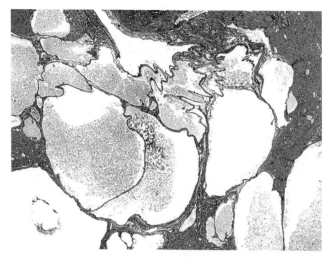

Figure 15.2 Adenomatoid tumor. Cystic pattern.

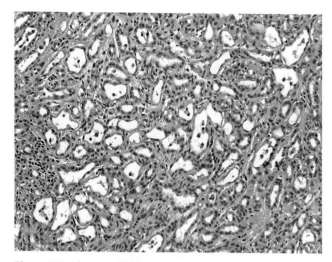

Figure 15.3 Adenomatoid tumor. Angiomatoid pattern.

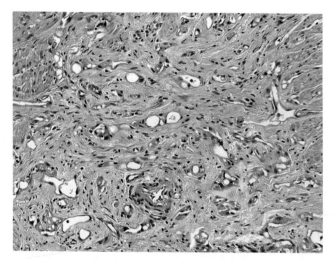

Figure 15.4 Adenomatoid tumor. Infiltrative pattern.

(A)

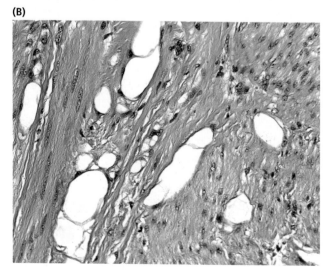

However, it may also occur in the corpus, typically in reproductive-aged women[9]. The histology and treatment are similar to typical yolk sac tumor (Figure 15.7). The differential diagnosis is carcinoma with yolk sac component (see ***Carcinoma with yolk sac tumor*** in Chapter 9) and carcinosarcoma (see Chapter 10).

TERATOMA

This is a very rare primary tumor in the uterus. Most reported cases consist of mature tissue and may represent heterotopias[13–16]. Immature teratoma has been reported in association with carcinoma[17].

(B)

Figure 15.5 (A, B) Adenomatoid tumor. Characteristic fine, thin strands of cytoplasm bridge the tubular spaces.

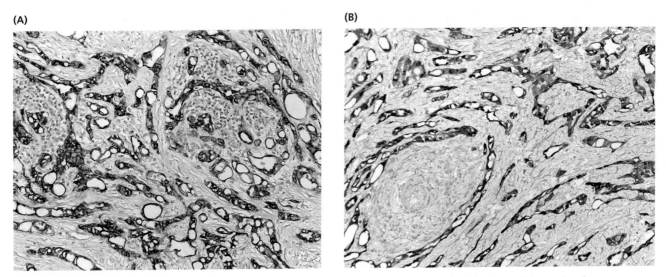

Figure 15.6 Adenomatoid tumor. (A) Cytokeratin expression is typically strong and diffuse. (B) Calretinin is a sensitive marker for adenomatoid tumor.

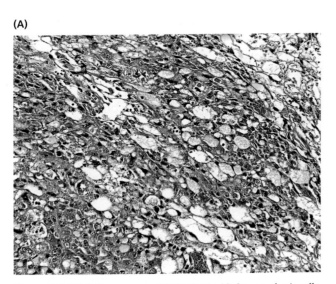

Figure 15.7 (A) Yolk sac tumor. (B) SALL4 highlights neoplastic cells.

CARCINOID

Two rare cases of uterine corpus carcinoid tumors have been described. Both were confined to the myometrium and consisted of nests of cytologically bland neuroendocrine cells[18,19]. When such cases are encountered, metastasis from another site should be excluded.

PIGMENTED NEUROECTODERMAL TUMOR OF INFANCY (RETINAL ANLAGE TUMOR)

There are only two reported uterine cases of retinal anlage tumor: one in the endocervix and one in the endometrium[20,21]. The cervical tumor featured immature-appearing neuroectodermal tissue with other areas of pigmented cells; while the endometrial tumor was associated with a carcinosarcoma. Whether or not these represent true retinal anlage tumors is unclear.

GLIOMA

Another very rare occurrence in the uterus, glioma is distinguished from primitive neuroectodermal tumor by the presence of a pure glial component in absence of the small round cell component[22].

(A)

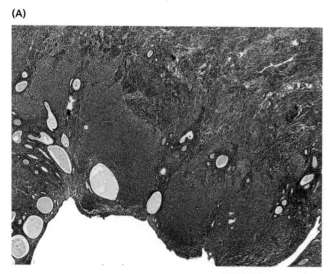

(B)

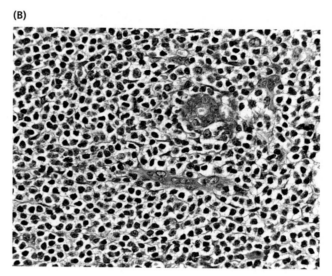

Figure 15.8 (A, B) Extranodal marginal zone lymphoma.

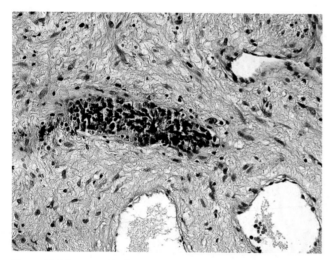

Figure 15.9 Intravascular lymphoma.

EXTRARENAL WILMS TUMOR

Wilms tumor is a very uncommon primary uterine tumor, but occurs in a wide age range (2–77 years). Involvement of endocervix, lower uterine segment, or endometrium may be present. Most patients present with abnormal bleeding and/or a mass[23–25]. The tumors exhibit typical Wilms tumor histology; skeletal muscle, smooth muscle, hyalin cartilage, and squamous epithelium may also be present. Peripheral primitive neuroectodermal tumors, carcinosarcoma, and teratoma should be excluded. Extrarenal Wilms tumor may have a better therapeutic response than peripheral primitive neuroectodermal tumors or carcinosarcoma.

LYMPHOMA AND LEUKEMIA

Most uterine lymphomas occur in the cervix; only about 10% involve the corpus primarily[26–33]. They occur over a wide age range, but most occur in the reproductive or postmenopausal years. Most have bleeding and/or a mass. The cervical tumors tend to form exophytic masses or involve the cervix in a circumferential, barrel-shaped manner. Corpus tumors are exophytic or infiltrative endomyometrial lesions. The most common type is diffuse B-cell lymphoma, followed by follicular cell lymphoma and Burkitt lymphoma. Other rare types include marginal zone lymphoma (Figure 15.8), intravascular lymphoma (Figure 15.9), mucosa-associated lymphoma, peripheral T-cell lymphoma, and NK/T-cell lymphomas[34–36]. Cervical tumors may have prominent stromal sclerosis. Lymphomas can be recognized on the basis of a mass lesion composed of a monomorphous population of neoplastic cells expressing CD45 and other lymphocyte markers. However, in limited samplings, the diagnosis often requires careful integration of clinical, histologic, immunohistochemical, and molecular studies.

The differential diagnosis is lymphoma-like lesion (Figure 15.10), lymphoepithelial carcinoma, leukemia, neuroendocrine carcinoma (small and large cell types), stromal sarcoma, and (the much more common) secondary involvement by disseminated lymphoma. Immunohistochemical stains can establish the diagnosis for almost all of these entities (Figure 15.11). Distinguishing lymphoma from lymphoma-like lesion can be more

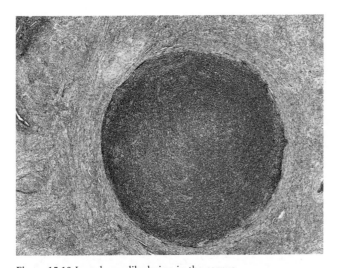

Figure 15.10 Lymphoma-like lesion in the corpus.

problematic, especially in limited specimens[37,38]. Most patients with lymphoma have symptoms and a mass lesion with evidence of infiltration into deep tissue, while most patients with lymphoma-like lesion are asymptomatic and have more limited, superficial involvement of cervical or endometrial tissue. Aberrant expression of lymphocyte markers may help differentiate reactive follicles from follicular lymphoma, as can gene rearrangement studies to determine clonality. However, clonal *IGH* rearrangements can be seen in lymphoma-like lesions, and correlation with the entire clinical, histologic, and immunohistologic picture is required before a definitive diagnosis of lymphoma is made on limited material[37].

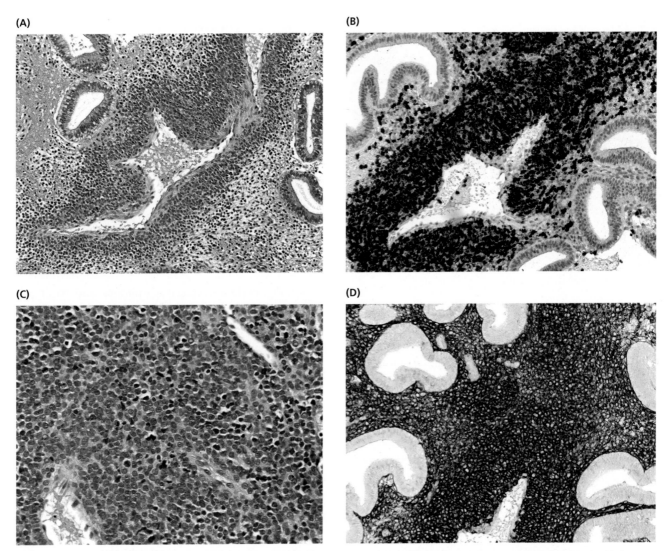

Figure 15.11 (A) Pre-B acute lymphoblastic leukemia in reproductive-aged woman with no prior diagnosis of leukemia. (B) TdT highlights the perivascular neoplastic cells. (C) Monomorphous population of cells may simulate endometrial stromal sarcoma. (D) Strong CD10 expression by the leukemic cells may add further confusion.

EXTRAMEDULLARY MYELOID TUMOR (GRANULOCYTIC SARCOMA)

Primary uterine involvement by myeloid leukemia (extramedullary myeloid tumor) is less common than primary lymphoma. Most cases occur in the cervix. Involvement of other genital and extragenital sites may be present. Most patients develop acute myeloid leukemia following detection of the uterine lesion. Secondary involvement by leukemia is more common. In both presentations, the leukemic cells form solid nodules and infiltrate normal structures, similar to extramedullary myeloid tumor elsewhere[27,30]. Immature eosinophils may provide a clue to the diagnosis. Confirmation can be made on the basis of a combination of CD43, myeloperoxidase, and/or lysozyme stains. Choroacetate esterase will stain most, but not all extramedullary myeloid tumors. Extramedullary hematopoiesis may also feature granulocytic precursors, but extramedullary hematopoiesis occurs as isolated foci within the endometrium or myometrium, and erythroid precursors are almost always also present; affected patients may have an underlying hematologic disorder, but in most cases patients have chronic anemia with no other recognizable hematologic abnormality[39].

OTHER TUMORS

Plasmacytomas may also occur in the uterus, but most plasma cell disorders in the uterine cervix and endometrium are inflammatory[31]. Rosai–Dorfman (sinus histiocytosis with massive lymphadenopathy) and Langerhans histiocytosis may rarely occur in the cervix and/or endometrium[40,41]. The diagnosis is established on the basis of their characteristic histologic and immunohistochemical features. A variety of inflammatory granulomatous and xanthogranulomatous disorders, including malakoplakia, should be excluded.

REFERENCES

1. Nogales FF, Isaac MA, Hardisson D, et al. Adenomatoid tumors of the uterus: an analysis of 60 cases. Int J Gynecol Pathol 2002; 21:34–40.
2. Otis CN. Uterine adenomatoid tumors: immunohistochemical characteristics with emphasis on Ber-EP4 immunoreactivity and distinction from adenocarcinoma. Int J Gynecol Pathol 1996;15:146–51.
3. Quigley J, Hart W. Adenomatoid tumors of the uterus. Amer J Clin Path 1981;76:627–35.
4. Carlier MT, Dardick I, Lagace AF, et al. Adenomatoid tumor of uterus: presentation in endometrial curettings. Int J Gynecol Pathol 1986;5:69–74.
5. Hes O, Perez-Montiel DM, Alvarado Cabrero I, et al. Thread-like bridging strands: a morphologic feature present in all adenomatoid tumors. Ann Diagn Pathol 2003;7:273–7.
6. Sangoi AR, McKenney JK, Schwartz EJ, et al. Adenomatoid tumors of the female and male genital tracts: a clinicopathological and immunohistochemical study of 44 cases. Mod Pathol 2009;22:1228–35.
7. Schwartz EJ, Longacre TA. Adenomatoid tumors of the female and male genital tracts express WT1. Int J Gynecol Pathol 2004; 23:123–8.
8. Copeland LJ, Sneige N, Ordonez NG, et al. Endodermal sinus tumor of the vagina and cervix. Cancer 1985;55:2558–65.
9. Clement PB, Young RH, Scully RE. Extraovarian pelvic yolk sac tumors. Cancer 1988;62:620–6.
10. Joseph MG, Fellows FG, Hearn SA. Primary endodermal sinus tumor of the endometrium. A clinicopathologic, immunocytochemical, and ultrastructural study. Cancer 1990;65:297–302.
11. Pileri S, Martinelli G, Serra L, et al. Endodermal sinus tumor arising in the endometrium. Obstet Gynecol 1980;56:391–6.
12. Spatz A, Bouron D, Pautier P, et al. Primary yolk sac tumor of the endometrium: a case report and review of the literature. Gynecol Oncol 1998;70:285–8.
13. Khoor A, Fleming MV, Purcell CA, et al. Mature teratoma of the uterine cervix with pulmonary differentiation. Arch Pathol Lab Med 1995;119:848–50.
14. Lim S, Kim Y, Kee Y, et al. Mature teratoma of the uterine cervix with lymphoid hyperplasia. Pathol Int 2003;53:327–31.
15. Martin E, Scholes J, Richart R, et al. Benign cystic teratoma of the uterus. Am J Obstet Gynecol 1979;135:429–31.
16. Tyagi SP, Saxena K, Rizvi R, et al. Foetal remnants in the uterus and their relation to other uterine heterotopia. Histopathology 1979;3:339–45.
17. Ansah-Boateng Y, Wells M, Poole D. Coexistent immature teratoma of the uterus and endometrial adenocarcinoma complicated by gliomatosis peritonei. Gynecol Oncol 1985;21:106–10.
18. Chetty R, Clark SP, Bhathal PS. Carcinoid tumour of the uterine corpus. Virchows Arch A Pathol Anat Histopathol 1993;422:93–5.
19. Gonzalez-Bosquet E, Gonzalez-Bosquet J, Garcia Jimenez A, et al. Carcinoid tumor of the uterine corpus. A case report. J Reprod Med 1998;43:844–6.
20. Schulz DM. A malignant, melanotic neoplasm of the uterus, resembling the retinal anlage tumors; report of a case. Am J Clin Pathol 1957;28:524–32.
21. Sobel N, Carcangui ML. Primary pigmented neuroectodermal tumor of the uterine cervix. Int J Surg Pathol 1994;2:31–6.
22. Young R, Kleinman G, Scully R. Glioma of the uterus. Report of a case with comments on histogenesis. Am J Surg Pathol 1981;5:695–9.
23. Benatar B, Wright C, Freinkel AL, et al. Primary extrarenal Wilms' tumor of the uterus presenting as a cervical polyp. Int J Gynecol Pathol 1998;17:277–80.
24. Garcia-Galvis OF, Stolnicu S, Munoz E, et al. Adult extrarenal Wilms tumor of the uterus with teratoid features. Hum Pathol 2009;40:418–24.
25. McAlpine J, Azodi M, O'Malley D, et al. Extrarenal Wilms' tumor of the uterine corpus. Gynecol Oncol 2005;96:892–6.
26. Ferry JA, Young RH. Malignant lymphoma, pseudolymphoma, and hematopoietic disorders of the female genital tract. Pathol Annu 1991;26:227–63.

27. Friedman HD, Adelson MD, Elder RC, *et al.* Granulocytic sarcoma of the uterine cervix – literature review of granulocytic sarcoma of the female genital tract. *Gynecol Oncol* 1992;**46**:128–37.

28. Harris N, Scully R. Malignant lymphoma and granulocytic sarcoma of the uterus and vagina. A clinicopathologic analysis of 27 cases. *Cancer* 1984;**53**:2530–45.

29. Kosari F, Daneshbod Y, Parwaresch R, *et al.* Lymphomas of the female genital tract: a study of 186 cases and review of the literature. *Am J Surg Pathol* 2005;**29**:1512–20.

30. Oliva E, Ferry JA, Young RH, *et al.* Granulocytic sarcoma of the female genital tract: a clinicopathologic study of 11 cases. *Am J Surg Pathol* 1997;**21**:1156–65.

31. Smith NL, Baird DB, Strausbauch PH. Endometrial involvement by multiple myeloma. *Int J Gynecol Pathol* 1997;**16**:173–5.

32. van de Rijn M, Kamel OW, Chang PP, *et al.* Primary low-grade endometrial B-cell lymphoma. *Am J Surg Pathol* 1997;**21**:187–94.

33. Vang R, Medeiros LJ, Ha CS, *et al.* Non-Hodgkin's lymphomas involving the uterus: a clinicopathologic analysis of 26 cases. *Mod Pathol* 2000;**13**:19–28.

34. Mehes G, Hegyi K, Csonka T, *et al.* Primary uterine NK-cell lymphoma, nasal-type: a unique malignancy of a prominent cell type of the endometrium. *Pathol Oncol Res* 2011; in press. doi: 10.1007/s12253-011-9360-4

35. Nakamura S, Kato M, Ichimura K, *et al.* Peripheral T/natural killer-cell lymphoma involving the female genital tract: a clinicopathologic study of 5 cases. *Int J Hematol* 2001;**73**:108–14.

36. Sur M, Ross C, Moens F, *et al.* Intravascular large B-cell lymphoma of the uterus: a diagnostic challenge. *Int J Gynecol Pathol* 2005;**24**:201–3.

37. Geyer JT, Ferry JA, Harris NL, *et al.* Florid reactive lymphoid hyperplasia of the lower female genital tract (lymphoma-like lesion): a benign condition that frequently harbors clonal immunoglobulin heavy chain gene rearrangements. *Am J Surg Pathol* 2010;**34**:161–8.

38. Young R, Harris N, Scully R. Lymphoma-like lesions of the lower female genital tract: a report of 16 cases. *Int J Gynecol Pathol* 1985;**4**:289–99.

39. Gru AA, Hassan A, Pfeifer JD, *et al.* Uterine extramedullary hematopoiesis: what is the clinical significance? *Int J Gynecol Pathol*, **29**:366–73.

40. Axiotis CA, Merino MJ, Duray PH. Langerhans cell histiocytosis of the female genital tract. *Cancer* 1991;**67**:1650–60.

41. Murray J, Fox H. Rosai-Dorfman disease of the uterine cervix. *Int J Gynecol Pathol* 1991;**10**:209–13.

INTRODUCTION

The most common mode of secondary tumor involvement of the uterine corpus or cervix is by direct extension, most often from a colorectal or bladder neoplasm. Most patients with such involvement also have concomitant invasion of other pelvic organs. Metastases to the uterus are not nearly as common, but the frequency and variety of metastatic tumors involving the uterus has increased in the last two decades due to improved imaging and improved chemotherapy for many solid tumors with consequent improved survival. Metastases occur secondary to other primary genital tract tumors as well as extragenital sources[1–4].

OTHER PRIMARY GENITAL TRACT TUMORS

Secondary involvement from other genital site primary tumors generally occurs as a result of direct spread from cervical, tubal, or ovarian cancers. However, implantation, either on the cervical mucosa or endometrium, is becoming recognized with increasing frequency (Figure 16.1). The cervical mucosal implants may be endometrial, tubal, or ovarian in origin, while the endometrial implants generally arise from tubal or ovarian sites[5–7]. In many instances, the site of origin is conjecture and, in some cases, simultaneous primary sites cannot be completely excluded. Although no single approach to this problem resolves these distinctions, a combination of the distributional pattern in conjunction with histologic and immunohistologic similarities (or differences) of tumors in different tumor sites can point to one or another diagnosis. Specific locational attributes may also be useful (i.e., WT1 tends to be expressed in pelvic (non-uterine) serous carcinomas, while uterine serous carcinomas usually do not express WT1).

EXTRAGENITAL TUMORS

Appendix

Appendiceal primary mucinous tumors (low-grade mucinous neoplasms) spread most commonly to the ovaries, but tubal, cervical, and endometrial mucosal involvement can be seen (Figure 16.2). In most such cases, the patient has clinical pseudomyxoma peritonei, and the question is whether or not there is a simultaneous mucinous tumor of the female genital tract, especially since endometrial and cervical mucosal involvement may not show direct invasion from the serosa or stroma. The characteristic bland histology, single or multifocal superficial involvement, and expression of both CK7 and CK20 will confirm secondary involvement by the appendiceal primary in most such cases[8]. However, since rare simultaneous primary mucinous tumors can occur in this setting, ancillary studies are warranted whenever there is a large volume of cervical or endometrial mucosal tumor or when there is apparent invasion from the mucosal tumor into the underlying cervical stroma or myometrium.

Goblet cell carcinoid is another tumor that may populate the mucosa of the cervix and endometrium. As with the low-grade mucinous tumors, there is usually evidence of disease spread elsewhere in the genital tract at the time of presentation. The presence of signet ring cells is highly unusual in endometrial cancers, although it can be seen in some primary cervical cancers. The presence of areas of more usual appearing endocervical adenocarcinoma is often a helpful diagnostic feature. The presence of numerous signet ring cells should also prompt consideration for a possible gastric or breast primary.

Bladder

Transitional cell carcinoma may secondarily involve the uterus by direct spread; the cervix is most commonly affected. Non-contiguous spread may also rarely occur,

(A)

(B)

(C)

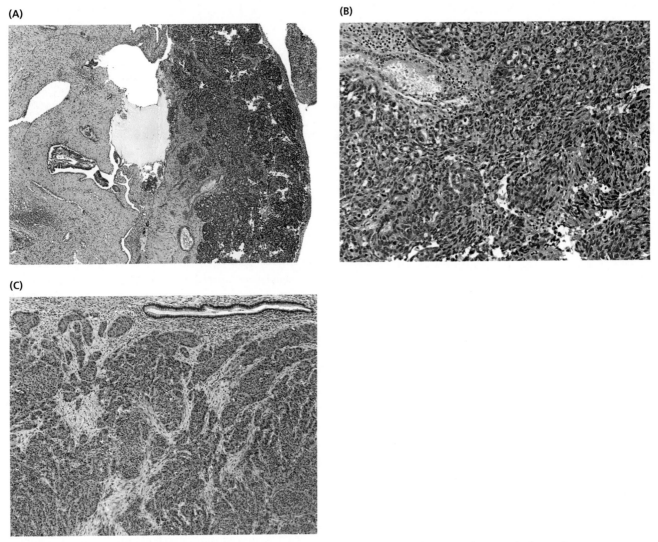

Figure 16.1 (A, B, C) Implant of ovarian high-grade serous carcinoma to endometrium. Implants may also occur in the cervix.

involving cervix or corpus. Primary cervical squamous cell carcinoma must always be excluded, especially in a premenopausal patient with a history of high-risk HPV and/or prior cervical dysplasia. This may be a difficult differential diagnosis, given the recent demonstration of high-risk HPV and/or overexpression of p16 in some bladder cancers[9,10].

Breast

Breast carcinoma is the most common tumor to metastasize to the uterus. Most, but not all patients have a prior history of breast cancer, although the clinical suspicion of a metastasis may be low[11,12]. Some cases are diagnosed during screening evaluation for tamoxifen therapy; others may be diagnosed in the evaluation of postmenopausal bleeding or suspected endometrial polyp. Lobular carcinoma is the most common type of breast cancer to spread to the female genital tract

(Figure 16.3), although duct-forming metastases have been reported. The differential diagnosis is stromal sarcoma and primary cervical adenocarcinoma, as well as a variety of other small cell malignancies. The malignant cells may form signet ring cells, which can be quite prominent[13]. The lobular cells tend to widely infiltrate the tissue, surrounding pre-existing glands; however, this gland preservation pattern is not specific for metastasis and may be seen on occasion with primary uterine tumors. A combination of PAX8 (positive in female genital tract primaries) and BRST2 (positive in breast primaries) should resolve most cases (Figure 16.4)[14,15].

Colorectum

Unlike colorectal metastases to the ovary, metastatic colorectal carcinoma involving the uterus is rare in absence of a known primary. However, the pathologist or the gynecologist

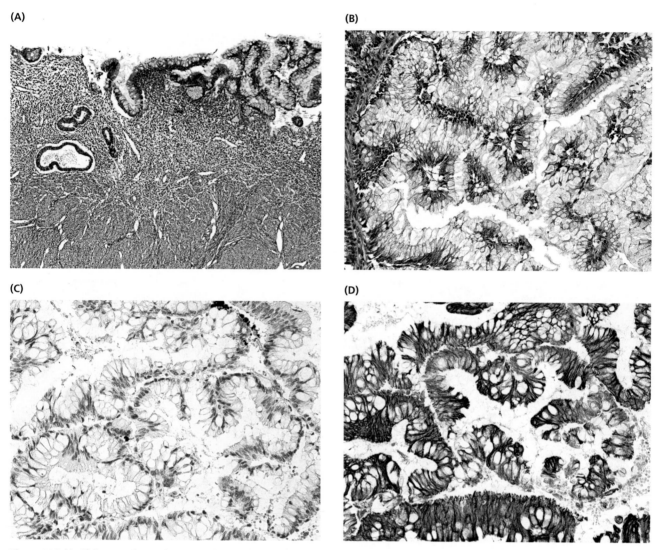

Figure 16.2 (A, B) Low-grade mucinous neoplasms of the appendix typically involve the ovary and fallopian tube, but endometrial colonization may also occur. (C) The CK7-negative, (D) CK20-positive phenotype suggests spread from an extra-uterine site.

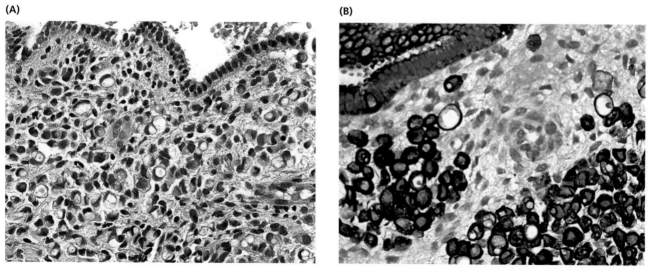

Figure 16.3 Metastatic breast cancer. (A) Lobular carcinoma replaces the endometrial stroma. When extensive, it may mimic an endometrial stromal neoplasm. (B) Cytokeratin highlights the lobular carcinoma cells. The cells are negative for PAX8 (not shown).

may not always have that history and, in these cases, misdiagnosis as endometrioid adenocarcinoma in an endometrial biopsy or curettage can occur. The presence of large amounts of necrotic material within the gland lumens (so-called dirty necrosis), cystic gland lumens, and a particularly well-developed cribriform gland pattern with goblet cells may suggest the diagnosis, although some types of endocervical adenocarcinomas may exhibit similar features (Figure 16.5). The neoplastic cells are almost always positive for CK20, with variable or absent staining for CK7, in colorectal metastases, while uterine primaries are positive for CK7 and not CK20 (Figure 16.6). CDX2 may be useful in this differential diagnosis[16], but caution should be exercised when using this

marker as primary uterine tumors with intestinal mucinous differentiation may also express CDX2.

Gallbladder and pancreas

This too is rare and typically occurs in the setting of a known primary carcinoma of the pancreatico-biliary tract[7,17,18]. The only clues to this diagnosis are prior history, microscopic features that are unusual for a primary uterine tumor, and apparent partial replacement of normal glands and/or surface mucosa. Unlike colorectal metastases, cytokeratin expression patterns may be similar to primary uterine tumors (Figure 16.7). CDX2 can be seen in

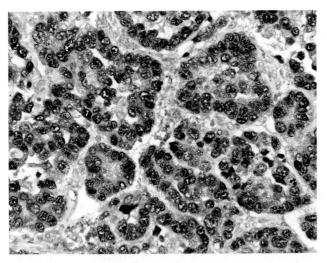

Figure 16.4 PAX8 in endometrial carcinoma.

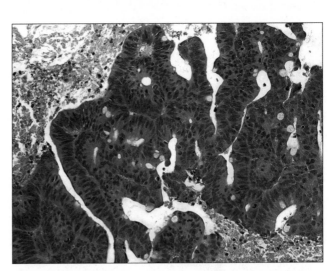

Figure 16.5 Metastatic colorectal carcinoma. Small intracellular mucin droplets and goblet cells are present, but this can easily be mistaken for endometrial adenocarcinoma in a curettage specimen.

(A)

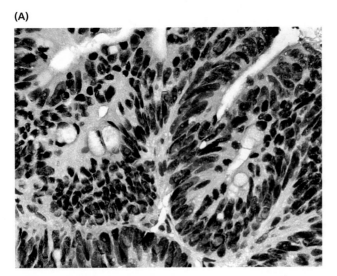

(B)

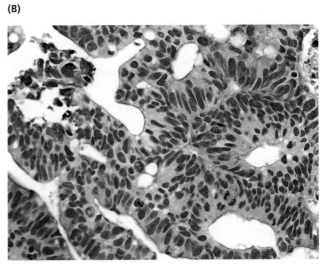

Figure 16.6 Metastatic colorectal carcinoma. (A) CDX2 highlights the malignant cells, but (B) CK7 and (C) CK20 are often more useful in confirming the diagnosis.

(C)

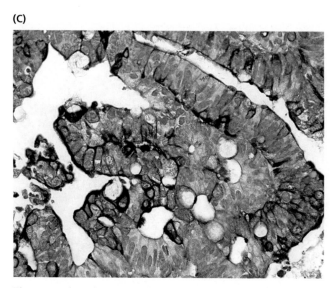

Figure 16.6 (cont.)

(A)

(B)

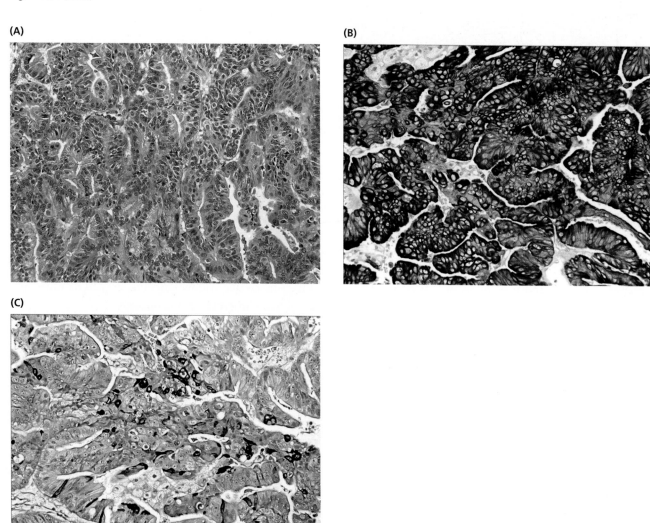

(C)

Figure 16.7 (A) Metastatic gallbladder carcinoma. Metastases from the biliary tract may be quite deceptive as they can mimic a variety of primary gynecologic carcinomas. (B) CK7 is strongly positive. (C) CK20 is focally positive.

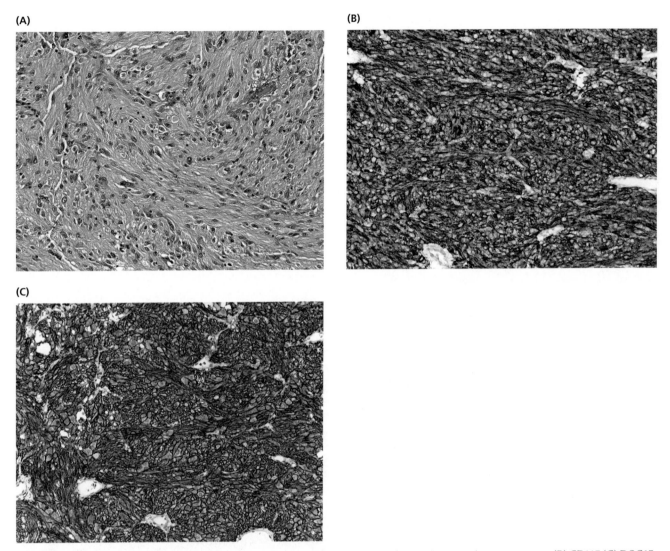

Figure 16.8 (A) Gastrointestinal stromal tumor involving the parauterine tissue may simulate a primary uterine corpus tumor. (B) CD117 (C) DOG17

biliary tract cancers and may, in absence of estrogen and progesterone hormone receptor expression suggest the diagnosis. Loss of DPC4 may be seen in approximately 50% of pancreatic primary adenocarcinomas.

Gastrointestinal stromal tumor

Extraintestinal gastrointestinal stromal tumors may mimic a primary uterine tumor[19], or secondarily involve the uterus either by extension from the bowel wall or an adjacent location (Figure 16.8). Metastases from intestinal gastrointestinal stromal tumors to the ovary have also been reported[20]. An immunohistochemical panel that includes CD117 (c-kit) and DOG1 will identify most cases of gastrointestinal stromal tumor, but care must be taken in the evaluation of uterine tumors, as strong CD117 expression in absence of a detectable c-kit mutation can occasionally

be seen in uterine leiomyosarcoma, as well as other primary uterine mesenchymal neoplasms[21].

Lymphoma/leukemia

Secondary involvement of the uterus by lymphoma or leukemia is more common than primary involvement[22–29]. The uterus is affected more commonly by chronic lymphocytic leukemia than any other type of leukemia or lymphoma. Patients with secondary uterine involvement by lymphoma range in age from 20 to greater than 75 years. The most common presenting feature is abnormal uterine bleeding, followed by a pelvic mass. In most cases, the uterus and cervix are involved, but isolated corpus or, less commonly, cervical involvement can be seen. Most are B-cell lymphomas, with diffuse large cell the most common type (Figure 16.9), but acute lymphoblastic leukemia (Figure 16.10) and marginal zone lymphoma (Figure 16.11)

(A)

(B)

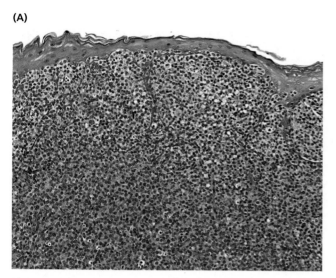

Figure 16.9 (A, B) Diffuse B-cell lymphoma secondarily involving cervix.

(A)

(B)

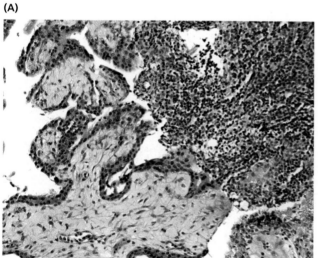
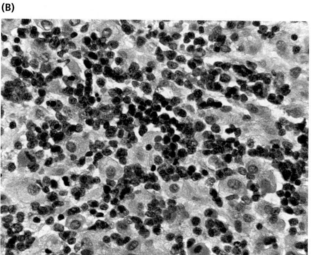

Figure 16.10 (A, B) Acute lymphoblastic leukemia involving placenta.

are also seen. T-cell lymphomas may also rarely secondarily involve the uterus. The differential diagnosis includes inflammatory conditions, other hematopoietic processes, undifferentiated carcinoma, small cell carcinoma, endometrial stromal tumors, melanoma, and Ewing/primitive neuroectodermal tumor. The clinical history of lymphoma or leukemia is the most helpful diagnostic clue.

Other carcinomas

Increasing use of positron emission tomography/computed tomography may lead to the discovery of occult uterine metastases masquerading as a second primary malignancy. Primary sites include lung, thyroid, kidney, and gastric cancer, as well as breast and colorectum[30-35]. The possibility

of metastasis should be included in the differential diagnosis of uterine masses that appear to be malignant, especially in patients with diffuse metastatic disease and in patients with a uterus in which the normal shape is preserved but in which involvement with a diffuse, heterogeneously enhancing infiltrative process is seen. Directed immunohistochemistry can be helpful in identifying lung and thyroid metastases; although TTF1 is occasionally expressed in ovarian cancer (<15%), this is less common in endometrial carcinomas.

Melanoma

Metastatic melanoma may present initially in the uterus or, more commonly, in the setting of known, pre-existing disease (Figure 16.12)[36-38]. The presence of melanin

(A)

(B)

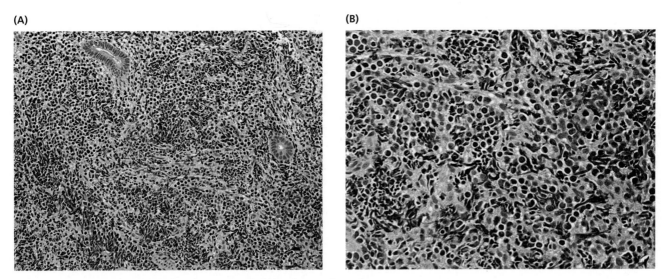

Figure 16.11 (A, B) Marginal zone lymphoma secondarily involving endometrium.

(A)

(B)

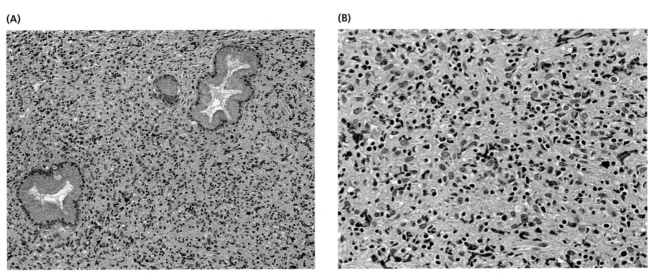

Figure 16.12 (A, B) Metastatic melanoma.

pigment may suggest the diagnosis. A panel of immuno-histochemical markers for undifferentiated neoplasms that includes S100 and, if necessary, other melanoma markers will establish the diagnosis. Primary cervical melanoma should be excluded; often, this is based entirely on absence of apparent primary tumor elsewhere, but occasionally an in situ component may be present.

REFERENCES

1. Kumar N, Hart W. Metastases to the uterine corpus from extragenital cancers. A clinicopathologic study of 63 cases. *Cancer* 1982;**50**:2163–9.
2. Lemoine NR, Hall PA. Epithelial tumors metastatic to the uterine cervix. A study of 33 cases and review of the literature. *Cancer* 1986;**57**:2002–5.
3. Mazur MT, Hsueh S, Gersell DJ. Metastases to the female genital tract. Analysis of 325 cases. *Cancer* 1984;**53**:1978–84.
4. Mulvany NJ, Nirenberg A, Oster AG. Non-primary cervical adeno-carcinomas. *Pathology* 1996;**28**:293–7.
5. Danielian PJ. Ovarian metastatic carcinoma presenting as a primary cervical carcinoma. *Acta Obstet Gynecol Scand* 1990; **69**:265–6.
6. Fanning J, Alvarez PM, Tsukada Y, *et al.* Cervical implantation meta-stasis by endometrial adenocarcinoma. *Cancer* 1991;**68**:1335–9.
7. McCluggage WG, Hurrell DP, Kennedy K. Metastatic carcinomas in the cervix mimicking primary cervical adenocarcinoma and ade-nocarcinoma in situ: report of a series of cases. *Am J Surg Pathol* 2010;**34**:735–41.
8. Moore WF, Bentley RC, Kim KR, *et al.* Goblet-cell mucinous epithe-lium lining the endometrium and endocervix: evidence of metastasis from an appendiceal primary tumor through the use of cytokeratin-7 and -20 immunostains. *Int J Gynecol Pathol* 1998;**17**:363–7.
9. Cioffi-Lavina M, Chapman-Fredricks J, Gomez-Fernandez C, *et al.* p16 expression in squamous cell carcinomas of cervix and bladder. *Appl Immunohistochem Mol Morphol*;**18**:344–7.
10. Husain E, Khawaja A, Shaikh T, *et al.* Transitional cell carcinoma of the urinary tract in renal transplant recipients. *Pathology* 2009;**41**:406–8.

11. Houghton JP, Ioffe OB, Silverberg SG, *et al.* Metastatic breast lobular carcinoma involving tamoxifen-associated endometrial polyps: report of two cases and review of tamoxifen-associated polypoid uterine lesions. *Mod Pathol* 2003;**16**:395–8.

12. Yazigi R, Sandstad J, Munoz AK. Breast cancer metastasizing to the uterine cervix. *Cancer* 1988;**61**:2558–60.

13. Kennebeck CH, Alagoz T. Signet ring breast carcinoma metastases limited to the endometrium and cervix. *Gynecol Oncol* 1998; **71**:461–4.

14. DiMaio M, Beck A, Montgomery K, *et al.* PAX8 and WT1 are superior to PAX2 and BRST2 in distinguishing mullerian tract tumors from breast carcinomas. *Mod Pathol* 2011;**24**:243A.

15. Laury AR, Perets R, Piao H, *et al.* A comprehensive analysis of PAX8 expression in human epithelial tumors. *Am J Surg Pathol* 2011;**35**:816–26.

16. Raspollini MR, Baroni G, Taddei A, *et al.* Primary cervical adenocarcinoma with intestinal differentiation and colonic carcinoma metastatic to cervix: an investigation using Cdx-2 and a limited immunohistochemical panel. *Arch Pathol Lab Med* 2003;**127**:1586–90.

17. Hall PA, Lemoine NR, Ryan JF. Carcinoma of the gall bladder metastatic to the cervix. Case report. *Br J Obstet Gynaecol* 1986;**93**:1187–90.

18. Martinez-Roman S, Frumovitz M, Deavers MT, *et al.* Metastatic carcinoma of the gallbladder mimicking an advanced cervical carcinoma. *Gynecol Oncol* 2005;**97**:942–5.

19. Peitsidis P, Zarganis P, Trichia H, *et al.* Extragastrointestinal stromal tumor mimicking a uterine tumor. A rare clinical entity. *Int J Gynecol Cancer* 2008;**18**:1115–18.

20. Irving JA, Lerwill MF, Young RH. Gastrointestinal stromal tumors metastatic to the ovary: a report of five cases. *Am J Surg Pathol* 2005;**29**:920–6.

21. Rushing RS, Shajahan S, Chendil D, *et al.* Uterine sarcomas express KIT protein but lack mutation(s) in exon 11 or 17 of c-KIT. *Gynecol Oncol* 2003;**91**:9–14.

22. Ferry JA, Young RH. Malignant lymphoma, pseudolymphoma, and hematopoietic disorders of the female genital tract. *Pathol Annu* 1991;**26**:227–63.

23. Friedman HD, Adelson MD, Elder RC, *et al.* Granulocytic sarcoma of the uterine cervix – literature review of granulocytic sarcoma of the female genital tract. *Gynecol Oncol* 1992;**46**: 128–37.

24. Harris N, Scully R. Malignant lymphoma and granulocytic sarcoma of the uterus and vagina. A clinicopathologic analysis of 27 cases. *Cancer* 1984;**53**:2530–45.

25. Kosari F, Daneshbod Y, Parwaresch R, *et al.* Lymphomas of the female genital tract: a study of 186 cases and review of the literature. *Am J Surg Pathol* 2005;**29**:1512–20.

26. Oliva E, Ferry JA, Young RH, *et al.* Granulocytic sarcoma of the female genital tract: a clinicopathologic study of 11 cases. *Am J Surg Pathol* 1997;**21**:1156–65.

27. Smith NL, Baird DB, Strausbauch PH. Endometrial involvement by multiple myeloma. *Int J Gynecol Pathol* 1997;**16**:173–5.

28. van de Rijn M, Kamel OW, Chang PP, *et al.* Primary low-grade endometrial B-cell lymphoma. *Am J Surg Pathol* 1997; **21**:187–94.

29. Vang R, Medeiros LJ, Ha CS, *et al.* Non-Hodgkin's lymphomas involving the uterus: a clinicopathologic analysis of 26 cases. *Mod Pathol* 2000;**13**:19–28.

30. Bozaci EA, Atabekoglu C, Sertcelik A, *et al.* Metachronous metastases from renal cell carcinoma to uterine cervix and vagina: case report and review of literature. *Gynecol Oncol* 2005; **99**:232–5.

31. Hollier LM, Boswank SE, Stringer CA. Adenocarcinoma of the lung metastatic to the uterine cervix: a case report and review of the literature. *Int J Gynecol Cancer* 1997;**7**:490–4.

32. Imachi M, Tsukamoto N, Amagase H, *et al.* Metastatic adenocarcinoma to the uterine cervix from gastric cancer. A clinicopathologic analysis of 16 cases. *Cancer* 1993;**71**:3472–7.

33. Treszezamsky A, Altuna S, Diaz L, *et al.* Metastases to the uterine cervix from a gastric carcinoma presenting with obstructive renal failure: a case report. *Int J Gynecol Cancer* 2003;**13**:555–7.

34. Yokoyama Y, Sato S, Futagami M, *et al.* Solitary metastasis to the uterine cervix from the early gastric cancer: a case report. *Eur J Gynaecol Oncol* 2000;**21**:469–71.

35. Zafrakas M, Papanikolaou AN, Venizelos ID, *et al.* A rare case of renal cell carcinoma metastasizing to the uterine cervix. *Eur J Gynaecol Oncol* 2009;**30**:239–40.

36. Berker B, Sertcelik A, Kaygusuz G, *et al.* Abnormal uterine bleeding as a presenting sign of metastasis to the endometrium in a patient with a history of cutaneous malignant melanoma. *Gynecol Oncol* 2004;**93**:252–6.

37. Fambrini M, Andersson KL, Buccoliero AM, *et al.* Late solitary metastasis of cutaneous malignant melanoma presenting as abnormal uterine bleeding. *J Obstet Gynaecol Res* 2008;**34**:731–4.

38. Wood C. Metastatic melanoma simulating a primary endometrial tumor. *Am J Obstet Gynecol* 1978;**131**:820–1.

17   GESTATIONAL TROPHOBLASTIC DISEASE

INTRODUCTION

The diagnosis and management of gestational trophoblastic disease has undergone significant changes in the past several years. The introduction of high-resolution ultrasound has led to the earlier detection of abnormal gestations and earlier evacuation of these abnormal gestations. As a result, the clinical and histologic features used to identify gestational trophoblastic disease are not as well developed, and diagnosing molar gestational disease is more challenging than ever.

The term "gestational trophoblastic disease" is used to refer to benign or malignant trophoblastic disease. Histologically, it is classified into hydatidiform mole, invasive mole (chorioadenoma destruens), choriocarcinoma, and placental site trophoblastic tumor (PSTT) as well as its close cousin, epithelioid trophoblastic tumor (ETT) (Table 17.1). Those gestational trophoblastic diseases that invade locally or metastasize are collectively known as gestational trophoblastic neoplasia. Most cases of gestational trophoblastic neoplasia are diagnosed when the serum β-hCG levels plateau or rise in patients being observed after the diagnosis of hydatidiform mole. If metastases are present, symptoms associated with the metastatic disease, such as hemoptysis or neurologic sudden onset seizure may be present. The FIGO and AJCC staging for gestational trophoblastic neoplasia is provided

Table 17.1 Classification of gestational trophoblastic disease[2]

Hydatidiform mole
- Complete, including early complete
- Partial

Invasive mole, including persistent or metastatic mole

Gestational choriocarcinoma

Placental site trophoblastic tumor, including epithelioid trophoblastic tumor

in Table 17.2[1,2]. All patients are also assigned a prognostic score, based on age, antecedent pregnancy, interval from index pregnancy, largest tumor size, sites of metastases, number of metastases, and previous failed chemotherapy (Table 17.3).

MOLAR GESTATIONS

Moles are classified as complete (classic and early complete) or partial. The estimated incidence of complete molar pregnancies is approximately 1/1000 of pregnancies, but has been reported as high as 2/1000 pregnancies in Japan and Southeast Asia. Risk factors are age under 15 years, age over 45 years, and history of prior mole[4]. Complete moles are also seen with increased frequency in patients with familial mole syndrome, which has an autosomal recessive pattern of inheritance. Increased incidence of molar gestations is historically seen in Asia, Latin America, and the Middle East, but this is gradually changing.

Table 17.2 Gestational trophoblastic neoplasia staging system (AJCC, 2010 and FIGO, 2000)[1,2]

AJCC[a]	FIGO	Description
T1	Stage I	Disease confined to the uterus
T2	Stage II	Gestational trophoblastic neoplasia extends outside of the uterus, but is limited to the genital structures (adnexa, vagina, broad ligament) by metastasis or direct extension
M1a	Stage III	Gestational trophoblastic neoplasia extends to the lungs, with or without known genital tract involvement
M1b	Stage IV	All other distant metastatic sites

[a] There is no regional lymph node designation in the staging of gestational trophoblastic neoplasia. Regional nodal metastases are classified as metastatic (AJCC M1 or FIGO stage III) disease.

Table 17.3 Modified WHO prognostic scoring index for gestational trophoblastic neoplasia[a] (FIGO, 2009)[3]

Scores[b]	0	1	2	4
Age	<40	≥40	—	—
Antecedent pregnancy	Hydatidiform mole	Abortion	Term pregnancy	—
Interval months from index pregnancy	<4	4–6	7–12	>2
Pretreatment serum β-hCG (IU/l)	$<10^3$	10^3 to $<10^4$	10^4 to 10^5	$\geq10^5$
Largest tumor size, including uterus (cm)	<3	3–4	≥5	—
Site of metastases	Lung	Spleen, kidney	Gastrointestinal tract	Liver, brain
Number of metastases	—	1–4	5–8	>8
Previous failed chemotherapy	—	—	Single drug	Two or more drugs

[a] Scores most accurately reflect risk for villous trophoblastic disease (invasive mole, gestational choriocarcinoma). This scoring system is not as well validated for extravillous trophoblastic disease (placental site trophoblastic tumor and epithelioid trophoblastic tumor).

[b] Low risk is a score of 6 or less. High risk is a score of 7 or greater. To stage and allot a risk factor score, a patient's diagnosis is allocated to a stage as represented by a Roman numeral I, II, III, and IV. This is then separated by a colon from the sum of all the actual risk factor scores expressed in Arabic numerals; for example stage II:4, stage IV:9. A stage and score are allotted for each patient.

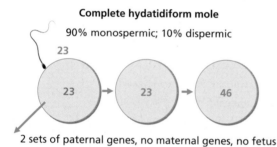

Complete hydatidiform mole

90% monospermic; 10% dispermic

2 sets of paternal genes, no maternal genes, no fetus

Diagram 17.1 Complete mole is formed as a result of fertilization of a functionally anucleate egg ("empty ovum") by a single sperm that undergoes reduplication (46XY), or rarely by two sperm (46XY or 46XX).

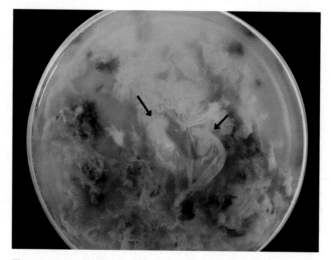

Figure 17.1 Complete mole. Tiny grape-like vesicles (arrows) are characteristic of complete mole.

It is difficult to provide an accurate ratio of complete mole versus partial mole, since the diagnosis of molar pregnancies, especially partial molar pregnancies, can be difficult and is subject to poor diagnostic reproducibility. In recent years, the identification of p57, a paternally imprinted, maternally expressed gene in villous stromal tissue, has changed the diagnostic evaluation of molar gestations[5–7]. p57 immunohistochemistry, in conjunction with other newly developed molecular studies has greatly enhanced our ability to (1) correctly identify moles, even at an early stage; and (2) distinguish complete moles from partial moles[7,8]. It is anticipated that data collected with these new techniques will yield more robust predictions for risk for persistent, recurrent, and subsequent trophoblastic disease.

Complete mole

The classic complete mole occurs as a result of fertilization of a functionally anucleate egg ("empty ovum") by a single sperm that undergoes reduplication (46XY), or rarely by two sperm (46XY or 46XX)[9,10]. The DNA content is diploid and is entirely paternal (Diagram 17.1). Patients present with excessive uterine enlargement; markedly elevated β-hCG; hyperemesis; hyperreactio luteinalis (multiple ovarian cysts); and passage of grape-like hydropic villi (Figure 17.1; Table 17.4). The curettings consist of an increased volume of tissue due to the presence of enlarged, edematous (hydropic) villi that are irregular and edematous on microscopic exam (Figure 17.2). Cisterns (formed by villous cavitation) are present (Figure 17.3), and there is circumferential or multifocal trophoblastic proliferation with trophoblastic atypia (Figure 17.4). Most complete moles are easily diagnosed (Table 17.5).

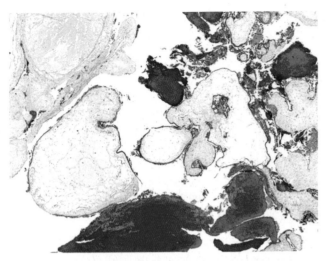

Figure 17.2 Complete mole. The villi are large and edematous, and often have a more basophilic stroma relative to the usual eosinophilic stroma seen in nonmolar chorionic villi.

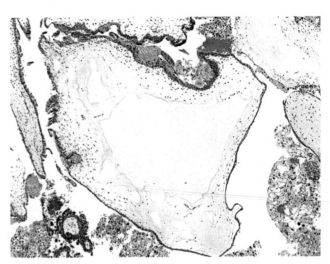

Figure 17.3 Complete mole. Cisterns are often present in the larger, more edematous chorionic villi.

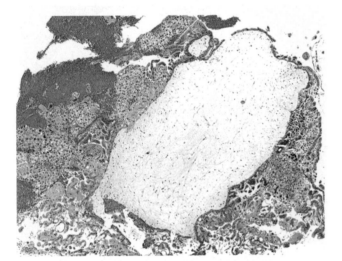

Figure 17.4 Complete mole. Trophoblastic proliferation, often with cytologic atypia, is a characteristic of complete mole.

Table 17.4 Clinical characteristics of classic complete mole[a]

Reproductive age
Excessive uterine enlargement
Vaginal bleeding, typically at 6–16 weeks gestation
Markedly elevated serum β-hCG (>100,000 mIU/ml)
Hyperemesis, pre-eclampsia, hyperthyroidism
Hyperreactio luteinalis (multiple ovarian cysts) – approximately 15%
Passage of grape-like hydropic villi
Failure of β-hCG to normalize following evacuation

[a] These findings may be muted or absent in early complete mole.

Table 17.5 Pathologic characteristics of complete mole, early complete mole, and partial mole

Complete mole (classic)	Early complete mole	Partial mole
Increased volume of tissue with macroscopic villous hydrops	No increased volume of tissue with no macroscopic villous hydrops	May or may not have increased volume with patchy villous hydrops
Enlarged, balloon-shaped villi	Bulbous, cauliflower-shaped villi	Dimorphic pattern with scalloped-shaped villi
Edematous villi	Villous edema focal or mild	Patchy villous edema
Cisterns	Cisterns often absent	Cisterns may be present
Hypocellular pink stroma	Hypercellular, blue stroma	Hypocellular pink stroma
Trophoblastic proliferation	Focal trophoblastic proliferation	Focal, mild trophoblastic proliferation
Inconspicuous vasculature; karyorrhectic debris may be present	Labyrinthine vasculature with karyorrhectic debris	Trophoblastic inclusions may be present
Trophoblast atypia	Trophoblast atypia	Stromal cell atypia may be present
Loss of p57	Loss of p57	Intact p57

Complete mole is associated with persistent disease (usually invasive mole) in 20–30% of cases, choriocarcinoma in 3–5% of cases, and recurrent mole in less than 2% of cases[7].

Early complete mole

Early complete mole arises in the same manner as that of the classic complete mole, but it is usually clinically unsuspected[11]. Since the early complete mole is evacuated in the first trimester, patients are asymptomatic, and elevations of serum β-hCG are modest at most[4]. The endometrial curetting tissue is not as voluminous as in the classic complete mole, and the appearance of the tissue is similar to that of a spontaneous abortion on gross exam. On microscopic examination, the classic histologic features of complete mole are absent or muted. Villous edema is mild and may be focal, often without cisterns (Figure 17.5). Focal trophoblastic proliferation may be present, but it is not as exuberant as in the classic complete mole (Table 17.5). However, pleomorphic and hyperchromatic intermediate trophoblast may be seen (Figure 17.6). The villi in early complete mole are bulbous in shape, resembling a cauliflower, and the stroma is hypercellular (Figure 17.7). A labyrinthine vascular network and nuclear karyorrhectic debris are additional features of the early complete mole

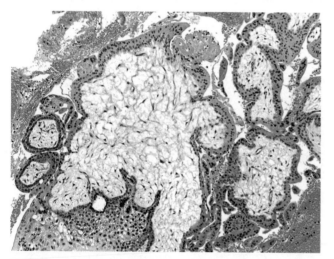

Figure 17.5 Early complete mole. Villous edema is mild and often focal, often without cisterns. Focal trophoblastic proliferation may be present, but it is not as exuberant as in the classic complete mole.

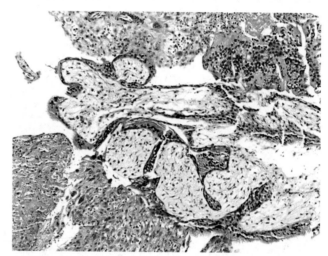

Figure 17.7 Early complete mole. The villi in early complete mole are bulbous in shape, resembling a cauliflower, and the stroma is hypercellular.

(A)

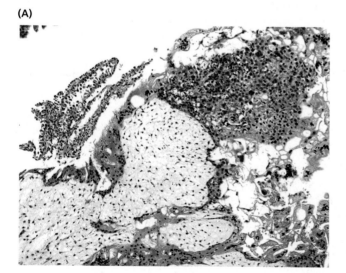

(B)

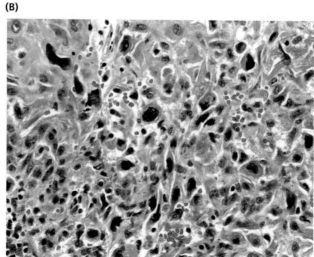

Figure 17.6 (A, B) Early complete mole. Like the classic mole, early complete mole may harbor pleomorphic and hyperchromatic intermediate trophoblast.

(A)   **(B)**

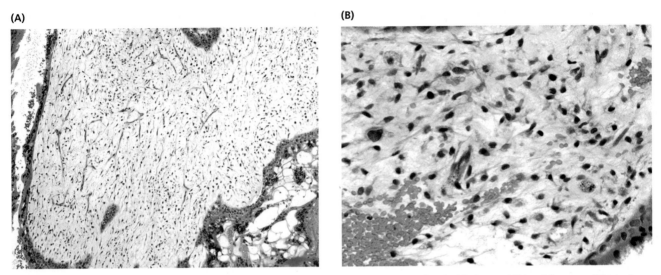

Figure 17.8 (A, B) Early complete mole. A labyrinthine vascular network and nuclear karyorrhectic debris are additional features of the early complete mole.

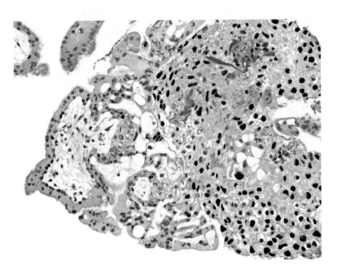

Figure 17.9 p57 is normally expressed by villous stromal cells, cytotrophoblast, and intervillous trophoblast, but not by syncytiotrophoblast. Note nuclear localization.

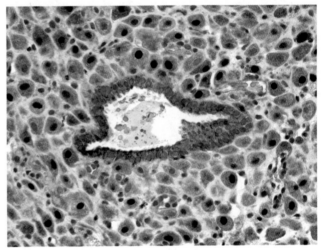

Figure 17.10 Nuclear p57 is normally expressed by decidual cells, but not endometrial secretory glandular epithelium.

(Figure 17.8). Nucleated red blood cells may rarely be seen, and do *not* militate against the diagnosis, provided all other diagnostic features are present[12].

p57 is a cell cycle inhibitor that is encoded by a paternally imprinted gene on chromosome 11p15.5 that is expressed almost exclusively in maternally derived tissues[6]. It is believed to be important in implantation and placental development. p57 is normally expressed in villous stromal cells, cytotrophoblast, intervillous trophoblast, and decidual cells, but not syncytiotrophoblast or gestational endometrial secretory glands (Figures 17.9 and 17.10). Both classic complete mole and early complete mole show loss of nuclear p57 expression in villous stromal cells and

cytotrophoblast (completely negative or, if positive, almost always <10%), since these moles are paternal in origin (Figure 17.11)[5]. In contrast, hydropic villi and partial moles retain nuclear p57 expression in the cytotrophoblast and villous stromal cells (Figure 17.12). Thus, p57 does not distinguish partial mole from hydropic abortus.

Although the staining pattern for p57 is straightforward in the majority of cases in clinical practice, occasional discordant or divergent p57 staining patterns may be seen[7]. In our experience, this is most commonly seen in twin pregnancy in which one is a complete mole and the other is a nonmolar abortus. In this case, two villous populations are usually seen: one in which the p57 is intact and the other in which p57 is lost. Chimeric or mosaic conceptions and retained maternal chromosome 11 are another potential source of confusion[7]. Mosaic conceptions may exhibit strong nuclear p57 expression in the cytotrophoblast but weak or completely absent expression in the villous cytotrophoblast. Retained expression of p57 is also seen in bi-parental complete hydatidiform moles associated with novel missense *NLRP7* gene mutations on chromosome 19q. Occasionally, weak nuclear p57 expression may be seen in the cytotrophoblast or villous stromal cells in complete moles (Figure 17.13); this staining pattern, which has been attributed to incomplete imprinting, does not usually pose a significant diagnostic problem as the surrounding intervillous trophoblast and decidual cells exhibit strong nuclear p57 expression, providing a strong internal positive control.

Patients with complete moles undergo complete suction curettage and weekly or biweekly measurement of serum β-hCG levels until three consecutive tests are normal, followed by monthly measurement of β-hCG levels for six months[4]. During this time the patients are instructed to avoid pregnancy. In addition, pathologic examination of the placenta and other products of conception and a six-week postpartum β-hCG level to establish normalization is recommended with all future pregnancies. Since many patients may wish to proceed with a new pregnancy, it is important that complete moles not be overdiagnosed. If there is any doubt, additional studies, such as p57 staining, should be pursued.

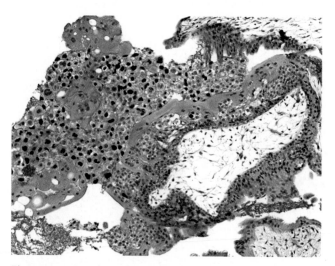

Figure 17.11 Complete mole. Nuclear p57 expression is lost in the villous stromal cells and cytotrophoblast, but preserved in intervillous trophoblast.

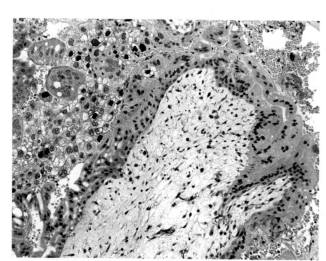

Figure 17.13 Weak p57 expression by cytotrophoblast and villous trophoblast has been attributed to partial imprinting.

(A)

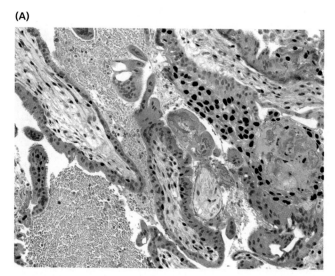

(B)

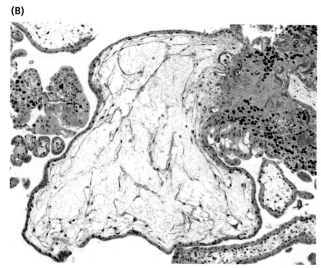

Figure 17.12 (A, B) Nuclear p57 is preserved in partial mole (depicted here), as well as in hydropic mole.

Partial hydatidiform mole

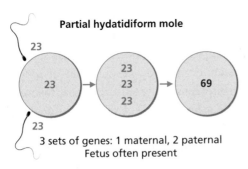

3 sets of genes: 1 maternal, 2 paternal
Fetus often present

Diagram 17.2 Partial mole is formed as a result of fertilization of an ovum by two or, less commonly, one duplicated spermatozoa, resulting in maternally and paternally derived triploid DNA content.

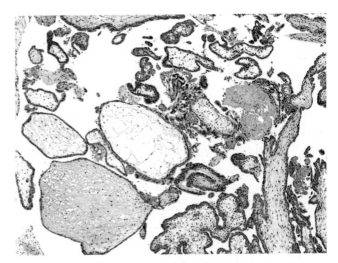

Figure 17.14 Partial mole. Dimorphic pattern consists of small, normal-sized villi and enlarged, edematous villi.

(A)

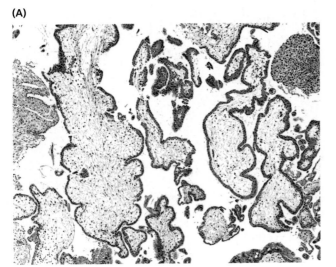

(B)

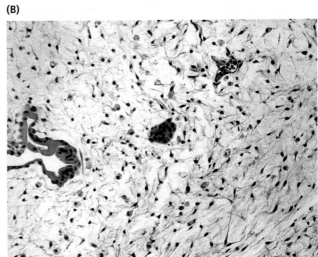

Figure 17.15 (A, B) Partial mole. The enlarged villi have scalloped borders with inclusions.

Partial mole

Partial moles arise as a result of fertilization of an ovum by two spermatozoa or, less commonly, one duplicated spermatozoon, resulting in maternally and paternally derived triploid DNA content (Diagram 17.2)[9,10,13]. A fetus is usually present, but rarely survives into the second trimester. Patients present with symptoms of incomplete or missed abortion. Less than 10% of patients with partial moles present with serum β-hCG levels >100,000 mIU/ml[4].

The villi in partial mole are variable in size and shape, imparting a dimorphic pattern (Figure 17.14). Villi are edematous (Figure 17.15), and the villous outlines are irregular, forming a scalloped appearance. Cisterns may be present, and there is focal, mild trophoblastic proliferation

(Figure 17.16). Trophoblastic inclusions can be seen. Atypical stromal cells may be present (Table 17.5). Fetal parts may be seen and, if present, are usually malformed.

Since p57 does not distinguish partial mole from hydropic abortus, molecular genotyping may be conducted to confirm suspected cases of partial mole[8]. However, it is not cost effective to perform molecular genotyping to guide patient management, since partial moles are rarely associated with persistent (<0.5%) or recurrent (<2%) disease. Progression to choriocarcinoma is also exceedingly rare[7], as many older reports of associations between partial mole and choriocarcinoma were based on the mistaken assumption that lesions we currently recognize as early complete mole were partial moles. Moreover, patients with

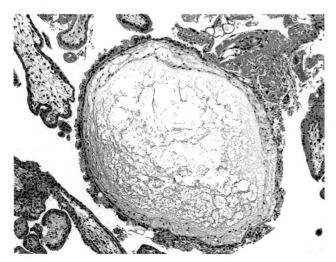

Figure 17.16 Partial mole. Villous edema is present, but trophoblastic proliferation is not as prominent as in complete mole.

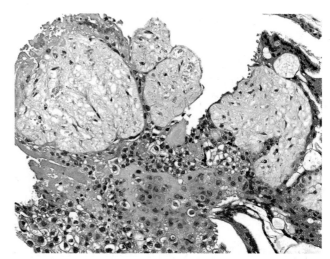

Figure 17.17 Early nonmolar gestation. Trophoblastic proliferation may be quite prominent, but the villi are small and non-edematous.

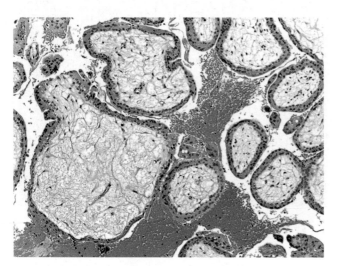

Figure 17.18 Hydropic abortus. The chorionic villi may be edematous, but there is no significant trophoblastic proliferation.

partial mole often need only a single follow-up β-hCG level to ensure decrease. Therefore, in practice, if there is uncertainty about whether a curetting specimen harbors a partial mole (versus a hydropic abortus), the pathologist should issue a note indicating the uncertainty, since no harm is done by asking the patient to return for a single follow-up β-hCG. If the β-hCG does not become undetectable on the follow-up assay, continued surveillance with additional evaluation can then be implemented.

Differential diagnosis of molar pregnancy

Early nonmolar pregnancy

Early nonmolar gestations (less than six weeks) may show circumferential trophoblastic proliferation and stromal basophilia, but the villi are usually not hydropic, cisterns are absent, and the degree of apoptosis and karyorrhexis is decreased relative to that seen in hydatidiform mole (Figure 17.17)[14].

Hydropic abortus

Grossly visible villous hydrops is very unusual in hydropic abortus. Tissue volume is scant. Villi in hydropic abortus are mildly enlarged and edematous, but are expanded in a uniform manner like a balloon (Figure 17.18). Cisterns are usually absent, but there may be focal trophoblastic proliferation – which is *usually* polar. Hydropic abortus may be associated with a fetus, but fetal parts are typically absent. DNA content may be diploid or triploid; karyotype abnormalities are often present. Tissue volume is scant, and no gross villous abnormalities are seen.

Trisomies

Trisomy 13, trisomy 18, and trisomy 21 may be associated with irregular villous enlargement (so-called abnormal villous morphology), hydrops and central cistern formation (Figure 17.19). Abnormal villous morphology may also occur in mosaic and chimeric conceptions[7].

Mesenchymal dysplasia

Mesenchymal dysplasia may mimic partial mole, but mesenchymal dysplasia is usually encountered late in pregnancy and has no trophoblastic proliferation. The associated gestations are usually chromosomally normal.

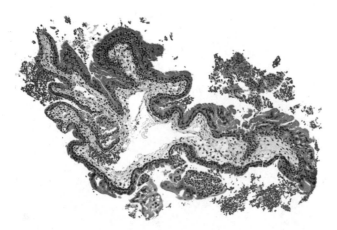

Figure 17.19 Trisomy 21 may be associated with abnormal villous morphology, hydrops and central cistern formation.

The placenta is enlarged and grossly abnormal due to multiple cysts and aneurysmally dilated chorionic plate vessels (Figure 17.20). Microscopically, mesenchymal dysplasia is characterized by enlarged stem villi in the region of the chorionic plate (Figure 17.21). The villous stroma exhibits prominent myxomatous change and inconspicuous vessels (Figure 17.22). The muscular wall of the fetal vessels is essentially replaced by collagen. Chorangiosis and extramedullary hematopoiesis is often present. Approximately 50% of cases are associated with Beckwith–Wiedemann syndrome (omphalocele, macroglossia, visceromegaly). Elevated maternal serum alpha-fetoprotein may be present.

(A)   **(B)**

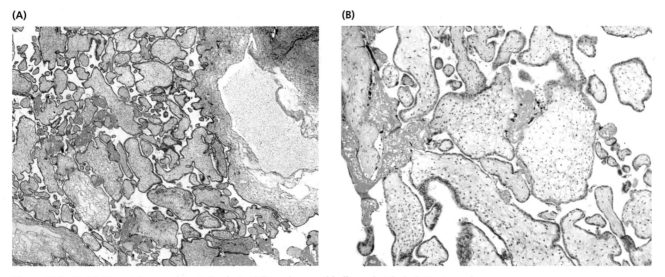

Figure 17.20 (A, B) Placental mesenchymal dysplasia. The cotyledons are distorted by cystic and polypoid masses. (Courtesy of Ann Folkins, MD, Stanford University.)

(A)   **(B)**

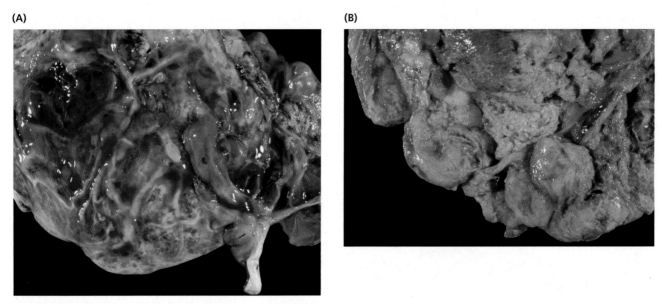

Figure 17.21 (A, B) Placental mesenchymal dysplasia. Villi are large and bulbous, but lack distinct vessels.

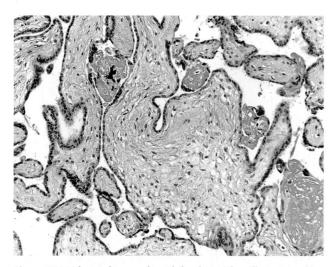

Figure 17.22 Placental mesenchymal dysplasia. The villous stroma is basophilic and lacks well-formed vessels.

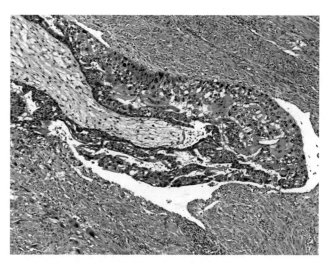

Figure 17.23 Invasive mole.

Invasive mole

Invasive mole is characterized by invasion into the myometrium or uterine vessels by molar villi. Approximately 10–15% of hydatidiform moles will result in invasive mole, and about 15% of these will metastasize to the lungs or vagina. Rarely is a pathologic diagnosis of an invasive mole made on an endometrial biopsy or curettage specimen, because this requires the identification of destructive invasion of the myometrium by the trophoblasts. Typically, scant or no myometrium is recovered on such a specimen. When myometrium is present in the sampling or if, for some reason, hysterectomy is performed, villi are seen juxtaposed to myometrium without an intervening layer of decidua, similar to the situation with placenta accreta (Figure 17.23).

Currently, in most cases of persistent trophoblastic disease (defined as persistent elevations of serum β-hCG following a tissue diagnosis of gestational trophoblastic disease), a presumptive diagnosis of invasive mole is made based on absence of chorionic villi on repeat curettage (to exclude incomplete evacuation), negative uterine ultrasound, and negative metastatic work-up. The diagnosis is usually not confirmed pathologically, as hysterectomy is no longer considered necessary to treat trophoblastic disease. Treatment consists of chemotherapy, typically methotrexate. Hysterectomy is sometimes performed after repeat curettage and chemotherapy, when the uterus is clinically considered to be a "sanctuary"; that is, there is persistent chemoresistant disease within the uterus. When examined microscopically in this setting, the villi often appear fibrotic or degenerate; an exaggerated placental site may also be seen.

RECURRENT GESTATIONAL TROPHOBLASTIC DISEASE

Recurrence is defined as the presence of gestational trophoblastic disease following complete remission (normalization of β-hCG) of treated gestational trophoblastic neoplasia. The diagnosis requires confirmation of persistent disease in addition to an elevated serum β-hCG.

When evaluating patients for possible persistent disease, it is important to understand that persistent low levels of β-hCG may occur in absence of pregnancy or gestational disease. Most common causes include false-positive β-hCG, low levels of β-hCG of pituitary origin, and so-called quiescent gestational trophoblastic disease. Treatment of these low levels in absence of documented neoplasia is ineffective: obviously a false-positive β-hCG and pituitary β-hCG will not respond to current chemotherapeutic regimens, and, to date, no treated cases of so-called quiescent gestational trophoblastic disease have fully responded to chemotherapy or to hysterectomy[15].

To determine whether an elevated β-hCG is biologically real, serum should be sent to a laboratory using tests that have not been reported to give false-positive results. Currently, all competitive β-hCG assays or radioimmunoassays have an inherent problem with false-positive β-hCG results. If an alternative test shows a similar β-hCG result, then it is probably a valid β-hCG. If the β-hCG is valid, the serum samples should then be sent to a specialist laboratory for measurement of β-hCG-H and β-hCG free β-subunit. If β-hCG-H is detectable (>1 ng/ml), then active gestational trophoblastic neoplasia may be present[16]. If β-hCG free β-subunit is more than one-third of the β-hCG result, then placental site trophoblastic tumor or non-trophoblastic malignancy should be considered. If neither β-hCG-H nor significant β-hCG free β-subunit is present, quiescent gestational trophoblastic disease should be considered. However, if the patient is perimenopausal or postmenopausal, or has had an oophorectomy, pituitary β-hCG is a likely source. In that case, the patient should take hormone replacement therapy or oral contraceptives. After two to three weeks, this should suppress β-hCG production if it is of pituitary origin. This recommended strategy applies to all patients with persistent low-level β-hCG, including those with a preceding hydatidiform mole or gestational trophoblastic neoplasia[15].

GESTATIONAL CHORIOCARCINOMA

Gestational choriocarcinoma occurs in approximately 1/40,000 pregnancies and 1/40 hydatidiform moles in North America. The incidence is higher in Japan (3.3/40,000) and Southeast Asia (9.2/40,000), as well as in Latin America and Africa, but as molar gestations decrease in these regions, it is highly likely that gestational choriocarcinoma will show a similar decrease. Approximately 50% develop after molar pregnancy (almost all are complete moles), 25% after abortion, and 2% after an ectopic pregnancy; the remaining occur after normal pregnancy. Rarely, choriocarcinoma may develop in an otherwise normal term placenta; most such tumors are without sequelae, but intrauterine demise has been reported secondary to massive hemorrhage. Pulmonary metastases are present in 90% of cases, and, in 20–60% of cases, the liver and brain are involved. Metastases to the pelvis and vagina, intestines, spleen, and kidney also occur. Rarely, metastases may be seen in a newborn. In some examples of metastatic gestational choriocarcinoma, the primary tumor is not identified, presumably due to tumor regression.

Patients with gestational choroicarcinoma present with vaginal bleeding and elevated serum β-hCG. Those with advanced disease may present with symptoms referable to the metastases (Table 17.6). A small proportion of patients may be asymptomatic; in most cases the disease is small volume and confined to the uterus. Gestational choriocarcinoma is highly sensitive to methotrexate-based chemotherapy. Overall survival rate is 90%. Causes of death include hemorrhage secondary to metastatic disease, multiorgan failure, and toxicity

Table 17.6 Clinical characteristics of gestational choriocarcinoma[a]

Reproductive age
Vaginal bleeding
Symptoms due to metastatic disease: hemoptysis, stroke, etc.
Markedly elevated serum β-hCG

[a] A small proportion of patients may be asymptomatic; in most cases the disease is small volume and confined to the uterus.

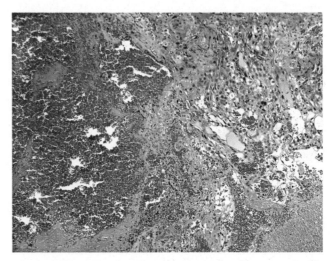

Figure 17.24 Gestational choriocarcinoma is typically associated with abundant hemorrhage and necrosis. One may have to search for the neoplastic tissue.

due to chemotherapy. Poor outcomes are particularly prevalent in HIV-infected women with low CD4 counts, due to poor tolerance to chemotherapy or poor performance status precluding administration of chemotherapy.

Gestational choriocarcinoma is an aggressive, highly malignant tumor. The tumor forms large, often polypoid invasive intrauterine masses with extensive hemorrhage and necrosis. Typically, the curettings also exhibit extensive hemorrhage and necrosis (Table 17.7). Often, the curetting consists almost entirely of blood and necrotic debris, and one has to search carefully for the diagnostic tissue (Figure 17.24). When it develops in the placenta, it is often quite small and may go undetected[17]. Microscopically, the diagnosis of choriocarcinoma is made on the basis of a malignant biphasic (or bilaminar) proliferation of cytotrophoblast and syncytiotrophoblast (Figure 17.25). Intermediate trophoblast may also be present, but is not required for the diagnosis. In some cases, one or another of the required elements (cytotrophoblast and syncytiotrophoblast) may be predominant (Figure 17.26). The term "atypical choriocarcinoma" has been applied to tumors that contain mostly cytotrophoblast and intermediate trophoblast; this pattern is often seen following chemotherapy, but may also be seen in treatment-naïve primary and metastatic tumors (Figure 17.27). Chorionic villi are almost always absent (with rare exceptions, such as choriocarcinoma occurring in a normal placenta, choriocarcinoma arising in twin gestation, etc.).

Syncytiotrophoblast cells are multinucleated with abundant, often glassy eosinophilic cytoplasm that is positive for cytokeratin, β-hCG, and inhibin (Figure 17.25). Cytotrophoblast cells are mononucleated and contain pale or clear cytoplasm (Figure 17.25). The nuclei are convoluted and hyperchromatic, often showing prominent macronucleoli. Mitotic figures are typically numerous, and atypical mitotic figures are often easily found.

Table 17.7 Pathologic characteristics of choriocarcinoma[a]

Large, polypoid uterine mass with necrosis and hemorrhage

Abundant hemorrhage and necrosis in curettings

Malignant, bilaminar proliferation of cytotrophoblast and syncytiotrophoblast

No chorionic villi – unless twin gestation or placental choriocarcinoma

[a] Often, the curetting consists almost entirely of blood and necrotic debris, and one has to search carefully for the diagnostic tissue.

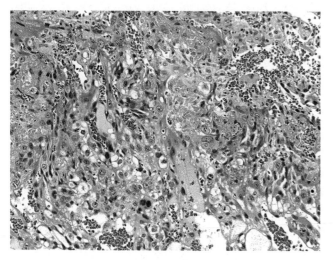

Figure 17.25 Gestational choriocarcinoma.

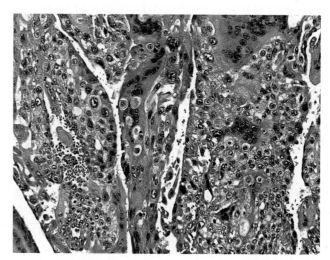

Figure 17.26 Gestational choriocarcinoma. Bilaminar cytotrophoblast and syncytiotrophoblast.

(A)

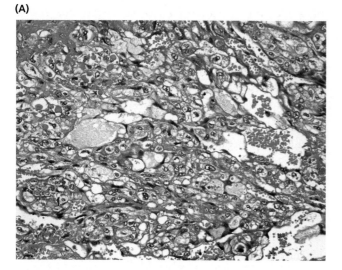

(B)

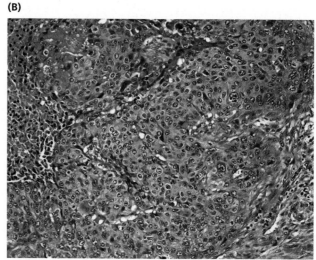

Figure 17.27 Atypical choriocarcinoma (A, B). Neoplastic cells, some of them vacuolated with hyperchromatic nuclei and attenuated cytoplasm, envelop larger mononuclear cells, imparting a nested appearance. The flattened cells are syncytiotrophoblast.

Differential diagnosis of gestational choriocarcinoma

Postabortion villous trophoblast

Curettages performed following spontaneous or induced incomplete abortion may contain trophoblastic tissue in absence of villi. The clinical history and review of the prior specimen, if available, will establish the correct diagnosis.

Post-molar curettings

Curettages performed for persistent trophoblastic neoplasia may contain markedly atypical trophoblastic tissue in absence of villi. If the curettage is obtained within the first six weeks of the initial diagnosis of a molar pregnancy, these cases are diagnosed and managed as persistent gestational trophoblastic neoplasia.

High-grade carcinoma

Some high-grade carcinomas feature enlarged, multinucleated giant cells and may have elevated β-hCG, but a distinct bilaminar arrangement of cytotrophoblast and syncytiotrophoblast is absent. Rarely, choriocarcinoma may occur in association with endometrioid carcinoma.

Very early gestation

In very early gestation, the trophoblastic tissue may exhibit marked cytologic atypia (Figure 17.17), but the volume of tissue is scant, the β-hCG is not abnormally elevated, and mitotic figures are absent or, if present, rare and of normal configuration. Villi may or may not be present.

PROLIFERATIONS OF THE EXTRAVILLOUS TROPHOBLAST (INTERMEDIATE TROPHOBLASTIC PROLIFERATIONS)

Proliferations of the extravillous trophoblast (intermediate trophoblastic proliferations) can be divided into non-neoplastic (placental site nodule and exaggerated placental site reaction) and neoplastic (placental site trophoblastic tumor and epithelioid trophoblastic tumor).

Placental site trophoblastic tumor

The typical patient with placental site trophoblastic tumor (PSTT) is premenopausal (Table 17.8). Patients may

Table 17.8 Clinical characteristics of placental site trophoblastic tumor and epithelioid trophoblastic tumor

Reproductive age or perimenopausal
Uterine or cervical mass
Serum β-hCG elevation (typically less than 10 000 units)[a]

[a] Occasional cases do not demonstrate serum β-hCG elevation.

experience abnormal vaginal bleeding, amenorrhea, or symptoms related to an enlarged uterus (i.e., a feeling of fullness, urinary urgency). Serum human chorionic gonadotropin (β-hCG) levels are elevated in at least three-quarters of patients, but in contrast to levels in choriocarcinoma patients, β-hCG levels in placental site trophoblastic tumor patients generally range from minimally elevated (i.e., more than 50 mIU/ml) to moderately elevated (usually not exceeding 8000 mIU/ml)[18]. The highest levels may be found in patients with metastatic disease and when the tumor is mixed with choriocarcinoma – a very rare event. The average serum β-hCG level in patients whose tumors lack these features is between 500 and 1000 mIU/ml[18].

The interval between diagnosis and antecedent pregnancy is, on average, approximately three years. Most placental site trophoblastic tumors occur in young women following term pregnancy of a girl[19]. Occasional placental site trophoblastic tumors are preceded by spontaneous or therapeutic abortions, and very rare cases develop after a diagnosis of a hydatidiform mole.

The tumors are usually based in the myometrium or endomyometrium; in approximately 85% of cases, the placental site trophoblastic tumor is organ confined, without evidence of metastasis. First-line therapy for disease limited to the uterus is hysterectomy and lymph node dissection, not chemotherapy. At least 85% of these patients survive without recurrence. Chemotherapy is reserved for patients with high-stage or recurrent disease. The most common sites of metastasis and recurrence include lung, liver, and vagina. While almost 100% of patients with organ-confined disease survive, approximately 50% of patients with metastases succumb to their disease[20]. There are anecdotal reports of highly toxic multi-agent chemotherapeutic regimens that have resulted in more favorable outcomes. Occasional patients with placental site trophoblastic tumor develop nephrotic syndrome.

The behavior of organ-confined placental site trophoblastic tumor is difficult to predict based on pathologic examination. A recent study, based on 55 cases[18] reported

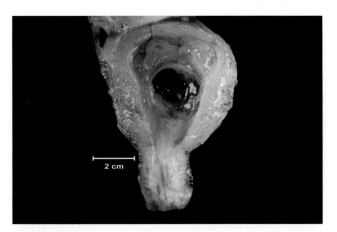

Figure 17.28 Placental site trophoblastic tumor forming a hemorrhagic mass in the uterine corpus.

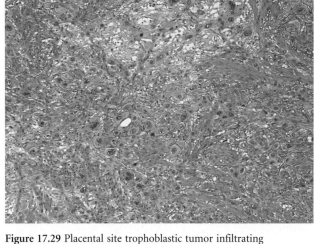

Figure 17.29 Placental site trophoblastic tumor infiltrating myometrium.

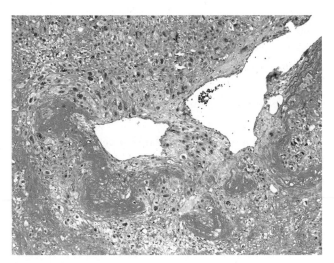

Figure 17.30 Placental site trophoblastic tumor with fibrinoid deposition around blood vessels.

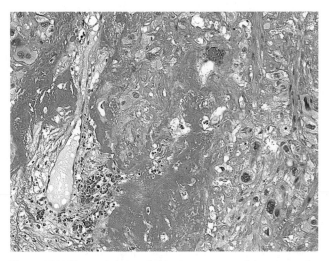

Figure 17.31 Placental site trophoblastic tumor containing scattered cells, some multinucleated, with enlarged nuclei. Examples with multinucleated cells can also be seen in Figures 17.28 and 17.29.

the following pathologic and clinical features to be associated with adverse outcomes: age over 35 years, interval before last pregnancy greater than 2 years, deep myometrial invasion, FIGO stage III or IV, maximum β-hCG level over 1000 mIU/ml, extensive coagulative necrosis, high mitotic index, and the presence of cells with clear cytoplasm.

Placental site trophoblastic tumors form polypoid or nodular masses, centered in the myometrium or endomyometrium (Figure 17.28), measuring, on average, approximately 5 cm in maximum dimension. About 10% arise in the cervix. The tumors are usually described as solid and fleshy, and yellow or tan. Hemorrhage and necrosis are common, and many invade deeply into the myometrium.

Placental site trophoblastic tumors are composed of large, predominantly monomorphic epithelioid cells,

with round nuclei and abundant amphophilic or eosinophilic cytoplasm; infiltration between preserved myometrial muscle fibers is often a useful diagnostic feature (Figure 17.29)[21]. The tumor cells characteristically colonize blood vessel walls, obliterating normal vascular architecture, and deposit bright, eosinophilic fibrinoid material (Figure 17.30). Scattered, rounded multinucleated trophoblastic cells can be found (Figure 17.31), but large amounts of syncytiotrophoblast, particularly if intimately associated with and wrapping around mononuclear trophoblastic cells, are more typical of choriocarcinoma (Figure 17.25). Histologic features reported to be associated with poor clinical outcome include cytoplasmic clearing, extensive necrosis, and greater than

(A) **(B)**

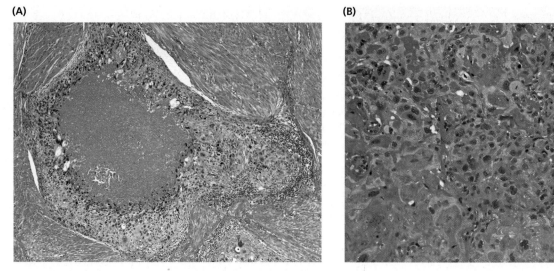

Figure 17.32 Epithelioid trophoblastic tumor forming nodules with central necrosis (A). High-power microscopy (B) reveals mononuclear epithelioid cells.

Table 17.9 Pathologic characteristics of placental site trophoblastic tumor

Polygonal eosinophilic or clear tumor cells infiltrating myometrium
Mitotic activity (usually less than 5 MF/10 HPF)
Rare, scattered, multinucleated cells
Fibrin deposition around blood vessel walls
No chorionic villi

6 MF/10 HPF, but data are limited[18]. Villi and features suggesting recent or concurrent pregnancy are lacking (Table 17.9).

Epithelioid trophoblastic tumor

Epithelioid trophoblastic tumor (ETT) is less common than placental site trophoblastic tumor[22]. Since epithelioid trophoblastic tumor is more recently described, the clinical features of this tumor subtype are not as well characterized. Based on review of only limited available data, it appears that the clinical presentation of epithelioid trophoblastic tumor, the rates of extrauterine disease at presentation, and relapse rates are broadly similar to placental site trophoblastic tumor[23]. The frequent cervical location of epithelioid trophoblastic tumor is one important difference[22,24]. Treatment algorithms are similar.

The gross appearance of epithelioid trophoblastic tumor is similar in many respects to placental site trophoblastic tumor, although there appear to be some important

differences. The majority have been reported to arise in the lower uterine segment or cervix, and some appear to have arisen in extragenital sites, including lung. Epithelioid trophoblastic tumors are, in general, smaller than placental site trophoblastic tumors, and may have a cystic appearance.

Despite many clinical similarities, epithelioid trophoblastic tumor and placental site trophoblastic tumor usually appear distinct on microscopy. Epithelioid trophoblastic tumors grow in a nodular, expansile fashion with central acellular, eosinophilic material and lymphocytic infiltrates at the advancing edge (Figure 17.32). This central eosinophilic material is obviously necrotic in many cases, but in others it resembles keratin or the fibrinoid material seen in placental site trophoblastic tumor[22]. Intact neoplastic cells are typically present in rounded nests and sheets at the periphery of the tumor, and track alongside vessels into the devitalized center, giving rise to the appearance of round, cellular islands with central vessels floating amidst the eosinophilic material. In rare cases, epithelioid trophoblastic tumors colonize cervical mucosa and simulate, to a striking degree, the appearance of squamous carcinoma in situ (Figure 17.33). Tumor cells are monomorphic and epithelioid in appearance and, in general, smaller in size than those found in placental site trophoblastic tumor. The mitotic rate seldom exceeds 5 MF/ 10 HPF. Admixtures of larger mononuclear trophoblastic cells and even multinucleated cells are common. Although multinucleated cells are usually scattered about, without the envelopment of mononuclear trophoblastic cells, some examples of mixed epithelioid trophoblastic tumor and

Table 17.10 Pathologic characteristics of epithelioid trophoblastic tumor

Nodular aggregates of epithelioid tumor cells with necrosis and fibrin in the nodules' centers[a]

Mitotic activity (usually less than 5 MF/10 HPF)

Rare, scattered, multinucleated cells[b]

No chorionic villi

[a] Rare epithelioid trophoblastic tumors demonstrate replacement of native cervical epithelium, resulting in resemblance to squamous dysplasia.

[b] Rare epithelioid trophoblastic tumors contain delimited foci resembling choriocarcinoma.

Table 17.11 Differential diagnosis of placental site trophoblastic tumor and epithelioid trophoblastic tumor

Placental site nodule

Exaggerated placental site

Choriocarcinoma

Squamous carcinoma and squamous intraepithelial lesion (squamous dysplasia)

Epithelioid smooth muscle tumor

Perivascular epithelioid cell tumor (PEComa)

Carcinoma of lung

(A)

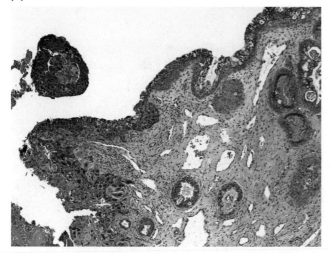

(B)

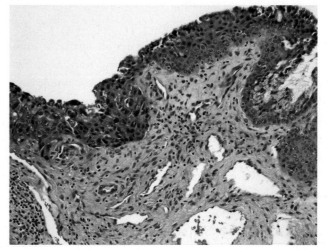

Figure 17.33 Epithelioid trophoblastic tumor colonizing cervix (A, B).

choriocarcinoma have been reported[22]. Villi and features suggesting recent or concurrent pregnancy are lacking (Table 17.10).

Differential diagnosis of extravillous trophoblastic disease

The differential diagnosis for extravillous trophoblastic tumors is listed in Table 17.11.

Placental site nodule

Placental site nodule is usually identified either in a curettage performed as part of a work-up for abnormal vaginal bleeding or amenorrhea, or incidentally in a hysterectomy specimen performed for an unrelated reason. Placental site nodule is occasionally found after an evaluation triggered by an abnormal Pap smear, abnormal vaginal bleeding,

retained products of conception, or infertility. These are benign lesions that do not require therapy.

When placental site nodules are found incidentally in a curettage specimen, specific gross features are seldom appreciated. In hysterectomies, approximately one-half are located in the endometrium or superficial myometrium, and one-half in the cervix. They are small lesions, typically measuring less than 5 mm. The appearance is generally described as a plaque or nodule that is tan to yellow in color.

Placental site nodules are small, rounded lesions of mononuclear trophoblastic cells set in hyalinized stroma (Figure 17.34). They may be single or multiple. As in epithelioid trophoblastic tumor, the central portion of the nodule tends to be acellular or paucicellular, while the trophoblastic cells are polarized towards the periphery. The nodules may be surrounded by a chronic inflammatory infiltrate. The trophoblastic cells are dispersed singly

(A)

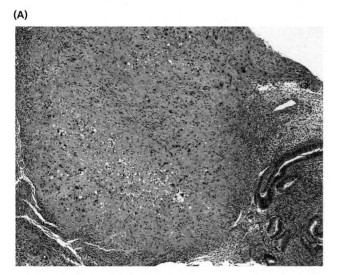

(B)

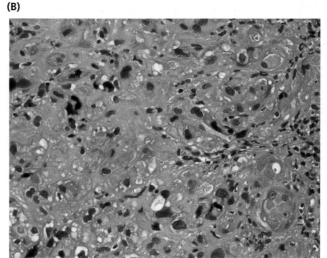

Figure 17.34 Placental site nodule (A, B).

or in small aggregates. Mitotic figures are sparse or non-existent. Rare tumors that display hybrid features of placental site nodule and epithelioid trophoblastic tumor have been described. These "atypical placental site nodules" are intermediate in size between typical placental site nodule and epithelioid trophoblastic tumor, have cohesive nests of cells, and, in some cases, detectable mitotic activity[22]. These lesions are benign; however it should be noted that atypical placental site nodules may accompany epithelioid trophoblastic tumors[22]. Careful clinical and pathologic assessment is therefore necessary to exclude epithelioid trophoblastic tumor in this scenario.

It should be difficult to find mitotic figures in a placental site nodule and, as such, the proliferative rate with Ki-67 (MIB1) should not exceed 10–15%. Placental site nodules also do not exhibit the geographic deposition of fibrinoid or eosinophilic necrotic debris. Serum β-hCG elevations have not been reported in placental site nodule. Placental site trophoblastic tumor is characterized by preferential expression of hPL and HLA-G, as opposed to placental alkaline phosphatase (PLAP) and p63 in placental site nodule[25,26].

Exaggerated placental site

Exaggerated placental site reactions are essentially always associated with a recent pregnancy, particularly a molar pregnancy. When unassociated with a molar pregnancy, these lesions are physiologic and benign, and do not warrant therapy. Molar pregnancies accompanied by an exaggerated placental site reaction are treated as molar pregnancies.

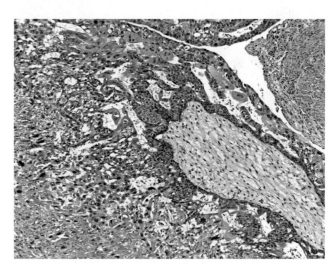

Figure 17.35 Exaggerated implantation site (lower left), associated with a molar pregnancy.

Exaggerated placental site reaction is characterized by an infiltrative proliferation of mononuclear trophoblastic cells associated with a placenta, a molar pregnancy, or changes attributed to a recent pregnancy (Figure 17.35). The trophoblastic cells splay apart myometrial fibers, but, in contrast to placental site trophoblastic tumor, expansile, tumor-like nodules of trophoblastic cells are not seen. The trophoblastic cells may also resemble those encountered in placental site trophoblastic tumor, including highly irregular and multiple nuclei, but a distinct mass lesion is absent. Mitotic figures are sparse or nonexistent in implantation sites from nonmolar gestations, but can be increased in molar pregnancies[27,28]. The association between molar pregnancy and exaggerated placental site reactions indicates that a diligent search for a molar pregnancy should

(A)

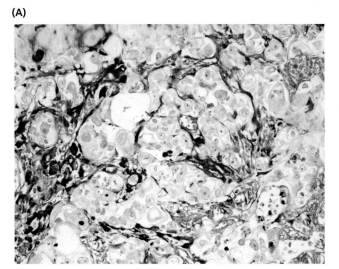

(B)

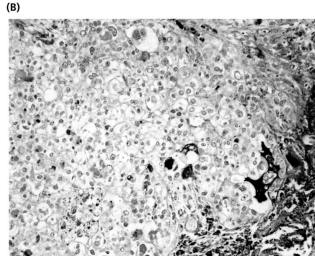

Figure 17.36 β-hCG immunostains in atypical choriocarcinoma (A) and epithelioid trophoblastic tumor (B). Characteristic attenuated syncytiotrophoblast surrounds aggregates of mononuclear trophoblast in choriocarcinoma.

be undertaken upon identification of exaggerated placental site reactions.

Unlike placental site trophoblastic tumor, exaggerated placental site reaction is generally found associated with chorionic villi, particularly those from a molar pregnancy. Placental site trophoblastic tumor, in contrast, typically forms a clinically detectable mass with proliferating trophoblastic cells, accompanied by serum elevations in β-hCG, without any villi.

Choriocarcinoma

Epithelioid trophoblastic tumor and placental site trophoblastic tumor can both contain syncytiotrophoblast and multinuclear intermediate trophoblastic cells. This leads to the inevitable problem of distinguishing them from choriocarcinoma. In typical cases, the multinucleated cells of epithelioid trophoblastic tumor and placental site trophoblastic tumor are round and haphazardly distributed (Figures 17.29–17.31), without the intimate admixture of numerous, elongate, multinuclear and mononuclear trophoblastic cells, characteristic of choriocarcinoma (Figure 17.25). Syncytiotrophoblast typically envelops the mononuclear trophoblastic cells in choriocarcinoma – a feature that is not usually encountered in epithelioid trophoblastic tumor or placental site trophoblastic tumor. However, some epithelioid trophoblastic tumors may contain areas that closely resemble classical choriocarcinoma[22,29]. When epithelioid trophoblastic tumors contain quantifiable foci of typical-appearing choriocarcinoma, a diagnosis of a mixed epithelioid trophoblastic tumor and choriocarcinoma should be considered. The typical

morphologic features of each entity should be obvious in such cases, and one component should be easily distinguished from the other. The serum β-hCG in these cases tends to be intermediate between those of pure epithelioid trophoblastic tumor and choriocarcinoma.

The problem posed by attenuated and sparse syncytiotrophoblast in choriocarcinoma is more difficult to resolve (Figure 17.27). This occurs most commonly in patients with a presumed choriocarcinoma or complete mole (serum β-hCG levels exceeding 10,000 units), who have been previously treated with chemotherapy. Residual lesions, particularly in the lung, may persist on imaging studies, and, while the peak serum β-hCG level has decreased, it is not normalized. Excision of the residual lesions typically shows a proliferation of neoplastic mononuclear trophoblastic cells without obvious syncytiotrophoblast[30]. This appearance may simulate that of metastatic epithelioid trophoblastic tumor or placental site trophoblastic tumor to a striking degree. The characteristic clinical history (history of chemotherapy and β-hCG too high for uncomplicated epithelioid trophoblastic tumor or placental site trophoblastic tumor), but not necessarily the morphologic appearance, should suggest the diagnosis of choriocarcinoma. Immunohistochemical β-hCG stains will show attenuated trophoblast surrounding aggregates of intermediate trophoblast in choriocarcinoma, whereas, in epithelioid trophoblastic tumor, β-hCG positive cells have a round shape and are sparse and haphazardly distributed (Figure 17.36). Proliferation rates using Ki-67 are also substantially higher in choriocarcinoma as compared to epithelioid trophoblastic tumor (Figure 17.37).

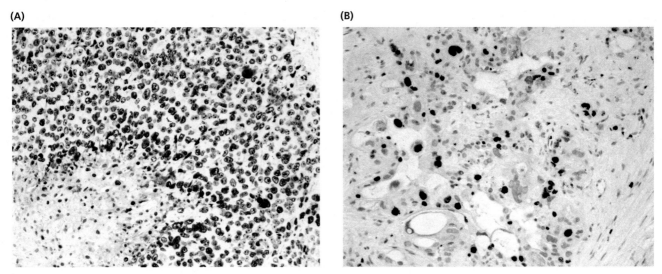

Figure 17.37 Ki-67 in atypical choriocarcinoma (A) and epithelioid trophoblastic tumor (B). Proliferation rates are significantly higher in choriocarcinoma.

A diagnosis of "persistent gestational trophoblastic disease" can be considered with the comment that, although the characteristic features of choriocarcinoma are absent, the combined clinical and pathologic findings are most compatible with that diagnosis.

Squamous carcinoma and squamous intraepithelial lesion (squamous dysplasia)

Epithelioid trophoblastic tumors are often confused with squamous dysplasia or squamous carcinoma because they are frequently located in the cervix and have an epithelioid, brightly eosinophilic appearance. The eosinophilic extracellular material often resembles keratin and, on occasion, epithelioid trophoblastic tumor can colonize and replace squamous epithelium (Figure 17.33), thereby resembling squamous dysplasia. Epithelioid trophoblastic tumor, placental site nodule, and squamous cell carcinoma share expression of cytokeratin and p63, but squamous cell carcinoma does not express the trophoblast-associated markers inhibin, CD10[22,31], CK18, and hydroxyl-δ-5-steroid dehydrogenase (HSD3B1)[22,31,32]. Moreover, epithelioid trophoblastic tumor lacks the p16 expression that is typical of HPV-associated squamous neoplasms[33]; HPV in situ studies should also be negative, although not all squamous cell carcinomas continue to express HPV by in situ analysis.

Epithelioid smooth muscle tumor

Placental site trophoblastic tumor is an epithelioid neoplasm that is frequently centered in the myometrium. With the exception of those similarities, these two lesions are

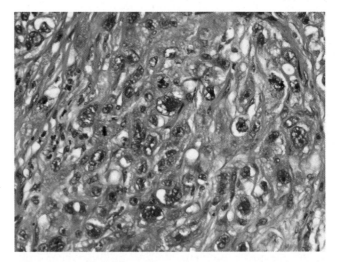

Figure 17.38 Epithelioid smooth muscle tumor resembling placental site trophoblastic tumor.

distinct. Placental site trophoblastic tumor patients are usually women in their reproductive years, whereas patients with epithelioid leiomyosarcoma (Figure 17.38) are usually perimenopausal or postmenopausal. Serum β-hCG elevations are typically seen with placental site trophoblastic tumor, but not with epithelioid smooth muscle tumors. Tumor cells in placental site trophoblastic tumor infiltrate between myometrial muscle fibers; whereas non-neoplastic myometrium is usually not seen within an epithelioid leiomyosarcoma, except in areas of infiltration into adjacent myometrium. In this last case, the pattern of invasion consists of a broad, pushing front or, on occasion, tongue-like fascicular infiltration. Placental site trophoblastic tumor frequently exhibits the characteristic

(A)

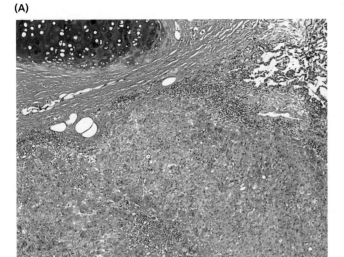

(B)

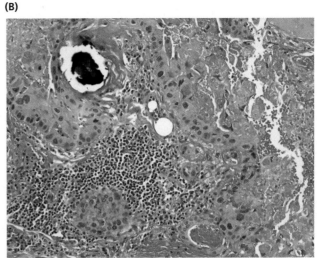

Figure 17.39 Primary pulmonary epithelioid trophoblastic tumor (A, B). Dystrophic calcification is seen in (B). A uterine primary was never documented.

replacement of blood vessel walls with fibrin deposition and, of course, has a strikingly different immunophenotype. The only markers that might be expressed in both lesions are pan-cytokeratin and CD10. An immunohistochemical panel that includes inhibin and desmin and/or h-caldesmon should permit discrimination in most cases. Some epithelioid smooth muscle tumors may not express these smooth muscle markers to the degree seen in the standard spindle smooth muscle tumor; in these instances, the possibility of a perivascular epithelioid cell tumor (PEComa) should also be considered. Perivascular epithelioid cell tumor can be identified on the basis of HMB45 and smooth muscle actin, in addition to other markers[34,35].

Epithelioid trophoblastic tumor versus placental site trophoblastic tumor

In their pure forms, epithelioid trophoblastic tumor and placental site trophoblastic tumor are histologically dissimilar lesions, as described in detail previously. In problematic cases, they can be separated with the use of immunohistochemistry as they are composed of different types of mononuclear trophoblast. Occasional cases, however, show overlapping features of both lesions. It is not certain whether important clinical differences exist, so the need to distinguish lesions with hybrid features remains more an academic matter than a practical one.

Extrauterine presentations

Gestational choriocarcinoma and extravillous trophoblastic tumors (tumors of intermediate trophoblast) very rarely arise in extrauterine locations (Figure 17.39).

Choriocarcinoma and placental site trophoblastic tumors have been reported in the fallopian tube, paratubal tissues, and ovary; regions that suggest tumor evolution from an ectopic pregnancy[36]. Choriocarcinoma and epithelioid trophoblastic tumor have been reported in the lung[22,29]. In some cases of extrauterine gestational choriocarcinoma, the primary tumor is not identified, presumably due to tumor regression (Figure 17.40). A uterine primary or morphologic mimic should be excluded before making a diagnosis of an extrauterine intermediate trophoblastic tumor. The differential diagnosis of primary pulmonary epithelioid trophoblastic tumor includes primary pulmonary non-small-cell carcinoma, such as squamous cell carcinoma and pleomorphic carcinoma, a primary or metastatic germ cell tumor with trophoblastic differentiation, and choriocarcinoma with treatment-related changes.

ANCILLARY DIAGNOSTIC TESTS

Trophoblastic cells, including cytotrophoblast, extravillous (intermediate) trophoblastic cells, and syncytiotrophoblast, stain strongly and diffusely with cytokeratins (AE1/AE3). Inhibin, CD10[25], CK18[32], and HSD3B1[37] are also pan-trophoblastic markers. Mel-CAM (also known as CD146), a membrane glycoprotein of the immunoglobulin gene superfamily involved in cell-to-cell interaction[38], is a general marker of intermediate trophoblastic cells, as is HLA-G[39]. Immunohistochemical algorithms to differentiate between trophoblastic lesions and distinguish trophoblastic

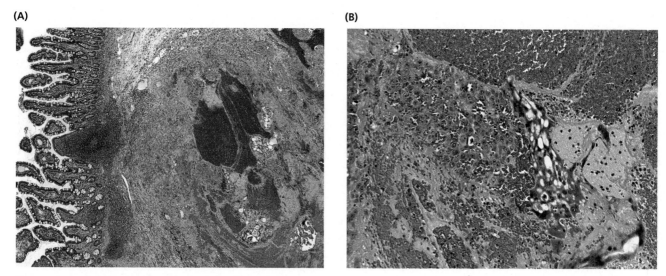

Figure 17.40   (A, B) Metastatic gestational choriocarcinoma in small intestine.

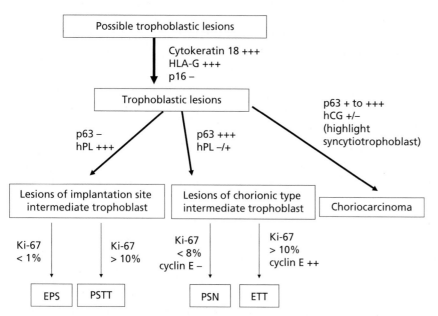

Diagram 17.3 Trophogram. Abbreviations: EPS = exaggerated placental site; PSN = placental site nodule. Adapted from Shih IM, Kurman RJ. p63 expression is useful in the distinction of epithelioid trophoblastic and placental site trophoblastic tumors by profiling trophoblastic subpopulations. *Am J Surg Pathol* 2004;**28**:1177–83, Fig. 3.

lesions from other tumors have been proposed, but, in most cases, the distinctions are best made on morphologic grounds (Diagram 17.3)[26,32]. Table 17.12 summarizes the relevant immunohistochemical markers used in gestational trophoblastic disease.

Molar pregnancy

This tumor is composed of neoplastic villi. Loss of normal expression of p57 is seen in complete moles, both classic and early types.

Choriocarcinoma

This tumor is composed of neoplastic trophoblast (syncytiotrophoblast and cytotrophoblast cells). In addition to the pan-trophoblastic markers mentioned above, β-hCG is typically expressed. The Ki-67 (MIB1) index in choriocarcinoma is quite high (>50%).

Placental site trophoblastic tumor

This tumor is composed of neoplastic invasive extravillous trophoblast (implantation site intermediate trophoblastic

Table 17.12 Ancillary diagnostic tests for gestational trophoblastic disease

Pan-trophoblastic markers

- Inhibin-α
- CD10
- CK18
- Hydroxyl-δ-5-steroid dehydrogenase (HSD3B1)

Markers supporting complete mole

- p57 (loss of normal expression)

Markers supporting choriocarcinoma

- β-hCG

Markers supporting epithelioid trophoblastic tumor and placental site nodule

- PLAP
- p63

Markers supporting placental site trophoblastic tumor and exaggerated placental site

- hPL
- HLA-G

Marker supporting placental site trophoblastic tumor or epithelioid trophoblastic tumor over placental site nodule

- Ki-67 (MIB1) greater than 15%

Marker supporting choriocarcinoma over placental site trophoblastic tumor and epithelioid trophoblastic tumor

- Ki-67 (MIB1) greater than 50%

cells). In addition to the pan-trophoblastic markers mentioned above, hPL and HLA-G are typically expressed. Based on one study, the reported Ki-67 (MIB1) proliferation index for placental site trophoblastic tumors is 14% (±7%)[28].

Epithelioid trophoblastic tumor

This tumor is composed of migratory extravillous trophoblast (chorionic site intermediate trophoblastic cells)[22]. Tumor cells express pan-trophoblastic markers as well as PLAP and p63; hPL and HLA-G are not expressed in epithelioid trophoblastic tumor[26,32].

Placental site nodule

Lesional cells express pan-trophoblastic markers, as well as the markers PLAP and p63 associated with chorionic intermediate trophoblast. The Ki-67 (MIB1) index in a placental site nodule should not exceed 10–15%[40].

Exaggerated placental site

This lesion, actually an exuberant, non-neoplastic physiologic finding that frequently accompanies molar pregnancies, is composed mostly of implantation site intermediate trophoblastic cells. The constituent cells express hPL and HLA-G[39]. In most cases, the Ki-67 (MIB1) index in an exaggerated placental site reaction should not exceed 10–15%[28].

REFERENCES

1. Edge SB, Byrd DR, Comptom CC, et al., eds. *AJCC Cancer Staging Manual*. New York: Springer; 2010.
2. Kohorn EI. The new FIGO 2000 staging and risk factor scoring system for gestational trophoblastic disease: description and critical assessment. *Int J Gynecol Cancer* 2001;**11**:73–7.
3. FIGO Committee on Gynecologic Oncology. Current FIGO staging for cancer of the vagina, fallopian tube, ovary, and gestational trophoblastic neoplasia. *Int J Gynaecol Obstet* 2009;**105**:3–4.
4. Lurain JR. Gestational trophoblastic disease I: epidemiology, pathology, clinical presentation and diagnosis of gestational trophoblastic disease, and management of hydatidiform mole. *Am J Obstet Gynecol* 2011;**203**:531–9.
5. Castrillon DH, Sun D, Weremowicz S, et al. Discrimination of complete hydatidiform mole from its mimics by immunohistochemistry of the paternally imprinted gene product p57KIP2. *Am J Surg Pathol* 2001;**25**:1225–30.
6. Chilosi M, Piazzola E, Lestani M, et al. Differential expression of p57kip2, a maternally imprinted cdk inhibitor, in normal human placenta and gestational trophoblastic disease. *Lab Invest* 1998;**78**:269–76.
7. Ronnett BM, DeScipio C, Murphy KM. Hydatidiform moles: ancillary techniques to refine diagnosis. *Int J Gynecol Pathol* 2011;**30**:101–16.
8. McConnell TG, Murphy KM, Hafez M, et al. Diagnosis and subclassification of hydatidiform moles using p57 immunohistochemistry and molecular genotyping: validation and prospective analysis in routine and consultation practice settings with development of an algorithmic approach. *Am J Surg Pathol* 2009;**33**:805–17.
9. Sebire NJ, Fisher RA, Rees HC. Histopathological diagnosis of partial and complete hydatidiform mole in the first trimester of pregnancy. *Pediatr Dev Pathol* 2003;**6**:69–77.
10. Sebire NJ, Makrydimas G, Agnantis NJ, et al. Updated diagnostic criteria for partial and complete hydatidiform moles in early pregnancy. *Anticancer Res* 2003;**23**:1723–8.
11. Keep D, Zaragoza MV, Hassold T, et al. Very early complete hydatidiform mole. *Hum Pathol* 1996;**27**:708–13.
12. Paradinas FJ, Fisher RA, Browne P, et al. Diploid hydatidiform moles with fetal red blood cells in molar villi. 1 – Pathology, incidence, and prognosis. *J Pathol* 1997;**181**:183–8.
13. Genest DR. Partial hydatidiform mole: clinicopathological features, differential diagnosis, ploidy and molecular studies, and gold standards for diagnosis. *Int J Gynecol Pathol* 2001;**20**:315–22.
14. Kim KR, Park BH, Hong YO, et al. The villous stromal constituents of complete hydatidiform mole differ histologically in very early

pregnancy from the normally developing placenta. *Am J Surg Pathol* 2009;**33**:176–85.

15. Cole LA, Khanlian SA, Giddings A, *et al.* Gestational trophoblastic diseases: 4. Presentation with persistent low positive human chorionic gonadotropin test results. *Gynecol Oncol* 2006;**102**:165–72.

16. Cole LA, Butler SA, Khanlian SA, *et al.* Gestational trophoblastic diseases: 2. Hyperglycosylated hCG as a reliable marker of active neoplasia. *Gynecol Oncol* 2006;**102**:151–9.

17. Ganapathi KA, Paczos T, George MD, *et al.* Incidental finding of placental choriocarcinoma after an uncomplicated term pregnancy: a case report with review of the literature. *Int J Gynecol Pathol* 2011;**29**:476–8.

18. Baergen RN, Rutgers JL, Young RH, *et al.* Placental site trophoblastic tumor: A study of 55 cases and review of the literature emphasizing factors of prognostic significance. *Gynecol Oncol* 2006;**100**:511–20.

19. Hui P, Martel M, Parkash V. Gestational trophoblastic diseases: recent advances in histopathologic diagnosis and related genetic aspects. *Adv Anat Pathol* 2005;**12**:116–25.

20. Lurain JR. Gestational trophoblastic disease II: classification and management of gestational trophoblastic neoplasia. *Am J Obstet Gynecol* 2011;**204**:11–18.

21. Young RH, Kurman RJ, Scully RE. Proliferations and tumors of intermediate trophoblast of the placental site. *Semin Diagn Pathol* 1988;**5**:223–37.

22. Shih IM, Kurman RJ. Epithelioid trophoblastic tumor: a neoplasm distinct from choriocarcinoma and placental site trophoblastic tumor simulating carcinoma. *Am J Surg Pathol* 1998;**22**:1393–403.

23. Palmer JE, Macdonald M, Wells M, *et al.* Epithelioid trophoblastic tumor: a review of the literature. *J Reprod Med* 2008;**53**:465–75.

24. Fadare O, Parkash V, Carcangiu ML, *et al.* Epithelioid trophoblastic tumor: clinicopathological features with an emphasis on uterine cervical involvement. *Mod Pathol* 2006;**19**:75–82.

25. Ordi J, Romagosa C, Tavassoli FA, *et al.* CD10 expression in epithelial tissues and tumors of the gynecologic tract: a useful marker in the diagnosis of mesonephric, trophoblastic, and clear cell tumors. *Am J Surg Pathol* 2003;**27**:178–86.

26. Shih IM. Trophogram, an immunohistochemistry-based algorithmic approach, in the differential diagnosis of trophoblastic tumors and tumorlike lesions. *Ann Diagn Pathol* 2007;**11**:228–34.

27. Montes M, Roberts D, Berkowitz RS, *et al.* Prevalence and significance of implantation site trophoblastic atypia in hydatidiform moles and spontaneous abortions. *Am J Clin Pathol* 1996;**105**:411–16.

28. Shih IM, Kurman RJ. Ki-67 labeling index in the differential diagnosis of exaggerated placental site, placental site trophoblastic tumor, and choriocarcinoma: a double immunohistochemical staining technique using Ki-67 and Mel-CAM antibodies. *Hum Pathol* 1998;**29**:27–33.

29. Lewin SN, Aghajanian C, Moreira AL, *et al.* Extrauterine epithelioid trophoblastic tumors presenting as primary lung carcinomas: morphologic and immunohistochemical features to resolve a diagnostic dilemma. *Am J Surg Pathol* 2009;**33**:1809–14.

30. Mazur MT. Metastatic gestational choriocarcinoma. Unusual pathologic variant following therapy. *Cancer* 1989;**63**:1370–7.

31. Shih IM, Kurman RJ. Immunohistochemical localization of inhibin-alpha in the placenta and gestational trophoblastic lesions. *Int J Gynecol Pathol* 1999;**18**:144–50.

32. Shih IM, Kurman RJ. p63 expression is useful in the distinction of epithelioid trophoblastic and placental site trophoblastic tumors by profiling trophoblastic subpopulations. *Am J Surg Pathol* 2004;**28**:1177–83.

33. Mao TL, Seidman JD, Kurman RJ, *et al.* Cyclin E and p16 immunoreactivity in epithelioid trophoblastic tumor – an aid in differential diagnosis. *Am J Surg Pathol* 2006;**30**:1105–10.

34. Folpe AL, Mentzel T, Lehr HA, *et al.* Perivascular epithelioid cell neoplasms of soft tissue and gynecologic origin: a clinicopathologic study of 26 cases and review of the literature. *Am J Surg Pathol* 2005;**29**:1558–75.

35. Vang R, Kempson RL. Perivascular epithelioid cell tumor ('PEComa') of the uterus: a subset of HMB-45-positive epithelioid mesenchymal neoplasms with an uncertain relationship to pure smooth muscle tumors. *Am J Surg Pathol* 2002;**26**:1–13.

36. Baergen RN, Rutgers J, Young RH. Extrauterine lesions of intermediate trophoblast. *Int J Gynecol Pathol* 2003;**22**:362–7.

37. Mao TL, Kurman RJ, Jeng YM, *et al.* HSD3B1 as a novel trophoblast-associated marker that assists in the differential diagnosis of trophoblastic tumors and tumorlike lesions. *Am J Surg Pathol* 2008;**32**:236–42.

38. Shih IM, Kurman RJ. Expression of melanoma cell adhesion molecule in intermediate trophoblast. *Lab Invest* 1996;**75**:377–88.

39. Singer G, Kurman RJ, McMaster MT, *et al.* HLA-G immunoreactivity is specific for intermediate trophoblast in gestational trophoblastic disease and can serve as a useful marker in differential diagnosis. *Am J Surg Pathol* 2002;**26**:914–20.

40. Shih IM, Seidman JD, Kurman RJ. Placental site nodule and characterization of distinctive types of intermediate trophoblast. *Hum Pathol* 1999;**30**:687–94.

18 OTHER PREGNANCY-RELATED ABNORMALITIES

INTRODUCTION

Pregnancy-related abnormalities can be divided into three groups of lesions: (1) normal pregnancy-related changes that pose diagnostic challenges either because they occur in an unusual site or unusual clinical setting or are clinically unsuspected; (2) abnormal pregnancy-related changes, usually associated with problems with placentation; this group of pregnancy-related abnormalities typically present with peripartum or, more commonly, postpartum bleeding; and (3) gestational trophoblastic disease. Gestational trophoblastic disease is discussed elsewhere (Chapter 17).

PHYSIOLOGIC PREGNANCY-RELATED CHANGES

Arias-Stella reaction

Arias-Stella reaction has been documented in endometrial glands during pregnancy (as early as 17 days following conception), in gestational trophoblastic disease, and in premenopausal and postmenopausal women treated with progestins, as well as in occasional women with no apparent source of progestin stimulation[1,2]. Gland involvement may be focal or extensive, and consists of large cells with voluminous, almost frothy, eosinophilic to clear cytoplasm and enlarged, irregular, often bulbous nuclei that may be hyperchromatic with smudged chromatin pattern or vesicular with intranuclear cytoplasmic pseudoinclusions (Figures 18.1–18.3). Intraglandular cellular tufting often imparts a pseudopapillary appearance to the involved glands. Other secretory changes, including subnuclear and/or supranuclear vacuoles, are common (Figure 18.4). Mitotic figures are infrequent or absent. Up to 10% of cases contained rare mitotic figures in Arias-Stella's series[3]; atypical mitotic figures have also been reported, but these are decidedly rare.

This glandular reaction may also develop in extraendometrial sites, such as the cervix (Figure 18.5) or fallopian tubes, and in foci of endometriosis[4–6]. Involvement of the cervix is seen in up to 10% of gravid uteri and occasionally in women with a history of oral contraceptive use.

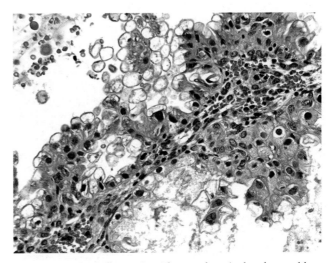

Figure 18.1 Arias-Stella reaction. The cytoplasm is abundant and has a frothy appearance.

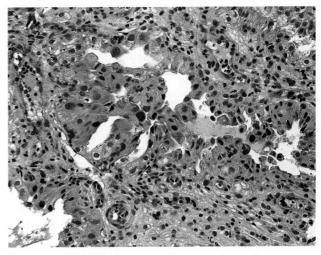

Figure 18.2 Arias-Stella reaction. The nuclei are hyperchromatic and the chromatin has a smudged appearance.

(A)

(B)

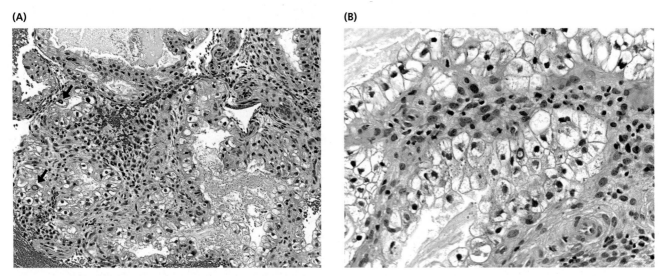

Figure 18.3 (A, B) Arias-Stella reaction. Intranuclear inclusions are present.

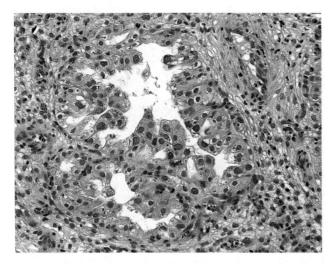

Figure 18.4 Arias-Stella reaction with subnuclear and supranuclear cytoplasmic vacuoles.

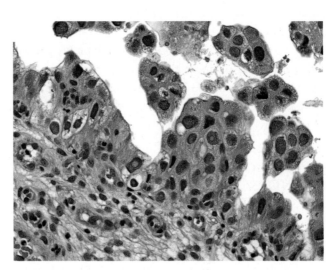

Figure 18.5 Arias-Stella reaction in cervix.

In the usual clinical setting, Arias-Stella reaction is a relatively straightforward diagnosis. However, diagnostic problems arise when sampling specimens are small and/or the clinical setting is unusual (e.g., patient, treating physician, and/or pathologist are unaware patient is pregnant; postmenopausal woman with no clear history of progestin treatment; etc.). In these situations, clear cell adenocarcinoma, either of cervical or endometrial origin, or cervical adenocarcinoma in situ are strong diagnostic considerations. In Arias-Stella reaction, the stroma is often deciduated (Figure 18.6) and the glands are not infiltrative; while clear cell carcinoma almost always features foci of hyalinized fibroblastic stroma, papilla with hyalinized cores, tubulocystic structures, or a solid, infiltrative

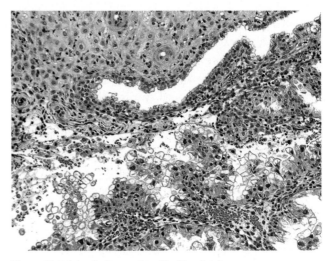

Figure 18.6 Arias-Stella reaction. Decidua is often present.

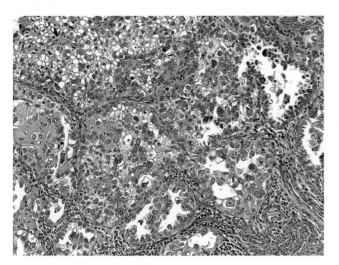

Figure 18.7 Clear cell carcinoma.

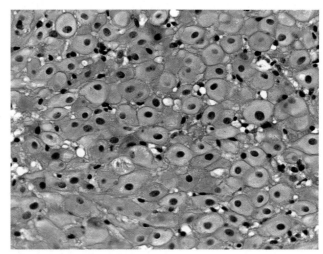

Figure 18.8 Decidual cells.

(A)

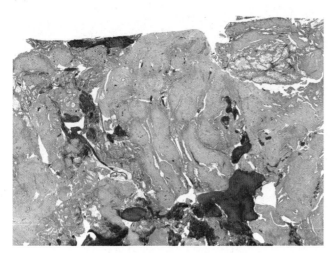

(B)

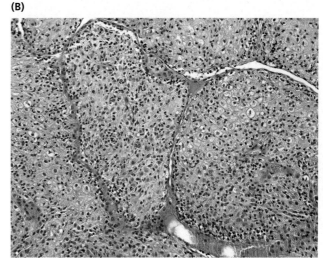

Figure 18.9 (A, B) Decidua with secondary myxoid change.

pattern (Figure 18.7). Mitotic figures are also more prominent in uterine and cervical clear cell carcinoma than in Arias-Stella reaction.

Ectopic decidua

Decidual tissue is usually seen during pregnancy and progestin treatment, but rare cases are seen in premenopausal and postmenopausal women in absence of any apparent cause. When particularly exuberant, the decidual tissue can form polypoid masses. Ectopic decidua can be seen in up to one-third of cervices from pregnant women; it is most prominent at term. Ectopic decidua is almost always an incidental finding, although rare cases have been biopsied due to cervical friability or cervical bleeding (Figure 4.1).

The unwary may mistake it for squamous cell carcinoma, particularly if there is an associated squamous intraepithelial lesion (cervical intraepithelial neoplasia). Most examples of decidua have abundant, pale eosinophilic cytoplasm, bland nuclei, and absent mitotic figures (Figure 18.8), but secondary changes, such as necrosis, nuclear atypia or signet ring–like changes may raise suspicion for malignancy (Figure 18.9). Epithelial malignancy can be excluded by negative cytokeratin staining. Sometimes the cellularity of a decidual reaction suggests endometrial stromal tumor with secondary deciduation (Figure 18.10). The absence of a distinct mass lesion, spiral arteriole-like vessels, and a delicate, arborizing capillary vascular pattern characteristic of endometrial stromal differentiation militate against that diagnosis.

Implantation site

Implantation site reaction consists of intermediate trophoblasts, cytotrophoblasts, and syncytial trophoblasts in varying numbers infiltrating myometrial tissue. Because the trophoblasts have enlarged, often atypical and mitotically active nuclei arranged in a syncytium, the resemblance to a malignant neoplasm can be striking, particularly if the infiltration is associated with invasion into blood vessels (Figure 18.11). Distinguishing implantation site from choriocarcinoma is based on the presence of chorionic villi in implantation site, and the presence of a bilaminar pattern of large numbers of cytotrophoblasts and syncytial trophoblasts and extensive hemorrhagic necrosis in choriocarcinoma (Figure 18.12). Sometimes implantation sites may exhibit florid trophoblastic proliferation, and these lesions have been referred to as exaggerated placental site (see Figure 17.35).

Placental site nodules or plaques

In contrast to implantation sites, placental site nodules or plaques are composed of nodular aggregates of intermediate trophoblasts embedded in a hyaline matrix. No cytotrophoblasts or syncytial trophoblasts are present. Typically, there is no histologic or clinical evidence of a recent pregnancy with placental site nodules. Placental site nodules are discussed in more detail elsewhere (see Chapter 17)[7–9].

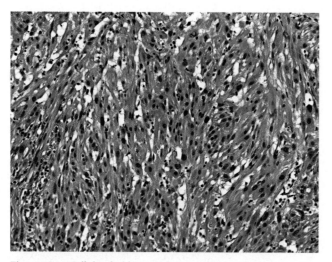

Figure 18.10 Cellular decidua may have spindled appearance resembling a mesenchymal stromal or smooth muscle process.

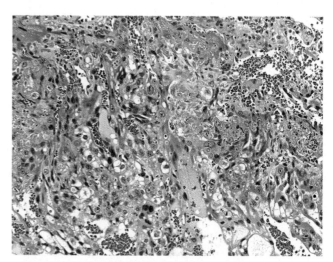

Figure 18.12 Choriocarcinoma. The degree of trophoblastic proliferation and atypia is more pronounced than in early implantation site.

(A)

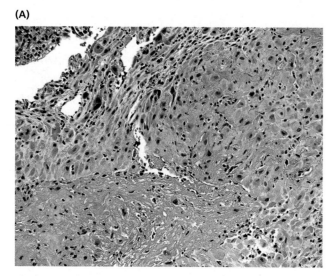

(B)

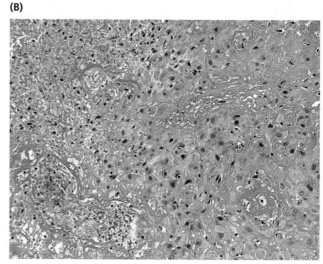

Figure 18.11 (A, B) Implantation site. The trophoblasts may simulate malignancy.

(A)

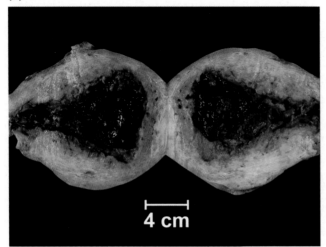

(B)

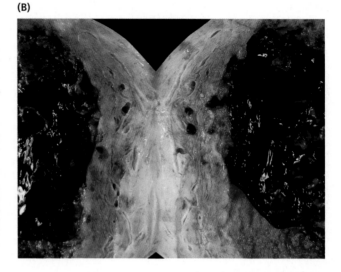

Figure 18.13 (A, B) Uterine atony (gross).

ABNORMAL PREGNANCY-RELATED CHANGES

Abnormal bleeding can occur anytime during and after pregnancy. Bleeding that occurs during pregnancy may be due to a variety of etiologic factors, including infection, inflammation, tumor, abnormal placentation, and abortion (Table 5.6). Abnormal bleeding that occurs following delivery is divided into primary postpartum hemorrhage and secondary postpartum hemorrhage. Primary postpartum hemorrhage is defined as hemorrhage occurring within the first 24 hours postpartum; whereas secondary postpartum hemorrhage is defined as hemorrhage occurring from 24 hours to up to 6 weeks postpartum. The causes of primary postpartum hemorrhage include uterine atony, placenta creta, retained products of conception, lower genital tract lacerations, uterine rupture or inversion, and congenital or acquired coagulopathy. Causes of secondary postpartum hemorrhage include retained products of conception, subinvolution of the placental implantation site, endometritis, dehiscence of a cesarean scar, fibroids, and, less commonly, malignancy (see Chapter 17).

Uterine atony

Uterine atony is the most common cause of postpartum hemorrhage. A recent review of hospital discharge ICD (International *Classification of Diseases, Ninth Revision, Clinical Modification*) codes throughout the United States showed a greater than 25% increase in postpartum hemorrhage from 1995 to 2004, primarily because of an increase

in the incidence of uterine atony. Risk factors for uterine atony include age <20 or ≥ 40 years, cesarean delivery, hypertensive diseases of pregnancy, polyhydramnios, chorioamnionitis, multiple gestation, retained placenta, and antepartum hemorrhage. Maternal age and cesarean delivery are the most common risk factors, but one-third or more cases occur in the absence of recognized risk factors[10]. Despite improved medical therapy for uterine atony, some patients require hysterectomy for uncontrolled postpartum hemorrhage.

Grossly, the atonic uterus is enlarged, flabby and may contain fresh clot (Figure 18.13). The pathologist should measure the average myometrial wall thickness, identify the site (anterior, low, etc.) and thinnest area of the placental bed, and describe any perforation, retained placental fragments, or other pathology present. Multiple leiomyomas predispose to atony, and their presence, size, and number should be specifically noted.

Microscopically, the uterine vessels may appear dilated in uterine atony (Figure 18.14), but this is a non-specific physiologic finding, and the pathologist should resist interpreting this as evidence of vascular malformation or neoplasm in absence of compelling radiographic support obtained via serial imaging studies prior to pregnancy and delivery. A variety of pathologic and non-pathologic conditions in the peripartum and postpartum uterus have imaging abnormalities that overlap with intrauterine vascular abnormality, and the positive predictive value is generally poor in this setting.

Since there are no specific pathologic findings of uterine atony, other potential causes of postpartum

(A)

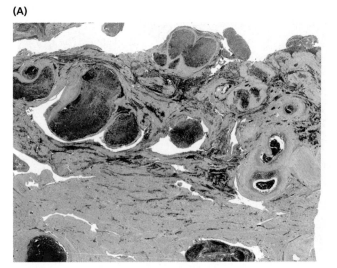

(B)

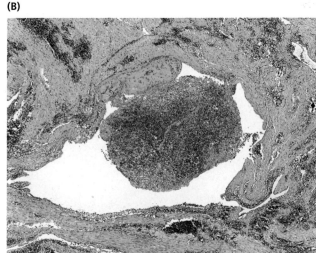

Figure 18.14 (A, B) Dilated vasculature in uterine atony.

(A)

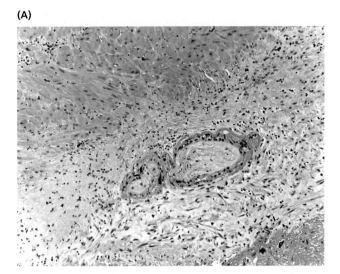

(B)

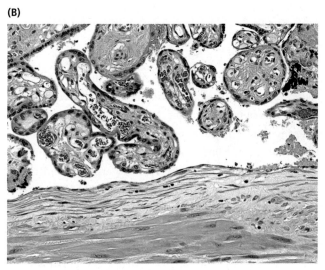

Figure 18.15 (A, B) Placenta accreta. The villi abut myometrium with no intervening intermediate trophoblast layer.

hemorrhage, including accreta, retained placenta, neoplasm, and, rarely, uterine rupture should be excluded. Vascular malformations and diffuse hemangiomas causing extensive postpartum hemorrhage are extremely rare; most are diagnosed on imaging studies prior to delivery and are initially managed by embolectomy before proceeding to hysterectomy (see Chapter 14).

Placenta creta

Placenta creta is due to inadequate or insufficient decidual tissue during implantation[11]. Risk factors include prior uterine surgery, and the risk increases with the number of prior cesarean sections[11]. Microscopically, the basal villi are in direct contact with the myometrium without intervening decidua in placenta creta. Fibrin and trophoblastic cells may be intermingled with the villi and myometrial tissue, but decidual cells are absent. There are three types, depending on the depth of myometrial involvement:

(1) placenta accreta: chorionic villi are adjacent to myometrium (Figure 18.15);
(2) placenta increta: chorionic villi invade myometrium (Figure 18.16);
(3) placenta percreta: chorionic villi invade the entire myometrial wall (Figure 18.17), possibly involving other organs.

Intermediate trophoblastic cells may mimic decidua, but can be identified by the presence of strong expression for

(A)

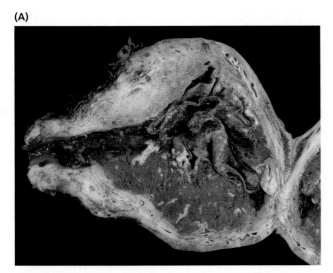

(B)

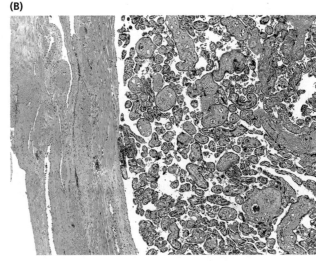

Figure 18.16 (A, B) Placenta increta.

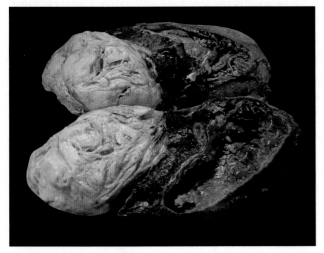

Figure 18.17 Placenta percreta.

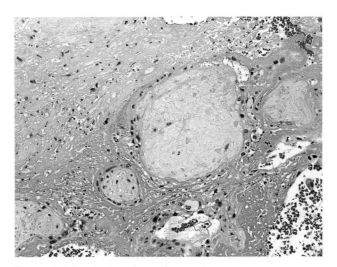

Figure 18.18 Retained products of conception.

cytokeratin. The uterus with suspected accreta should be sampled along the placental bed to document the presence and depth of myometrial involvement. The threshold for increta (as opposed to accreta) is poorly defined. We diagnose placenta increta whenever we encounter chorionic villi intermingled with myometrial tissue, and reserve the diagnosis of accreta for those that appear to show superficial myometrial involvement only (Figures 18.15 and 18.16, respectively). Percreta may be associated with extension onto the outer uterine serosa and, in extreme cases, with involvement of adjacent organs, especially bladder.

Retained products of conception

Retained products of conception can occur following any intrauterine pregnancy, including spontaneous pregnancy loss (miscarriage) and planned pregnancy termination, in addition to preterm/term delivery. The presence of retained products after a spontaneous pregnancy loss distinguishes an incomplete from a complete miscarriage. The diagnosis of retained products of conception requires pathologic documentation of the presence of placental and/or fetal tissue in the uterus. Decidual tissue is often also present, but is insufficient for the diagnosis. In most instances, the pathologic diagnosis is not difficult. However, in some cases, chorionic villi are sparse or necrotic, and positive identification can be more problematic. Often, the only evidence of residual pregnancy is occasional "ghost" outlines of villi enmeshed in fibrin and coagulated blood (Figure 18.18); trichrome stain can demarcate these "ghost" villi from the surrounding fibrin and coagulum if there is uncertainty about their identity. Often, there is associated chronic endometritis.

Subinvolution of implantation site

When the implantation site reaction does not promptly regress after abortion or delivery, it is designated subinvolution. Subinvolution of the placental site may be an anatomic cause of delayed postpartum uterine bleeding. Delayed bleeding occurs typically within the second week of delivery, but bleeding can develop anytime between one week and several months postpartum. Subinvolution is recognized by (1) the presence of superficial dilated and clustered myometrial arteries that are partially occluded by thrombi of various ages; and (2) extravillous interstitial or endovascular trophoblasts (Figure 18.19)[12].

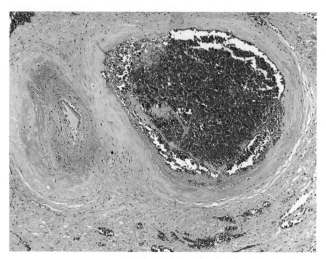

Figure 18.19 Subinvolution of myometrial vessels.

The diagnosis of subinvolution should only be rendered in the clinical setting of delayed (secondary) postpartum bleeding. Physiologic patency of uteroplacental arteries will be seen in the immediate postpartum period (<24 hours) and should not be interpreted as subinvolution (see *Uterine atony*, above).

Postpartum endometritis

Endometritis is the most common cause of postpartum fever. Risk factors are cesarean section, instrumental delivery, internal fetal monitoring, frequent vaginal examinations, preterm labor, premature rupture of membranes, manual removal of the placenta, and meconium. Postpartum endometritis can occur up to six weeks following delivery.

Postpartum endometritis is typically a polymicrobial infection involving a mixture of aerobes and anaerobes from the genital tract[13]. In early postpartum endometritis, Group B streptococcus is an important contributor, as is *Escherichia coli*. Although endometrial biopsy is often obtained to diagnose chronic endometritis in the non-obstetric population, biopsy is seldom performed for diagnosis in the postpartum setting, as patients are treated on the basis of clinical findings. When biopsies are obtained, the findings consist of a dense acute neutrophilic infiltrate involving glands and stroma, often with microabscesses (Figure 18.20). Necrosis is often also present. When severe, necrotizing myometritis has been reported; this is particularly common with Group A streptococcus infection.

(A)

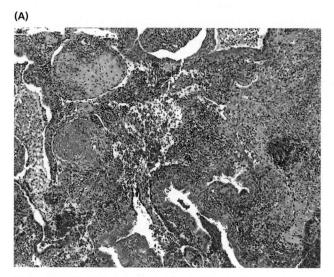

(B)

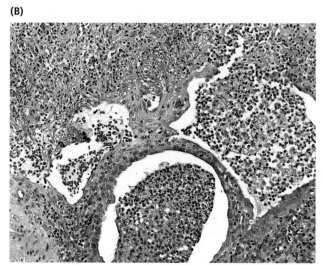

Figure 18.20 (A, B) Postpartum endometritis.

Uterine rupture

Uterine rupture is a catastrophic event requiring emergent surgery. Most cases are now managed by suture over the rupture. Hysterectomy is performed in instances of suspected accreta or underlying anatomic abnormality not amenable to surgical repair (e.g., pseudoaneurysm of uterine artery).

REFERENCES

1. Arias-Stella J. The Arias-Stella reaction: facts and fancies four decades after. *Adv Anat Pathol* 2002;**9**:12–23.
2. Huettner PC, Gersell DJ. Arias-Stella reaction in nonpregnant women: a clinicopathologic study of nine cases. *Int J Gynecol Pathol* 1994;**13**:241–7.
3. Arias-Stella J, Jr., Arias-Velasquez A, Arias-Stella J. Normal and abnormal mitoses in the atypical endometrial change associated with chorionic tissue effect [corrected]. *Am J Surg Pathol* 1994;**18**:694–701.
4. Milchgrub S, Sandstad J. Arias-Stella reaction in fallopian tube epithelium. A light and electron microscopic study with a review of the literature. *Am J Clin Pathol* 1991;**95**:892–5.
5. Nucci MR, Young RH. Arias-Stella reaction of the endocervix: a report of 18 cases with emphasis on its varied histology and differential diagnosis. *Am J Surg Pathol* 2004;**28**:608–12.
6. Sakaki M, Hirokawa M, Sano T, *et al.* Ovarian endometriosis showing decidual change and Arias-Stella reaction with biotin-containing intranuclear inclusions. *Acta Cytol* 2003;**47**:321–4.
7. Huettner PC, Gersell DJ. Placental site nodule: a clinicopathologic study of 38 cases. *Int J Gynecol Pathol* 1994;**13**:191–8.
8. Shih IM, Seidman JD, Kurman RJ. Placental site nodule and characterization of distinctive types of intermediate trophoblast. *Hum Pathol* 1999;**30**:687–94.
9. Young RH, Kurman RJ, Scully RE. Placental site nodules and plaques. A clinicopathologic analysis of 20 cases. *Am J Surg Pathol* 1990;**14**:1001–9.
10. Bateman BT, Berman MF, Riley LE, *et al.* The epidemiology of postpartum hemorrhage in a large, nationwide sample of deliveries. *Anesth Analg* 2010;**110**:1368–73.
11. Tantbirojn P, Crum CP, Parast MM. Pathophysiology of placenta creta: the role of decidua and extravillous trophoblast. *Placenta* 2008;**29**:639–45.
12. Weydert JA, Benda JA. Subinvolution of the placental site as an anatomic cause of postpartum uterine bleeding: a review. *Arch Pathol Lab Med* 2006;**130**:1538–42.
13. Cox SM, Gilstrap LC, 3rd. Postpartum endometritis. *Obstet Gynecol Clin North Am* 1989;**16**:363–71.

19 LYNCH SYNDROME (HEREDITARY NON-POLYPOSIS COLORECTAL CANCER SYNDROME)

INTRODUCTION

Lynch syndrome (also known as hereditary non-polyposis colorectal cancer syndrome [HNPCC]), confers a predisposition to developing certain types of cancers, including endometrial and ovarian carcinomas. Although adenocarcinoma of the colon is the most common tumor type diagnosed in men with the syndrome, endometrial carcinoma is the most common tumor in women diagnosed with the syndrome. It is not valid to assume that screening modalities useful for detecting Lynch syndrome–associated endometrial cancers should be the same as for colorectal carcinoma, because Lynch syndrome–associated endometrial carcinomas differ significantly from syndromic colon cancers. In Lynch syndrome–associated endometrial cancer, the average age of onset is older, the spectrum of DNA mismatch repair gene mutation types is wider, and the association with microsatellite instability (MSI) is more variable (Table 19.1).

Endometrial cancer has been characterized as a "sentinel" cancer, because its diagnosis can prompt detection and diagnosis of other Lynch syndrome–associated carcinomas, such as colon cancer – and screening for colon cancer in Lynch syndrome kindreds can reduce by 65% the risk of death from that disease. Lynch syndrome–associated endometrial cancers differ significantly from sporadic endometrial cancers: they present at a younger age; their association with obesity and hyperestrinism appears to be weaker; and there is some evidence that these tumors may be relatively more aggressive (Table 19.2). At least 2–5% of endometrial cancers are due to Lynch syndrome–defining mutations, but this is probably a low estimate due to few large-scale population-based studies[1,2]. Despite the relative rarity of these tumors, there has been recent interest in studying their genetic, molecular, morphologic, and clinical attributes. An appreciation of these features can be used to devise schemes for detecting endometrial cancer–associated Lynch syndrome, which is one of the major themes of this chapter.

LYNCH SYNDROME DEFINITION, GENETICS AND PATHOPHYSIOLOGY

Lynch syndrome is an autosomal-dominant inherited cancer-susceptibility syndrome featuring high rates of colorectal, endometrial, ovarian, gastric, urinary, and biliary cancers, among others (Table 19.3). The syndrome is almost always characterized by a mutation in one, of the DNA mismatch repair (DNA MMR) genes, listed in order of decreasing frequency in Lynch syndrome–associated endometrial cancer: *hMSH6*, *hMSH2*, *hMLH1*, or *hPMS2*[2].

Table 19.1 Comparison of Lynch syndrome-associated endometrial and colorectal carcinoma

	Endometrial carcinoma	Colorectal carcinoma
Age at presentation (years)	45–55	35–45
DNA MMR mutations	*hMSH6 > hMSH2>hMLH1*	*hMLH1 = hMSH2>hMSH6*
MSI-H[a] rate (%)	70	99

[a] MSI-H = Microsatellite instability-high; see the section on **Microsatellite instability**.

Table 19.2 Comparison of Lynch syndrome–associated and sporadic endometrial carcinoma

	Lynch syndrome endometrial cancer	Sporadic endometrial cancer
Age at presentation (years)[a]	45–55	65
Body mass index[a]	Low	High
Clinical behavior[a]	Possibly aggressive	Baseline

[a] Wide variations occur; these figures are meant to provide a snapshot to facilitate comparison.

Table 19.3 Sites of Lynch syndrome–associated carcinomas[a]

(1) Colorectum[b]

(2) Endometrium[b]

(3) Renal pelvis and ureter

(4) Ovary

(5) Stomach

(6) Small intestine

(7) Brain, skin, prostate

[a] Listed in rough order of decreasing incidence in men and women

[b] Endometrial cancer rates exceed those of colorectal cancers in women. Some investigators have estimated that endometrial cancer rates may be twice those of colon cancer rates in women[3].

Table 19.4 Amsterdam Criteria[12,13]

Amsterdam Criteria I

Three or more family members with a confirmed diagnosis of colorectal cancer; one of whom is a first-degree (parent, child, sibling) relative of the other two

Two successive affected generations

One or more colon cancers diagnosed under the age of 50 years

Familial adenomatous polyposis (FAP) has been excluded

Amsterdam Criteria II

Three or more family members with Lynch syndrome–related cancers; one of whom is a first-degree relative of the other two

Two successive affected generations

One or more of the Lynch syndrome–related cancers diagnosed under the age of 50 years

Familial adenomatous polyposis (FAP) has been excluded

Lynch syndrome mutation carriers possess one wild-type allele and one mutated allele in somatic tissues. A second "hit," such as loss of heterozygosity, promoter methylation or a second mutation, is present in the genome of Lynch syndrome tumors. In general, proteins derived from mutated genes cannot bind their obligate dimerization partners, which abrogates the normal function of the DNA mismatch repair system, allowing neoplasms to arise. Under physiologic conditions, MLH1 binds PMS2, and MSH2 binds MSH6. A breakdown in the normal functioning of the DNA mismatch repair system usually, but not always, leads to accumulation of repeated sequences of DNA, called microsatellite instability (MSI).

Lynch syndrome significance

The lifetime cumulative risk of developing an endometrial cancer for a patient with Lynch syndrome varies from 27% to 71%, depending upon which DNA mismatch repair gene is mutated[1,2,4,5]. The highest risk is in the setting of *hMSH6* mutation, and the lowest is with *hMLH1* mutation. Lynch syndrome–associated endometrial cancers differ from sporadic tumors in several significant ways (Table 19.2). The average age of onset of endometrial cancer in a Lynch syndrome patient is between 45 and 55 years of age[5]: at least a decade earlier than sporadic endometrial cancer. Approximately 10% of patients who develop endometrial cancer before age 50 have Lynch syndrome[6,7]. Affected patients are also less frequently obese, particularly in studies of very young patients with Lynch syndrome–associated endometrial cancers. There is some evidence that Lynch syndrome–associated tumors may be relatively more aggressive than sporadic ones, with significantly increased rates of deep myometrial invasion,

lymphovascular invasion, high FIGO grade, and high FIGO stage[8,9,10].

It is important to recognize which endometrial cancer patients have Lynch syndrome. Diagnosing a Lynch syndrome–associated endometrial cancer provides the patient with the opportunity to be screened for the development of other Lynch syndrome–associated tumors, particularly colon cancer, and it allows blood relatives to undergo screening for Lynch syndrome. Surveillance for colon cancer has led to improved survivals of patients in Lynch syndrome families. In one study, colon cancer screening reduced mortality by almost 65%[11]. There have been comparatively fewer studies regarding endometrial cancer screening, and the ones that have been performed have not yielded comparable results.

Lynch syndrome diagnosis

A diagnosis of Lynch syndrome can only be established by documentation of a germline mutation in a mismatch repair gene. However, it is impractical to perform mutational analysis on all patient samples. Detection of patients at risk for Lynch syndrome has therefore relied upon assessment of a variety of associated features such as young age, and family and personal history of Lynch syndrome–associated tumors (Tables 19.4–19.7). Individually and as a group, these features are neither specific nor sensitive for detecting potential Lynch syndrome patients with endometrial cancer[16]. According to one large recent study, age-based screening would fail to detect 6 of 10 patients with Lynch syndrome–defining mutations;

Table 19.5 The Revised Bethesda Guidelines for testing colorectal tumors for microsatellite instability (MSI)[14]

Tumors from individuals should be tested for microsatellite instability in the following situations:

- Colorectal cancer diagnosed in a patient who is less than 50 years of age
- Presence of synchronous or metachronous colorectal, or other Lynch syndrome–associated tumors[a], regardless of age
- Colorectal cancer with the MSI-H[b] histology[c] diagnosed in a patient who is less than 60 years of age
- Colorectal cancer diagnosed in one or more first-degree relatives with a Lynch syndrome–related tumor, with one of the cancers being diagnosed under the age of 50 years
- Colorectal cancer diagnosed in two or more first-degree or second-degree relatives with Lynch syndrome–related tumors, regardless of age

[a] Lynch syndrome–related tumors include colorectal, endometrial, stomach, ovarian, pancreas, ureter and renal pelvis, biliary tract, and brain (usually glioblastoma as seen in Turcot syndrome) tumors, sebaceous gland adenomas and keratoacanthomas in Muir–Torre syndrome, and carcinoma of the small bowel.
[b] Microsatellite instability-high (MSI-H) in tumors refers to changes in two or more of the five National Cancer Institute–recommended panels of microsatellite markers.
[c] Presence of tumor-infiltrating lymphocytes, Crohn's-like lymphocytic reaction, mucinous/signet ring differentiation, or medullary growth pattern

Table 19.7 Southwest Gynecologic Oncology Criteria (5–10% risk)[15]

Patients with endometrial or colorectal cancer diagnosed prior to the age of 50

Patient with endometrial or ovarian cancer with a synchronous or metachronous colon or other Lynch/HNPCC-associated tumor at any age

Patients with synchronous or metachronous ovarian and colorectal cancer with the first cancer diagnosed prior to the age of 50

Patients with colorectal or endometrial cancer diagnosed at any age with two or more first-degree or second-degree relatives with Lynch/ HNPCC-associated tumors, regardless of age

Patients with a first-degree or second-degree relative who meets the above criteria

Table 19.6 Southwest Gynecologic Oncology (SGO) Criteria (20–25% risk)[15]

Patients with endometrial or colorectal cancer who meet the revised Amsterdam Criteria

Patients with synchronous or metachronous endometrial and colorectal cancer with the first cancer diagnosed prior to the age of 50

Patients with synchronous or metachronous ovarian and colorectal cancer with the first cancer diagnosed prior to the age of 50

Patients with colorectal or endometrial cancer with evidence of a mismatch repair defect (i.e., MSI or dMMR)

Patients with a first or second degree relative with a known mismatch repair gene mutation

Abbreviations: MSI = microsatellite instability; dMMR = mismatch repair protein deficiency.

are, apparently, many DNA mismatch repair mutations that have not been fully characterized. Supplementary methods that can be used to stratify patients into groups that are high- and low-risk for Lynch syndrome include assays for MSI, methylation of the *hMLH1* promoter, and immunohistochemical expression of DNA mismatch repair gene products (Diagram 19.1).

Microsatellite instability

Microsatellite instability analysis is accomplished by polymerase chain reaction using five primers as defined by the international workshop on Lynch syndrome in Bethesda – two mononucleotide (BAT25 and BAT26) and three dinucleotide repeats (D2S123, D5S346, and D17S250). Mononucleotide markers may be better than dinucleotides for microsatellite instability identification and a panel that uses 5 mononucleotide markers is being used increasingly. Tumors are classified as MSI-high (MSI-H) when two or more of the five markers show microsatellite instability, MSI-low (MSI-L) when one of the markers shows microsatellite instability, and MS-stable (MSS) if none of the markers show microsatellite instability. It is well known that microsatellite instability testing, in general, is not specific for Lynch syndrome, since high-level microsatellite instability occurs in two settings – genetic and epigenetic. High-level microsatellite instability is present in approximately 20% of endometrial cancers and, in more than 80% of those cases, high-level microsatellite instability results from methylation (epigenetic inactivation) of *hMLH1* promoter. The remaining MSI-H cases are due to germline mutations in one, or occasionally more, of the DNA mismatch repair genes; affected patients have Lynch

while screening based on family history would fail to detect 7 of 10 such patients[2].

Gene sequencing

The most direct method of documenting a Lynch syndrome–defining mutation is gene sequencing, but this method is costly and only marginally sensitive, since there

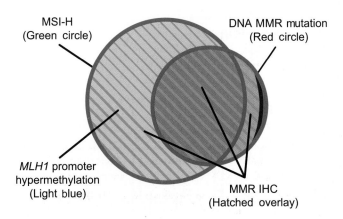

MSI-H
(Green circle)

DNA MMR mutation
(Red circle)

MLH1 promoter
hypermethylation
(Light blue)

MMR IHC
(Hatched overlay)

Diagram 19.1 Relationship between DNA mismatch repair gene mutation, microsatellite instability, and DNA mismatch repair immunohistochemistry in endometrial carcinoma. Endometrial carcinoma patients with Lynch syndrome/hereditary non-polyposis colorectal cancer have mutations in one of the DNA mismatch repair genes, represented by the area inside the red circle. In endometrial cancer, mutations in *MSH6* or *MSH2* far outnumber those involving *MLH1*. Approximately 80% of cases with gene mutations can be indirectly detected with microsatellite instability testing, indicated by the area inside the green circle (MSI-H). Microsatellite instability testing, however, is not specific for DNA mismatch repair gene mutation, as most MSI-H cases, indicated by areas shaded light blue, arise secondary to *MLH1* promoter methylation, not gene mutation. These patients have MSI-H cancers that are sporadic, and the affected patients do not have Lynch syndrome/hereditary non-polyposis colorectal cancer. Microsatellite instability testing is also somewhat insensitive for gene mutations in general, and *MSH6* mutations specifically (i.e., microsatellite instability testing does not recognize all mutated cases). These cases are represented by the sliver of orange shading within the red circle between the green and blue lines. Abnormalities with immunohistochemical testing for DNA mismatch repair expression (IHC; areas underneath the hatched overlay) detect a greater percentage of gene mutation cases than does microsatellite instability testing, including many *MSH6* mutated cases, but, similar to microsatellite instability testing, immunohistochemistry recognizes many sporadic cases as well. Finally, there are rare mutations that cannot be recognized by either microsatellite instability testing or immunohistochemistry testing (red sliver outside the blue line).

syndrome. In one large study, high-level microsatellite instability was present in 18% of endometrial cancers; while only 2% of patients had Lynch syndrome[2]. Microsatellite analysis also failed to identify 3 of 10 patients with Lynch syndrome, indicating that, as regards endometrial cancer, microsatellite instability analysis is not only non-specific, but also relatively insensitive. Rates of microsatellite instability vary with the type of DNA mismatch repair gene mutation present. Microsatellite instability is a feature that is present only variably in tumors that arise in patients with *hMSH6* mutation[2], the most common mutation seen in Lynch syndrome–associated endometrial cancer.

Methylation of hMLH1 promoter

Because assays that detect methylation of the *hMLH1* promoter can recognize epigenetic mechanisms that lead to high-level microsatellite instability, one can derive information regarding DNA mismatch repair gene mutation if a methylation assay is performed along with a microsatellite instability assay or immunohistochemistry for DNA mismatch repair[17]. A patient whose tumor is MSI-H, but lacks *hMLH1* promoter methylation likely has Lynch syndrome, whereas one whose tumor is MSI-H with *hMLH1* promoter methylation probably does not. Unlike colon cancer, *hMLH1* methylation cannot be detected by *BRAF* mutational analysis (Diagram 19.2).

Immunohistochemistry for DNA mismatch repair

Immunohistochemistry has been shown to be a sensitive and specific method to detect mismatch repair, and is a powerful, albeit indirect, modality for detecting germline mutation. In a recent report, immunohistochemistry with MLH1 and MSH2 antibodies had a sensitivity of 69% and a specificity of 100% in detecting high-level microsatellite instability[18]. When the panel was expanded to include PMS2 and MSH6 antibodies, the sensitivity for detection of high-level microsatellite instability improved to 91%, but the specificity decreased to 83%[18]. The decreased specificity was primarily due to a lack of correlation between loss of MSH6 expression and high-level microsatellite instability. The positive predictive value of immunohistochemistry for detecting a germline mutation, particularly with absent MSH2 or MSH6 staining, is very high. It has been suggested that loss of these specific proteins by immunohistochemistry, even in the absence of detectable germline mutations, may be sufficient evidence of Lynch syndrome, since current germline testing for MSH2 and MSH6 mutations is relatively insensitive. Compared to microsatellite instability analysis, immunohistochemistry is a convenient test and is readily performed in most pathology laboratories. Immunohistochemistry is also advantageous as it can pinpoint the affected gene or genes, leading to an ability to target specific genes for sequencing. However, since some DNA mismatch repair gene mutations cannot be detected by immunohistochemistry, some investigators still recommend using both immunohistochemistry and microsatellite instability testing in combination to maximize the ability to detect every patient at risk for Lynch syndrome.

DNA mismatch repair proteins MLH1, MSH2, MSH6, and PMS2 are found to be absent in tumor cell nuclei by

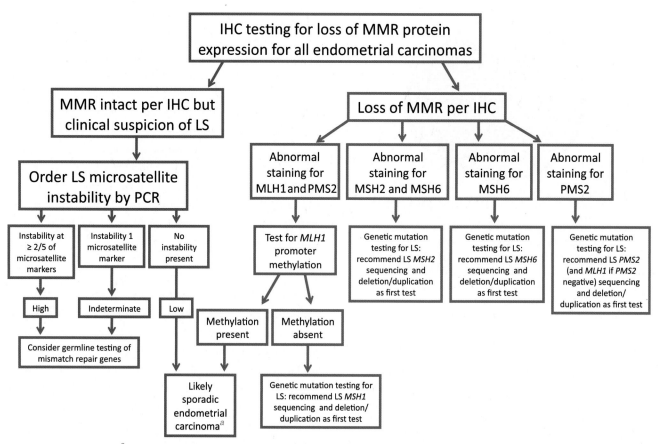

Diagram 19.2 Algorithm for testing endometrial carcinomas for possible Lynch syndrome based on mismatch repair protein deficiency. LS = Lynch syndrome. Another cost effective approach entails initial screening for MSH6 and PMS2 expression, followed by MSH2 or MLH1 if an abnormality is detected.

immunohistochemistry in up to one-third of endometrioid adenocarcinomas[18,19]. The vast majority of endometrial cancers with abnormal DNA mismatch repair expression have epigenetic silencing of *hMLH1* due to methylation of its promoter. Since MLH1 and PMS2 are obligate dimerization partners, as are MSH2 and MSH6, loss of MLH1 is usually coupled with concurrent loss of PMS2, and loss of MSH2 is accompanied by MSH6 loss. Isolated loss of PMS2 may be due to *hPMS2* mutation or *hMLH1* mutation that yields an intact MLH1 protein. Isolated loss of MSH6 is almost always due to *hMSH6* mutation.

Despite the relative ease of performing the assays, the interpretation of DNA mismatch repair immunohistochemistry can be problematic, particularly with MLH1 and MSH6. In general, only complete loss of expression in the setting of a valid positive internal control is considered interpretable (Figure 19.1). Valid internal controls include non-neoplastic endometrial stroma, lymphocytes,

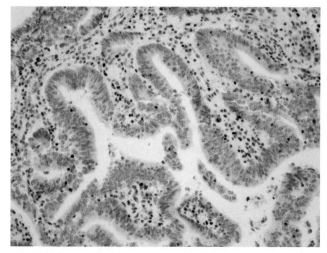

Figure 19.1 Well-differentiated endometrioid adenocarcinoma without expression of MLH1 in tumor cell nuclei. Non-neoplastic cells, including lymphocytes, stromal cells, and endothelial cells, show retained expression, which is evidence of a positive internal control. This tumor is likely to be unrelated to Lynch syndrome and requires methylation analysis to determine its methylation status.

(A)

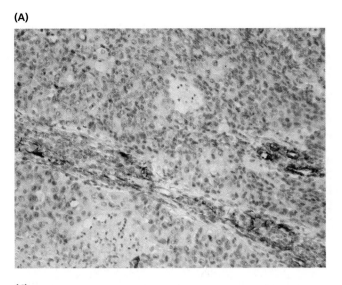

(B)

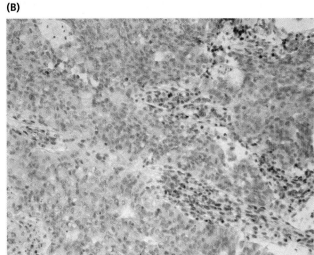

(C)

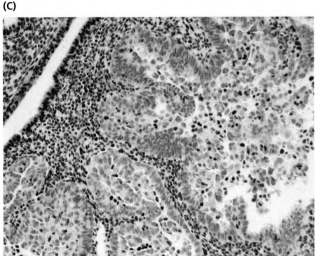

Figure 19.2 Clear cell carcinoma with difficult-to-interpret DNA mismatch repair immunohistochemical stains. The patient has a provisional diagnosis of Lynch syndrome. Panel A shows intact expression of MLH1, while panel B shows loss of MSH2 with intact positive internal controls. Panel C shows focal MSH6 expression in tumor cell nuclei, which is commonly encountered. To classify a tumor as deficient in MSH6, the tumor should be completely devoid of nuclear MSH6 nuclear expression.

and normal glands with reproducibly stained nuclei. Care should be taken to ensure that the lesion being assessed is adenocarcinoma, not hyperplasia. Common pitfalls (Figures 19.2 and 19.3) in interpreting these stains are discussed in a recent review[20]. When such problematic cases are encountered, they should be reviewed by at least two pathologists with experience in the interpretation of immunohistochemistry for DNA mismatch repair. If no consensus is reached, the stain should be repeated. There are rare cases that remain uninterpretable and are deemed inconclusive.

Lynch syndrome tumor morphology and topography (Table 19.8)

It has been proposed that many Lynch syndrome–associated endometrial cancers have specific features that allow recognition[21]. In a study of Lynch syndrome–associated endometrial cancers, the authors reported that 86% of tumors were endometrioid (and 14% were nonendometrioid)[17]: rates that are comparable to sporadic endometrial cancers. Significantly, another recent study showed that rates of nonendometrioid carcinomas were higher in Lynch syndrome–associated endometrial cancers (44%) when compared to age-matched control cases that were not associated with Lynch syndrome. The average age of presentation for nonendometrioid, Lynch syndrome–associated carcinomas was 44 years[10]. This suggests that nonendometrioid carcinoma diagnosed in a patient before 50 or 55 years of age is at high risk for being associated with Lynch syndrome, but this has not been substantiated in other studies. Nonendometrioid carcinomas that have been reported include clear cell carcinoma, serous carcinoma, carcinosarcoma, and small cell carcinoma. Undifferentiated and dedifferentiated carcinomas[22–24] are also included in the spectrum.

(A)

(B)

(C)

(D)

(E)

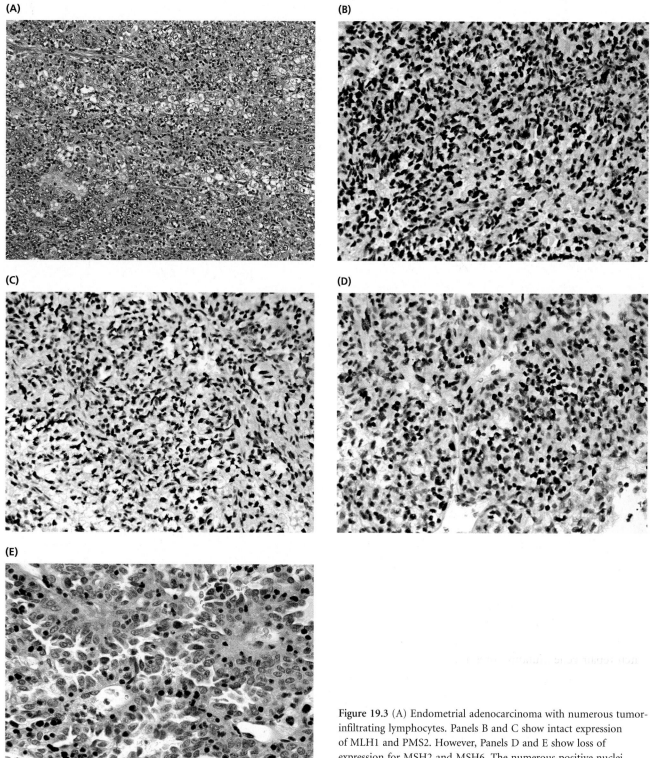

Figure 19.3 (A) Endometrial adenocarcinoma with numerous tumor-infiltrating lymphocytes. Panels B and C show intact expression of MLH1 and PMS2. However, Panels D and E show loss of expression for MSH2 and MSH6. The numerous positive nuclei represent the infiltrating lymphocytes. This tumor was initially misclassified as mismatch repair protein proficient (i.e., intact for all markers) due to the numerous infiltrating lymphocytes.

Table 19.8 Lynch syndrome tumor morphology and topography

Nonendometrioid carcinoma[a] in young women
Endometrioid carcinoma[b] with numerous tumor-infiltrating lymphocytes (more than 42 per 10 high power fields)
Lower uterine segment localization
Synchronous ovarian clear cell carcinoma

[a] Clear cell carcinoma, undifferentiated carcinoma, dedifferentiated carcinoma, carcinosarcoma, and rare serous carcinomas.
[b] Many are poorly differentiated and may be impossible to distinguish from undifferentiated carcinoma.

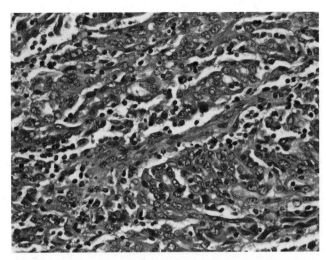

Figure 19.4 Poorly differentiated tumors in Lynch syndrome, such as depicted here, can be difficult to subclassify.

Endometrioid carcinomas predominate in Lynch syndrome families despite the reported incidence of nonendometrioid carcinomas in young patients with Lynch syndrome. As noted earlier, these tumors tend to be more poorly differentiated as compared to sporadic tumors, and, anecdotally, the poorly differentiated tumors can be difficult to subclassify (Figure 19.4). Many are high-grade tumors with a mix of glandular, papillary, and solid architecture, with variable components including cells with clear or mucinous cytoplasm and spindle cells. Many MSI-H[21] and Lynch syndrome–associated endometrial cancers contain dense peritumoral lymphocytes and high numbers of tumor-infiltrating lymphocytes (TILs) (Figure 19.5) that are statistically less frequently observed in sporadic, non-methylated tumors. A cutoff of 42 lymphocytes per 10 high-power fields has been proposed as a value that balances sensitivity and specificity for use as a screening modality[21]. This value is higher than that recommended for colon cancer screening, since the density of lymphoid infiltrates appears to be generally higher in endometrial cancer when compared to colon cancer. Rates of nonendometrioid histology and density of tumor-infiltrating lymphocytes may vary according to the type of DNA mismatch repair gene mutation present.

As in the colon (where right-sided cancers are overly represented in Lynch syndrome patients), endometrial carcinoma topography also appears related to Lynch syndrome status. Origin in the lower uterine segment and the presence of certain types of synchronous and metachronous carcinomas in the pelvis have been associated with Lynch syndrome. According to one study, nearly 30% of patients with an endometrial cancer based in the lower uterine segment had Lynch syndrome[25]. Synchronous and metachronous ovarian clear cell carcinomas and carcinomas arising in endometriosis have been reported as part of the spectrum as well[8]. That being said, it is important to remember that most synchronous endometrial and ovarian carcinomas, particularly in patients younger than 40 years of age, are not related to Lynch syndrome[26,27]. Sporadic tumors that arise in this setting are almost always well differentiated and endometrioid in both sites.

SCREENING ENDOMETRIAL CANCERS FOR LYNCH SYNDROME

As discussed previously, screening based on age and a personal or family history of Lynch syndrome–associated cancers is insufficiently sensitive and specific to detect Lynch syndrome patients. In an effort to increase screening sensitivity and specificity, a variety of screening protocols have been implemented in some high-volume cancer centers.

One approach involves use of immunohistochemistry for DNA mismatch repair to evaluate endometrial cancers in patients under 50 years of age, when tumor morphology or topography is suggestive of Lynch syndrome, and when there is a family or personal history of Lynch syndrome–associated tumors[8]. In this paradigm (Table 19.9), immunohistochemistry for DNA mismatch repair is triggered by the pathologist in the former two instances, and it is usually requested by clinicians in the latter instance. Any abnormal immunohistochemical result alerts the clinician to arrange a genetic counseling session during which there is a discussion about the need to perform supplementary tests, such as methylation assay, microsatellite instability

(A)

(B)

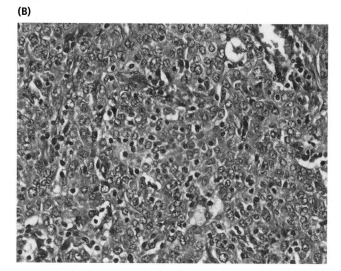

(C)

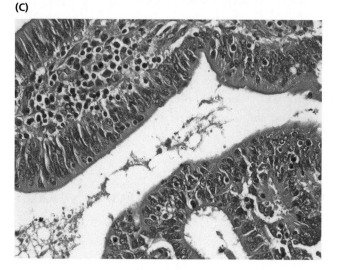

Figure 19.5 Tumor-infiltrating lymphocytes. Panel A shows dense peritumoral and tumor-infiltrating lymphocytes at low-power magnification. Panel B, a poorly differentiated carcinoma with an undifferentiated appearance, and panel C, a well-differentiated endometrioid carcinoma, show prominent tumor-infiltrating lymphocytes.

Table 19.9 Algorithm for detecting endometrial cancer patients at increased risk for Lynch syndrome

Perform immunohistochemistry for DNA mismatch repair proteins (MLH1, PMS2, MSH2, and MSH6) when any of the following is present.

- Personal or family history of Lynch syndrome–associated tumors (information usually supplied by clinician)
- Age under 50 years
- Morphology
  - Tumor-infiltrating lymphocytes
  - Dedifferentiated and undifferentiated endometrial carcinoma
- Topography
  - Lower uterine segment
  - Synchronous or metachronous tumors (ovarian clear cell, colorectal)

assay, and/or DNA mismatch repair gene sequencing. Preliminary results using endometrioid carcinomas rich in tumor-infiltrating lymphocytes, lower uterine segment

tumors, and dedifferentiated carcinomas as criteria for tumor morphology and topography, along with age and clinical history criteria, led to enrichment of patient numbers at risk for Lynch syndrome in a recent study[8]. Of patients' tumors that met criteria, 60% showed abnormal DNA mismatch repair expression, as compared to a comparison group in which only 20% of tumors had DNA mismatch repair abnormalities. Since Lynch syndrome may initially present in women over 50 years of age, and the cost of two immunohistochemical stains is relatively low compared to the benefit of identifying a patient (and kindred) with Lynch syndrome, some institutions test all endometrial cancers with immunohistochemistry using MSH6 and PMS2 as initial screening antibodies, followed by MLH1 or MSH2 if an abnormality is detected. (Diagram 19.2); in other centers, testing is performed only at the discretion of the patient's gynecologist or clinical geneticist.

(A)

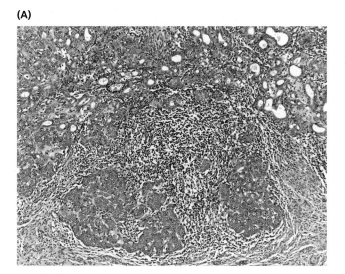

(B)

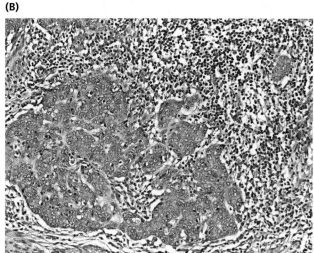

Figure 19.6 (A, B) Occult adenocarcinoma arising in lower uterine segment of risk-reducing hysterectomy specimen in patient with Lynch syndrome.

Regardless of the screening method that is used, there should be a method in place that ensures that all eligible endometrial cancers are tested, and all patients with abnormal results are (1) offered genetic counseling, and (2) sent for proper cancer screening studies.

RISK-REDUCING HYSTERECTOMY

Occult malignancy at the time of risk-reducing (prophylactic) hysterectomy is occasionally detected in individuals with Lynch syndrome (Figure 19.6). Because of the risk of occult malignancy, in either the endometrium or the ovaries at the time of risk-reducing surgery, all patients should undergo preoperative endometrial biopsy, preferably by a gynecologic oncologist in case staging is required. The pathologist should be aware that the patient has Lynch syndrome in order to conduct a careful, thorough examination of both the endometrium (with attention to the lower uterine segment) and ovaries. Any suspicious masses should be submitted for frozen section evaluation. Although there is currently no standardized protocol for processing the surgical specimens from prophylactic surgery in patients with Lynch syndrome, we recommend complete evaluation of all endometrial and ovarian tissue.

REFERENCES

1. Gruber SB, Thompson WD. A population-based study of endometrial cancer and familial risk in younger women. Cancer and Steroid Hormone Study Group. *Cancer Epidemiol Biomarkers Prev* 1996;**5**:411–17.

2. Hampel H, Frankel W, Panescu J, *et al.* Screening for Lynch syndrome (hereditary nonpolyposis colorectal cancer) among endometrial cancer patients. *Cancer Res* 2006;**66**:7810–17.

3. Resnick KE, Hampel H, Fishel R, *et al.* Current and emerging trends in Lynch syndrome identification in women with endometrial cancer. *Gynecol Oncol* 2009;**114**:128–34.

4. Dunlop MG, Farrington SM, Carothers AD, *et al.* Cancer risk associated with germline DNA mismatch repair gene mutations. *Hum Mol Genet* 1997;**6**:105–10.

5. Vasen HF, Wijnen JT, Menko FH, *et al.* Cancer risk in families with hereditary nonpolyposis colorectal cancer diagnosed by mutation analysis. *Gastroenterology* 1996;**110**:1020–7.

6. Berends MJ, Wu Y, Sijmons RH, *et al.* Toward new strategies to select young endometrial cancer patients for mismatch repair gene mutation analysis. *J Clin Oncol* 2003;**21**:4364–70.

7. Lu KH, Schorge JO, Rodabaugh KJ, *et al.* Prospective determination of prevalence of lynch syndrome in young women with endometrial cancer. *J Clin Oncol* 2007;**25**:5158–64.

8. Garg K, Leitao MM, Jr., Kauff ND, *et al.* Selection of endometrial carcinomas for DNA mismatch repair protein immunohistochemistry using patient age and tumor morphology enhances detection of mismatch repair abnormalities. *Am J Surg Pathol* 2009;**33**:925–33.

9. Garg K, Shih K, Barakat R, *et al.* Endometrial carcinomas in women aged 40 years and younger: tumors associated with loss of DNA mismatch repair proteins comprise a distinct clinicopathologic subset. *Am J Surg Pathol* 2009;**33**(12):1869–77.

10. Carcangiu ML, Radice P, Casalini P, *et al.* Lynch syndrome–related endometrial carcinomas show a high frequency of nonendometrioid types and of high FIGO grade endometrioid types. *Int J Surg Pathol* 2010;**18**(1):21–6.

11. Jarvinen HJ, Mecklin JP, Sistonen P. Screening reduces colorectal cancer rate in families with hereditary nonpolyposis colorectal cancer. *Gastroenterology* 1995;**108**:1405–11.

12. Vasen HF, Mecklin JP, Khan PM, *et al.* The International Collaborative Group on Hereditary Non-Polyposis Colorectal Cancer (ICG-HNPCC). *Dis Colon Rectum* 1991;**34**:424–5.

13. Vasen HF, Watson P, Mecklin JP, *et al.* New clinical criteria for hereditary nonpolyposis colorectal cancer (HNPCC, Lynch syndrome)

proposed by the International Collaborative group on HNPCC. *Gastroenterology* 1999;**116**:1453–6.

14. Umar A, Boland CR, Terdiman JP, *et al.* Revised Bethesda Guidelines for hereditary nonpolyposis colorectal cancer (Lynch syndrome) and microsatellite instability. *J Natl Cancer Inst* 2004;**96**:261–8.

15. Lancaster JM, Powell CB, Kauff ND, *et al.* Society of Gynecologic Oncologists Education Committee statement on risk assessment for inherited gynecologic cancer predispositions. *Gynecol Oncol* 2007;**107**:159–62.

16. Mills AM, Liou S, Ford JM *et al.* Lynch syndrome screening should be considered for all patients with newly diagnosed endometrial cancer. *Mod Pathol* 2011;**24**:260A.

17. Broaddus RR, Lynch HT, Chen LM, *et al.* Pathologic features of endometrial carcinoma associated with HNPCC: a comparison with sporadic endometrial carcinoma. *Cancer* 2006;**106**:87–94.

18. Modica I, Soslow RA, Black D, *et al.* Utility of immunohistochemistry in predicting microsatellite instability in endometrial carcinoma. *Am J Surg Pathol* 2007;**31**:744–51.

19. Vasen HF, Hendriks Y, de Jong AE, *et al.* Identification of HNPCC by molecular analysis of colorectal and endometrial tumors. *Dis Markers* 2004;**20**:207–13.

20. Shia J. Immunohistochemistry versus microsatellite instability testing for screening colorectal cancer patients at risk for hereditary nonpolyposis colorectal cancer syndrome. Part I. The utility of immunohistochemistry. *J Mol Diagn* 2008;**10**:293–300.

21. Shia J, Black D, Hummer AJ, *et al.* Routinely assessed morphological features correlate with microsatellite instability status in endometrial cancer. *Hum Pathol* 2008;**39**:116–25.

22. Altrabulsi B, Malpica A, Deavers MT, *et al.* Undifferentiated carcinoma of the endometrium. *Am J Surg Pathol* 2005;**29**:1316–21.

23. Silva EG, Deavers MT, Bodurka DC, *et al.* Association of low-grade endometrioid carcinoma of the uterus and ovary with undifferentiated carcinoma: a new type of dedifferentiated carcinoma? *Int J Gynecol Pathol* 2006;**25**:52–8.

24. Tafe LJ, Garg K, Chew I, *et al.* Endometrial and ovarian carcinomas with undifferentiated components: clinically aggressive and frequently underrecognized neoplasms. *Mod Pathol* 2010;**23**:781–9.

25. Westin SN, Lacour RA, Urbauer DL, *et al.* Carcinoma of the lower uterine segment: a newly described association with Lynch syndrome. *J Clin Oncol* 2008;**26**:5965–71.

26. Shannon C, Kirk J, Barnetson R, *et al.* Incidence of microsatellite instability in synchronous tumors of the ovary and endometrium. *Clin Cancer Res* 2003;**9**:1387–92.

27. Soliman PT, Broaddus RR, Schmeler KM, *et al.* Women with synchronous primary cancers of the endometrium and ovary: do they have Lynch syndrome? *J Clin Oncol* 2005;**23**:9344–50.

20 CYTOLOGY OF PERITONEUM AND ABDOMINAL WASHINGS

C. Haynes and C. S. Kong

INTRODUCTION

Peritoneal wash cytology has classically been used during exploratory laparotomy to detect occult serosal involvement by a neoplastic process or to demonstrate persistent or recurrent malignancy. In the past, peritoneal wash cytology has had significant therapeutic and prognostic impact, especially for ovarian and endometrial carcinomas. The current FIGO recommendations have eliminated the results of cytologic evaluation of peritoneal washing specimens from the staging criteria for endometrial carcinoma, which de-emphasizes the role of wash cytology in uterine corpus cancer[1,2]. This change is based on the long-observed undetermined clinical significance of isolated positive peritoneal wash cytology in low-grade, organ-confined endometrial carcinoma (previously considered FIGO stage IIIA). In addition, a positive wash cytology does not correlate with the histologic subtype of endometrial carcinoma, grade, depth of invasion, or the presence of vascular invasion. Positive peritoneal wash cytology does impact survival, but only if other adverse prognostic factors are present[3]. Despite the updated recommendations, continued collection of cytology may provide useful information for making postoperative treatment decisions or in future research studies. The clinical significance of positive wash cytology for cervical carcinoma is less clear[4]. Since we continue to receive peritoneal wash specimens on some patients with corpus cancer either during a staging or exploratory procedure for suspected gynecologic malignancy of unknown primary site, the discussion in this chapter focuses on the interpretation of these specimens.

In the presence of disease, serosal membranes become irritated and damaged, which leads to eventual disruption of the dynamic balance between the formation and resorption of serous fluid. The presence of an effusion is associated with reactive changes in mesothelial cells that can sometimes be difficult to distinguish from neoplastic cells.

Mechanical disruption of the mesothelial lining cells, via peritoneal wash/lavage, increases sensitivity by producing a more cellular sample of mesothelial cells. Cells that spontaneously exfoliate occur as three-dimensional clusters, while mechanical disruption leads to flat sheets arranged in an orderly mosaic pattern (Figure 20.1). Occasionally, the flat sheets can be folded and give the appearance of papillary clusters. Nuclear and chromatin detail are optimal on Papanicolaou-stained fixed slides, while cytoplasmic detail and extracellular material (e.g., mucin) are better appreciated on air-dried, Romanowsky-stained slides.

The majority of the discrepancies of peritoneal wash cytology are due to sampling error, with a minority of discrepancies due to interpretive error. Reported sensitivity ranges from 49 to 88%; specificity, from 95.5 to 100%[4]. With second-look operations, the false-negative rate can be as high as 86%[4,7,8]. Small sample size accounts for more than 70% of the false-negative results[9]. At least 30–50 ml of fluid should optimally be evaluated to provide adequate sensitivity and specificity for the detection of metastatic disease. A commonly encountered problem is the infrequent exfoliation of malignant cells in a background of numerous mesothelial cells or macrophages, which can lead to difficulty in rendering a definitive diagnosis. In these cases, centrifugation of the fluid to yield cell block material can be helpful by providing architectural detail and material for immunohistochemical evaluation.

Benign conditions

Benign mesothelial cells

Normally, mesothelial cells form a flat, single layer of cells that line the body cavities, but inflammation, previous surgery, peritoneal inflammatory disease, tubo-ovarian abscess, ruptured ectopic pregnancy, ruptured ovarian cyst, or endometriosis can all lead to proliferative changes

(A)

(B)

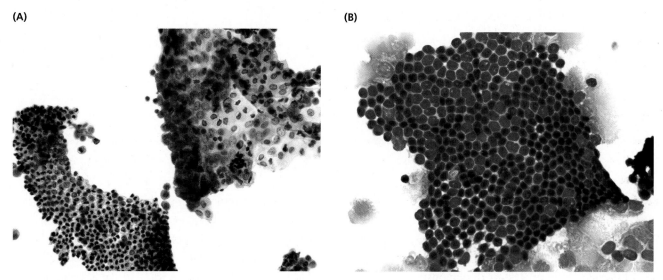

Figure 20.1 (A, B) Flat sheets of non-overlapping mesothelial cells are characteristic of peritoneal wash specimens.

within mesothelial cells that can be difficult to distinguish from malignancy[10]. The presence of many singly dispersed or a uniform regular arrangement of cells usually indicates benign origin. Mesothelial cells can also form occasional cell balls or papillary clusters. These clusters have scalloped borders, as opposed to the community borders that are commonly seen with carcinomas. Benign cells usually have a single nucleus, but occasional binucleation or multinucleation can be seen. Mesothelial cells are separated from each other by a clear space often referred to as a "window" or "skirt" (Figure 20.2). The nuclei are centrally placed and round to oval, with one or more nucleoli and a nuclear-to-cytoplasmic ratio of 1:2–3. Benign mesothelial cell nuclei have smooth nuclear outlines, evenly distributed fine chromatin, and perinuclear zonal pallor. The nucleoli may be large and prominent but uniform in size and shape. The cytoplasm is typically homogeneous and dense around the nucleus, and lighter along the periphery due to the presence of long microvilli. In contrast, the cytoplasm of adenocarcinomas is typically lighter around the nucleus and denser at the periphery of the cell (Figure 20.3).

Degenerative changes can result in cytoplasmic blebs or vacuoles and nuclear changes such as pyknosis or karyorrhexis that can cause the chromatin to appear coarse or clumped. Reactive changes can cause nuclear enlargement, prominent nucleoli, and pleomorphism that ranges from mild to marked. These changes usually affect the cells more or less uniformly, resulting in the "sibling image" characteristic of benign cells (Figure 20.4). Occasionally, estrogenic effects, especially at mid-cycle, can lead to the presence of diffuse nuclear grooves or scalloping of the

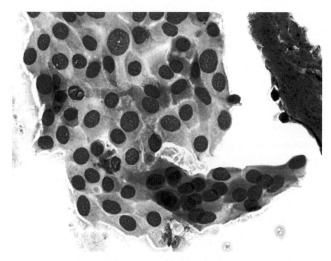

Figure 20.2 Mesothelial cells have long microvilli leading to the presence of a clear space (or window) between cells.

nuclei within otherwise benign-appearing mesothelial cells (Figure 20.5)[11]. Mitotic figures may also be present. However, abnormal mitotic figures, glandular or acinar arrangements, and numerous large clusters of mesothelial cells are extremely uncommon in benign fluids, and should raise suspicion for a malignant process. Immunohistochemical stains performed on cell block sections can be helpful in these cases (see **Ancillary diagnostic tests**).

Non-neoplastic conditions

Non-neoplastic conditions that can be detected in peritoneal wash specimens include endosalpingiosis (mullerian inclusions), benign fallopian tube epithelium, endometriosis, collagen balls, and post-radiation changes[12].

(A)

(B)

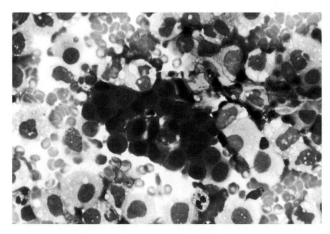

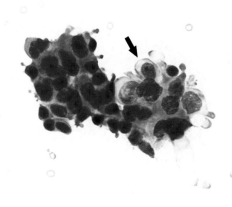

Figure 20.3 (A) Benign mesothelial cells with cytoplasm that is dense around the nucleus and lighter at the cell edges contrast with (B) adenocarcinoma cells with cytoplasm that is lighter around the nucleus and denser at the periphery (arrow).

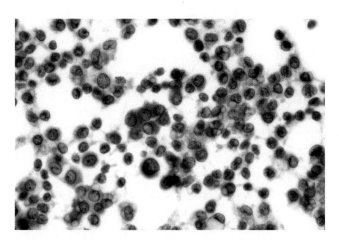

Figure 20.4 Reactive mesothelial cells have enlarged nuclei and prominent nucleoli, but the cells appear relatively uniform and lack nuclear crowding.

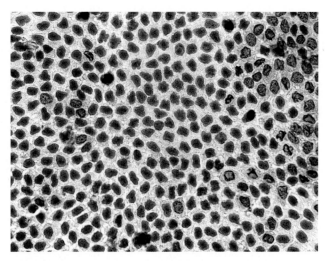

Figure 20.5 Estrogen effect can cause benign mesothelial cell nuclei to scallop and groove.

Endosalpingiosis

The presence of ectopic epithelium resembling that of normal endosalpinx (endosalpingiosis) can be seen on the surfaces of the ovaries, uterine serosa, omentum, and pelvic nodes, and at times is seen in association with calcifications. Derived from metaplastic proliferations of mesothelial cells or coelomic epithelium, they are composed of papillary/tubular structures lined by benign-appearing ciliated epithelial cells often forming concentric layers of tightly cohesive epithelial cells surrounding psammoma bodies[9]. The epithelial cells are cuboidal to columnar in shape, with slightly pleomorphic, round to oval nuclei containing finely granular, evenly distributed chromatin, and occasional small nucleoli. Single cells are rare, and the presence of cilia aids with diagnosis of

endosalpingiosis (Figure 20.6). A false-positive diagnosis may alter staging and subsequent patient management. The major neoplastic entities to consider in the differential diagnosis are a serous tumor of low malignant potential (borderline tumor) and well-differentiated serous carcinoma of the mullerian tract. Benign fallopian tube epithelium can also become detached from the tubal fimbriae and, in contrast to endosalpingiosis, will appear as a few flat sheets of ciliated columnar epithelium.

Endometriosis

The diagnosis of endometriosis requires identifying endometrial glands and stroma in addition to admixed hemosiderin-laden macrophages (Figure 20.7). The glandular

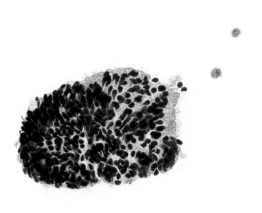

Figure 20.6 Endosalpingiosis resembles normal endosalpinx with cytologically bland, ciliated columnar cells.

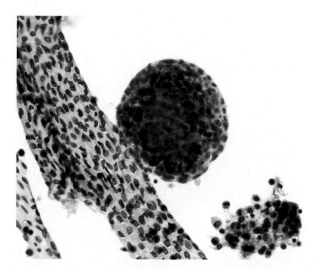

Figure 20.7 Diagnosing endometriosis in fluid cytology requires the identification of endometrial glands and hemosiderin-laden macrophages.

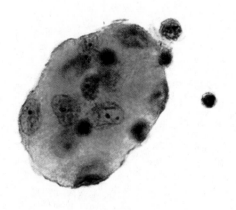

Figure 20.8 Collagen balls are benign tissue fragments with a central core of collagen covered by a flattened layer of mesothelial cells.

cells have round to oval nuclei, and are often arranged in three-dimensional clusters, tubular structures, or sheets. The stromal cells have round or bean-shaped nuclei with fine chromatin, rare nucleoli, and scant, vacuolated cytoplasm. The most sensitive finding is the presence of admixed hemosiderin-laden macrophages[10,12–14]. However, if present alone, hemosiderin-laden macrophages are non-specific and may be indicative of prior hemorrhage due to causes other than endometriosis.

Collagen balls

Collagen balls are tissue fragments composed of a three-dimensional spheroid collagen core covered with benign-appearing mesothelial cells (Figure 20.8)[10]. The Papanicolaou stain highlights the collagenous connective tissue, which appears as a smoothly contoured, homogeneous, pale-green body covered by a flattened layer of mesothelial cells. Collagen balls are most frequently seen in peritoneal washings obtained at the time of gynecologic surgery or in culdocentesis specimens[12].

Radiation change

With post-radiation changes, the cells undergo enlargement with retention of normal nuclear-to-cytoplasmic ratios. In addition, the cytoplasm often becomes vacuolated, and the enlarged cells have smudgy chromatin.

Other findings that can be mistaken for neoplastic conditions include the presence of psammoma bodies, muscle, and adipose tissue; the latter two commonly arise from the surgical incision site.

Malignant conditions

The presence of malignant cells in a peritoneal wash sample signifies the spread of disease beyond the organ of origin, and is often associated with a worse prognosis. When evaluating peritoneal wash samples, it is important to review histologic sections of the primary tumor to confirm that the neoplastic cells in the wash specimen appear morphologically similar to the primary. Performing cytologic–histologic correlation at the time of initial evaluation will help prevent false-positive diagnoses, especially with cases of low-grade carcinomas.

The primary site and histologic subtype of tumor have an impact on the detection rate of peritoneal involvement by peritoneal wash cytology. Ovarian carcinomas are the most likely to lead to positive effusions, followed by endometrial carcinoma, then cervical carcinoma[5].

Adenocarcinoma not otherwise specified

Identification of a dual population of cells that are easily distinguished from surrounding benign mesothelial cells is often helpful (Figure 20.9). Reactive processes usually create a spectrum of changes that make it difficult to distinguish a distinct "foreign" population. Tumor cells frequently aggregate in clumps or cell balls, and sometimes show gland-like formation. It is important to remember

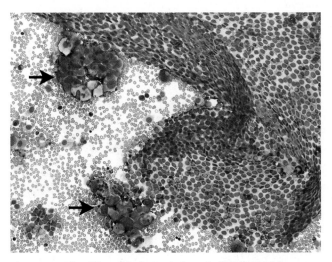

Figure 20.9 Identifying a dual population of cells is helpful for diagnosing malignancy in fluid cytology. Arrows indicate clusters of adenocarcinoma adjacent to a flat sheet of benign mesothelial cells.

that no single cytologic or architectural feature is diagnostic of malignancy, and a combination of features including marked cellular enlargement, high nuclear-to-cytoplasmic ratios, irregular nuclear contours, abnormal chromatin, prominent nucleoli, and the presence of abnormal mitotic figures is helpful. When sloughed, malignant cells continue to divide and consequently form large, three-dimensional groups of cells known as proliferation spheres. The proliferation spheres form smooth outer contours and appear to have "community borders" (Figure 20.10). A useful tool to aid with the diagnosis of malignancy is to compare cell characteristics to the surrounding mesothelial cells. One potential pitfall is when an entire population of malignant cells is present; thereby leading to difficulty in identifying a second "foreign" population. One of the great mimics of benign mesothelial cells is metastatic lobular breast carcinoma, because it often presents as a population of single cells that can be mistaken for benign mesothelial cells or histiocytes.

Serous neoplasms

High-grade serous carcinomas are characterized by three-dimensional balls or papillary clusters of tumor cells with irregular and randomly located cytoplasmic vacuoles and marked nuclear pleomorphism (Figure 20.11). Papillary formations are commonly found, and acinar structures with hollow centers can also be seen. Psammoma bodies occur with all types of serous neoplasms (Figure 20.12) but are not specific for a neoplastic process, as they are also associated with benign mesothelial hyperplasia.

(A)

(B)

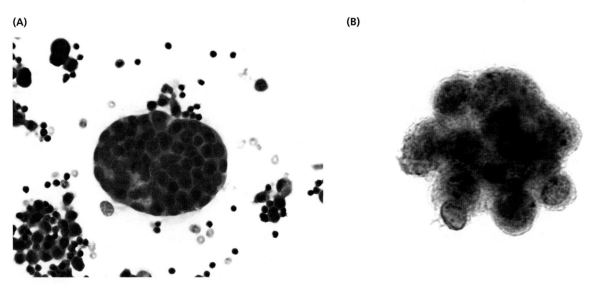

Figure 20.10 (A) Clusters of malignant glandular cells with community borders contrast with the (B) scalloped borders of benign mesothelial cells.

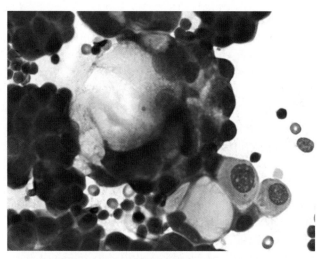

Figure 20.11 High-grade serous carcinomas have markedly pleomorphic nuclei with large cytoplasmic vacuoles.

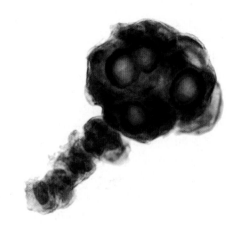

Figure 20.12 Psammoma bodies, lamellated calcifications surrounded by epithelial cells, in a case of serous tumor of low malignant potential.

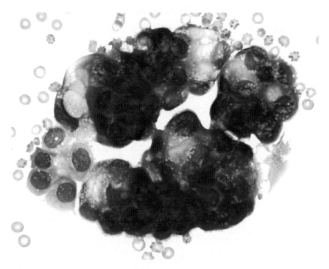

Figure 20.13 Serous tumor of low malignant potential with large cytoplasmic vacuoles and cytologically bland nuclei.

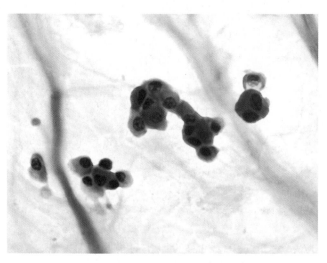

Figure 20.14 Mucinous neoplasms are characterized by clusters of tumor cells floating in pools of abundant extracellular mucin.

Serous tumor of low malignant potential (LMP) (also known as serous borderline tumor) can be virtually impossible to distinguish from a well-differentiated serous carcinoma based on cytologic features alone. Correlation with the surgical resection specimen is critical in these cases to avoid an overdiagnosis of malignancy. However, if the resection specimen is not available for review, a diagnosis of "involved by serous neoplasm" can be issued with definitive classification deferred to the surgical specimen. Serous tumors of low malignant potential can be distinguished from mesothelial cells by the presence of large papillary fragments with cellular overlap and lack of mesothelial windows (Figure 20.13)[10,15,16]. Immunohistochemical stains can be helpful in difficult cases. (See *Ancillary diagnostic tests.*)

Mucinous neoplasms

The presence of abundant extracellular mucin that dissects through connective tissues and fills the peritoneal cavity is pathognomonic for pseudomyxoma peritonei[17]. The peritoneal findings are primarily composed of extracellular mucin with occasional vacuolated histiocytes. If present, the tumor cells may occur singly or in small groups and are characterized by well-differentiated columnar cells with abundant apical mucin (Figure 20.14).

Squamous cell carcinoma

Squamous cell carcinoma is rarely seen in peritoneal wash specimens. When present, the cells occur singly or in loosely cohesive groups, and the keratinizing type has

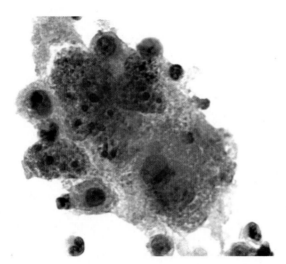

Figure 20.15 Carcinosarcoma with single malignant epithelial cells with marked nuclear pleomorphism.

dense orangeophilic cytoplasm with hyperchromatic nuclei that have irregular contours and coarse chromatin. The nuclei range from small and pyknotic to large and pleomorphic. Keratin pearls and abnormally shaped cells can also be seen. Non-keratinizing squamous cell carcinoma occurs as loosely cohesive groups and occasional cell balls, which may also undergo degenerative vacuolization, mimicking adenocarcinoma.

Small cell carcinoma

Small cell undifferentiated carcinoma appears as single cells or cohesive clusters of cells with nuclear molding. The neoplastic cells have scant cytoplasm, stippled chromatin and indistinct nucleoli.

Other

With carcinosarcoma, the epithelial component usually metastasizes as markedly pleomorphic, malignant epithelial cells (Figure 20.15). When the sarcomatous component spreads, the cytology specimen is typically paucicellular with rare malignant spindle cells[18].

ANCILLARY DIAGNOSTIC TESTS

Immunohistochemistry is intended to complement, not replace, morphologic evaluation, and is used as an adjunct to improve the accuracy of the cytologic diagnosis in difficult cases. Stains are most often used to distinguish benign mesothelial cells and histiocytes from metastatic carcinoma, or to help determine the cell lineage and the type of tumor present. As a general rule, it is best to perform at least one stain that is expected to be positive and one stain that is expected to be negative. Interpretation of results based on a single stain can be misleading.

Immunostains can be performed on direct smears, cytospins, ThinPrep slides and cell block sections. However, FFPE cell block sections are the best for immunoperoxidase stains. By spinning down the fluid, the residual sediment can be used to make a formalin-fixed, paraffin-embedded (FFPE) block. Since most pathology laboratories optimize these stains for FFPE material, it is best to use this preparation so that there will be no need to adjust the staining conditions for cell block material. If immunostains are performed on cytologic preparations, the controls should reflect the preparation method (i.e., cytospin control slide, ThinPrep control slide, etc.); the methodology should also be validated for the different preparation types. With cytologic preparations, a proteinaceous background can lead to high background and non-specific staining; three-dimensional cell clusters can trap stain, leading to false-positive results[19].

In distinguishing benign reactive mesothelial cells from metastatic carcinoma, a stain for a mesothelial marker (i.e., calretinin, WT1, D2-40) should be performed along with a general carcinoma marker (i.e., MOC-31, Ber-EP4)[20]. If the cells appear vacuolated, a histiocytic marker (e.g., CD163) may also be useful. Histiocytes are usually present in effusions, and may be difficult to distinguish from reactive mesothelial cells or metastatic adenocarcinoma.

For calretinin, the human recombinant form must be used for best results. Positive staining is characterized by diffuse and strong cytoplasmic reactivity. Focal strong staining is less specific. Calretinin is the most sensitive mesothelial marker. WT1 is a nuclear stain, which makes it easier to interpret than calretinin. It is positive in mesothelial cells, but is also positive in ovarian and primary peritoneal serous carcinomas. If paired with a general carcinoma marker, the finding of WT1 reactivity can be helpful in pointing towards a mullerian tract seras primary[14,23]. Mesothelial cells are also positive for CK5/6 but this stain is less specific, as virtually all squamous cell carcinomas are also positive.

Both Ber-EP4 and MOC-31 are carcinoma markers consisting of monoclonal antibodies against epithelial cell adhesion molecules (Ep-CAM). They are positive in a majority of adenocarcinomas; MOC-31 is more frequently

Table 20.1 Distinguishing features of metastatic adenocarcinoma and reactive mesothelial cells

	Metastatic adenocarcinoma	Reactive mesothelial cells
Cell types	Two distinct populations of cells	Spectrum of changes within single cell type, ranging from bland to atypical; histiocytes may also be present, giving impression of two populations of cells
Cytoplasm	Lighter around nucleus, denser around periphery	Denser around nucleus, lighter at edges
Cell borders	Indistinct	Clear space (windows) between cells
Shape of clusters	Three-dimensional balls with smooth borders	Clusters with scalloped borders

positive in squamous cell carcinomas. There is no consensus on which is the best epithelial marker (Table 20.1).

The final diagnosis should never be made on the basis of immunohistochemical results alone, and should encompass the cytologic findings, as well as morphologic correlation with the surgically resected specimen.

REFERENCES

1. Kim HS, Song YS. International Federation of Gynecology and Obstetrics (FIGO) staging system revised: what should be considered critically for gynecologic cancer? *J Gynecol Oncol* 2009;**20**:135–6.
2. Mariani A, Dowdy SC, Podratz KC. New surgical staging of endometrial cancer: 20 years later. *Int J Gynaecol Obstet* 2009;**105**:110–11.
3. Takeshima N, Nishida H, Tabata T, Hirai Y, Hasumi K. Positive peritoneal cytology in endometrial cancer: enhancement of other prognostic indicators. *Gynecol Oncol* 2001;**82**:470–3.
4. Walts AE. Optimization of the peritoneal lavage. *Diagn Cytopathol* 1998;**18**:265–9.
5. Zuna RE, Behrens A. Peritoneal washing cytology in gynecologic cancers: long-term follow-up of 355 patients. *J Natl Cancer Inst* 1996;**88**:980–7.
6. Zuna RE, Hansen K, Mann W. Peritoneal washing cytology in cervical carcinoma. Analysis of 109 patients. *Acta Cytol* 1990;**34**:645–51.
7. Ohwada M, Suzuki M, Suzuki T, et al. Problems with peritoneal cytology in second-look laparotomy performed in patients with epithelial ovarian carcinoma. *Cancer* 2001;**93**:376–80.
8. Rubin SC, Dulaney ED, Markman M, et al. Peritoneal cytology as an indicator of disease in patients with residual ovarian carcinoma. *Obstet Gynecol* 1988;**71**:851–3.
9. Sneige N, Fanning CV. Peritoneal washing cytology in women: diagnostic pitfalls and clues for correct diagnosis. *Diagn Cytopathol* 1992;**8**:632–40; discussion 40–2.
10. Shield P. Peritoneal washing cytology. *Cytopathology* 2004;**15**:131–41.
11. McGowan L, Davis RH. Peritoneal fluid cellular patterns in obstetrics and gynecology. *Am J Obstet Gynecol* 1970;**106**:979–95.
12. Selvaggi SM. Diagnostic pitfalls of peritoneal washing cytology and the role of cell blocks in their diagnosis. *Diagn Cytopathol* 2003;**28**:335–41.
13. Stowell SB, Wiley CM, Perez-Reyes N, Powers CN. Cytologic diagnosis of peritoneal fluids. Applicability to the laparoscopic diagnosis of endometriosis. *Acta Cytol* 1997;**41**:817–22.
14. Lin O. Challenges in the interpretation of peritoneal cytologic specimens. *Arch Pathol Lab Med* 2009;**133**:739–42.
15. Weir MM, Bell DA. Cytologic identification of serous neoplasms in peritoneal fluids. *Cancer* 2001;**93**:309–18.
16. Gammon R, Hameed A, Keyhani-Rofagha S. Peritoneal washing in borderline epithelial ovarian tumors in women under 25: the use of cell block preparations. *Diagn Cytopathol* 1998;**18**:212–14.
17. Pai RK, Longacre TA. Appendiceal mucinous tumors and pseudomyxoma peritonei: histologic features, diagnostic problems, and proposed classification. *Adv Anat Pathol* 2005;**12**:291–311.
18. Valente PT, Schantz HD, Edmonds PR, Hanjani P. Peritoneal cytology of uncommon ovarian tumors. *Diagn Cytopathol* 1992;**8**:98–106.
19. Fetsch PA, Simsir A, Brosky K, Abati A. Comparison of three commonly used cytologic preparations in effusion immunocytochemistry. *Diagn Cytopathol* 2002;**26**:61–6.
20. Ordonez NG. Value of immunohistochemistry in distinguishing peritoneal mesothelioma from serous carcinoma of the ovary and peritoneum: a review and update. *Adv Anat Pathol* 2006;**13**:16–25.
21. Ordonez NG. The diagnostic utility of immunohistochemistry and electron microscopy in distinguishing between peritoneal mesotheliomas and serous carcinomas: a comparative study. *Mod Pathol* 2006;**19**:34–48.
22. Ordonez NG. D2-40 and podoplanin are highly specific and sensitive immunohistochemical markers of epithelioid malignant mesothelioma. *Hum Pathol* 2005;**36**:372–80.
23. Acs G, Pasha T, Zhang PJ. WT1 is differentially expressed in serous, endometrioid, clear cell, and mucinous carcinomas of the peritoneum, fallopian tube, ovary, and endometrium. *Int J Gynecol Pathol* 2004;**23**:110–18.

INDEX